Fazlul H. Sarkar
Editor

Nutraceuticals and Cancer

Springer

Editor
Fazlul H. Sarkar, Ph.D.
Distinguished Professor
Departments of Pathology and Oncology
Karmanos Cancer Institute
Wayne State University
740 HWCRC
4100 JohnR Street
Detroit, Michigan 48201
USA
fsarkar@med.wayne.edu

ISBN 978-94-007-2629-1 e-ISBN 978-94-007-2630-7
DOI 10.1007/978-94-007-2630-7
Springer Dordrecht Heidelberg London New York

Library of Congress Control Number: 2011941667

Printed on acid-free paper

Springer is part of Springer Science+Business Media (www.springer.com)

Preface

I would like to thank the publisher to entrust me with organizing the special topic on the emerging role and molecular concepts of nutraceutical (natural agents) in human health especially the value of nutraceuticals for the prevention and/or treatment of human malignancies. This book illustrates the role of several dietary agents, collectively called nutraceuticals or natural agents in the prevention and/or treatment of human malignancies known to be mediated through alterations in multiple molecular targets. This book contains sixteen chapters which begin with historical perspective on the value of natural agents in the prevention of human malignancies followed by a series of current topics on multiple nutraceuticals targeting multiple cancers. This collection would likely be useful for bringing newer generations with broader perspectives in launching cutting-edge innovative molecular research, which would certainly help in designing targeted clinical trials in order to realize the dream of customize strategies for the prevention and/or treatment of human malignancies without causing any systemic toxicity. Moreover, the knowledge gained would allow novel utilization of nutraceuticals as adjunct to both conventional chemotherapy and radiation therapy in order to improve the overall quality of life and survival of patients diagnosed with cancers. I would like to thank all the authors for their cooperation, hard work and talented contributions to bring this book to the readers in a timely fashion. I would like to thank the publisher and the entire publishing group for their dedication and professionalism. Finally, I would like to dedicate this book to my lovely wife, Arfatun H. Sarkar and my wonderful children, Sarah, Sanila and Shaan for their understanding and sacrifice in allowing me to work harder and spend time away from them rather than with them which they rightly deserved.

Contents

Contributors

Vaqar M. Adhami Department of Dermatology, University of Wisconsin-Madison, Madison, WI 53706, USA, vmadhami@wisc.edu

Farrukh Afaq Department of Dermatology, Comprehensive Cancer Center, University of Alabama at Birmingham, Birmingham, AL 35294, USA, fafaq@uab.edu

Aamir Ahmad Department of Pathology, Barbara Ann Karmanos Cancer Institute, Wayne State University School of Medicine, Detroit, MI, USA, ahmada@karmanos.org

Shrikant Anant Department of Molecular and Integrative Physiology, Cancer Center, University of Kansas Medical Center, Kansas City, KS 66160, USA, sanant@kumc.edu

Sanjeev Banerjee Department of Pathology, Barbara Ann Karmanos Cancer Institute, Wayne State University School of Medicine, Detroit, MI 48201, USA, sbanerjee@wayne.edu

Bin Bao Department of Pathology, Barbara Ann Karmanos Cancer Institute, Wayne State University School of Medicine, Detroit, MI, USA, baob@karmanos.org

Christopher Blair Departments of Urology and Pharmaceutical Sciences, University of California, Irvine, Orange, CA 92868, USA, cblair1@uci.edu

Ajay Bommareddy Department of Pharmaceutical Sciences, Nesbitt School of Pharmacy & Nursing, Wilkes University, Wilkes-Barre, PA, USA, ajay.bommareddy@wilkes.edu

James A. Cardelli Department of Microbiology and Immunology and the Feist-Weiller Cancer Center, Louisiana State University Health Sciences Center, Shreveport, LA 71130, USA, JCarde@lsuhsc.edu

Steven Carmella Masonic Cancer Center, University of Minnesota, Minneapolis, MN 55455, USA, carme001@umn.edu

David T. Coleman Department of Microbiology and Immunology and the Feist-Weiller Cancer Center, Louisiana State University Health Sciences Center, Shreveport, LA 71130, USA, dcole1@lsuhsc.edu

Animesh Dhar Department of Cancer Biology, Cancer Center, University of Kansas Medical Center, Kansas City, KS 66160, USA, adhar@kumc.edu

Laura Fogt Department of Molecular and Integrative Physiology, University of Kansas Medical Center, Kansas City, KS 66160, USA, lfogton@olethaschools.com

Simone Fulda Institute for Experimental Cancer Research in Pediatrics, Goethe-University Frankfurt, 60528 Frankfurt, Germany, simone.fulda@kgu.de

Vay Liang W. Go Department of Medicine, David Geffen School of Medicine, UCLA Center for Excellence in Pancreatic Diseases, University of California, Los Angeles, CA 90095-1786, USA, vlwgo@ucla.edu

Sanjay Gupta Department of Urology, Case Comprehensive Cancer Center, University Hospitals Case Medical Center, Case Western Reserve University, Cleveland, OH 44106, USA, sanjay.gupta@case.edu

Diane M. Harris Department of Medicine, David Geffen School of Medicine, UCLA Center for Excellence in Pancreatic Diseases, University of California, Los Angeles, CA 90095-1786, USA, dmharris@ucla.edu

Stephen S. Hecht Masonic Cancer Center, University of Minnesota, Minneapolis, MN 55455, USA, hecht002@umn.edu

Yi-Wen Huang Department of Obstetrics and Gynecology, Medical College of Wisconsin, Milwaukee, WI 53220, USA, ywhuang@mcw.edu

Qing Jiang Department of Nutrition Science, Purdue University, West Lafayette, IN 47907, USA, qjiang@purdue.edu

Santosh K. Katiyar Department of Dermatology, Comprehensive Cancer Center, Nutrition Obesity Research Center, University of Alabama at Birmingham, Birmingham, AL 35294, USA; Birmingham VA Medical Center, Birmingham, AL, USA, skatiyar@uab.edu

Robert Keyes Division of Hematology and Oncology, Department of Medicine, Medical College of Wisconsin, Milwaukee, WI 53220, USA, rkeyes@mcw.edu

Ah-Ng Tony Kong Department of Pharmaceutics, Ernest-Mario School of Pharmacy, Center for Cancer Prevention Research, Rutgers, The State University of New Jersey, Piscataway, NJ 08854, USA, KongT@pharmacy.rutgers.edu

Dejuan Kong Department of Pathology, Barbara Ann Karmanos Cancer Institute, Wayne State University School of Medicine, Detroit, MI, USA, dkong@med.wayne.edu

Chieh-Ti Kuo Division of Hematology and Oncology, Department of Medicine, Medical College of Wisconsin, Milwaukee, WI 53220, USA, ckuo@mcw.edu

Yiwei Li Department of Pathology, Barbara Ann Karmanos Cancer Institute, Wayne State University School of Medicine, Detroit, MI, USA, yiweili@med.wayne.edu

Silvia Y. Moya-Camarena Centro de Investigación en Alimentación y Desarrollo, A. C., Hermosillo, Sonora, 83000, Mexico, moyas@ciad.mx

Hasan Mukhtar Department of Dermatology, University of Wisconsin-Madison, Madison, WI 53706, USA, hmukhtar@wisc.edu

Subhash Padhye Abeda Inamdar Senior College, Azam Campus, Pune 411 001, Maharashtra, India, sbpadhye@hotmail.com

Mansi A. Parasramka Department of Pathology, Barbara Ann Karmanos Cancer Institute, Wayne State University School of Medicine, Detroit, MI 48201, USA, parasramkamansi@gmail.com

Anna A. Powolny Department of Pharmacology and Chemical Biology, University of Pittsburgh School of Medicine, University of Pittsburgh Cancer Institute, Pittsburgh, PA, USA, apowolny@spelman.edu

Ashok K. Saluja Department of Surgery, University of Minnesota, Minneapolis, MN, USA, asaluja@umn.edu

Veena Sangwan Department of Surgery, University of Minnesota, Minneapolis, MN, USA, sang0001@umn.edu

Fazlul H. Sarkar Departments of Pathology and Oncology, Karmanos Cancer Institute, Wayne State University, 740 HWCRC, Detroit, Michigan 48201, USA, fsarkar@med.wayne.edu

Constance Lay-Lay Saw Department of Pharmaceutics, Ernest-Mario School of Pharmacy, Center for Cancer Prevention Research, Rutgers, The State University of New Jersey, Piscataway, NJ 08854, USA, constancesaw@gmail.com

Sanjeev Shukla Department of Urology, University Hospitals Case Medical Center, Case Western Reserve University, Cleveland, OH 44106, USA, sanjeev.shukla@case.edu

Imtiaz A. Siddiqui Department of Dermatology, University of Wisconsin-Madison, Madison, WI 53706, USA, iasiddiqui@wisc.edu

Shivendra V. Singh Department of Pharmacology and Chemical Biology, University of Pittsburgh School of Medicine, University of Pittsburgh Cancer Institute, Pittsburgh, PA, USA, singhs@upmc.edu

Priya Srihari Department of Medicine, David Geffen School of Medicine, UCLA Center for Excellence in Pancreatic Diseases, University of California, Los Angeles, CA 90095-1786, USA, priya.srihari.89@gmail.com

Gary D. Stoner Division of Hematology and Oncology, Department of Medicine, Medical College of Wisconsin, Milwaukee, WI 53220, USA, gstoner@mcw.edu

Dharmalingam Subramaniam Department of Molecular and Integrative Physiology, Cancer Center, University of Kansas Medical Center, Kansas City, KS 66160, USA, dsubramaniam@kumc.edu

Li-Shu Wang Division of Hematology and Oncology, Department of Medicine, Medical College of Wisconsin, Milwaukee, WI 53220, USA, liswang@mcw.edu

Xiaolin Zi Departments of Urology and Pharmaceutical Sciences, Chao Family Comprehensive Cancer Center, University of California, Irvine, Orange, CA 92868, USA, xzi@uci.edu

Chapter 1
Global Overview of the Role of Nutraceuticals in Cancer

Vay Liang W. Go, Diane M. Harris, and Priya Srihari

Abstract Cancer is a chronic disease of the genome that is influenced by nutritional factors at many stages of carcinogenesis, promotion and progression. A number of studies have demonstrated that dietary factors affect cancer risk. Previously these investigations have focused on macro- and micronutrients but more recent studies have explored the actions of non-nutritional phytochemicals and nutraceuticals. Investigations of the mechanisms of action of phytonutrients have led to pre-clinical studies with promising results. In the post-genomic era, the application of "omic" technologies provides further advances in nutraceutical research by utilizing integrative systems biology. In the future, well-designed clinical trials will help elucidate the role of nutraceuticals in the therapy and prevention of cancer and the role of complementary and alternative medicine (CAM) therapies in cancer management.

Abbreviations

AICR	American Institute for Cancer Research
CAM	Complementary and Alternative Medicine
CARDS	Computer Access to Research on Dietary Supplements
CDC	Centers for Disease Control and Prevention
DGA	Dietary Guidelines for Americans
DSHEA	Dietary Supplement Health and Education Act
FIM	The Foundation for Innovation in Medicine
NCI	National Cancer Institute
USDA	United States Department of Agriculture
USFDA	United States Food and Drug Administration
USDHHS	United States Department of Health and Human Services
NIH	National Institutes of Health

V.L.W. Go (✉)
Department of Medicine, David Geffen School of Medicine, UCLA Center for Excellence in Pancreatic Diseases, University of California, Los Angeles, CA 90095-1786, USA
e-mail: vlwgo@ucla.edu

F.H. Sarkar (ed.), *Nutraceuticals and Cancer*, DOI 10.1007/978-94-007-2630-7_1,

1.1 Introduction

Cancer is a chronic disease of the genome that is influenced at many stages of carcinogenesis, promotion and progression by environmental factors; thus the cancer metabolic phenotype is the result of the interaction between the genome and environmental factors. Perhaps the strongest environmental component is diet and related lifestyle factors. In fact, it has been estimated that some 35% of all cancer deaths are caused by diet, although depending on cancer site, the estimates of cancer deaths attributable to diet can range from 10 to 70% (World Cancer Research Fund 2007).

The distribution of cancer incidence and mortality rates varies geographically due to the influences of various environmental and cultural factors. In economically developing countries such as those in Asia, Africa, and Latin America, cancers of the upper aerodigestive tract, stomach, liver, and cervix are common, but in developed countries, such as those in Europe and North America, colorectal and hormone-related (breast, ovary, endometrium, and prostate) cancers predominate (World Cancer Research Fund 2007). Many of the cancers of still-developing countries are those promoted by infectious diseases, while cancers common in "Western" countries are those strongly influenced by other environmental factors such as diet and lifestyle (Harris and Go 2006). The 2007 expert report by the World Cancer Research Fund and the American Institute for Cancer Research (AICR) examines the role of food, diet, nutrition, and related lifestyle factors in geographic differences of cancer incidence (World Cancer Research Fund 2007). Epidemiological studies of diet and cancer in the U.S. have explored the impact on cancer risk of a myriad of different dietary and lifestyle factors, including dietary patterns, whole foods, nutrients and phytochemicals, body mass, growth and weight gain, physical activity and more. Whether associations are identified between these factors and cancer risk depends on cancer type, geographic region or population studied, how diet in subjects is analyzed, and many other issues related to study design. To generalize, a number of studies show that fruit and vegetable intake is strongly associated with a decrease in cancer risk. Additionally, other dietary factors such as whole grains, dietary fiber, some macronutrients, and *n*-3 fatty acids may decrease risk. Conversely, some factors increase risk, including high intake of total fat, saturated fat, alcohol, grilled meats and more. In addition, physical activity is shown to decrease cancer risk, whereas obesity (high body mass index) will increase risk (Harris and Go 2006). The U.S. National Cancer Institute (NCI) has sponsored many clinical intervention trials to evaluate the cancer-preventive properties of macronutrients and micronutrients (vitamins and minerals) (NCI 2011; Greenwald et al. 2002). The data compiled from these studies has resulted in dietary recommendations for cancer prevention. The AICR has released a set of guidelines for primary prevention to reduce cancer risk based upon the results of review of the epidemiological and clinical literature (World Cancer Research Fund 2007). In addition, the recently released Dietary Guidelines for Americans (DGA), 2010 from the U.S. Departments of Agriculture (USDA) and Health and Human Services (USDHHS) consider cancer prevention when determining the dietary guidelines, a focus that began with DGA, 2005 (USDA and USDHHS 2005, 2010). While the DGA, 2010 makes no conclusion on the relationship between diet and cancer risk, it acknowledges that certain diet factors are associated with cancer risk, and thus incorporates them into the guidelines (Harris et al. 2011; DeFelice 2002; USDA and USDHHS 2010).

1.2 Nutraceuticals and Bioactive Dietary Components

There is no clear definition for the term "nutraceutical". The first definition came from the Foundation for Innovation in Medicine (FIM): "A nutraceutical is any substance that is a food or a part of a food and provides medical or health benefits, including the prevention and treatment of disease" (DeFelice 2002). Under this definition, nutraceutical categories could include dietary supplements, including botanicals, functional foods, and medicinal foods (National Nutraceutical Center 2011). The distinctions between these categories are largely driven by marketing, but some do have regulatory definitions.

In the U.S., dietary supplements are defined in the Dietary Supplement Health and Education Act (DSHEA) of 1994 as "a product taken by mouth that includes a 'dietary ingredient' intended to supplement the diet" (USFDA 2011). These "dietary ingredients" may include: vitamins, minerals, herbs or other botanicals, amino acids, substances for use by man to supplement the diet by increasing the total dietary intake (e.g., enzymes or tissues from organs or glands), or a concentrate, metabolite, constituent or extract. Dietary supplements can be delivered in many forms, such as tablets, capsules, liquids, or powders. DSHEA stipulates that dietary supplements are in a special category and are generally regulated as foods and not drugs by the U.S. Food and Drug Administration (FDA). It also requires dietary supplements be labeled as such with nutrition labeling in the form of a "Supplement Facts" panel. In addition, the manufacturer of a dietary supplement may make a health, nutrient, or structure/function claim for the product as long as no drug claims are made, such that the product can diagnose, cure, treat, or prevent disease (Office of Dietary Supplement). DSHEA stipulates that only manufacturers are responsible for determining the safety of dietary supplements before they are marketed, and a firm does not have to provide FDA with evidence to support safety or effectiveness to market a dietary supplement (USFDA 2011). In addition, although the FDA has issued Good Manufacturing Practices for dietary supplements, there is no legal or regulatory definition for standardization of dietary supplement products (Office of Dietary Supplements 2011).

The definitions of functional foods and medicinal foods are not distinct and are still evolving; currently the FDA has no regulatory authority over functional foods. In fact, Japan is the only country that has a regulatory framework for functional foods, known there as Foods for Specified Health Use (Hasler and Brown 2009). The American Dietetic Association in its position statement on functional foods notes that all foods are functional at some physiological level, as they provide nutrients and other substances that are necessary to support life. However, functional foods provide additional health benefits in that they reduce disease risk and/or promote optimal health. The ADA defines categories of functional foods to include conventional foods (whole foods, such as garlic, nuts, and tomatoes); modified foods, including fortified (e.g. calcium-fortified orange juice), enriched (e.g. folate-enriched bread) or enhanced (such as snacks enhanced with bioactive components); medical foods (must be administered under the supervision of a physician for management of a disease or condition with distinct nutritional requirements; examples include oral supplements free of phenylalanine given to patients with phenylketonuria); and foods for special dietary use (foods that supply a special dietary need and are sold at the retail level; e.g. infant foods or gluten-free foods) (Hasler and Brown 2009).

The term "phytochemicals" applies to a wide variety of plant-derived compounds produced by plants which can be used as nutraceuticals. Bioactive phytochemicals possess anticarcinogenic, antimutagenic, antiinflammatory, and antioxidant properties. There may be as many as 100,000 different compounds found in a variety of fruits, vegetables, and other plants, including carotenoids, flavonoids, organosulfur compounds, isothiocyanates, indoles, monoterpenes, phenolic acids, and chlorophyll; the activity of many of these nutraceuticals on cancer prevention and treatment are discussed comprehensively in subsequent chapters (Harris and Go 2006; USDA and USDHHS 2010). Substantial research has previously been conducted on the intake and actions of individual or a few polyphenols at one time; however, a recent study evaluated the dietary intake of a large number of polyphenols in French adults (Pérez-Jiménez et al. 2011). This study used the Phenol-Explorer database, which contains data on 502 polyphenols in 452 foods, to find that a total of 337 polyphenols were consumed in a large group of French adults. This was one of the first studies to evaluate the comprehensive dietary intake of a large group of nutraceuticals. It demonstrates the wide variety of polyphenols present in plant-derived foods as well as how many of these are regularly consumed. Further studies are needed to define the intake of phytonutrients in the diets of many different populations in a variety of geographic areas.

In addition to studies on macro- and micronutrients in cancer risk, the NCI has sponsored clinical studies testing efficacy of phytochemicals. Some concerns have been raised about the potential negative interactions of complementary and alternative modalities with traditional therapies, but a review of cancer studies found that antioxidants and other nutraceuticals usually do not interfere with, and in some cases can even enhance the effects or decrease the side effects of conventional cancer treatments (Simone et al. 2007). Food sources of naturally produced phytochemicals usually contain multiple bioactive compounds. Most studies only focus on activity of a single compound, and combined effects of phytochemicals are mostly unknown. Studies have shown that whole food intake might increase efficacy and decrease toxicity of individual phytochemicals as opposed to high doses of a single bioactive compound itself, and as a result, U.S. organizations involved with nutrition and cancer prevention (e.g. the NCI and the AICR) and the DGA, 2010 advocate increasing daily intake of whole plant-based foods, including fruits, vegetables and whole grains, to decrease cancer risk rather than providing guidelines on the intake of individual phytochemicals themselves (World Cancer Research Fund 2007; Harris and Go 2006; Harris et al. 2011).

1.3 Historical Perspectives

The use of dietary-related CAM is common among cancer patients; CAM is generally used in support of traditional treatments to manage symptoms and improve quality of life, although often it is promoted as an alternative to mainstream therapies. Reports show that CAM usage is rising, both in cancer patients and the general public (van Tonder et al. 2009). One survey conducted in the U.S. found that between 1990 and 1997, use of at least one of sixteen CAM therapies increased from 33.8 to 42.1% in the U.S. adult population (Eisenberg et al. 1998). Reports of the use of CAM therapies are varied, but overall interest has increased as a result of the limits of mainstream treatments, increased media coverage of CAM, and a trend towards holistic and natural therapies. Data from the 2007 National Health Interview Survey (NHIS) show that natural products are the most common form of CAM therapy among all adults (Barnes et al. 2008). Figure 1.1 shows that natural products represent 17.7% of adult CAM usage, the most common among the

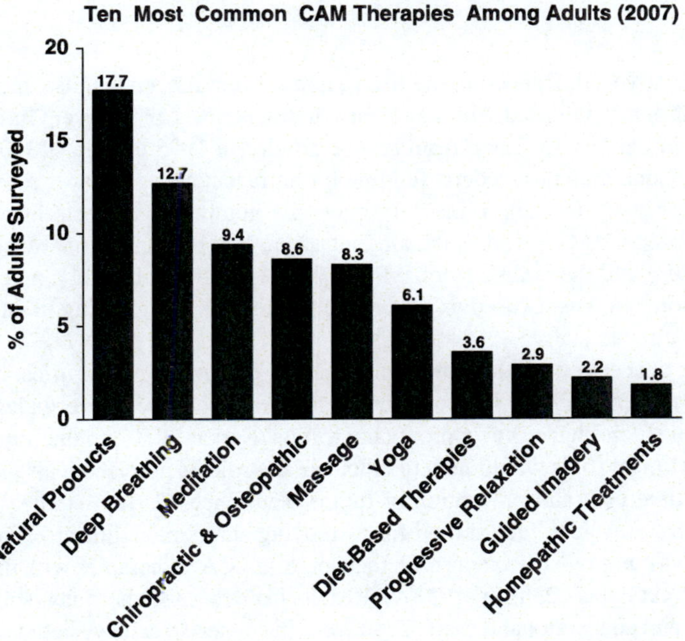

Fig. 1.1 The ten most common CAM therapies among adults. Data from the 2007 National Health Interview Survey (NHIS) (Barnes et al. 2008)

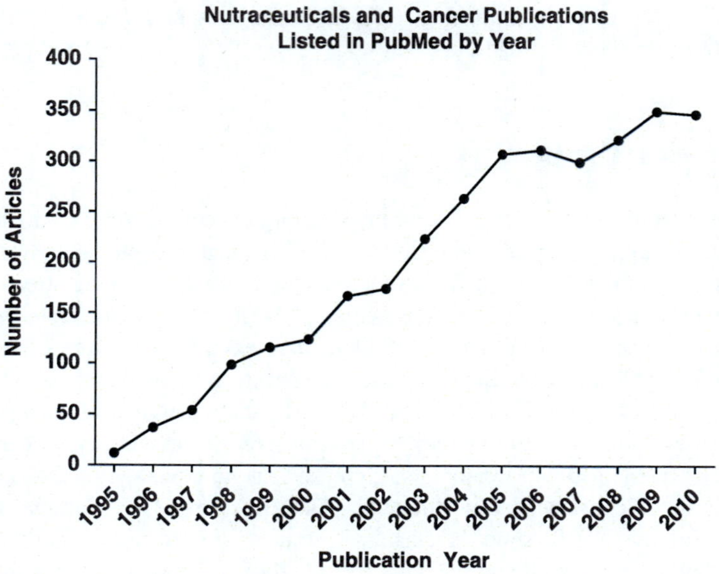

Fig. 1.2 The number of published articles per year in PubMed determined using the keyword search of "nutraceuticals and cancer" for each year from 1995 to 2010

modalities surveyed. Reflecting the rise in interest in nutraceutical use, the number of publications in PubMed with keywords "nutraceuticals and cancer" has steadily increased in the last 15 years, from twelve articles in 1995 to almost 350 in 2010 (Fig. 1.2). Concomitantly, federal funding for nutraceutical and cancer research has increased as well. Data in Table 1.1 shows the number of projects investigating dietary-related CAM as well as the amount of funding by the National Institutes of Health (NIH) and the USDA from 1999 to 2007 (Regan et al. 2011); much of this research portfolio has focused on cancer, and again, reflects growing interest in the action of nutraceuticals.

Certain concerns over the safety and efficacy of nutraceuticals in cancer treatment and prevention have lead to controversy over their use. Nevertheless, many pre-clinical studies have shown promising results (Sarkar 2010). In the future, well-designed clinical trials would help to elucidate the role of nutraceuticals as therapy in cancer treatment and prevention of tumor recurrence. Current studies in CAM management of cancer have shifted from studying single modalities to "integrative oncology," a comprehensive approach that combines CAM therapies with more conventional treatments (Deng et al. 2009). Results from these studies may demonstrate that CAM and conventional therapies can work in concert to achieve better symptom management and improvements in quality of life and treatment efficacy.

Table 1.1 The total number of projects and funding for the NIH and USDA top 10 dietary supplements, 1999–2007 (Regan et al. 2011)

	NIH		USDA	
Ingredient	Projects, *n*	Funding, *USD, millions*	Projects, *n*	Funding, *USD, millions*
Vitamins and minerals	3197	1093	1443	294
Botanicals	1583	439	592	87
Phytochemicals	1470	415	697	123
Fatty acids and lipids	1051	304	685	130
Unspecified	1015	266	81	21
Proteins and amino acids	597	156	229	45
Antioxidants	528	142	290	82
Dietary fiber and carbohydrates	196	79	165	24
Hormones/precursors	185	57	10	1
Other	196	63	64	9

1.4 Current Research and Future Directions

Much of the current research has been in the mechanisms of action of phytonutrients in the various steps of carcinogenesis. Potential molecular targets for chemopreventive actions of dietary components include inhibition of cellular replication, promotion of anti-growth signals, stimulation of differentiation, enhancement of apoptosis, induction of senescence, inhibition of angiogenesis and metastasis, and regulation of epigenetic events (Harris and Go 2006). Much progress has been accomplished in these areas related to development of various solid tumors, as discussed in the following chapters. The gains made in in vitro investigations and the use of animal models for in vivo experimentation on the mechanisms of action of various phytochemicals and their bioavailability provide the foundation for pre-clinical and clinical trials.

The paradigm of a rigorous systematic research approach to access the health benefits of nutraceuticals and their recommendation has been proposed by Dr. Mary Frances Picciano and colleagues (Table 1.2) (Picciano et al. 2006). The paradigm begins with preclinical in vitro and in vivo studies and epidemiological evidence, before human clinical trials are conducted. All available evidence must be reviewed thoroughly and objectively to determine whether data on efficacy and safety justifies proceeding to human studies. Clinical trials usually proceed in three stages: human safety trials, efficacy trials, and large-scale trials. The gold standard of scientific clinical trials are double-blind, randomized, placebo control trials. The results of such studies ultimately will inform evidence-based clinical recommendations. However, to date only a limited number of clinical trials on CAM have reached the final stage of this paradigm (Barnes et al. 2008; NCI 2011).

Table 1.2 Evaluating dietary supplements: a research approach (Picciano et al. 2006)

BASIC BIOMEDICAL LABORATORY RESEARCH
(*In vitro* experiments and *in vivo* animal experiments)

↓

HUMAN OBSERVATIONAL EPIDEMIOLOGICAL STUDIES
(Identify possible links between dietary supplements and cancer prevention)

↓

HYPOTHESIS DEVELOPMENT
(Evaluation of existing laboratory and epidemiological evidence on dietary supplement safety and effectiveness: as related to cancer prevention and therapy)

↓

DECISION POINT → DO NOT PROCEED

↓

PROCEED

↓

HUMAN SAFETY TRIALS
(Identify adverse side effects: safe dosage: and potential interactions)

↓

SMALL TRIALS IN DEFINED POPULATIONS
(Measure supplement effectiveness at various safe doses)

↓

LARGE-SCALE: DOUBLE-BLIND: PLACEBO-CONTROLLED: RANDOMIZED CLINICAL INTERVENTION TRIALS
(Test whether supplementation has the hypothesized human health benefit)

↓

DEVELOP SUPPLEMENTAL RECOMMENDATION

Basic researchers and clinical investigators, in addition to investigating the potential mechanisms of action of dietary supplements, are studying other factors that might influence the use of nutraceuticals in the treatment and prevention of cancer, such as timing of use, optimal dosages, bioavailability, efficacy and interaction with other therapeutic modalities. To address some of the challenges of poor bioavailability of certain nutraceuticals, new systems for delivery of these compounds have been developed, including use of nanotechnology to increase their bioavailability (Huang et al. 2010). Recently nanoemulsion-based delivery systems have proven to be the best platform to enhance the oral bioavailability and biologic efficacies of different phytochemicals (Huang et al. 2010).

One key achievement in biological science and nutrition research over the last century has been the elucidation of the biochemical pathways in nutrient metabolism in relation to human health. This has been accelerated in the last half of the past century after the discovery of the structure of DNA by Watson and Crick, which heralded the beginning of a genomic era and development of new technologies in genomics, proteomics, metabolomics and bioinformatics. These new "omic" technologies permit assessing multiple molecular pathways from genome to phenotype and nutrient metabolism as a network of metabolic genotype-phenotype relationships. These "omics" have now been used in molecular nutrition research in nutrient-gene interaction and biomarkers research related to specific chronic diseases. Advances in biomarker studies evaluating nutrient-gene interactions have evolved from reductionist to more holistic approaches using functional genomics and metabolic profiling (Go et al. 2004, 2005; Lee et al. 2010).

1.5 Conclusion and Implications

Cancer is a genetic disease resulting from multiple genetic defects, many of which can be caused by various environmental factors, including diet. The implications of our broadening knowledge of cancer biology and the influence of nutrient and phytochemical intake and metabolism is that nutritional interventions may potentially be used to prevent and/or slow the progression of tumor development and metastasis.

In the post-genomic era, new opportunities are arising from advances in nutrition sciences to understand the integrative systems biology of living organisms. The complexities of the interactions among genotype, diet, and environment are unraveling and new knowledge gained from these investigations will facilitate personalized nutrition recommendations. Although the DGA, 2010 provides the framework for prevention of chronic diseases including cancer for the general population, we hope that in the near future, a new paradigm and recommendations will be developed for diet and lifestyle changes as a prevention strategy based on individual metabolic genotypes and phenotypes. This effort should begin with early childhood and continue through all stages of the life cycle. Additionally, cancer risk management must include public health programs that will target primary prevention in the population as well as clinical programs that focus on individual risk management. Simultaneously, agricultural and food sciences must continue to consider levels of beneficial nutrients and phytochemicals in plant products grown and processed for food. The ability of nutraceuticals to aid in cancer prevention and/or treatment could be both non-toxic and cost-effective, but given the complexity of the human diet, the individuality of cancer progression, and the intricacies of therapy interactions, continuing research in the field of nutraceuticals and cancer prevention and treatment is warranted (Harris and Go 2006).

References

Barnes PM, Bloom B, Nahin R (2008) Complementary and alternative medicine use among adults and children: United States, 2007. CDC National Health Statistics Report #12

DeFelice SL (2002) FIM rationale and proposed guidelines for the Nutraceutical Research & Education Act – NREA. Foundation for Innovation of Medicine. http://www.fimdefelice.org/archives/arc.researchact.html. Accessed May 5 2011

Deng GE, Frenkel M, Cohen L et al (2009) Evidence-based clinical practice guidelines for integrative oncology: complementary therapy and botanicals. J Soc Integr Oncol 7:85–120

Eisenberg DM, Davis RB, Ettner SL et al (1998) Trends in alternative medicine use in the United States, 1990–1997: results from a follow up national survey. JAMA 280:1569–1575

Go VLW, Wong DA, Wang Y et al (2004) Diet and cancer prevention: evidence-based medicine to genomic medicine. J Nutr 134:3513S–3516S

Go VLW, Nguyen CTH, Harris DM et al (2005) Nutrient-gene interaction: metabolic genotype-phenotype relationship. J Nutr 135:3016S–3020S

Greenwald P, Milner JA, Anderson DE et al (2002) Micronutrients in cancer chemoprevention. Cancer Metastasis Rev 21(3–4):217–230

Harris DM, Go VLW (2006) How dietary components protect from cancer. In: Awad AB, Bradford PG (eds) Nutrition and cancer prevention. CRC Press, Boca Raton, FL, pp. 27–74

Harris DM, Srihari P, Go VLW (2011) Pancreatic cancer prevention and the 2010 dietary guidelines for Americans. Pancreas 40(5):641–643

Hasler CM, Brown AC (2009) Position of the American Dietetic Association: functional foods. J Am Diet Assoc 109:735–746

Huang Q, Yu H, Ru Q (2010) Bioavailability and delivery of nutraceuticals using nanotechnology. J Food Sci 75(1):R50–R57

Lee WNP, Wahjudi PN, Xu J et al (2010) Tracer-based metabolomics: concepts and practices. Clin Biochem 43:1269–1277

National Cancer Institute (2011) Nutrition in Cancer Care (PDQ) Nutrition therapy. National Cancer Institute. http://www.cancer.gov/cancertopics/pdq/supportivecare/nutrition/HealthProfessional/Page4#Section_49. Accessed May 6, 2011

National Nutraceutical Center (2011) What are nutraceuticals? http://www.clemson.edu/NNC/what_are_nutra.html. Accessed June 20 2011

Office of Dietary Supplements, National Institutes of Health (2011) Dietary supplements: background information. http://ods.od.nih.gov/factsheets/DietarySupplements/. Retrieved 20 June 2011

Pérez-Jiménez J, Fezeu L, Touvier M et al (2011) Dietary intake of 337 polyphenols in French adults. Am J Clin Nutr 93:1220–1228

Picciano MF, Cohen BE, Thomas PR (2006) Dietary supplements in cancer prevention and therapy. In: Heber D, Blackburn GL, Go VLW et al (eds) Nutritional oncology, 2nd edn. Elsevier, San Diego, CA, pp. 507–579

Regan KS, Wambogo EA, Haggans CJ (2011) NIH and USDA funding of dietary supplement research, 1999–2007. J Nutr 141:1–3

Sarkar FH (2010) Preface. Cancer Metastasis Rev 29:381–382. doi:10.1007/s 1055-010-9243-2

Simone CB II, Simone LM, Simone V et al (2007) Antioxidants and other nutrients do not interfere with chemotherapy or radiation therapy and can increase kill and increase survival, part 2. Altern Ther Health Med 13:40–47

U.S. Department of Agriculture and U.S. Department of Health and Human Services (2005) Dietary guidelines for Americans, 2005, 6th edn. Government Printing Office, Washington, DC

U.S. Department of Agriculture and U.S. Department of Health and Human Services (2010) Dietary guidelines for Americans, 2010, 7th edn. Government Printing Office, Washington, DC

U.S. Food and Drug Administration (2011) Overview of dietary supplements. U.S. Food and Drug Administration. http://www.fda.gov/Food/DietarySupplements/ConsumerInformation/ucm110417.htm#what. Accessed 5 May 2011

van Tonder E, Herselman MG, Visser J (2009) The prevalence of dietary-related complementary and alternative therapies and their perceived usefulness among cancer patients. J Hum Nutr Diet 22:528–535

World Cancer Research Fund/American Institute for Cancer Research (2007) Food, nutrition, physical activity, and the prevention of cancer. AICR, Washington, DC

Chapter 2
Cancer Stem Cells: Novel Target Using Dietary Components for Prevention and Treatment

Animesh Dhar, Laura Fogt, Dharmalingam Subramaniam, and Shrikant Anant

Abstract Cancer is the second leading cause of mortality in the United States and no significant treatment is currently available. Although an increasing number of therapeutic options exist for patients with advanced disease, their efficacy is time limited and non-curative. Presently approximately close to 60% of cancer patients in the United States are believed to utilize therapies derived from plants, herbs, flowers, or nutrients either exclusively or concurrently with traditional chemotherapy or radiation therapy. A growing body of evidence suggests that cancer stem cells within a solid tumor initiate and sustain tumor growth and could be quiescent even after therapeutic intervention by common anti-cancer drugs. Identification of important signaling pathways that regulate cancer stem cells could lead to novel targets for drug intervention. Dietary compounds have been shown to interfere in cancer stem cell related pathways and therefore offer a promising approach for prevention.

2.1 Introduction

Cancer, second only to heart disease, is the leading cause of death in the United States. Although progress has been made in the early detection of cancer and in improvements of cancer therapies, the ability to provide long-term survival has been limited. Increasing evidence suggests that a minute, biologically unique population of cancer stem cells (CSCs) exists in most neoplasms and may be responsible for tumor initiation, progression, metastasis, and relapse. Characterization of CSCs has led to the identification of key cellular activities that may make CSCs vulnerable to therapeutic interventions that target drug-effluxing capabilities, stem cell pathways, anti-apoptotic mechanisms, and induction of differentiation (Kawasaki et al. 2008) Dietary compounds made from fruits, vegetables, and grains possess anti-cancer properties and represent a promising therapeutic approach for the prevention and treatment of many cancers.

S. Anant (✉)
Department of Molecular and Integrative Physiology, Cancer Center, University of Kansas Medical Center, Kansas City, KS 66160, USA
e-mail: sanant@kumc.edu

F.H. Sarkar (ed.), *Nutraceuticals and Cancer*, DOI 10.1007/978-94-007-2630-7_2,

Cancerous tumors are defined by uncontrolled proliferating cells that have lost their ability to be regulated by the host. Malignant tumors may remain localized for a time, but eventually they spread into the surrounding environment, enter into the circulatory system, and invade other tissues. Tumors are comprised of heterogeneous populations of cells that have varying degrees of tumorigenic potential. Only subsets of tumor cells are thought to initiate and promote tumorigenesis, and recent evidence has implicated a pluripotent subset of cells that have the capacity to seed the cellular heterogeneity seen in tumors (Kawasaki et al. 2008; Clarke and Fuller 2006). These CSCs are the earliest undifferentiated progenitors with an unlimited capacity to propagate. Given their potential role in tumorigenesis, CSCs are important targets for therapy. Here, we begin with a discussion of the role of CSCs and the relevance of these cells to tumorigenesis. We will then discuss the biological processes relevant to stem gene pathways and drug effluxing capability, in turn, emphasize cellular differentiation and the importance of dietary compounds that show promise in attempts to target CSCs. Possible chemopreventive and therapeutic action of dietary components are summarized in Figs. 2.1 and 2.2.

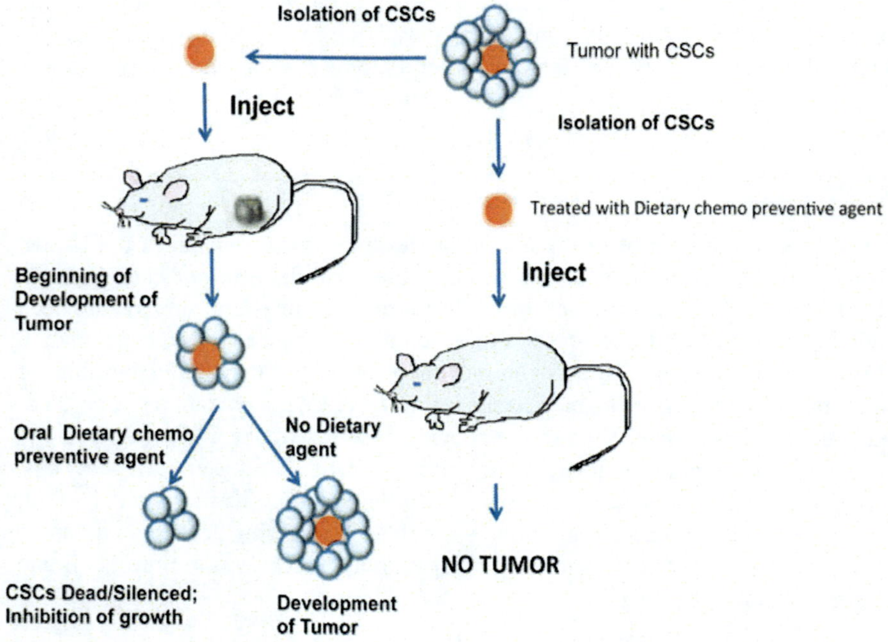

Fig. 2.1 Targeting CSCs by dietary compounds: Cancer stem cells (CSCs) can be isolated from population of tumor cells using surface markers that could be inoculated through small population of CSCs, which develop tumors to immunologically permissive mice (nude or NOD/SCID mice). Targeting CSCs through dietary components could prevent the development of tumor of those mice

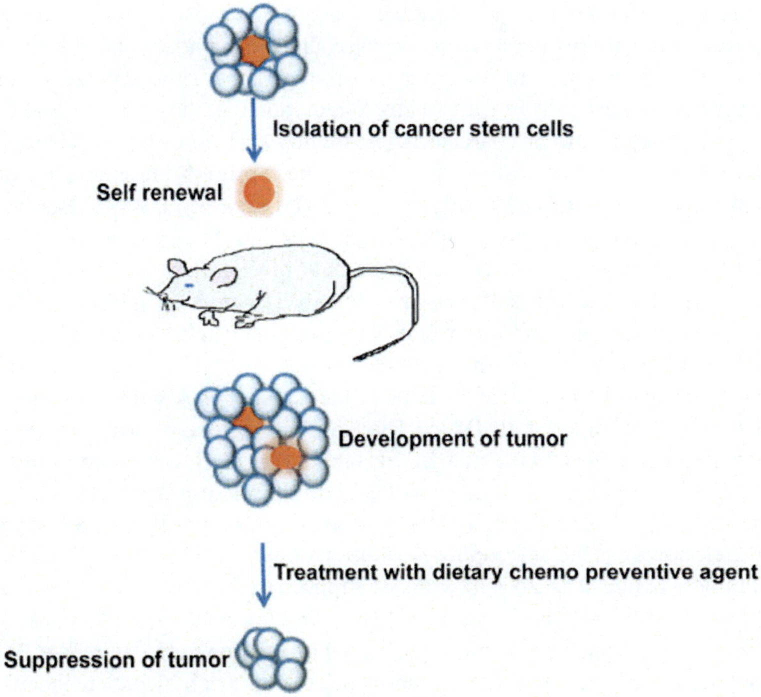

Fig. 2.2 Possible therapeutic action of dietary agents on CSCs: CSCs are capable of self-renewal and differentiation in immunologically permissive mice. Dietary agents could be therapeutic target for those CSCs

2.2 Cancer Stem Cells

CSCs are a small subset of cells that have the capacity to generate the heterogeneous population of cells that constitute a tumor. Furthermore, these cells are believed to be resistant to a number of chemotherapeutic agents (Dean et al. 2005). In contrast, the bulk of the tumor (consisting of non-CSCs) does not possess these qualities. From a clinical standpoint, the CSC provides a compelling explanation for cancer patients who often relapse after treatment (radiation, surgery, and/or chemotherapy). Thus, if CSCs are resistant to therapy, then it may be the CSCs that promote the regrowth of tumor cells following withdrawal from chemotherapy (Huntley and Gilliland 2005; Pardal et al. 2003). CSCs may arise as a result of mutations in early stem cell progenitors; however, it is equally possible that they are derived from mature, more differentiated cells. It is now widely believed that long-lived, uncommon cells are tissue stem cells (SCs) or cells derived from them that acquire the ability to self–renew. Self-renewal, one of the defining characteristics of stem cells, is a cell division in which one or both of the resulting daughter cells remain undifferentiated, retaining the ability to give rise to another stem cell with the same capacity to proliferate as the parental cell (Lapidot et al. 1994; Bonnet and Dick 1997). In addition to self-renewal, stem cells have the capacity to differentiate, generating new cells in each organ. When mutated, they can become CSCs. CSCs are defined by similar characteristics, mainly their abilities to self-renew, a characteristic that drives tumorigenesis, and to (aberrantly) differentiate, a property that generates the bulk of cells within a tumor (Lapidot et al. 1994; Bonnet and Dick 1997). These self-renewing 'cancer stem cells' might constitute only a small fraction of the cells within a tumor, with the bulk of the tumor composed of more differentiated cells that lack self-renewal capacity (Dean et al. 2005). CSCs may account for only a small fraction of cells (approximately 1%) in any given tumor (Huntley and Gilliland 2005; Pardal et al. 2003).

CSCs were first identified and characterized in patients with acute myeloid leukemia (AML) (Lapidot et al. 1994). The CSC theory asserts that many types of cancer are initiated from and maintained by a minor population of tumorigenic cells that are capable of continuous self-renewal and differentiation (Korkaya et al. 2009; Liu et al. 2005). This cell population undergoes unlimited proliferation and gives rise to differentiated cells, developing new tumors phenotypically recapitulating the original tumors (Zhou et al. 2009). Evidence supporting the CSC model was initially obtained from acute myeloid leukemia (Bednar and Simeone 2009; Ischenko et al. 2008). Dick et al. isolated a cell subpopulation with surface marker CD34+CD38−, which was able to recapitulate the phenotypes of the original patient neoplasms along serial passaging through multiple NOD/SCID recipient mice (Bonnet and Dick 1997; Lapidot et al. 1994; Zhang and Tang 2007). Subsequent studies support that solid tumors, including breast (Al-Hajj et al. 2003; Ginestier et al. 2007), pancreatic (Li et al. 2007; Hermann et al. 2007), brain (Singh et al. 2003; Son et al. 2009), colon (Ricci-Vitiani et al. 2007; Dalerba et al. 2007a; O'Brian et al. 2007a), liver (Yang et al. 2008a), head/neck (Prince et al. 2007), ovarian (Bapat et al. 2005; Schatton et al. 2008) and melanoma (Fang et al. 2005; Hirsch et al. 2009), are also driven and sustained by CSCs (Ischenko et al. 2008). The isolation and characterization of CSCs in solid tumors was conducted by Al-Hajj et al. using breast cancer patient sample (Bonnet and Dick 1997). In the study, a breast cancer cell population expressing the surface marker, $CD44^{+}CD24^{-/low}$ Lin^{-}, was able to form tumors with the same heterogeneity as the primary tumor with as few as 100 cells in NOD/SCID breast cancer mice model (Bonnet and Dick 1997). Similarly, enzymatic activity of aldehyde dehydrogenase 1 (ALDH 1) was also demonstrated to be a selective marker to enrich for breast cancer stem/progenitor cells (Ginestier et al. 2007). These two phenotypes, $ALDH^{+}$ and $CD44^{+}CD24^{-/low}$ Lin^{-}, were identified as possessing a small overlap that has the highest tumorigenic capacity, generating tumors from as few as 20 cells (Ginestier et al. 2007). Recently, the $CD44^{+}CD24^{+}ESA^{+}$ (epithelial specific antigen positive) and $CD133^{+}$ subpopulations were found to harbor putative pancreatic CSCs (Al-Hajj et al. 2003; Hermann et al. 2007), and an overlap was suggested to exist between these two populations (Hermann et al. 2007). These cell markers have been widely used to evaluate the ability of drugs to target cancer stem/progenitor cells (Hermann et al.

2007; Hirsch et al. 2009). Another technique that has been developed to isolate and characterized cancer stem/progenitor cells is tumorisphere structure culture (Dontu et al. 2003; Charafe-Jauffret et al. 2008; Marshall et al. 2007; Hemmati et al. 2003). This is based on the ability of stem/progenitor cells to grow in serum-free, non-adherent suspension as spherical clusters, while differentiated cells fail to survive under the same condition (Dontu et al. 2003; Charafe-Jauffret et al. 2008). Cancer stem/progenitor cells are capable of yielding secondary spheres and differentiating along multiple lineages (Dontu et al. 2003). Decreases in tumorisphere formation in primary culture in the presence of drug treatment and in subsequent passages that are cultured in the absence of drugs indicate an inhibitory effect of the drug on self-renewal capacity of cancer stem/progenitor cells (Dontu et al. 2003; Li et al. 2010). This is a reliable model that is increasingly being used to evaluate the drug efficacy against CSCs (Al-Hajj et al. 2003; Visvader and Lindeman 2008; Dick 2003). Another method that is also being used involves implanting human cancer cells or human primary tumors into immunodeficient mice. After treatment, the dissociated tumor cells are analyzed for CSC population based on their specific cell markers, and the same number of living tumor cells from control and treated mice are reimplanted to a second group of mice that do not receive any treatment (Korkaya et al. 2009). Tumorigenicity is then monitored in the recipient mice. For example, the ability of breast cancer cells from the primary NOD/SCID xenografts to regenerate tumors upon re-implantation in the mammary fat pads of secondary mice reflects the inhibitory effect of the treatment on CSCs (Korkaya et al. 2009). Failure of tumor initiation indicates the effectiveness of the treatment against breast CSCs.

A hallmark feature of breast CSCs is the formation of large, floating spheres, termed mammospheres, that can be serially passaged (Gupta et al. 2003). These mammospheres are highly tumorigenic and capable of forming colonies in vitro. Similar findings have been reported for brain tumor SCs (neurospheres) and prostate CSCs (prostatospheres) (Singh et al. 2003; Gupta et al. 2003). Treatment of mammospheres with soluble hedgehog (Hh) showed 100% more secondary spheres and a 67% increase in the number of cells per sphere (Choudhuri et al. 2002), suggesting Hh is an important regulator of SC self-renewal. CSCs have three unique properties that make them particularly important to tumor initiation, growth, and metastasis: self-renewal, multipotency, and a high proliferative capacity (Stockler et al. 2000). Self-renewal is the ability of an SC to undergo symmetrical or asymmetrical division. Symmetrical division allows the cancer SCs to form either two differentiated daughter cells or two SCs. Asymmetric division results in one differentiated cell and one stem cell. The biological properties of self-renewal enable the SC to maintain its pluripotency while giving rise to differentiated progeny (Gupta et al. 2003). Current methods of measuring self-renewal require the putative CSC to be serially transplantable (2–3 generations) into immunocompromised mice (Li et al. 2011). O'Brien et al. demonstrated that primary colon cancer cells expressing CD133 were the putative CSCs. The $CD133^+$ cells formed tumors in NOD/SCID mice, whereas the $CD133^-$ cells (which comprised the bulk of the tumor) did not. $CD133^+$ cells were subsequently isolated from the parental mouse tumor and serially transplanted back into NOD/SCID mice. Secondary and tertiary transplantation of the CD133$^+$ cells continued to form tumors, demonstrating self-renewal capacity of the CSCs. Each tumor that formed from the serial transplantation appeared histologically similar to the parental mouse tumor. Multipotency is the ability of CSCs to differentiate into the heterogeneous population of cells that form the tumor. This can be demonstrated by inducing putative CSCs toward a more differentiated cell fate. For example, Hurt et al. showed that LNCaP prostate cancer cells expressing CD44$^+$CD24$^-$ behaved as prostate CSCs (Gupta et al. 2003). Progress in stem cell research and the identification of potential CSCs in different cancers provides hope for the use of stem cells in regenerative medicine and treatments for disease (Prince et al. 2007; Bapat et al. 2005; Li et al. 2011).

2.3 Stem Cells Signaling Pathways

Little is known about the molecular mechanisms that control self-renewal of CSCs, an essential element of tumor survival and propagation. Genes expressed in embryonic SCs, encoding proteins involved in Hedgehog (Hh), Wnt/β-catenin, and Notch signaling, are key factors in regulating self-renewal. Although these genes are expressed in normal SCs, they are frequently mutated or aberrantly activated in cancers, thus making them potential therapeutic targets. Possible signaling pathways involved in CSCs are described in Fig. 2.3.

2.3.1 Hedegehog

Hedgehog (Hh) is a secreted protein involved in a number of vertebrate developmental processes, including polarity in the central nervous system, left-right asymmetry, organogenesis and spermatogenesis (Hammerschmidt et al. 1997). Liu et al. (2006) have demonstrated that the hedgehog pathway plays a crucial role in regulating self-renewal of normal and malignant human mammary stem cells by utilizing both in vitro and mouse model systems. Hedgehog-Gli signaling has also been shown to control the self-renewal behavior of human glioma CSCs and tumorigenicity (Clement et al. 2007). Hedgehog signals through binding to its transmembrane receptor Patched (Ptch). In the absence of hedgehog ligands (Sonic Hedgehog, Desert Hedgehog and Indian Hedgehog), Ptch associates with Smoothened (Smo) and blocks Smo function (Liu et al. 2005; Cohen 2003; Lewis and Veltmaat 2004). When hedgehog binds to Ptch, Smo is released, triggering dissociation of transcription factors, Gli1, Gli2 and Gli3 from Fused (Fu) and suppressor of Fused (SuFu), leading to transcription of an array of genes, such as cyclin D, cyclin E, Myc and elements of EGF pathway (Liu et al. 2005; Cohen 2003; Lewis and Veltmaat 2004; Pasca and Hebrok 2003). Sonic hedgehog pathway is also linked to transcription factor NF-κB signaling. It was suggested that overexpression of sonic hedgehog is activated by NF-κB in pancreatic cancer resulting in increased cell proliferation (Nakashima et al. 2006). Kasperczyk et al. characterized sonic hedgehog as a novel

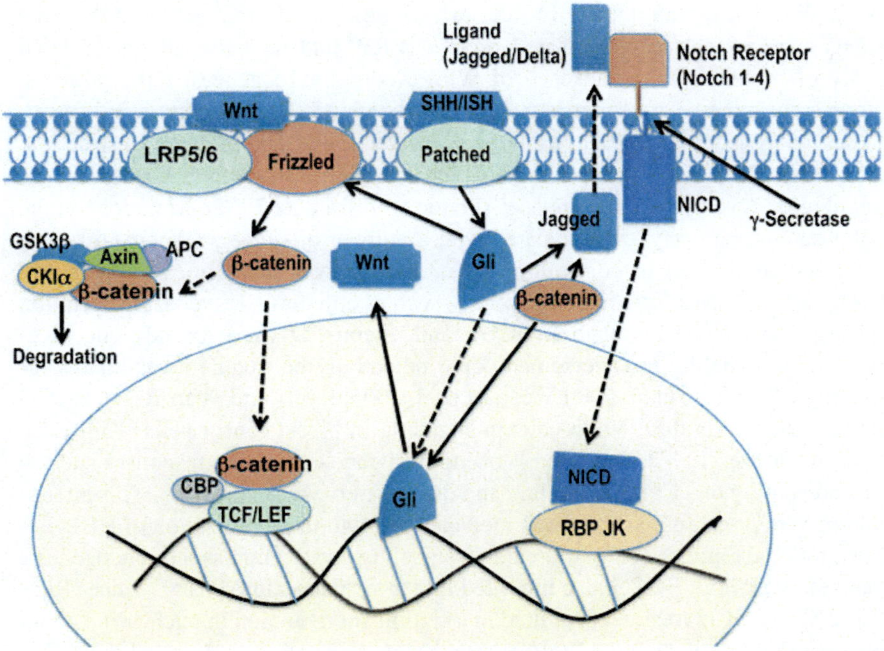

Fig. 2.3 Signaling pathways (Wnt, Hedgehog [SHH/ISH] and Notch) of CSCs interfered by dietary components: Wnt signal transmits through interactions with Frizzled and low-density lipoprotein related receptors (LRP) to initiate β-catenin signaling pathway. Then β-catenin phosphorylated by Wnt complexes and translocated to the nucleus, in turn, regulates the expression of target genes through making complexes with CREB binding protein (CBP) and T cell factor/lymphoid enhancer factor (TCF/LEF). β-catenin can also bind to axis inhibition protein (Axin), adenomatous polyposis coli (APC), phosphorylated glycogen synthase kinase (GSK-3β) and casein kinase Iα (CKIα) in the absence of Wnt ligands and then undergoes proteasome degradation. Sonic (SHH) and Indian (IHH) hedgehog (Hh) ligands bind to Patched cell surface receptor that subsequently activate glioma-associated oncogene family zinc finger (Gli) transcription factor that acts as an effector in Hh pathway. Notch signaling initiated through binding of surface bound ligands (Jagged/Delta) to Notch receptors (Notch1 to Notch4) and that triggers serial cleavage events at Notch proteins by ADAM protease family and γ-secretase. Intracellular domain of Notch (NICD) is released and is translocated to nucleus where it acts as a transcription co-activator by binding with recombination signal sequence-binding protein J (RBP-J) to activate downstream target genes. Dietary components can interfere of these three signaling mechanisms of CSCs either by inhibiting the binding of ligands or preventing translocation of transcription factors to nucleus

NF-κB target gene and mapped minimal NF-κB consensus site to position +139 of sonic hedgehog promoter (Kasperczyk et al. 2009).

2.3.2 Wnt/β-Catenin

Wnt/β-catenin signaling is involved in a wide range of developmental processes including maintenance of stem cell compartments in adult tissue (Blank et al.

2008). Wnt is a protein tethered to the extracellular matrix that activates the low-density lipoprotein receptor–related protein (LRP) and receptors of the Frizzled family of proteins. In the absence of Wnt, a complex of at least three proteins, cytoplasmic enzyme glycogen synthase kinase-3β (GSK- 3β), axin, and adenomatous polyposis coli (APC) destabilizes β-catenin and targets it for destruction. Activation of Wnt stabilizes β-catenin, which acts as a transcriptional coactivator for a number of developmental responses (Fodde and Brabletz 2007). Mutations in the Wnt/β-catenin pathway are associated with a number of cancers (Woodward et al. 2007) and implicated in controlling CSCs self-renewal capabilities (Taipale and Beachy 2011). Several dietary compounds, such as curcumin, resveratrol, selenium, (–)-epigallocatechin- 3-gallate (EGCG), and vitamin D were recently shown to inhibit Wnt signaling in cancers and could potentially be excellent candidates for targeting CSCs (Rao et al. 2000; Reguart et al. 2005; Byers and Shah 2007). EGCG has been shown to alter Wnt/β-catenin signaling in breast cancer cells (Kim et al. 2006). Moreover, EGCG inhibited Wnt-induced gene expression responses such as reduced activity of TCF/LEF binding and decreased c-Myc expression. This attenuation of Wnt/β -catenin activity was mediated through the stabilization of HBP-1, a transcriptional repressor of Wnt/β-catenin signaling and a suppressor of oncogenesis (Yang et al. 2008b). EGCG also inhibited tumor formation in $APC^{min/+}$ mice (Bose et al. 2007). EGCG treatment resulted in a significant reduction in nuclear β-catenin levels, further implicating the Wnt/β -catenin signaling pathway. Apart from EGCG, soy isoflavones, curcumin, green tea polyphenols, 3,3'-diindolylmethane, resveratrol, lycopene, vitamin D, etc. have been found to prevent, reverse, or delay the carcinogenic process. Interestingly, these agents have also shown to prevent or delay the progression of cancer, which could in part be due to their ability to attack CSCs or EMT-type cells by attenuating the Wnt signaling pathway in prostate cancer (Sarkar et al. 2010).

2.3.3 Notch

Notch signaling is known to control cell proliferation and apoptosis to modulate the development of many organs (Li et al. 2011; Wang et al. 2009). A number of recent studies have demonstrated that Notch-activated genes and pathways can drive tumor growth through the expansion of CSCs (Huntley and Gilliland 2005; Wang et al. 2009; Wilson and Radtke 2006; Peacock and Watkins 2008; Fan and Eberhart 2008; Kakarala and Wicha 2008; Scoville et al. 2008). Notch pathway is believed to be dysregulated in CSCs, ultimately leading to uncontrolled CSC self-renewal (Li et al. 2011; Wang et al. 2009). For example, Notch pathway was shown to play an important role in the self-renewal function of malignant breast cancer CSCs (Farnie and Clarke 2007; Androutsellis-Theotokis et al. 2006). Four Notch proteins, Notch-1 to Notch-4, have been identified to express as transmembrane receptors in a variety of stem/progenitor cells (Mumm and Kopan 2000). Binding of surface-bound ligands (Jagged1, Jagged2, Delta-like1, Delta-like3 and Delta-like4) triggers serial cleavage events at the Notch proteins by ADAM protease family and γ-secretase (Mumm and Kopan 2000; Wu and Rao 1999; Borggrefe and Oswald 2009). Notch signaling is initiated when a ligand interacts with a notch transmembrane receptor on adjacent cells. This process usually initiates the ADAM-mediated cleavage of the extracellular domain leading to the γ-secretase mediated proteolytic release of the Notch intracellular domain (NICD), which, in turn, translocates into the nucleus of the cells. The NICD in the nucleus interacts with cofactors such as the C promoter-binding factor-1 (CBF1) transcriptional cofactor and transactivates target genes including the hairy and enhancer of split (Hes) and Hes related with YRPW motif (Hey) families. Similarly, Notch has been shown to interact with signal sequence-binding protein Jκ (RBP-J) to activate downstream target genes, c-Myc, cyclin D1, p21, NF-κB (Borggrefe and Oswald 2009; Weng et al. 2006; Satoh et al. 2004; Palomero et al. 2006; Ronchini and Capobianco 2001; Rangarajan et al. 2001; Oswald et al. 1998). Notch1 has also been reported to cross talk with NF-κB pathway in diverse cellular situations (Oswald et al. 1998; Jang et al. 2004; Nickoloff et al. 2002; Wang et al. 2001, 2006a; Chen et al. 2007). Specifically, Notch-1 is necessary for expression of several NF-κB subunits (Jang et al. 2004; Cheng et al. 2001; Shin et al. 2006) and stimulates NF-κB promoter activity (Jang et al. 2004).

2.4 Cancer Stem Cell Markers

Several molecules have been proposed as CSC markers, including CD133, CD44, Musashi-1 (Msi-1), DCLK-1 and aldehyde dehydrogenase-1 (ALDH-1).

2.4.1 CD133

CD133 is a 5-transmembrane glycoprotein of 865 amino acids that is expressed on the apical plasma membrane protrusions of embryonical epithelial structures surface (Corbeil et al. 2000; Papailiou et al. 2011). Initially, the role of organizer of the plasma membrane topology was credited to CD133 due to its location (Corbeil et al. 2001), but, to date, its function remains unclear (Haraguchi et al. 2006). Brain (Singh et al. 2004a), gut (Papailiou et al. 2011), and pancreatic (Hermann et al. 2007) tumor CSCs have been isolated with the help of CD133 antibodies, but it has also been confined to multiple differentiated cells like acinar and islet cells in the pancreas, and goblet and columnar epithelial cells lining the colon (Zhu et al. 2009). CD133 is known to be present at various locations both in the cell membrane and the cytoplasm, indicating its various functions. Immervoll et al. (2008) showed that the apical/ endoluminal membranous staining characterized as well polarized, differentiated cells, whereas cytoplasmic CD133 staining in cancer cells may be indicative of putative CSCs. In residual tumor cells post-chemoradiotherapy (CRT), both apical/endoluminal membrane and cytoplasmic CD133 staining were detected, with some cells not being stained by cytokeratin 20 (CK20) (Saigusa et al. 2009). The tumorigenic potential of CD133 positive ($CD133^+$) cells has been demonstrated in studies that used freshly dissociated tumor cells injected into immunocompromised mice (Hermann et al. 2007). Injection of isolated CD133^{+} cells from primary colorectal cancer and colorectal cancer metastases gave rise to tumors in mice that displayed the same morphologic features of the parental tumor. Neither CD133 negative (CD133^{-}) nor CD133 low cell populations showed evidence of this CSC ability. Furthermore, these results were reproducibly maintained upon serial transplantation, whereas CD133^{-} were able to do so even after serial transplantation (Cohen 2003). Nevertheless, CD133^{+} has limitations as a CSC marker, since it appears not to predict tumor initiation potential in stage A tumors (Papailiou et al. 2011; Hermann et al. 2007).

2.4.2 *CD44*

CD44 is a class I transmembrane glycoprotein that can act as a receptor for extracellular matrices such as hyaluronic acid, and is a known downstream target of the Wnt/β–catenin pathway (Singh et al. 2004a; Subramaniam et al. 2010). It was the first marker identified for a solid tumor stem cell found in a study of tumorigenic breast cancer (Al-Hajj et al. 2003). Currently, it is not known whether all CD44 positive cells are stem cells, because a large population of cells within a tumor expresses CD44. Given that CD44 has many splice variants, the possibility exists that a specific splice variant is expressed in the stem cells. Colorectal cancer stem cells were similarly shown to express CD44 and the epithelial cell adhesion molecule EpCAM, and in several colorectal tumors CD166 could be used for further enrichment of colon cancer stem cells within the EpCAM/CD44^{+} population (Dalerba and Clarke 2007; Dalerba et al. 2007b). CD44^{+}CD24$^{-/low}$ESA^{+} formed a tumor in NOD/SCID mice with as few as 100 cells, whereas their depleted counterparts required 200-fold more (Kawasaki et al. 2008; Bonnet and Dick 1997). In a recent study, they have identified CD44 as a gastric cancer stem cell marker. CD44^{+} murine cells formed spheroid colonies, xenograft tumors, and also gave rise to CD44^{-} cells and exhibited differentiation. The CD44^{+} gastric cancer cells demonstrated properties of chemo- and radio-resistance, which likely accounts for the resistance of this tumor type to standard treatment protocols. Moreover, CD44 expression correlated with the presence of dysplasia in murine and human gastric cancer (Papailiou et al. 2011). This stem cell marker emphasizes the necessity of novel therapeutic approaches to target a better clinical outcome for patients with cancer.

2.4.3 *Lgr5*

Lgr5 refers to a leukine-rich repeat containing G protein coupled receptor, also known as Gpr49 that encodes a seven-transmembrane protein with a large extracellular domain for ligand binding and a short cytoplasmic tail for coupling G proteins (Papailiou et al. 2011). It is exclusively expressed in cycling crypt base columnar cells of the intestine that represent colon CSC (Papailiou et al. 2011), and it has been demonstrated that single sorted Lgr5 positive cells can also initiate long-term culture by generating crypt–villus organoid in which all differentiated cell lines are present. These self-organizing structures can be accomplished by exposing a single cell to a uniform set of growth signals, without any requirement for niche presence (Sato et al. 2009). In the mouse colon, Lgr5 expressing cells are restricted to cycling columnar cells at the base of the crypt, intermingled with goblet cells, divide every day and differentiate into the expected functional lineages of the colonic epithelium (Barker et al. 2009). In a later study, researchers observed that β-catenin high/Lgr5$^+$ cells formed microadenomas in the mouse colon within 3 weeks of induction and adenomas of a considerable size within 36 days, and that transformation of SC through loss of APC is an efficient way. Moreover, Haegebarth and Clevers (Haegebarth and Clevers 2009) demonstrated the origin of intestinal cancer from Lgr5+ crypt base columnar cells by showing that deletion of APC in these SCs leads to their transformation within days. These transformed cells remain in the bottom of the crypt, giving growth to a microadenoma that shortly develops to a macroscopic adenoma within 3–5 weeks (Sato et al. 2009).

2.4.4 Doublecortin Calmodulin Like Kinase-1

Doublecortin and Ca2$^+$/calmodulin-dependent kinase-like-1 (DCLK-1) was identified to be a stem cell marker by May et al. DCLK1 has been shown to be a marker for quiescent stem cells in the colonic mucosa and in colon cancer tissues. In the normal intestine, DCLK-1 positive cells were identified to be in the +3 to +6 position and in occasional colon-based columnar (CBC) epithelial cells (May et al. 2010). Many previous studies have demonstrated that the stem cell is located in the +3 to +6 position (Giannakis et al. 2008). The adenomatous polyposis coli (APC)/multiple intestinal neoplasia (APC$^{Min/+}$) mouse has an autosomal dominant heterozygous nonsense mutation of the mouse APC gene and exhibit spontaneous gastrointestinal tumors similarly found in humans with germ line and somatic APC mutations (Su et al. 1992). When expression of DCLK-1 was examined in the adenomas in the APC$^{Min/+}$ mice, DCLK-1-expressing cells were negative for proliferating cell nuclear antigen and nuclear β-catenin in normal appearing intestine. However, β -catenin was nuclear in DCLK-1-positive cells in adenomas. Thus, nuclear translocation of β-catenin distinguishes normal and adenoma stem cells. Targeting DCLK-1 may therefore represent a strategy for developing novel chemotherapeutic agents (May et al. 2008). DCLK-1 has been shown to be a novel putative stem/progenitor marker that can be used to isolate normal pancreatic stem/progenitors, and potentially regenerates pancreatic tissues (Mwangi and Srinivasan 2010). Recently it has been shown that DCLK-1 regulates epithelial-mesenchymal transition (EMT) in human pancreatic cells through a miR-200a-dependent mechanism (Sureban et al. 2011).

2.4.5 Musashi-1

Musashi-1 (Msi-1) is an RNA-binding protein marker expressed in CNS stem cells (Kaneko et al. 2000) and has been recently proposed as the first intestinal stem cell marker due to its expression in developing adult small intestinal crypts and its expanded expression throughout the entire clonogenic region in the small intestine after irradiation (Booth and Potten 2000). Immunohostochemical analysis of normal human colonic crypts revealed that the majority of cells expressing Msi-1 reside in the base of the crypt in accordance with the expected CSC position, but immunoreactivity was also observed in higher places of the crypt, implying that Msi-1 is still expressed by early transient-amplifying progenitor cells (Nishimura et al. 2003).

2.4.6 *Aldehyde Dehydrogenase*

ALDH-1 has been proposed lately as a promising new marker for normal and malignant human CSCs. Isolation of ALDH-1$^+$ cancer cells and implantation in mice generated tumor xenografts, while further isolation of cancer cells using a second biological marker (CD44 or CD133) only modestly increased enrichment based on tumor-initiating ability (Huang et al. 2009). ALDH-1 has been demonstrated as a specific marker in lung adenocarcinoma (Liang and Shi 2011) and in breast cancers (Morimoto et al. 2009). Although, it is not clear whether ALDH1 is expressed only in the stem cells or also in other progenitor cells within a tumor. Nevertheless, ALDH1 can be used in fluorescence activated cell sorting as a method to enrich stem cells. There are several members in the ALDH family. They catalyze the oxidation of a wide variety of aldehydes to carboxylic acids, and are known to play an important role in endobiotic and xenobiotic metabolism (Mwangi and Srinivasan 2010).

2.5 Diet and Cancer Stem Cells

The ability of dietary compounds to inhibit tumor formation both in vitro and in vivo is well documented (Ichikawa et al. 2007). Many of these compounds have anti-oxidant, anti-proliferative, and pro-apoptotic effects on a variety of cancers, including leukemia, prostate, breast, colon, brain, melanoma, and pancreatic (Ichikawa et al. 2007; Lev-Ari et al. 2007; Christensen and LeBlanc 1996; Karmakar et al. 2007). The benefit of many of these compounds is that they are well tolerated and are found in many food products that can be added to one's diet (Aggarwal et al. 2007). Furthermore, dietary compounds could be taken on a long-term basis to either prevent primary tumor formation or tumor recurrence (Aggarwal et al. 2007). Indeed, there are a number of dietary compounds that have been evaluated in preventing disease targeting CSCs (Table 2.1). Their sources of those dietary components are described in Fig. 2.4.

2.5.1 *EGCG*

Mixture of green tea catechins was used in a chemoprevention trial on patients with high-grade prostate intraepithelial neoplasia (HG-PIN), the main premalignant

Table 2.1 List of potential CSC targets by natural compounds

Natural Compounds	Cancers	CSC Targets
Curcumin (Turmeric)	Colon, Pancreas, Breast	DCLK-1. Notch-1
ECGC (Green Tea)	Breast, Prostate	β-Catenin, Wnt, Notch-1
Sulforaphane (Broccoli)	Pancreas, Breast	β-Catenin, Notch-1, Notch-2, Wnt-9
Genistein (Soy isoflavone)	Prostate, Breast, Bladder	β-Catenin, Wnt-5a, Notch-2, CSK-3β
Resveratrol (Red wine)	Colon, Prostate	β-Catenin, Notch-1, CSK-3β
Lycopene (Tomato)	Breast	β-Catenin
Vitamin D3 (Fish, Egg)	Colon	E-Cadherin, TCF-4

lesion of prostate cancer (Bettuzzi et al. 2006). Preclinical data had shown that green tea catechins, particularly (–)-epigallocatechin- 3-gallate (EGCG), have anti-cancer activities (Kawasaki et al. 2008). Patients were given three daily treatments (600 mg/day) of the mixed catechins extracted from the aqueous layer ethyl acetate following ethanol extraction procedure in HPLC using C18 reverse phase column eluted with acetonitrile/ethyl acetate/0.05% H_3PO_4 in water as mobile phase. After

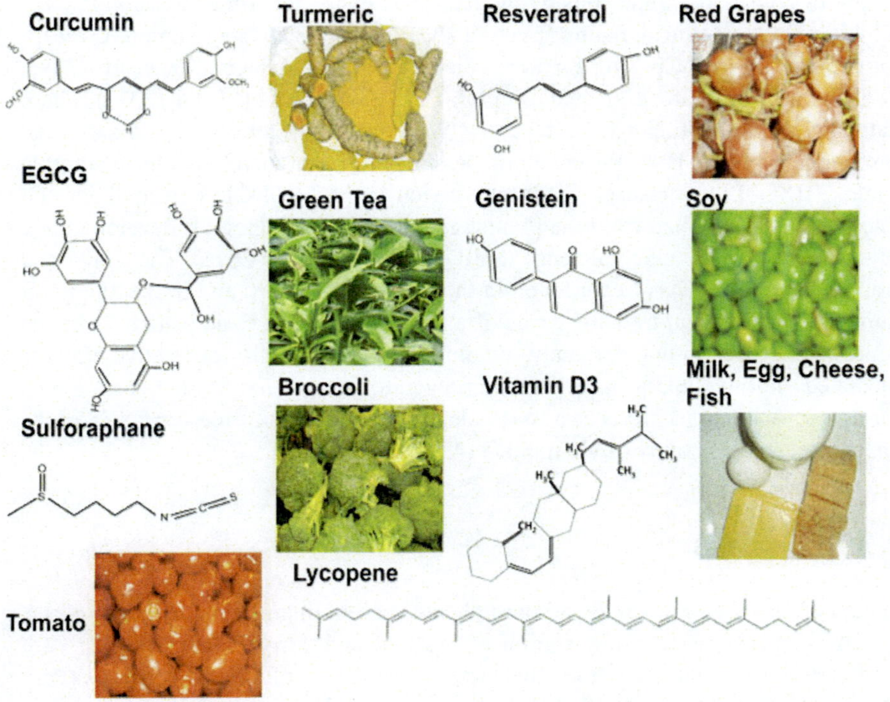

Fig. 2.4 Selected chemopreventive dietary components and its sources: the structure of dietary components and its sources are described here

1 year, the conversion rate from HG-PIN to prostate cancer was 3% in the experimental group and 30% in the placebo group. The inhibitory effects of Wnt and hedgehog (Hh) signaling by EGCG have been demonstrated in various cancers (Sarkar et al. 2010). EGCG has been shown to inhibit β-catenin expression and TCF-4 reporter activity in lung cancer suggesting inhibitory effect of EGCG on Wnt signaling pathway. In colon cancer cells, EGCG treatment inhibited GSK-3α and GSK-3β activity (Gao et al. 2009). EGCG also reduced breast cancer cell proliferation and invasiveness by inhibiting of Wnt signaling through the induction of HBP1 transcriptional repressor (Kim et al. 2006). EGCG also inhibited Hh signaling through downregulation of Gli-1 mRNA expression and GLI reporter activity in prostate cancer. (Slusarz et al. 2010). EGCG also inhibited Indian Hh pathway through down regulation of PTCH and GLI-1 expression in human chondrosarcoma cells (Tang et al. 2010).

2.5.2 Vitamin D3

Vitamin D3 has been shown to reduce the incidence of human breast, prostate and colon cancers (Shin et al. 2002; Grant and Garland 2002; Guyton et al. 2003) and induce apoptosis and cell cycle arrest of various cancer cells (Danilenko and Studzinski 2004). It has been demonstrated that vitamin D3 promoted the differentiation of colon carcinoma cells by the induction of E-cadherin expression and the inhibition of β-catenin signaling (Li et al. 2011). Ligand-activated vitamin D receptor competed with TCF-4 for β-catenin binding, thereby reducing levels of c-Myc, peroxisome proliferator-activated receptor, TCF-1 and CD 44 (Li et al. 2011). These data suggest that vitamin D3 affects the Wnt signaling pathway and a stem cell associated protein CD44. Recent study demonstrated that novel Gemini vitamin D analog, BXL0124, represses CD44 expression in MCF10DCIS.com cells, a cell line that was developed from the premalignant MCF10A xenograft developed in a severe combined immunodeficiency (SCID) mouse (So et al. 2011). The compound was able to inhibit CD44 expression in the cells both in vitro and in the xenograft tumors, suggesting an inhibitory role of a Gemini vitamin D3 derivative on breast cancer stem cells. In another study, Vitamin D3 induced anti-proliferative effect is mediated via Interleukin-1 a in prostate progenitor/stem cells (Maund et al. 2011). Further investigations are necessary to clearly demonstrate a role for CSCs in the chemopreventive activity of vitamin D3 (43).

2.5.3 Curcumin

Curcumin is a well-known dietary polyphenol present in an Indian spice, turmeric, which is usually used in preparation of mustard and curry (Li et al. 2011; Park et al. 2005). Curcumin possesses anti-inflammatory and antioxidant activities (Park et al. 2005; Satoskar et al. 1986) and has been studied as a chemoprevention agent in several cancer models (Miquel et al. 2002; Shao et al. 2002). Jaiswal et al.

suggested that curcumin induced caspase-3-mediated cleavage of β-catenin, leading to inactivation of Wnt/β-catenin signaling in HCT116 intestinal cancer cells. Park et al. strengthened the point that curcumin decreased β-catenin/TCF transcription activity in all tested cancer cell lines, including gastric, colon and intestinal cancer cells, which was attributed to the reduced amount of nuclear β-catenin and TCF-4 proteins. Moreover, analysis of the gene transcription profile revealed the expression of Wnt receptor Frizzled-1 was potently suppressed by curcumin (Yan et al. 2005). Curcumin was also shown to be able to attenuate response of β-catenin to Wnt-3a in colon cancer cells through down-regulation of p300, a positive regulator of Wnt/ β-catenin signaling (Ryu et al. 2008). In addition, Wang et al. (2006b) demonstrated that curcumin down-regulated Notch-1 mRNA level in pancreatic cancer cells, indicating a transcriptional inactivation of Notch-1 by curcumin. Curcumin-induced inactivation of NF-κB DNA binding activity was potentially mediated by Notch-1 signaling pathway (Wang et al. 2006c). Kakarala et al. demonstrated that curcumin was able to target breast stem/progenitor cells, as evidenced by suppressed mammosphere formation along serial passage and by a decrease in the percent of ALDH-positive cells. On the contrary, curcumin had little impact on differentiated cells (Kakarala et al. 2010). By utilizing a TCF-LEF reporter assay system in MCF7 cells, these authors confirmed that the effect of curcumin on breast cancer stem/progenitor cells was mediated through its potent inhibitory effect on ENT/b-catenin signaling. Colon CSCs have been shown to express surface markers CD44, CD166, CD133, and ESA (Saigusa et al. 2009). 5-Fluorouracil or FOLFOX, which remains the backbone of colorectal cancer chemotherapeutics, has shown limited success in the treatment of colon cancers (Patel et al. 2008). Recent studies have demonstrated that curcumin enhances the effects of 5-FU and oxaliplatin in mediating growth inhibition of colon cancer cells by modulating EGFR and IGF-R (Patel et al. 2008). Also, curcumin by itself or in combination with the conventional colon cancer chemotherapeutic regimen could be an effective therapeutic strategy to prevent the emergence of chemoresistant colon cancer cells by reducing/eliminating the CSCs (Yu et al. 2009). Recent studies in breast cancer cells demonstrated that curcumin and piperine inhibited Wnt signaling. Curcumin and piperine separately, and in combination, inhibit breast cancer stem cell self-renewal but do not cause toxicity to differentiated cells. Both curcumin and piperine inhibited mammosphere formation, serial passaging, and percent of ALDH$^+$ cells by 50% in normal and malignant breast cells. There was no effect on cellular differentiation. These compounds could be potential cancer preventive agents. Mammosphere formation assays may be a quantifiable method to assess cancer preventive agent efficacy and Wnt signaling assessment can be a mechanistic biomarker for use in human clinical trials (Kakarala et al. 2010). Curcumin inhibited Notch and Wnt signaling pathways in CSCs suggesting inhibition of cancer growth (64). It was reported that curcumin could decrease ALDH$^+$ cells in breast cancer cells through inhibition of Wnt signaling. Curcumin significantly reduced the nuclear expression of disheveled and β-catenin proteins (Sarkar et al. 2010). The expression levels of GSK-3β and E-cadherin were also altered by curcumin treatment. In colon cancer, curcumin inhibited tansactivation of β-catenin/TCF/LEF complex and decreased

DNA binding activity if the complex resulting decreases of growth of colon cancer (Subramaniam et al. 2010; Jaiswal et al. 2002). Curcumin and its analogue DiFiD inhibited Notch signaling pathways by inhibiting expression of Notch-1 receptor and its ligand Jagged and γ-secretase complex in pancreatic cancer (Subramaniam et al. 2010; Subramaniam et al. A novel curcumin derivative DiFiD prevents pancreatic cancer growth *in vivo* by suppressing Notch, unpublished observation). In prostate cancer, curcumin inhibited Hh signaling both in vitro and in vivo by decreasing Gli-1 mRNA expression and Gli-1 receptor activity. Curcumin could also reduce or delay prostate cancer growth in vivo in TRAMP mice (Sarkar et al. 2010; Slusarz et al. 2010). These data indicate that curcumin can interfere with Wnt, Hh and Notch signaling pathways for the prevention of cancer by inhibiting CSCs.

2.5.4 Sulforaphane

Extensive number of studies has substantiated the chemopreventive property of high consumption of cruciferous vegetables (e.g., broccoli and broccoli sprouts). The chemopreventive activity has been mostly attributed to the activity of isothiocyanates that are enzymatically hydrolyzed from glucosinolates contained in these vegetables (Li et al. 2011). In particular, sulforaphane, which is converted from a major glucosinolate in broccoli/broccoli sprouts (Zhang et al. 1992; Clarke et al. 2008), has been demonstrated to be not only effective in preventing chemically induced cancers in animal models (Fahey et al. 1997; Fahey et al. 2002; Zhang et al. 1994; Chung et al. 2000), but also in inhibiting the growth of established tumors (Singh et al. 2004b; Jackson and Singletary 2004). In a very recent report, Kallifatidis et al. suggested that sulforaphane could abrogate the resistance of pancreatic tumor initiating cells (TICs) to TRAIL (tumor necrosis factor-related apoptosis-inducing ligand) by interfering with TRAIL-activated NF-κB signaling. Based on this study, they concluded that combination of sulforaphane with TRAIL would be a promising strategy for targeting pancreatic TICs (Kallifatidis et al. 2009). The down-regulation of NF-κB function by sulforaphane treatment has been reported in prostate and colon cancer cells as well (Choi et al. 2007; Xu et al. 2005; Jeong et al. 2004; Khor et al. 2006). In addition, expression of Wnt-9-a was shown to be significantly suppressed in $Apc^{Min/+}$ mouse adenomas treated with sulforaphane (Khor et al. 2006). Sulforaphane was previously shown to induce down-regulation of β-catenin in human cervical carcinoma HeLa and hepatocarcinoma HepG2 cells (Park et al. 2007). On the other hand, several studies have reported the activity of sulforaphane to down-regulate Akt pathway in ovarian, prostate and colorectal cancers (Shen et al. 2007; Chaudhuri et al. 2007; Chung et al. 2000). PI3K/Akt pathway was demonstrated to play an important role in regulating breast stem/progenitor cells by promoting β-catenin downstream signaling pathway. It has been shown that sulforaphane is effective in targeting breast cancer stem/progenitor cells in vitro and in vivo (Shao et al. 2002). Sulforaphane inhibits breast CSCs at concentrations (0.5–5 μM) approximately 10-fold lower of that exhibiting anti-proliferative effect on cancer cell culture. It has been demonstrated that sulforaphane can inhibit breast

CSCs in vivo (Shao et al. 2002). The data showed that recipient NOD/SCID mice inoculated with tumor cells derived from sulforaphane-treated primary xenografts failed to develop tumor regrowth up to 33 days, whereas control tumor cells quickly gave rise to large tumors. This study demonstrated a down-regulation of Wnt/β-catenin self-renewal pathway in breast cancer cells (Li et al. 2011).

2.5.5 Genistein

High consumption of soy-rich food has shown an inverse correlation with the incidence of breast cancer (Li et al. 2011; Ziegler et al. 1993). Increased plasma concentration of genistein (one of the most active soy isoflavones) is associated with reduced risk of breast cancer in recent studies (Iwasaki et al. 2008, Verheus et al. 2007). Soy isoflavones, especially genistein, exhibit potent antiproliferative effects on various cancers (Li et al. 2011; Barnes 1995). These isoflavones inhibit the phosphorylation of Akt and FOXO3a, and enhance the expression of GSK3β, thereby leading to increased phosphorylation of β-catenin in prostate cancer cells (Li et al. 2008, Sarkar et al. 2009). Genistein was reported to attenuate β-catenin-mediated expression of Wnt downstream target genes in mammary epithelial cells by up-regulating E-cadherin (Su and Simmen 2009). Using gene microarray technique, a study revealed that dietary exposure to genistein down-regulated Wnt signaling through inhibiting Wnt-5a expression and enhancing Sfrp-2 (secreted frizzled-related protein-2, an extracellular Wnt receptor antagonist) expression and reduced Notch-2 expression in rat mammary epithelial cells in vivo (Su et al. 2007; Wang et al. 2006b). It has been demonstrated that genistein inhibited Notch-1 signaling, thereby down-regulating NF-κB activity, eventually leading to cell growth inhibition and apoptosis in pancreatic cancer cells. The inactivation of NF-κB by genistein in several cancers (Wang et al. 2006c; Davis et al. 1999; Chen et al. 2000) provides a basis for further investigation in the impact on the hedgehog pathway. It has been reported that genistein could inactivate Notch signaling as well as hedgehog signaling (Li et al. 2011), suggesting that genistein could be a novel agent for the treatment of pancreatic cancer by targeting multiple pathways simultaneously including Akt and NF-κB signaling pathways, and by eliminating EMT and CSC phenotypic cells (Li et al. 2011; Sarkar et al. 2010). It was found that genistein could decrease Gli-1 mRNA concentration and down-regulate Gli-1 reporter activity with significant inhibition of prostrate cancer cell growth (Slusarz et al. 2010). Based on all these data, future studies on the effect of soy isoflavone, particularly genistein, on CSCs is justified.

2.5.6 Resveratrol

Resveratrol, a polyphenol derived from a wide variety of plants such as grapes, berries, plums and peanuts (Harikumar and Aggarwal 2008), has been shown to possess chemopreventive and chemotherapeutic potential against human cancers

(Aggarwal et al. 2004). Resveratrol exhibited an inhibitory effect on the proliferation of various human cancer cells and on the carcinogenesis in animal models (Aggarwal et al. 2004; Bishayee 2009). Low concentrations of resveratrol were shown to significantly decrease the nuclear localization of β-catenin in colon cancer cells (Hope et al. 2008). The inhibitory effects of resveratrol on Waldenstrom's macroglobulinemia cells were suggested to be mediated through the down-regulation of Akt and Wnt signaling pathways (Sarkar et al. 2009; Roccaro et al. 2008). Cecchinato et al. (2007) reported that resveratrol inhibited the PI3K/Akt pathway, thereby activating GSK3β in acute lymphoblastic leukemia cells. Furthermore, these authors showed for the first time that escalating doses of resveratrol led to a progressive decrease in Notch-1 protein level, as well as the mRNA levels of its downstream effectors (Cecchinato et al. 2007). Resveratrol also inhibited sonic hedgehog signaling pathway in prostate cancer in both in vivo and in vitro models by impairing Gli-1 expression and GLI reporter activity that in turn significantly inhibited of cancer cell growth (Sarkar et al. 2010; Slusarz et al. 2010). Therefore, the potential impacts of resveratrol against CSCs need to be studied in the future.

2.5.7 *Lycopene*

Lycopene, one of the most extensively studied carotenoids in tomatoes, possesses potent anti-oxidant activity due to its extended conjugated hydrocarbon chain (Li et al. 2011; van Breemen and Pajkovic 2008). Lycopene has been shown to induce apoptosis and inhibit cell cycle progression in various cancer cells (Nahum et al. 2006; Nahum et al. 2001; Hantz et al. 2005; Salman et al. 2007; Lian et al. 2007; Fornelli et al. 2007; Gunasekera et al. 2007). The efficacy of lycopene against xenograft tumors was reported in a number of in vivo studies (Salman et al. 2007; Gunasekera et al. 2007; Tang et al. 2005; Nagasawa et al. 1995; Sharoni et al. 1997). In colon cancer cells, lycopene suppressed Akt activation and nonphosphorylated β-catenin protein level, and augmented the phosphorylated form of β-catenin, which were associated with reduced protein expression of cyclin D1 (Tang et al. 2008). Hence, lycopene may inhibit Wnt/β-catenin signaling via the connection along Akt/GSK3β/ β-catenin. These data suggest that studies on CSCs in response to lycopene would perhaps be promising.

2.6 Drug Resistance and Cancer Stem Cells

A primary characteristic of CSCs is their ability to differentiate into heterogeneous cells with differing rates of proliferation. Until recently, most cancers were treated using anti-proliferation agents that affected cells at various points in the cell cycle (Kawasaki et al. 2008; Subramaniam et al. 2010). Several treatment cycles are required to ensure that tumor cells at all stages of the cell cycle are affected. Despite many rounds of chemotherapy, the patient often relapses, suggesting this approach does not effectively target the quiescent CSC (Subramaniam et al. 2010). Therefore, inducing CSCs to differentiate into proliferative stages that would be labile to chemotherapeutics may be an effective step in combating cancer.

Although chemotherapy can reduce tumor mass, an aggressive population of CSCs within the tumor may be capable of resisting chemotherapeutic drugs (Dean et al. 2005), leading to relapse and multidrug resistance (MDR) (193). For example, CSCs from brain tumors express the neural stem cell surface marker $CD133^+$ (Singh et al. 2003). CSCs isolated from patient glioblastomas were more resistant to chemotherapeutic agents (e.g., temozolomide, carboplatin, paclitaxel, and etoposide) than were their non-cancer SC counterparts ($CD133^-$). Additionally, CD133 expression was higher in recurrent glioblastomas as compared to these newly diagnosed patients, suggesting the $CD133^+$ CSCs was better able to survive therapy. Finally, it has been demonstrated a close association between CD133 and MDR expression in glioblastoma tissue (Gottesman 2002) that in turn, indicated resistance to chemotherapeutics. Greater MDR expression has also been associated with CSCs from melanomas, pancreas, and breast cancers (Shervington and Lu 2008; Keshet et al. 2008; Zhou et al. 2007, 2008). The major mechanism of drug efflux in MDR is carried out by energy- dependent transporter proteins belonging to the ATP-binding cassette (ABC) family. Members of this group of transporter proteins include P-glycoprotein (P-gp), multidrug resistant-associated proteins (MRPs), and mitoxantrone resistance protein (MXR or ABCG2). Although clinical trials have yet to assess the role of natural products against MDR, a variety of natural products interact with ABC transport proteins and reverse the MDR phenotype in vitro. Specifically, plant polyphenols and the phytochemical curcumin (found in the spice turmeric) have been extensively studied. Polyphenol compounds are active agents in green tea and include EGCG and epigallocatechin (EGC), the most biologically active catechins. In Chinese hamster ovary (P-gp+) cells, green tea–derived polyphenols inhibited P-gp transport activities, as evidenced by the accumulation of rhodamine-123 dye within the cells (Jodoin et al. 2002). EGCG enhanced anticancer activity of vinblastine (an anti-mitotic drug) or doxorubicin (a DNA-interacting anthracycline antibiotic), suggesting EGCG facilitated a reduction in drug efflux and a reversal of the MDR phenotype (Mei et al. 2003; Sadzuka et al. 2000; Zhu et al. 2001). It was demonstrated that certain polyphenols (i.e., quercetin, silymarin, resveratrol, naringenin, daidzein, and hesperetin) inhibited the MRP1, 4, and 5 ABC transporters (Wu et al. 2005). The investigators measured efflux inhibition using fluorescent substrate or radiolabeled-vinblastine accumulation in MRP1- expressing HEK293 cells. Sonic Hh signaling increases resistance to multiple structurally unrelated chemotherapeutic agents in part through promotion of drug efflux by the regulating of MDR1 and BCRP expression suggesting a role of MDR in regulation by Hh signaling pathway in breast cancer (Kawasaki et al. 2008). It has been observed that Gli1 plays a dominant role in chemoresistance of glioma cells in sonic Hh pathway, and that suppression of Gli1 expression might be a valid therapeutic option for overcoming MDR and for increasing the success of chemotherapy (Kawasaki et al. 2008; Sarkar et al. 2010).

Treatment of L1210/ Adr cells (a multidrug-resistant mouse leukemia cell line) with curcumin and observed decreased expression of mdr1b gene, mediated by the phosphoinositide-3′ kinase (PI3K), Akt, and nuclear factor-kappaB (NF-κB) pathways (Zhou et al. 2008). Curcumin also inhibited the activity of the transporter ABCG2 (Zhou et al. 2007). Addition of curcumin reversed MDR in ABCG2-expressing HEK cells and facilitated the accumulation of doxorubicin and mitoxantrone in cells, thereby increasing the cells sensitivity to the chemotherapeutic drugs. CSCs may exploit MDR to lower the cellular accumulation of chemotherapeutic drugs and thereby sustain tumor growth. Natural products show great promise as anti-MDR agents, and given the strong link between CSCs and MDR, may reflect the feasibility of targeting CSCs to fight disease (Gottesman 2002).

2.7 Concluding Remarks and Future Directions

Dietary compounds are natural products that have been shown to have efficacy in preventing cancers in animal models. More recently, clinical trials are being pursued to demonstrate their efficacy in humans. Studies also are starting to demonstrate that these compounds can be used to target CSCs. However, dietary compounds are not without their disadvantages. The chemicals in the diet can alter drug pharmacokinetics by modulating the activity of P-gp and CYP3A4, an enzyme that oxidizes many anti-cancer drugs (Hermann et al. 2007). The net result is a reduction in oral absorption and elimination of the therapeutic drug. Given the clinical implications and the widespread use of these chemicals, rigorous testing for possible adverse interactions are required as well as stringent quality control protocols. Even with these caveats, however, dietary chemicals still represent a promising addition to standard therapy. The advantages of dietary chemicals are: (1) they target CSCs by interfering Wnt, hedgehog and Notch signaling pathways that are keys for CSCs self-renewal; (2) they show significant promise as a complement to current chemotherapy through inhibition of CSCs and (3) they are safe and could be used over time after conventional therapy, ostensibly to keep CSCs in check and limit relapse. These novel dietary agents probably target highly resistant CSCs thereby preventing cancer. Investigating the properties of phytochemicals and their role in targeting CSCs will further enhance our understanding of how CSCs contribute to a growing tumor and enable us to develop treatment strategies. An additional challenge will also be in protecting normal stem cells and ultimately targeting these CSCs in different cancers.

Acknowledgements Work cited from our laboratory was supported by the US PHS grant CA109269 and CA135559, awarded by the National Cancer Institute. Contributions of the present and past members of the TOSA and CA151727 to AD Anant laboratory are greatly appreciated.

References

Aggarwal BB, Bhardwaj A, Aggarwal RS et al (2004) Role of resveratrol in prevention and therapy of cancer: preclinical and clinical studies. Anticancer Res 24:2783–2840

Aggarwal BB, Sethi G, Baladandayuthapani V (2007) Targeting cell signaling pathways for drug discovery: an old lock needs a new key. J Cell Biochem 102:580–592

Al-Hajj M, Wicha MS, Benito-Hernandez A et al (2003) Prospective Identification of tumorigenic breast cancer cells. Proc Natl Acad Sci USA 100:3983–3988

Androutsellis-Theotokis A, Leker RR, Soldner F et al (2006) Notch signaling regulates stem cell numbers in vitro and in vivo. Nature 442:823–826

Bapat SA, Mali AM, Koppikar CB et al (2005) Stem and progenitor-like cells contribute to the aggressive behavior of human epithelial ovarian cancer. Cancer Res 65:3025–3029

Barker N, Ridgway RA, van Es JH et al (2009) Crypt stem cells as the cells-of-origin of intestinal cancer. Nature 457:608–612

Barnes S (1995) Effect of genistein on in vitro and in vivo models of cancer. J Nutr 125:777S–783S

Bednar F, Simeone DM (2009) Pancreatic cancer stem cells and relevance to cancer treatments. J Cell Biochem 107:40–45

Bettuzzi S, Brausi M, Rizzi F (2006) Chemoprevention of human prostate cancer by oral administration of green tea catechins in volunteers with high-grade prostate intraepithelial neoplasia: a preliminary report from a one-year proof-of principle study. Cancer Res 66:1234–1240

Bishayee A (2009) Cancer prevention and treatment with resveratrol: from rodent studies to clinical trials. Cancer Prev Res 2:409–418

Blank U, Karlsson G, Karlsson S (2008) Signaling pathways governing stem-cell fate. Blood 111:492–503

Bonnet D, Dick JE (1997) Human acute myeloid leukemia is organized as a hierarchy that originates from a primitive hematopoietic cell. Nat Med 3:730–737

Booth C, Potten CS (2000) Gut instincts: thoughts on intestinal epithelial stem cells. J Clin Invest 105:1493–1499

Borggrefe T, Oswald F (2009) The Notch signaling pathway: transcriptional regulation at Notch target genes. Cell Mol Life Sci 66:1631–1646

Bose M, Hao X, Ju J et al (2007) Inhibition of tumorigenesis in ApcMin/+ mice by a combination of (-)-epigallocatechin-3-gallate and fish oil. J. Agric. Food Chem 55:7695–7700

Byers S, Shah S (2007) Vitamin D and the regulation of Wnt/beta-catenin signaling and innate immunity in colorectal cancer. Nutr Rev 65:S118–S120

Cecchinato V, Chiaramonte R, Nizzardo M et al (2007) Resveratrol-induced apoptosis in human T-cell acute lymphoblastic leukaemia MOLT-4 cells. Biochem Pharmacol 74:1568–1574

Charafe-Jauffret E, Monville F, Ginestier C et al (2008) Cancer stem cells in breast: current opinion and future challenges. Pathobiology 75:75–84

Chaudhuri D, Orsulic S, Ashok BT (2007) Antiproliferative activity of sulforaphane in Akt-overexpressing ovarian cancer cells. Mol Cancer Ther 6:334–345

Chen CC, Sun YT, Chen JJ et al (2000) TNF-alpha-induced cyclooxygenase-2 expression in human lung epithelial cells: involvement of the phospholipase C-gamma 2, protein kinase C-alpha, tyrosine kinase, NF-kappa B-inducing kinase, and I-kappa B kinase 1/2 pathway. J Immunol 165:2719–2728

Chen Y, Shu W, Chen W et al (2007) Curcumin, both histone deacetylase and p300/CBP-specific inhibitor, represses the activity of nuclear factor kappa B and Notch 1 in Raji cells. Basic Clin Pharmacol Toxicol 101:427–433

Cheng P, Zlobin A, Volgina V et al (2001) Notch-1 regulates NF-kappaB activity in hemopoietic progenitor cells. J Immunol 167:4458–4467

Choi S, Lew KL, Xiao H et al (2007) D,L-Sulforaphane-induced cell death in human prostate cancer cells is regulated by inhibitor of apoptosis family proteins and Apaf-1. Carcinogenesis 28:151–162

Choudhuri T, Pal S, Agwarwal ML, Das T et al (2002) Curcumin induces apoptosis in human breast cancer cells through p53-dependent Bax induction. FEBS Lett 512:334–340
Christensen JG, LeBlanc GA (1996) Reversal of multidrug resistance *in vivo* by dietary administration of the phytochemical indole-3-carbinol. Cancer Res 56:574–581
Chung FL, Conaway CC, Rao CV et al (2000) Chemoprevention of colonic aberrant crypt foci in Fischer rats by sulforaphane and phenethyl isothiocyanate Carcinogenesis 21:2287–2291
Clarke MF, Fuller M (2006) Stem cells and cancer: two faces of eve. Cell 125:1111–1115
Clarke JD, Dashwood RH, Ho E (2008) Multi-targeted prevention of cancer by sulforaphane. Cancer Lett 269:291–304
Clement V, Sanchez P, de Tribolet N et al (2007) HEDGEHOG GLI1 signaling regulates human glioma growth, cancer stem cell self-renewal, and tumorigenicity. Curr Biol 17:165–77
Cohen Jr MM (2003) The hedgehog signaling network. Am J Med Genet 123A:5–28
Corbeil D, Roper K, Hellwig A et al (2000) The human AC133 hematopoietic stem cell antigen is also expressed in epithelial cells and targeted to plasma membrane protrusions. J Biol Chem 275:5512–5520
Corbeil D, Roper K, Fargeas CA et al (2001) Prominin: a story of cholesterol, plasma membrane protrusions and human pathology. Traffic 2:82–91
Dalerba P, Clarke MF (2007) Cancer stem cells and tumor metastasis: first steps into uncharted territory. Cell Stem Cell 1:241–242
Dalerba P, Dylla SJ, Park IK et al (2007a) Phenotypic characterization of human colorectal cancer stem cells. Proc Natl Acad Sci USA 104:10158–10163
Dalerba P, Cho RW, Clarke MF (2007b) Cancer stem cells: models and concepts. Annu Rev Med 58:267–284
Danilenko M, Studzinski GP (2004) Enhancement by other compounds of the anticancer activity of vitamin D(3) and its analogs. Exp Cell Res 298:339–358
Davis JN, Kucuk O, Sarkar FH (1999) Genistein inhibits NF-kappa B activation in prostate cancer cells. Nutr Cancer 35:167–174
Dean M, Fojo T, Bates S (2005) Tumor stem cells and drug resistance. Nat Rev Cancer 5:275–284
Dontu G, Abdallah WM, Foley JM et al (2003) In vitro propagation and transcriptional profiling of human mammary stem/progenitor cells. Genes Dev 17:1253–1270
Dick JE (2003) Breast cancer stem cells revealed. Proc Natl Acad Sci USA 100:3547–3549
Fahey JW, Zhang Y, Talalay P (1997) Broccoli sprouts: an exceptionally rich source of inducers of enzymes that protect against chemical carcinogens. Proc Natl Acad Sci USA 94:10367–10372
Fahey JW, Haristoy X, Dolan PM et al (2002) Sulforaphane inhibits extracellular, intracellular, and antibiotic-resistant strains of Helicobacter pylori and prevents benzo[a]pyrene-induced stomach tumors. Proc Natl Acad Sci USA 99:7610–7615
Fan X, Eberhart CG (2008) Medulloblastoma stem cells. J Clin Oncol 26:2821–2827
Fang D, Nguyen TK, Leishear K et al (2005) A tumorigenic subpopulation with stem cell properties in melanomas. Cancer Res 65:9328–9337
Farnie G, Clarke RB (2007) Mammary stem cells and breast cancer – role of Notch signalling. Stem Cell Rev 3:169–175
Fodde R, Brabletz T (2007) Wnt/beta-catenin signaling in cancer stemness and malignant behavior. Curr Opin Cell Biol 19:150–158
Fornelli F, Leone A, Verdesca I et al (2007) The influence of lycopene on the proliferation of human breast cell line (MCF-7). Toxicol In Vitro 21:217–223
Gao Z, Xu Z, Hung MS et al (2009). Promoter demethylation of WIF-1 by epigallocatechin-3-gallate in lung cancer cells 15. Anticancer Res 29:2025–2030
Giannakis M, Chen SL, Karam SM et al (2008) Helicobacter pylori evolution during progression from chronic atrophic gastritis to gastric cancer and its impact on gastric stem cells. Proc Natl Acad Sci USA 105:4358–4363
Ginestier C, Hur MH, Charafe-Jauffret E et al (2007) ALDH1 is a marker of normal and malignant human mammary stem cells and a predictor of poor clinical outcome. Cell Stem Cell 1: 555–5566

Gottesman MM (2002) Mechanisms of cancer drug resistance. Annu Rev Med 53:615–627
Grant WB, Garland CF (2002) Evidence supporting the role of vitamin D in reducing the risk of cancer. J Intern Med 252:178–179
Gunasekera RS, Sewgobind K, Desai S et al (2007) Lycopene and lutein inhibit proliferation in rat prostate carcinoma cells. Nutr Cancer 58:171–177
Gupta S, Hussain T, Mukhtar H (2003) Molecular pathway for (−)-epigallocatechin-3-gallate-induced cell cycle arrest and apoptosis of human prostate carcinoma cells. Arch Biochem Biophys 410:177–185
Guyton KZ, Kensler TW, Posner GH (2003) Vitamin D and vitamin D analogs as cancer chemopreventive agents. Nutr Rev 61:227–238
Haegebarth A, Clevers H (2009) Wnt signaling, Lgr5, and stem cells in the intestine and the skin. Am J Pathol 174:715–721
Hammerschmidt M, Brook A, McMahon AP (1997) The world according to hedgehog. Trends Genet 13:14–21
Hantz HL, Young LF, Martin KR (2005) Physiologically attainable concentrations of lycopene induce mitochondrial apoptosis in LNCaP human prostate cancer cells. Exp Biol Med 230: 171–179
Haraguchi N, Utsunomiya T, Inoue H et al (2006) Characterization of a side population of cancer cells from human gastrointestinal system. Stem Cells 24:506–513
Harikumar KB, Aggarwal BB (2008) Resveratrol, a multitargeted agent for age associated chronic diseases. Cell Cycle 7:1020–1035
Hemmati HD, Nakano I, Lazareff JA et al (2003) Cancerous stem cells can arise from pediatric brain tumors. Proc Natl Acad Sci USA 100:15178–15183
Hermann PC, Huber SL, Herrler T et al (2007) Distinct populations of cancer stem cells determine tumor growth and metastatic activity in human pancreatic cancer. Cell Stem Cell 1:313–323
Hirsch HA, Iliopoulos D, Tsichlis PN et al (2009) Metformin selectively targets cancer stem cells, and acts together with chemotherapy to block tumor growth and prolong remission. Cancer Res 69:7507–7511
Hope C, Planutis K, Planutiene M et al (2008) Low concentrations of resveratrol inhibit Wnt signal throughput in colon-derived cells: implications for colon cancer prevention. Mol Nutr Food Res 52(Suppl 1):S52–S61
Huang EH, Hynes MJ, Zhang T et al (2009) Aldehyde dehydrogenase 1 is a marker for normal and malignant human colonic stem cells (SC) and tracks SC overpopulation during colon tumorigenesis. Cancer Res 69:3382–3389
Huntley BJ, Gilliland DJ (2005) Leukemia stem cells and the evolution of cancer-stem-cell research. Nat Rev Cancer 5:311–321
Ichikawa H, Nakamura Y, Kashiwada Y et al (2007) Anticancer drugs designed by mother nature: Ancient drugs but modern targets. Curr Pharm Des 13:3400–3416
Immervoll H, Hoem D, Sakariassen PO et al (2008) Expression of the "stem cell marker" CD133 in pancreas and pancreatic ductal adenocarcinomas. BMC Cancer 8:48–62
Ischenko I, Seeliger H, Schaffer M et al (2008) Cancer stem cells: how can we target them? Curr Med Chem 15:3171–3184
Iwasaki M, InoueM, Otani T et al (2008) Plasma isoflavone level and subsequent risk of breast cancer among Japanese women: a nested case-control study from the Japan Public Health Center-based prospective study group. J Clin Oncol 26:1677–1683
Jackson SJ, Singletary KW (2004) Sulforaphane inhibits human MCF-7 mammary cancer mitotic progression and tubulin polymerization. J Nutr 134:2229–2236
Jaiswal AS, Marlow BP, Gupta N et al (2002) Beta-catenin-mediated transactivation and cell–cell adhesion pathways are important in curcumin (diferuylmethane)- induced growth arrest and apoptosis in colon cancer cells. Oncogene 21:8414–8427
Jang MS, Miao H, Carlesso N et al (2004) Notch-1 regulates cell death independently of differentiation in murine erythroleukemia cells through multiple apoptosis and cell cycle pathways. J Cell Physiol 199:418–433

Jeong WS, Kim IW, Hu R et al (2004) Modulatory properties of various natural chemopreventive agents on the activation of NF-kappaB signaling pathway. Pharm Res 21:661–670

Jodoin J, Demeule M, Beliveau R (2002) Inhibition of the multidrug resistance P-glycoprotein activity by green tea polyphenols. Biochim Biophys Acta 1542:149–159

Kakarala M, Wicha MS (2008) Implications of the cancer stem-cell hypothesis for breast cancer prevention and therapy. J Clin Oncol 26:2813–2820

Kakarala M, Brenner DE, Korkaya H et al (2010) Targeting breast stem cells with the cancer preventive compounds curcumin and piperine. Breast Cancer Res Treat 122:777–785

Kallifatidis G, Rausch V, Baumann B et al (2009) Sulforaphane targets pancreatic tumour-initiating cells by NF-kappaB-induced antiapoptotic signalling. Gut 58:949–963

Kaneko Y, Sakakibara S, Imai T et al (2000) Musashi1: an evolutionally conserved marker for CNS progenitor cells including neural stem cells. Dev Neurosci 22:139–153

Karmakar S, Banik NL, Ray SK (2007) Molecular mechanism of inositol hexaphosphate-mediated apoptosis in human malignant glioblastoma T98G cells. Neurochem Res 32:2094–2102

Kasperczyk H, Baumann B, Debatin KM (2009) Characterization of sonic hedgehog as a novel NF-kappaB target gene that promotes NF-kappaB-mediated apoptosis resistance and tumor growth in vivo. FASEB J 23:21–33

Kawasaki BT, Hurt EM, Mistree T et al (2008) Targeting cancer stem cells with phytochemicals. Mol Interven 8:174–183

Keshet GI, Goldstein I, Itzhaki O et al (2008) MDR1 expression identifies human melanoma stem cells. Biochem Biophys Res Commun 368:930–936

Khor TO, Hu R, Shen G et al (2006) Pharmacogenomics of cancer chemopreventive isothiocyanate compound sulforaphane in the intestinal polyps of ApcMin/+mice. Biopharm Drug Dispos 27:407–420

Kim J, Zhang X, Rieger-Christ KM et al (2006) Suppression of Wnt signaling by the green tea compound (-)-epigallocatechin 3-gallate (EGCG) in invasive breast cancer cells. Requirement of the transcriptional repressor HBP1. J Biol Chem 281:10865–10875

Korkaya H, Paulson A, Charafe-Jauffret E et al (2009) Regulation of mammary stem/progenitor cells by PTEN/Akt/beta-catenin signaling. PLoS Biol e1000121:7

Lapidot T, Sirard C, Vormoor J et al (1994) A cell initiating human acute myeloid leukemia after transplantation into SCID mice. Nature 367:645–648

Lev-Ari S, Vexler A, Starr A (2007) Curcumin augments gemcitabine cytotoxic effect on pancreatic adenocarcinoma cell lines. Cancer Invest 25:411–418

Lewis MT, Veltmaat JM (2004) Next stop, the twilight zone: hedgehog network regulation of mammary gland development. J Mammary Gland Biol Neoplasia 9:165–181

Li C, Heidt DG, Dalerba P et al (2007) Identification of pancreatic cancer stem cells. Cancer Res 67:1030–1037

Li Y, Wang Z, Kong D, Li R et al (2008) Regulation of Akt/FOXO3a/GSK- 3beta/AR signaling network by isoflavone in prostate cancer cells. J Biol Chem 283:27707–27716

Li Y, Zhang T, Korkaya H et al (2010) Sulforaphane, a dietary component of broccoli/broccoli sprouts, inhibits breast cancer stem cells. Clin Cancer Res 16:2580–2590

Li Y, Wicha MS, Schwartz SJ et al (2011) Implications of cancer stem cell theory for cancer chemoprevention by natural dietary compounds. J Nutr Chem (Epub ahead of print)

Lian F, Smith DE, Ernst H et al (2007) Apo-19′-lycopenoic acid inhibits lung cancer cell growth in vitro, and suppresses lung tumorigenesis in the A/J mouse model in vivo. Carcinogenesis 28:1567–1574

Liang D, Shi, Y (2011) Aldehyde dehydrogenase-1 is a specific marker for stem cells in human lung adenocarcinoma. Med Oncol (Epub ahead of print)

Liu S, Dontu G, Wicha MS (2005) Mammary stem cells, self-renewal pathways, and carcinogenesis. Breast Cancer Res 7:86–95

Liu S, Dontu G, Mantle ID et al (2006) Hedgehog signaling and Bmi-1 regulate self-renewal of normal and malignant human mammary stem cells. Cancer Res 66:6063–6071

Marshall II, GP, Reynolds BA, Laywell ED (2007) Using the neurosphere assay to quantify neural stem cells in vivo. Curr Pharm Biotechnol 8:141–145

Maund SL, Barclay WW, Hover LD et al (2011) Interleukin alpha mediates the anti-proliferative effects of 1, 25dihydroxyvitamin D3 in prostate progenitor/stem cells. Cancer Res (Epub ahead of print)

May R, Riehl TE, Hunt C (2008) Identification of a novel putative gastrointestinal stem cell and adenoma stem cell marker, doublecortin and CaM kinase-like-1, following radiation injury and in adenomatous polyposis coli/multiple intestinal neoplasia mice. Stem Cells 26:630–637

May R, Sureban SM, Lightfoot SA et al (2010) Identification of a novel putative/pancreatic stem cell marker DCAMKL-1 in normal mouse pancreas. Am J Physiol Gastrointest Liver Physiol 299:G303–G310

Mei Y, Wei D, Liu J (2003) Reversal of cancer multidrug resistance by tea polyphenol in KB cells. J. Chemother 15:260–265

Miquel J, Bernd A, Sempere JM et al (2002) The curcuma antioxidants: pharmacological effects and prospects for future clinical use. A review. Arch Gerontolal Geriatr 34:37–46

Morimoto K, kim SJ, Tanei T et al (2009) Stem cell marker aldehyde dehydrogenase 1-positive breast cancers are characterized by negative estrogen receptor, positive human epidermal growth factor receptor type 2, and high Ki67 expression. Cancer Sci 100:1062–1068

Mumm JS, Kopan R (2000) Notch signaling: from the outside in. Dev Biol 228:151–65

Mwangi SM, Srinivasan S (2010) DCAMKL-1: a new horizon for pancreatic progenitor identification (Comment). Am J Physiol Gastrointest Liver Physiol 299:G303–G310

Nagasawa H, Mitamura T, Sakamoto S et al (1995) Effects of lycopene on spontaneous mammary tumour development in SHN virgin mice. Anticancer Res 15:1173–1178

Nahum A, Hirsch K, Danilenko M et al (2001) Lycopene inhibition of cell cycle progression in breast and endometrial cancer cells is associated with reduction in cyclin D levels and retention of p27(Kip1) in the cyclin E–cdk2 complexes. Oncogene 20:3428–3436

Nahum A, Zeller L, Danilenko M et al (2006) Lycopene inhibition of IGF-induced cancer cell growth depends on the level of cyclin D1. Eur J Nutr 45:275–282

Nakashima H, Nakamura M, Yamaguchi H et al (2006) Nuclear factor-kappaB contributes to hedgehog signaling pathway activation through sonic hedgehog induction in pancreatic cancer. Cancer Res 66:7041–7049

Nickoloff BJ, Qin JZ, Chaturvedi V et al (2002) Jagged-1 mediated activation of notch signaling induces complete maturation of human keratinocytes through NF-kappaB and PPAR gamma. Cell Death Differ 9:842–855

Nishimura S, Wakabayashi N, Toyoda K et al (2003) Expression of Musashi-1 in human normal colon crypt cells: a possible stem cell marker of human colon epithelium. Dig Dis Sci 8: 1523–1529

O'Brian CA, Pollen A, Galinger S et al (2007) A human colon cancer cell capable of initiating tumor growth in immunodeficient mice. Nature 445:106–110

Oswald F, Liptay S, Adler G, Schmid RM (1998) NF-kappaB2 is a putative target gene of activated Notch-1 via RBP-Jkappa. Mol Cell Biol 18:2077–2088

Palomero T, Lim WK, Odom DT et al (2006) NOTCH1 directly regulates c-MYC and activates a feed-forward-loop transcriptional network promoting leukemic cell growth. Proc Natl Acad Sci USA 103:18261–18266

Papailiou J, Bramis KJ, Gazouli M et al (2011) Stem cells ion colon cancer: a new era in cancer theory begins. Int J Colorectal Dis 26:1–11

Pardal R, Clarke MF, Morrison SJ (2003) Applying the principles of stem-cell biology to cancer. Nat Rev Cancer 3:895–902

Park CH, Hahm ER, Park S et al (2005)The inhibitory mechanism of curcumin and its derivative against beta-catenin/Tcf signaling. FEBS Lett 579:2965–2971

Park SY, Kim GY, Bae SJ et al (2007) Induction of apoptosis by isothiocyanate sulforaphane in human cervical carcinoma HeLa and hepatocarcinoma HepG2 cells through activation of caspase-3. Oncol Rep 18:181–187

Pasca, DM, Hebrok, M (2003) Hedgehog signalling in cancer formation and maintenance. Nat Rev Cancer 3:903–911

Patel BB, Sengupta R, Qazi S et al (2008) Curcumin enhances the effects of 5-fluorouracil and oxaliplatin in mediating growth inhibition of colon cancer cells by modulating EGFR and IGF-1R. Int J Cancer 122:267–273

Peacock CD, Watkins DN (2008) Cancer stem cells and the ontogeny of lung cancer. J Clin Oncol 26:2883–2889

Prince ME, Sivanandan R, Kaczorowski A et al (2007) Identification of a subpopulation of cells with cancer stem cell properties in head and neck squamous cell carcinoma. Proc Natl Acad Sci USA 104:973–978

Rangarajan A, Talora C, Okuyama R et al (2001) Notch signaling is a direct determinant of keratinocyte growth arrest and entry into differentiation. EMBO J 20:3427–3436

Rao CV, Cooma I, Rodriguez JG et al (2000) Chemoprevention of familial adenomatous polyposis development in the APC(min) mouse model by 1,4-phenylene bis(methylene) selenocyanate. Carcinogenesis 21:617–621

Reguart N, He B, Taron MR (2005) The role of Wnt signaling in cancer and stem cells. Future Oncol 1:787–797

Ricci-Vitiani L, Lombardi DG, Pilozzi E et al (2007) Identification and expansion of human colon-cancer-initiating cells. Nature 445:111–1115

Roccaro AM, Leleu X, Sacco A et al (2008) Resveratrol exerts antiproliferative activity and induces apoptosis in Waldenstrom's macroglobulinemia. Clin Cancer Res 14:1849–1858

Ronchini C, Capobianco AJ (2001) Induction of cyclin D1 transcription and CDK2 activity by Notch(ic): implication for cell cycle disruption in transformation by Notch (ic). Mol Cell Biol 21:5925–5934

Ryu MJ, Cho M, Song JY et al (2008) Natural derivatives of curcumin attenuate the Wnt/beta-catenin pathway through down-regulation of the transcriptional coactivator p300. Biochem Biophys Res Commun 377:1304–1308

Sadzuka Y, Sugiyama T, Sonobe T (2000) Efficacies of tea components on doxorubicin induced antitumor activity and reversal of multidrug resistance. Toxicol. Lett 114:155–162

Saigusa S, Tanaka K, Toiyama Y et al (2009) Correlation of CD133, OCT4, and SOX2 in rectal cancer and their association with distant recurrence after chemoradiotherapy. Ann Surg Oncol 6:3488–3498

Salman H, Bergman M, Djaldetti M et al (2007) Lycopene affects proliferation and apoptosis of four malignant cell lines. Biomed Pharmacother 61:366–369

Sarkar FH, Li Y, Wang Z et al (2009) Cellular signaling perturbation by natural products. Cell Signal 21:1541–1547

Sarkar FH, LI Y, Wang Z et al (2010) The role of nutriceuticals in the regulation of Wnt and Hedgehog signaling in cancer. Cancer Metasta Rev 29:383–394

Sato T, Vries RG, Snippert HJ et al (2009) Single Lgr5 stem cells build crypt-villus structures in vitro without a mesenchymal niche. Nature 459:262–265

Satoh Y, Matsumura I, Tanaka H et al (2004) Roles for c-Myc in self-renewal of hematopoietic stem cells. J Biol Chem 279:24986–24993

Satoskar RR, Shah SJ, Shenoy SG (1986) Evaluation of anti-inflammatory property of curcumin (diferuloyl methane) in patients with postoperative inflammation. Int J Clin Pharmacol Ther Toxicol 24:651–6544

Schatton T, Murphy GF, Frank NY et al (2008) Identification of cells initiating human melanomas. Nature 451:345–349

Scoville DH, Sato T, He XC et al (2008) Current view: intestinal stem cells and signaling. Gastroenterology 134:849–864

Shao ZM, Shen ZZ, Liu CH et al (2002) Curcumin exerts multiple suppressive effects on human breast carcinoma cells. Int J Cancer 98:234–240

Sharoni Y, Giron E, Rise M (1997) Effects of lycopene-enriched tomato oleoresin on 7,12-dimethyl-benz[a]anthracene-induced rat mammary tumors. Cancer Detect Prev 21:118–123

Shen G, Khor TO, Hu R et al (2007) Chemoprevention of familial adenomatous polyposis by natural dietary compounds sulforaphane and dibenzoylmethane alone and in combination in ApcMin/+ mouse. Cancer Res 67:9937–9944

Shervington A, Lu C (2008) Expression of multidrug resistance genes in normal and cancer stem cells. Cancer Invest 26:535–542

Shin MH, Holmes MD, Hankinson SE et al (2002) Intake of dairy products, calcium, and vitamin D and risk of breast cancer. J Natl Cancer Inst 94:1301–1311

Shin HM, Minter LM, Cho OH et al (2006) Notch1 augments NF-kappaB activity by facilitating its nuclear retention. EMBO J 25:129–138

Singh SK, Clarke ID, Teraski M et al (2003) Identification of a cancer stem cell in human brain tumors. Cancer Res 63:5821–5828

Singh SK, Hawkins C, Clarke ID et al (2004a) Identification of human brain tumour initiating cells. Nature 432:396–401

Singh AV, Xiao D, Lew KL et al (2004b) Sulforaphane induces caspasemediated apoptosis in cultured PC-3 human prostate cancer cells and retards growth of PC-3 xenografts in vivo. Carcinogenesis 25:83–90

Slusarz A, Shenouda NS, Sakla MS et al (2010) Common botanical compounds inhibit the hedgehog signaling pathway in prostate cancer. Cancer Res70:3382–3390

So JY, Lee HJ, Smolarek AK et al (2011) A novel Gemini vitamin D analog represses the expression of a stem cell marker CD44 in breast cancer. Mol Pharmacol 79:360–367

Son MJ, Woolard K, Nam DH et al (2009) SSEA-1 is an enrichment marker for tumor-initiating cells in human glioblastoma. Cell Stem Cell 4:440–452

Stockler M, Wilcken NR, Ghersi D et al (2000) Systematic reviews of chemotherapy and endocrine therapy in metastatic breast cancer. Cancer Treat Rev 26:151–168

Su Y, Simmen RC (2009) Soy isoflavone genistein upregulates epithelial adhesion molecule E-cadherin expression and attenuates beta-catenin signaling in mammary epithelial cells. Carcinogenesis 30:331–339

Su LK, Kinzler KW, Vogelstein B et al (1992) Multiple intestinal neoplasia caused by a mutation in the murine homolog of the APC gene. Science 256:668–670

Su Y, Simmen FA, Xiao R, Simmen RC (2007) Expression profiling of rat mammary epithelial cells reveals candidate signaling pathways in dietary protection from mammary tumors. Physiol Genomics 30:8–16

Subramaniam D, Ramalingam S, Houchen CW et al (2010) Cancer stem cells: a novel paradigm for cancer prevention and treatment. Mini Rev Med Chem 10:359–371

Sureban S, May R, Lightfoot et al (2011) DCAMKL-1 regulates epithililial-mesenchymal transition in human pancreatic cells through a miR-200a-dependent mechanism. Cancer Res 71:2328–2338

Taipale J, Beachy PA (2011) The Hedgehog and Wnt signalling pathways in cancer. Nature 411:349–354

Tang L, Jin T, Zeng X, Wang JS (2005) Lycopene inhibits the growth of human androgenindependent prostate cancer cells in vitro and in BALB/c nude mice. J Nutr 135:287–290

Tang FY, Shih CJ, Cheng LH et al (2008) Lycopene inhibits growth of human colon cancer cells via suppression of the Akt signaling pathway. Mol Nutr Food Res 52:646–654

Tang GQ, Yan TQ, Guo W et al (2010) (−)- Epigallocatechin-3-gallate induces apoptosis and suppresses proliferation by inhibiting the human Indian Hedgehog pathway in human chondrosarcoma cells. J Cancer Res Clin Oncology 136:1179–1185

van Breemen RB, Pajkovic N (2008) Multitargeted therapy of cancer by lycopene. Cancer Lett 269:339–351

Verheus M, van Gils CH, Keinan-Boker L et al (2007) Plasma phytoestrogens and subsequent breast cancer risk. J Clin Oncol 25:648–655

Visvader JE, Lindeman GJ (2008) Cancer stem cells in solid tumours: accumulating evidence and unresolved questions. Nat Rev Cancer 8:755–768

Wang J, Shelly L, Miele L (2001) Human Notch-1 inhibits NF-kappa B activity in the nucleus through a direct interaction involving a novel domain. J Immunol167:289–295
Wang Z, Banerjee S, Li Y (2006a) Down-regulation of notch-1 inhibits invasion by inactivation of nuclear factor-kappaB, vascular endothelial growth factor, and matrix metalloproteinase-9 in pancreatic cancer cells. Cancer Res 66:2778–2784
Wang Z, Zhang Y, Li Y et al (2006b) Down-regulation of Notch-1 contributes to cell growth inhibition and apoptosis in pancreatic cancer cells. Mol Cancer Ther 5:483–493
Wang Z, Zhang Y, Banerjee S et al (2006c) Inhibition of nuclear factor kappab activity by genistein is mediated via Notch-1 signaling pathway in pancreatic cancer cells. Int J Cancer 118: 1930–1936
Wang Z, Li Y, Banerjee S, Sarkar FH (2009) Emerging role of Notch in stem cells and cancer. Cancer Lett 279:8–12
Weng AP, Millholland JM, Yashiro-Ohtani Y et al (2006) c-Myc is an important direct target of Notch1 in T-cell acute lymphoblastic leukemia/lymphoma. Genes Dev 20:2096–2109
Wilson A, Radtke F (2006) Multiple functions of Notch signaling in self-renewing organs and cancer. FEBS Lett 580:2860–2568
Woodward WA, Chen MS, Behbod F et al (2007) WNT/beta-catenin mediates radiation resistance of mouse mammary progenitor cells. Proc Natl Acad Sci USA 4:618–623
Wu JY, Rao Y (1999) Fringe: defining borders by regulating the notch pathway. Curr Opin Neurobiol 9:537–543
Wu CP, Calcagno AM, Hladky SB et al (2005) Modulatory effects of plant phenols on human multidrug-resistance proteins 1, 4 and 5 (ABCC1, 4 and 5). FEBS J 272:4725–4740
Xu C, Shen G, Chen C et al (2005) Suppression of NF-kappaB and NFkappaB- regulated gene expression by sulforaphane and PEITC through Ikappa-B alpha, IKK pathway in human prostate cancer PC-3 cells. Oncogene 24:4486–4495
Yan C, Jamaluddin MS, Aggarwal B et al (2005) Gene expression profiling identifies activating transcription factor 3 as a novel contributor to the proapoptotic effect of curcumin. Mol Cancer Ther 4:233–241
Yang ZF, Ho DW, Ng MN et al (2008a) Significance of CD90+ cancer stem cells in human liver cancer. Cancer Cell 13:153–66
Yang W, Yan HX, Chen L et al (2008b) Wnt/beta-catenin signaling contributes to activation of normal and tumorigenic liver progenitor cells. Cancer Res 68:4287–4295
Yu Y, Kanwar SS, Patel BB et al (2009) Elimination of colon cancer stem-like cells by the combination of curcumin and FOLFOX. Transl Oncol 2:321–328
Zhang Y, Tang L (2007) Discovery and development of sulforaphane as a cancer chemopreventive phytochemical. Acta Pharmacol Sin 28:1343–1354
Zhang Y, Talalay P, Cho CG et al (1992) A major inducer of anticarcinogenic protective enzymes from broccoli: isolation and elucidation of structure. Proc Natl Acad Sci USA 89:2399–2403
Zhang Y, Kensler TW, Cho CG et al (1994) Anticarcinogenic activities of sulforaphane and structurally related synthetic norbornyl isothiocyanates. Proc Natl Acad Sci USA 91:3147–3150
Zhou, J, Zhang, H, Gu, P et al (2007) NF-kappa B pathway inhibitors preferentially inhibit breast cancer stemlike cells. Breast Cancer Res Treat 111:419–427
Zhou J, Wang CY, Liu T et al (2008) Persistence of side population cells with high drug efflux capacity in pancreatic cancer. World J. Gastroenterol 14:925–930
Zhou BB, Zhang H, Damelin M et al (2009) Tumour-initiating cells: challenges and opportunities for anticancer drug discovery. Nat Rev Drug Discov 8:806–823
Zhu A, Wang X, Guo Z (2001) Study of tea polyphenol as a reversal agent for carcinoma cell lines' multidrug resistance (study of TP as a MDR reversal agent). Nucl Med Biol 28:735–740
Zhu L, Gibson P, Currle DS et al (2009) Prominin1 marks intestinal stem cells that are susceptible to neoplastic transformation. Nature 457:603–607
Ziegler RG, Hoover RN, Pike MC et al (1993) Migration patterns and breast cancer risk in Asian-American women. J Natl Cancer Inst 85:1819–1827

Chapter 3
Polyphenols as Receptor Tyrosine Kinase Inhibitors and Anti-cancer Agents

David T. Coleman and James A. Cardelli

Abstract Historically, there has been a great deal of interest in the use of natural products to promote human health. A large number of publications have demonstrated that phytochemicals, especially polyphenols, have biological activities that suggest they could positively impact a variety of health problems including cancer. The number of polyphenols is extremely large and we are just now learning the vast number of cellular molecular targets they affect to act as chemopreventive and anti-cancer agents. An important problem yet to be resolved is to identify those key molecular targets impacted by polyphenols that are most critical in cancer progression. Receptor tyrosine kinases (RTKs) are important proteins that couple extracellular signals with intracellular signaling pathways that can contribute to all stages of cancer development. This review will focus on the various ways in which a number of polyphenols can inhibit RTKs. We will discuss the possibility that the inhibition of a multitude of RTKs, often impacted by single polyphenols, can be explained by a few molecular mechanisms. We will discuss the current clinical trials that have been done using polyphenols and approaches that are being used to overcome the issue of bioavailability. Finally, we will also discuss the challenges and possible solutions to advancing polyphenols for actual clinical use as anti-cancer agents.

3.1 Introduction

There is an increasing interest in the use of plant derived compounds (phytochemicals) as chemopreventive and anti-cancer agents (Surh 2003). Much of this interest is the result of the huge cost to develop anti-cancer drugs and the high frequency at which drugs are either never approved or are pulled from the market because of a lack of efficacy or unexpected toxicity. Also, many population studies support the idea that a diet rich in plant-derived, biologically active substances can have a dramatic effect on health and carcinogenesis (Scalbert et al. 2005). Cell culture

J.A. Cardelli (✉)
Department of Microbiology and Immunology and the Feist-Weiller Cancer Center, Louisiana State University Health Sciences Center, Shreveport, LA 71130, USA
e-mail: JCarde@lsuhsc.edu

F.H. Sarkar (ed.), *Nutraceuticals and Cancer*, DOI 10.1007/978-94-007-2630-7_3,

and animal studies have demonstrated that dietary agents can suppress all stages of carcinogenesis, from cellular transformation to metastasis; although many of these animal studies do not fully recapitulate the complexity of human cancer progression and cellular studies often use unachievable levels of polyphenols (Gupta et al. 2010).

Progress in the commercialization of these agents as anti-cancer therapeutics has been slowed for a variety of reasons. For instance, much of the research involves in vitro approaches using cultured cell lines and concentrations of agents that are not achievable in vivo. Also, many of the better studied components appear to impact multiple cellular processes and proteins, compounding the attempts at defining molecular mechanisms and thereby limiting clinical predictability. Critically, as discussed below, there is a paucity of human clinical trials using plant-derived compounds and demonstration that these agents work to slow or stop the progression of cancer in patients is of utmost importance. Finally, even if these trials were successful, there is a lack of patent space for most phytochemicals, so drug company-sponsored research, development, and marketing is wanting.

The goal of this chapter will be to review the evidence that phytochemicals, known as polyphenols, act as anti-cancer agents and to explore the idea that these agents might share common mechanisms of action although their molecular targets may vary. Polyphenols are defined as substances found in plants that are characterized by the presence of at least one hydroxylated phenol group. They can be classified as belonging to the flavonoid, chalcone, stilbene or phenolic acid/alcohol subclasses (Kang et al. 2011). This review will primarily focus on polyphenols that belong to the flavonoid class which includes a bewildering array of chemicals found in a large number of fruits and vegetables. These substances can be further divided into the anthocyanins (e.g. malvidin and cyanidin), flavan-3-ols (e.g. catechins EGCG and theaflavin), flavanones (e.g. taxifolin and hesperetin), flavones (e.g. luteolin and apigenin), isoflavones (e.g. genistein) and flavonols (e.g. quercetin and myricetin). We will also briefly discuss 3 of the better studied non-flavonoid polyphenols, curcumin, ellagic acid and resveratrol (Fig. 3.1). Most polyphenols are potent anti-oxidants which could in part explain how they affect cancer cells, but this review will focus more on their effects on growth factor receptors, specifically receptor tyrosine kinases (RTKs) implicated in cancer progression.

RTKs regulate important signaling pathways in cancer cells that play key roles in cellular proliferation, survival, motility, invasion and metastasis. RTKs are activated by specific ligands (growth factors and cytokines) which results in recruitment and activation of a variety of downstream signaling pathways. Many RTKs are constitutively activated by mutation or overexpressed in tumor cells and they are thought to play a major role in cancer progression. This is consistent with a number of targeted agents developed by drug companies to inhibit the activity of specific receptors, often with some clinical efficacy. Unfortunately, single modality approaches appear to have a smaller success rate then multimodality approaches.

A large number of studies have implicated various polyphenols in targeting not only RTKs but also some of the downstream players including MAP kinase, PI-3-Kinase and NF-B (Kang et al. 2011). Most of these polyphenols appear to act in

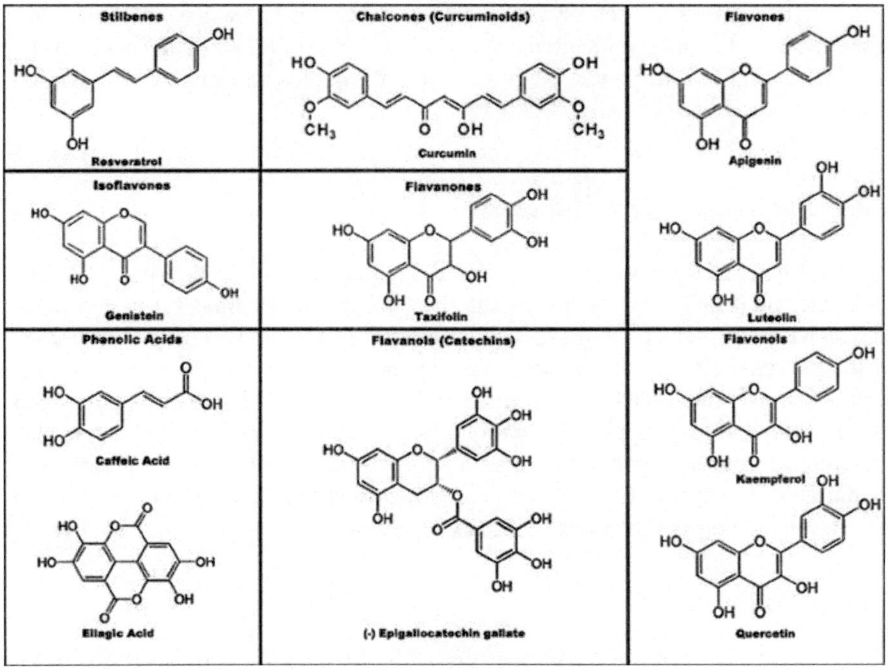

Fig. 3.1 The chemical structures of the polyphenols discussed in this review

a multimodality fashion to inhibit more than one RTK. The focus of this review will be to discuss research to explore how different polyphenols can prevent the activation of RTKs. We will limit our discussion to the following receptors: Insulin-like growth factor-1 receptor (IGF-1R), epidermal growth factor receptor (EGFR) family, vascular endothelial growth factor receptor (VEGF-R), and the hepatocyte growth factor receptor (HGFR or MET). We will explore the idea that a "common" mechanism of action could explain how so many polyphenols can prevent activation of a large number of different RTKs. Finally, we will discuss the evidence supporting the clinical relevance of polyphenols as anti-cancer agents and the future directions.

3.2 Flavonoid Family of Polyphenols

Flavonoids are one of the largest groups of anti-oxidants and are responsible for the vibrant colors found in petals of flowers and fruits. Their distribution is wide spread and includes apples, grapes, walnuts, onions, blueberries, soybeans, citrus fruits and many vegetables. Flavonoids are polyphenol compounds characterized by two or more aromatic rings with at least one hydroxyl group. Within this subclass, individual flavonoids are distinguished by extent of hydroxylation and saturation

(Fig. 3.1). Members in each of the subclasses described below have been demonstrated to be potent inhibitors often against a wide range of RTKs (Kang et al. 2011). In this section, we will review the best studied flavonoids and summarize research that demonstrates their anti-RTK activity.

3.2.1 Flavanols – Tea Catechins

There are 4 main catechins found in green tea, epigallocatechin gallate (EGCG), epigallocatechin (EGC), epicatechin gallate (ECG) and epicatechin (EC), and of these EGCG has been studied the most. The chemopreventive and anti-cancer properties of tea polyphenols have been extensively characterized in a large number of cell culture animal studies (Khan and Mukhtar 2008). The results are compelling and demonstrate that tea polyphenols inhibit a large number of processes and enzymes important in cancer progression. This section will focus on the ability of catechins to inhibit RTK activity. This area was recently covered in an excellent review from the Bisson laboratory (Larsen et al. 2010).

3.2.1.1 MET

MET is a disulphide-linked heterodimer consisting of an entirely extracellular α-domain and a β-chain including a short ectodomain, followed by a transmembrane and a cytoplasmic domain. The cytoplasmic domain contains a juxtamembrane and kinase domain and a carboxy-terminus. Activation of the MET pathway occurs following the binding of its only known ligand hepatocyte growth factor (HGF). Phosphorylation of two cytoplasmic tyrosine residues act as docking sites for a variety of adaptors, including Gab1, Grb2, PI3K, PLCγ, Src, and Shp2 (Schaeper et al. 2000). Gab1 has been shown to play an important role in Met signaling by relaying signals to Shp2, Crk, PI3K and others (Gu and Neel 2003; Rosário and Birchmeier 2003) to activate the PI3K and Ras-Raf-MAPK pathways (reviewed in (Gao and Woude 2005; Schaeper et al. 2000). These major pathways (and others) are responsible for increases in proliferation, survival, motility, invasion and metastasis of tumor cells. MET is often over-expressed or mutated in human tumors, leading to activation in the absence of HGF (Benvenuti and Comoglio 2007; Tulasne and Foveau 2007).

It has been demonstrated that EGCG and ECG inhibited activation of MET in multiple breast cancer cell lines at physiologically relevant concentrations (Bigelow and Cardelli 2006). The non-galloyated catechins were much less effective, suggesting a role for the gallate group. The Dashwood laboratory also found that ECG and EGCG effectively blocked HGF activation of MET in a variety of colon cancer cell lines (Larsen and Dashwood 2010). EGCG also blocks MET activation in prostate cancer cells (Duhon et al. 2010), lung cancer cells (Milligan et al. 2009), glioma cancer cells (Cardelli, unpublished), oral cancer cells (Koh et al. 2011) and hypopharyngeal (FADU) cancer cells (Lim et al. 2008), demonstrating the generality of these findings. Most of these studies used physiologically relevant (low micromolar) concentrations of EGCG. The potential mechanisms of action for EGCG with regard to RTKs (discussed in greater detail below) include disruption of lipid rafts (Duhon et al. 2010) and binding to the ATP pocket of the kinase activity domain (Larsen et al. 2010).

Interestingly, we published that EGCG lowered serum levels of HGF in patients with prostate cancer and decreased production of HGF in cancer associated fibroblasts (McLarty et al. 2009), suggesting this polyphenol can act on both tumor cells and fibroblasts found in the stroma to inhibit the HGF-MET signaling axis.

3.2.1.2 EGFR Family

The EGFR family of receptors is important in the regulation of cancer cell proliferation and survival and consists of 4 members: EGFR (ErbB1), EGFR-2 (HER-2), EGFR-3 (HER-3) and EGFR-4 (HER-4). A variety of ligands have been identified that activate these receptors, including EGF, TGF, heregulin and others (Foley et al. 2010). The EGF receptors mediate their effects via homo- and heterodimerization, transphosphorylation, and subsequent activation of downstream signaling pathways, which include the PI3K and the MAPK pathways. HER2 is overexpressed or mutated in 20–30% of breast cancer patients, leading to a more invasive outcome concomitant with resistance to common chemotherapeutic regimens (Sebastian et al. 2006). No natural ligand has been discovered for HER2; therefore, signaling by this receptor requires heterodimerization with other EGFR family members, including EGFR and HER3, which are also overexpressed in a high proportion of breast cancer patients (reviewed in (Sebastian et al. 2006)).

It was first reported in 1997 that EGCG blocked the activation of EGFR in epidermal carcinoma cell lines and might do so by preventing binding of EGF to its receptor (Liang et al. 1997). Another laboratory proposed that inactivation of EGFR was the result of an oxidative byproduct of EGCG although this has been disputed (Dashwood et al. 2002; Hou et al. 2005). Comparable to what was observed for MET, it has been reported that EGCG disrupts lipid rafts to prevent signaling through EGFR (Adachi et al. 2007). It has also been demonstrated that EGCG can lower levels of EGFR by both inhibiting transcription of the encoding gene (Fu and Chen 2006) and inducing internalization followed by degradation (Adachi et al. 2008).

HER2 has also been demonstrated to be a target for EGCG. EGCG was demonstrated to inhibit growth of HER2 overexpressing mouse mammary carcinoma cell line, NF639, at the level of receptor phosphorylation (Pianetti et al. 2002) consistent with results found using the BT474 cell-line (Masuda et al. 2003). EGCG acted to reduce basal activity and to block ligand mediated increases in phosphorylation.

The humanized monoclonal antibody Trastuzumab was developed to target HER2 and has shown benefit as a first line treatment for HER2 positive breast cancer (Callahan and Hurvitz 2011). However, resistance to Trastuzumab therapy and subsequent cancer progression are common. A recent report provides evidence that

EGCG can also inhibit growth and survival of Trastuzumab-resistant breast cancer cells (Eddy et al. 2007). Similar results have been found for other cancer cell lines. A small percentage of non-small cell lung cancer patients respond to the EGFR inhibitor erlotinib, although acquired resistance is almost inevitable (Moran 2011). Milligan et al. demonstrated that EGCG increased the effects of erlotinib in resistant lung cancer cells (Milligan et al. 2009). Together, these studies suggest that EGCG may prove to be a useful adjuvant combinatorial agent increasing the effectiveness of targeted therapeutics.

3.2.1.3 VEGFR

The VEGF signaling pathway consists of two transmembrane receptors, VEGFR1 and VEGFR2 and a soluble form of VEGFR1, sVEGFR. VEGF-A, -B, -C and D- are capable of binding all forms of the receptor. Activation of the pathway in endothelial cells leads to endothelial growth and subsequent increased tumoral microvessel density, invasion and metastasis (Koch et al. 2011). High serum and intratumoral levels of VEGF are associated with poor prognosis, high recurrence, and increased risk of metastatic disease (Fox et al. 2007).

It has been found that EGCG blocks the VEGF signaling axis. Lee et al. reported that micromolar concentrations of EGCG inhibited the activation of VEGF-R1 and –R2 (Lee et al. 2004). EGCG, versus the other catechins, was most effective at inhibiting angiogenesis perhaps by preventing the binding of VEGF to its receptor (Kondo et al. 2002). EGCG blocked VEGF secretion from both HUVEC and MDA-MB-231 breast carcinoma cells most likely by reducing transcription of the encoding gene (Sartippour et al. 2002). EGCG reduced levels of the AP-1 transcription factors, c-FOS and c-JUN (Sartippour et al. 2002), and since the VEGF gene contains AP-1 sites in its promoter, this is consistent with EGCG lowering VEGF levels by decreasing AP-1 transcription factor availability. EGCG also reduced expression of VEGF from prostate cancer associated fibroblasts and lowered VEGF in prostate cancer patients consuming high levels of tea extract (McLarty et al. 2009).

3.2.1.4 IGF-1R

IGF-I or IGF-II can activate IGF-1R stimulating downstream proteins including PI-3K/AKT, Ras/Raf and MAPK/ERK. Activation of these signaling pathways leads to increased proliferation, transformation and survival. Of interest, this pathway is associated with prostate and breast cancer development and poor prognosis (Shimizu et al. 2008). EGCG has been reported to inhibit IGF-1R kinase activity in cell-free systems (Li et al. 2007), perhaps by directly binding to the receptor to inhibit downstream activation of AKT and ERK, thus inhibiting IGF-1 stimulation of proliferation. Another report demonstrated EGCG blocked activation of IGF-1R in hepatoma cells and reduced levels of IGF-1 and IGF-2.

3.2.2 Flavones: Apigenin and Luteolin

Flavones, although less commonly found than the other flavonoids, are found in red peppers, celery, broccoli, and apples. The flavones apigenin and luteolin are characterized by a C-ring 2–3 double bond with the B ring connected to the C ring at the second carbon. The flavone structure provides these compounds with a slightly more lipophilic nature than the similar flavonol class of flavonoids. Increased lipophilicity suggests flavones have greater membrane permeability and thus, greater potential cellular activity (Beecher 2003; Scalbert and Williamson 2000; Walle 2004). Importantly, in skin penetration studies with human volunteers, flavones were shown to penetrate into deep skin layers, not just absorbed at the surface (Merfort et al. 1994). This information provides merit for the use of this class of polyphenols in topical therapeutics.

IGF stimulation is a major player in the progression of prostate cancer. As such, it is highly significant that recent reports reveal both luteolin and apigenin inhibit IGF-1 induced activation of EGFR and IGF-1R in prostate cancer cells DU145 and PC-3 (Fang et al. 2006). These compounds are effective in the lower micromolar range in vitro and have also shown effective at lowering active IGF-1R levels in tumor xenograft tissue samples (Shukla and Gupta 2009).

Apigenin has been shown to inhibit the growth promoting effects of Her2 overexpression in breast cancer cells via multiple mechanisms. Firstly, the compound appears to shutdown the major downstream signaling pathway of PI3K both by direct inhibition of this protein as well as by blocking the docking of PI3K with Her2. Secondly, it has been shown that apigenin causes degradation of Her2 by dissociating its complex with the chaperone protein GRP4 leading to polyubiquitination and proteasomal degradation. Ultimately these effects on Her2 signaling lead to apoptosis of breast cancer cells that are addicted to oncogenic Her2 overexpression (Way et al. 2004; Way et al. 2005). Comparable results were observed with head and neck carcinoma cell lines (Masuelli et al. 2011). Similarly, luteolin downregulates Her2 protein levels in breast and ovarian cancer cell lines by dissociating the receptor from its chaperone Hsp90 leading to proteasomal degradation (Chiang et al. 2007). Interestingly, the effect of these two compounds is most profound when applied to cells with aberrant receptor overexpression. Direct inhibitory effects of flavones on EGFR activation have also been reported (Huang et al. 1999; Lee et al. 2002).

The HGF/MET signaling axis is another target of both apigenin and luteolin. Work of the Cardelli research group has shown that, along with Luteolin, apigenin downregulates the expression of MET in a number of cell lines (Coleman et al. 2009). Although the specific mechanism of this action for apigenin has not yet been delineated, by structural comparison it is suspected that effects on fatty acid synthase activity cause the posttranslational downregulation of c-Met. It has been reported that at much higher concentrations luteolin can inhibit activation of the c-Met receptor (Lee et al. 2006). Apigenin does not appear to directly inhibit HGF-induced activation of MET; however, HGF-induced invasion and migration are prevented most likely due to direct inhibition of PI3K, similar to luteolin (Agullo et al. 1997; Lee et al. 2008).

Luteolin and apigenin have both been shown to affect angiogenesis associated receptor tyrosine kinases through a number of mechanisms as well. PDGFR signaling is involved in promoting the migration of smooth muscle cells required for the stabilization of tumor-associated neovasculature. These two flavones are reported to block PDGF-induced activation of PDGFR-β thereby impairing smooth muscle cell migration. In addition, by blocking PDGFR signaling, these compounds reduced smooth muscle cell-derived VEGF secretion at the level of transcription. In this report, luteolin and apigenin had potent effects at 15 μM while sample flavonol compounds, kaempferol and myricetin had no effect. However, for reasons not mentioned, the effects of the flavones required 18 h of preincubation but did not cause decreased receptor levels. The antiangiogenic potential of these compounds was demonstrated by inhibition of vessel formation in an in vivo mouse Matrigel plug assay (Lamy et al. 2008).

3.2.3 Flavonols: Quercetin and Kaempferol

Flavonols are much more abundant in food sources than the flavones. This class of compounds including quercetin and kaempferol is found in most fruits, vegetables, and grains but is especially rich in citrus fruits, tea leaves, and onions. These compounds are characterized, much like flavones, by a 2–3 double bond in the C ring as well as a B-C ring connection at the second C ring carbon; however, these two classes are distinguished by the flavonols having a c-ring hydroxyl group in addition to the double bonded oxygen (Beecher 2003; Scalbert and Williamson 2000; Walle 2004).

Quercetin has been shown in multiple studies to inhibit activation of ErB family receptors in different cancer cells lines and through different mechanisms. In multiple cell lines the mechanism of receptor downregulation is through ATP-binding site competition in heat-shock proteins followed by polyubiquitination and degradation of the receptor. This action of quercetin has been implicated for degradation of EGFR and Her2 (Jeong et al. 2008; Jung et al. 2010). In HT-29 colon cancer cells, quercetin inhibited Her2 and Her3 expression at the level of transcription, resulting in apoptosis (Kim et al. 2005b). Researchers have also demonstrated that quercetin can block the phosphorylation of EGFR in colon and pancreatic cell lines (Fridrich et al. 2008; Huang et al. 1999; Lee et al. 2002).

A number of studies have reported the effects of quercetin on angiogenesis. In human gastric cancer cells, quercetin was shown to reduce both the expression of VEGFR as well as its ligand VEGF although the mechanism was not reported (Yu et al. 2009). In the lung cancer cell line H157, quercetin was reported to decrease expression of VEGF; however, in this cell line it was specifically in a HIF1-α independent manner (Ansó et al. 2010).

Researchers have determined that the flavonols quercetin and kaempferol can inhibit HGF-induced MET activation in a cell line model of the highly invasive medulloblastoma at lower micromolar ranges (Labbe et al. 2009). In addition, as mentioned earlier with luteolin and apigenin, quercetin was shown to downregulate

MET protein expression in prostate cancer cell lines, possibly by inhibition of fatty acid synthase activity (Coleman et al. 2009).

In another report, quercetin and kaempferol were shown to block the anti-apoptotic and growth promoting effects of IGF in rat prostate cancer cell lines at concentrations between 25 and 40 μM (Wang et al. 2003). Using an ex vivo kinase activity assay, researchers determined the receptor tyrosine kinases most potently affected by quercetin were PDGFR and FGFR at 2 μM (Boly et al. 2011).

3.2.4 Flavanones: Taxifolin

Flavanones are characterized by a saturated C-ring (Beecher 2003; Scalbert and Williamson 2000; Walle 2004). In comparison with other flavonoids, the flavanones, taxifolin specifically, often have the least biological activity in cell-based assays, with respect to receptor tyrosine kinases. In fact, the only report of taxifolin affecting receptor tyrosine kinases at micromolar concentrations is that of the Chen laboratory, showing it downregulates VEGF expression in ovarian cancer cells, albeit less than any other flavonoid class tested (Luo et al. 2008). However, what studies of taxifolin do provide is a structural comparison to more effective compounds. Consistently in cell based assays, flavonoid compounds without an unsaturated 2–3 bond within the C ring, including taxifolin, show very minimal efficacy thereby, implicating biological importance to the saturation status of this bond.

3.2.5 Isoflavones: Genistein

Isoflavones are unique in that the B-C ring connection is formed at the third carbon of the C ring, but like the flavones and flavonols the 2–3 bond of the C ring is unsaturated. Soy foods and legumes are enriched in genistein and other isoflavones. Because of the high content in Asian diets, genistein is proposed as an explanation for lower rates of breast cancer in Asian women (Beecher 2003; Scalbert and Williamson 2000; Walle 2004). Based on previous studies, genistein is often considered to be a general tyrosine kinase inhibitor with little or no activity toward serine/threonine kinases. The authors of this chapter feel it necessary to suggest caution when considering the use of genistein as a tool to inhibit tyrosine kinase activity in cell-based assays. As made clear in this review, many classes of polyphenols have pleiotropic biological activities within a cellular context that would make interpretation of supposed specific effects very difficult. With this said, whether specific or not, a multitude of papers have revealed effects of genistein on cancer-associated receptor tyrosine kinases.

The Ellington laboratory reported that treatment of immortalized non-neoplastic breast epithelial cells with submicromolar concentrations of genistein downregulated the MET receptor suggesting chemopreventive potential (Singletary and Ellington 2006). Using the transgenic adenocarcinoma of mouse prostate (TRAMP) model, researchers used a diet containing genistein at 250 mg/kg, starting at 5 weeks of age and lasting for 12 weeks. Genistein in the diet resulted in downregulation of both EGFR and IGF-1R among other mitogenic proteins (Wang et al. 2004). In other reports, genistein prevents the basal and hypoxia-induced expression of VEGF in prostate cancer cells as well as HUVECs. This downregulation was shown to be, at least in part, through inhibition of HIF-1α nuclear accumulation (Guo et al. 2007). The Sarkar laboratory reported that genistein was able to ameliorate the increase in MMP secretion endowed by transfection of MDA-MB-435 cells with erbb2 (Li et al. 1999). Another report indicates Genistein can both inhibit IGF-1 activation of IGF-1R as well as downregulate total IGF-1R protein expression in colon cancer cells (Kim et al. 2005a).

3.3 Non-flavonoid Family of Polyphenols

3.3.1 Curcumin

Curcumin is a polyphenol found at high levels in the Indian spice turmeric and has been used for centuries to treat anti-inflammatory diseases. More recently, a large number of studies have revealed that curcumin might have anti-cancer properties. Several review articles cover in detail the myriad number of molecular targets and pathways impacted by this polyphenol in cancer cells (Goel et al. 2008; Shehzad et al. 2010). This section will focus on curcumin as an inhibitor of RTK activity.

A number of studies have revealed that curcumin has an impact on the EGR family of receptors. Chen et al. reported that like EGCG, curcumin lowered EGFR levels by suppressing activity of the transcription factor egr-1 (Chen et al. 2005). Another report demonstrated that curcumin inhibited AP-1 activity resulting in a reduction in transcription of MET (Seol et al. 2000). It was also reported that curcumin blocked activation of EGFR by EGF although no mechanism for this repression was presented (Korutla et al. 1995; Zhou et al. 2007). Another interesting study revealed that curcumin disrupted the physical interaction of α6β4 with EGFR perhaps by disrupting lipid rafts (Soung and Chung 2011). This integrin is known to couple to EGFR and other RTKs to enhance signaling in cancer cells. The mechanism for this action has yet to be discovered.

3.3.2 Resveratrol

Resveratrol is a polyphenol found in a variety of different plants but most notably in high concentrations in the skin of red grapes. Interest in this polyphenol is primarily due to its anticarcinogenic, anti-inflammatory, and cardioprotective properties (Kundu and Surh 2008). A large number of targets have also been proposed for resveratrol to explain its health benefits. Compared to curcumin and EGCG, much less research has been published regarding the role of resveratrol as an RTK inhibitor. Resveratrol has been reported to block EGFR and IGFR activation (Stewart and O'Brian 2004; Tang et al. 2008). An interesting study also reported that resveratrol lowered ROS-mediated invasion of hepatoma cells perhaps by reducing the expression of HGF (Miura et al. 2004). Resveratrol was also shown to block Met activation in tumor cells in vitro (De Ledinghen et al. 2001).

3.3.3 Ellagic Acid

Ellagic acid is metabolically derived following ingestion of polyphenols named ellagitannins, found in fruits and nuts, including pomegranates. Ellagic acid impacts a number of molecular targets involved in inflammation, most notably NF-κB (Heber 2008). This polyphenol has been demonstrated to lower levels of VEGF in an in vivo model.

We have determined that ellagic acid, consisting of two gallic acid groups in a ring structure, is 100 times more potent than EGCG at inhibiting HGF-induced motility of prostate tumor cells. We have also determined that ellagic acid does not directly prevent activation of MET by HGF but instead appears to "attenuate" activity perhaps by activating phosphatases that remove phosphates from the receptor tail (manuscript in preparation). A range of largely unstudied plant polyphenols (hydrolysable tannins), especially punicafolin, effectively blocked HGF-induced tumor cell invasion (Tanimura et al. 2005). As described above, the C-ring gallate group was demonstrated to be critical for the activity of tea polyphenols, since epicatechin and epigallocatechin were much less effective in breast and prostate tumor cells. Together this suggests that a range of chemicals containing attached gallate groups could be potent MET inhibitors.

3.4 Are There Common Mechanisms of Action?

As described above, it is apparent that different polyphenols can inactivate the same RTKs. In addition, individual polyphenols can inactivate multiple RTKs. In this section, we will discuss the possible mechanisms of action of flavonoid polyphenols and if there is a common theme that emerges. We will primarily focus on EGCG and discuss how a single agent can inactivate so many different RTKs. Some of the possible proposed mechanisms of action of polyphenols on RTK activity include: (1) competitive inhibition of binding of growth factor ligands or ATP binding sites, (2) inhibition of RTK transcription or translation, (3) generation of ROS or oxidative products, (4) inhibition of fatty acid synthase (FASN) and (5) disruption of lipid rafts and plasma membrane organization (Fig. 3.2).

Studies have reported that EGCG directly binds to and/or prevents interaction of EGF and VEGF with their cognate receptors (Kondo et al. 2002; Liang et al. 1997). An additional study demonstrated that EGCG might bind to the ATP binding site of

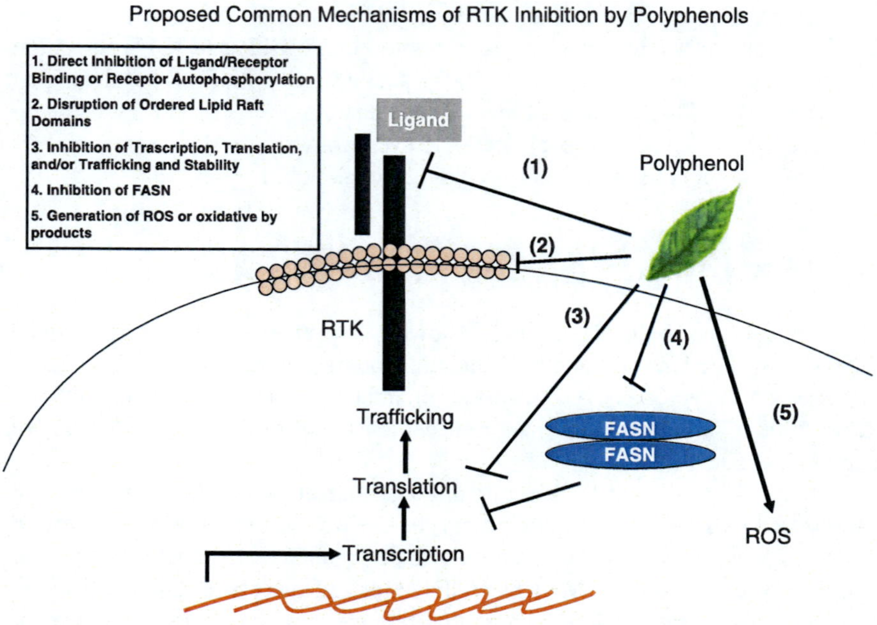

Fig. 3.2 Schematic representation of the various ways in which polyphenols can act to inhibit RTK activity or levels

MET. Given the relative simple structure of this catechin and the diverse structures of these putative targets, these studies are difficult to interpret at a molecular level.

EGCG can inactivate ERK activity directly, leading to inactivation transcription factors like EGR-1 which regulates expression of RTKs. Three studies have in fact demonstrated that EGCG lowers the transcription of EGFR, VEGF and IL-8 perhaps via ERK inhibition (Fu and Chen 2006; McLarty et al. 2009; Sartippour et al. 2002).

EGCG is quickly oxidized under normal cell culture condition and it has been proposed that this oxidized derivative is responsible for inactivation of EGFR (Hou et al. 2005), since the addition of superoxide dismutase reduces the effectiveness of EGCG. Also, high concentrations of EGCG can generate intracellular ROS, and this could inactivate receptors; however this has been disputed in a subsequent study (Dashwood et al. 2002).

Another common mechanism of action seems to be the ability of flavanoids to inhibit the activity of FASN. Swinnen et al. published a report revealing the effects of flavanoids including luteolin, apigenin, quercetin, and EGCG on FASN activity (Brusselmans et al. 2003; Brusselmans et al. 2005). FASN is the sole enzyme responsible for de novo fatty acid synthesis and has been shown to commonly be hyperactive in cancer. In cancer, these fatty acids are utilized exceptionally for phospholipids partitioning into lipid rafts, as well as for post-translational modifications of signaling proteins (Menendez and Lupu 2007). The work of Ruth Lupu and

Javier Menendez has shown that FASN inhibition can downregulate Her2 through PEA-3 mediated transcriptional repression (Menendez et al. 2005). Conversely, overexpression of FASN has been shown to drive expression and activity of erbB family receptors (Vazquez-Martin et al. 2008). Our laboratory has established a link between c-Met expression and FASN activity (Coleman et al. 2009). Furthermore, numerous studies have emphasized the importance of palmitoylation of signaling proteins downstream of receptor tyrosine kinase activity (reviewed in (Linder and Deschenes 2007; Resh 2006)). FASN inhibition by flavonoids can prevent this posttranslational modification, thereby repressing the activity of multiple signaling pathways.

Lipid rafts are highly ordered domains of the plasma membrane, rich in sphingolipids and cholesterol, surrounded by unordered phospholipids. These structures are important mediators of cellular signaling and several RTKs reside within lipid rafts. RTKs move in and out of these domains, resulting in either stimulation or inhibition of signaling pathways. These lipid rafts provide a scaffolding environment for anchorage of receptors and their downstream mediators resulting in activation of signaling (reviewed in (Pike 2009)).

A study published over 10 years ago used surface plasmon resonance imaging to demonstrate that EGCG bound to lipid rafts on the surface of KU812 cells and inhibited the IgE receptor, Fcε-RI (Fujimura et al. 2004). Also, EGCG binds with high affinity to the laminin receptor which localizes primarily to lipid rafts (Tachibana et al. 2004).

EGFR localizes to lipid rafts and the Weinstein laboratory reported that the non-activated form of EGFR was localized in the soluble non-lipid raft fraction, whereas the phosphorylated, active form moved to the insoluble lipid rafts (Adachi et al. 2007). EGCG and Polyphenon E inhibited EGF-induced movement of EGFR into lipid rafts, and thereby, the formation of an active EGFR dimer and EGF binding. EC demonstrated no inhibitory activity. EGCG blocked the intercalation of DiIC16 into lipid rafts which is consistent with an alteration in ordered lipid rafts.

A recent study also demonstrated that active MET resided in lipid rafts (Duhon et al. 2010). Furthermore, agents that removed or lowered cholesterol levels blocked HGF-induced signaling in prostate cancer cells and prostate cancer associated fibroblasts. Finally, the addition of cholesterol partially blocked the inhibitory activity of EGCG which is consistent with this polyphenol altering the position of cholesterol (Duhon et al. 2010). In support of these combined observations, several biochemical studies have revealed the tendency of plant flavonoids, including catechins, to incorporate into hydrophobic regions or the polar membrane interface of synthetic membranes.

Adachi reported that EGCG altered the gramicidin transport channel and we have demonstrated HGF-activation of lysosome trafficking is dependent on the sodium proton transporters NHE1 and NHE3 (Adachi et al. 2007; Steffan et al. 2010). These data suggest that a target for EGCG and perhaps other polyphenols could be ion transport channels. It seems reasonable to propose that RTK activity could be coupled to ion channels that represent a primary target for polyphenols.

Finally, studies performed over 40 years ago revealed that the plasma membranes of cancer cells were biochemically distinct from normal cells in terms of glycoproteins, glycolipids, lipids and other plasma membrane moieties (Nicolson 1982). Lipid rafts in tumor cells represent a site for protein complex formation leading to downstream activation of various RTK-mediated cellular signaling pathways, resulting in increased tumor growth and aggressiveness. It is an intriguing possibility that EGCG and other flavonoids inactivate or disrupt lipid rafts or other regions of the plasma membrane to inhibit the activation of RTKs localized at the cell surface.

3.5 Clinical Relevance and Future Directions

3.5.1 Evidence of Clinical Impact of Polyphenols

3.5.1.1 Bioavailability

A conundrum that has plagued the study of polyphenols as anti-cancer agents not only includes identifying the *key* molecular targets for these agents but also involves the physiological relevance of in vitro studies. Many of the published reports demonstrating an effect of a particular polyphenol use concentrations 10–100 times that observed in vivo. This disconnect has slowed progress in developing these agents for clinical use. For instance, micromolar concentrations of curcumin have routinely been used in vitro but recent studies in humans have shown that consumption of very large doses of this polyphenol, although well tolerated, leads to submicromolar levels of curcumin in the serum (Goel et al. 2008; Shehzad et al. 2010). This does not mean curcumin is inactive as a human anti-cancer agent, but does argue that targets in vivo may not be directly predictable based on in vitro studies. The same conclusion can be drawn for other polyphenols, such as resveratrol. Low bioavailability is the result of many factors including poor adsorption, rapid metabolism and ways to improve bioavailability are discussed below.

3.5.1.2 Clinical Trials

EGCG – Data on biological efficacy of polyphenols can only be drawn from clinical trials and this area of research has only recently begun to be explored. The most data we have is from the study of EGCG. Earlier phase I trials demonstrated that EGCG was well tolerated and that serum levels of more than 1 micromolar were achievable (Chow et al. 2003; Chow et al. 2005), in line with concentrations that have been demonstrated to work in vitro. There have been 4 published clinical trials using EGCG or extracts from tea enriched in this polyphenol. An open label Phase II study using a tea extract demonstrated no clinical efficacy in men with advanced prostate cancer (Jatoi et al. 2003). A second trial in men with hormone refractory prostate cancer also demonstrated no effects but the dose of EGCG was 5 times lower than used in the two trials described next (Choan et al. 2005). A third trial involved treating men with high grade prostatic intraepithelial neoplasia (HG-PIN) with green tea extract (Bettuzzi et al. 2006). The authors observed a significant reduction in the rate at which HG-PIN progressed to prostate cancer in the treated group. A final phase II single arm trial done by our group examined the effectiveness of Polyphenon E (containing 800 mg of EGCG and lesser amounts of catechins) on reduction of a number of serum markers predictive of prostate cancer progression (McLarty et al. 2009). Decreases in the serum levels of HGF, VEGF, IGF-1 and PSA were observed over an average dose period of 43 days. To our knowledge no clinical studies using tea extracts have measured levels of active receptors, although our preliminary results suggest that men involved in the trial who consumed Polyphenon E demonstrated a significant reduction in phosphorylated MET in prostate cancer tissue.

Curcumin – Several studies have examined the safety and pharmacokinetics of curcumin and they have demonstrated that doses as high as 8 gram per day are well tolerated (reviewed in (Goel et al. 2008; Shehzad et al. 2010). Demonstrations that curcumin acts as a anticancer agent in humans is in its early stages and bioavailability still remains an issue.

Genistein and isoflavones – A few phase-I/II trials have been published using isoflavone supplementation. In a phase I studies it was demonstrated that micromolar levels of genistein was reached in patients given high doses of isoflavones and this was not associated with any toxicity (reviewed in (Banerjee et al. 2008)). A phase II trial was also done supplementing prostate cancer patients (androgen-sensitive or –insensitive) with Novasoy containing high levels of genistein. The authors reported a significant reduction in the rise rate of PSA in both groups of patients (Hussain et al. 2003).

3.5.2 More Effective Use of Polyphenols

A recent study summarized nearly 100 papers that examined bioavailability of 18 major polyphenols (Manach et al. 2005). The conclusions were that most of the polyphenols reached submicromolar concentrations in the serum, levels that would be inactive in vitro. This issue has largely been ignored but needs to be addressed in future studies. In this section, we will present some ideas regarding approaches that either raise the working concentration of polyphenols in serum or allow them to be more effective at lower concentrations.

3.5.2.1 Nanoparticles to Deliver Polyphenols

Research efforts have increased dramatically in the area of nanoparticle technology to deliver chemicals, sometimes in a directed fashion, to treat human cancer. A recent review does an excellent job of summarizing the use of nanotechnology to more effectively deliver polyphenols and other nutraceuticals that have poor solubility and low bioavailability (Nair et al. 2010). The list of nanoparticles containing nutraceuticals generated using a variety of platforms include EGCG, curcumin, ellagic acid, eugenol, genistein, quercetin, resveratrol and others. Studies have demonstrated that nanoparticles containing curcumin improve oral bioavailability by at least 9-fold compared to ingestion of curcumin alone, and others have found that encapsulation enhances the anticancer activity of this polyphenol (Bansal et al. 2011). Another study used layer by layer technology to generate nanoparticles loaded with EGCG (Shutava et al. 2009) and demonstrated an increased effect in vitro while another group used PLA-PEG nanoparticles to enhance chemoprevention in animal models (Siddiqui and Mukhtar 2010). Perhaps even more intriguing is the reported generation of nanoparticles that can be targeted to cell surface proteins overexpressed in tumor cells (Sanna et al. 2011). We envision that these nanoparticles loaded with polyphenols could be targeted to RTKs such as MET and EGFR overexpressed in many types of cancers.

Many of these in vivo studies administered the polyphenol-nanoparticle by i.v injection. Future research will need to generate nanoparticles that can be administered orally and still increase the serum levels of the active polyphenol.

3.5.2.2 Combination Therapy

Another way to increase the effectiveness of polyphenols as RTK inhibitors is to combine them with each other or with targeted agents. We published a report demonstrating that EGCG increased the responsiveness of lung cancer cells in vitro and in vivo to the EGFR inhibitor erlotinib (Milligan et al. 2009). Many of these cell lines were completely resistant to this targeted agent in the absence of EGCG. Other reports have appeared demonstrating that polyphenols can enhance the effectiveness of chemotherapy and radiotherapy, although the molecular targets have not been defined (Suganuma et al. 2011; Yunos et al. 2011).

It is conceivable that combinations of polyphenols could be more effective at inhibiting RTKs and acting as anti-cancer agents than single polyphenols at the same concentration. This would be important since bioavailability is an issue, and low serum/tissue levels of polyphenols might not be limiting if multiple polyphenols were present and combinations were more effective than single agents. Relatively few studies have been published demonstrating additivity and/or synergy of combinations of phytochemicals but we predict this will be an increasingly important area of future research.

3.5.3 The Long Road to Clinical Use

Although in vitro and in vivo studies have demonstrated repeatedly that polyphenols possess anti-cancer and potentially other health benefits, the clinical use of these agents has languished. We propose it is time to change this and shift emphasis of polyphenol research from cell culture based towards clinical trials, development and eventual commercialization. There are many reasons for the delay in implementing this phase of research including, difficulty gaining approval for use of polyphenols as anti-cancer agents given the high cost, time and effort for clinical trials, lack of access to drug development facilities, problems in changing the established paradigms that polyphenols will never be as efficacious as "true" cancer therapies and last but not least, the general lack of interest by drug companies in advancing development of natural products. This last problem is generally thought to be due to the lack of patent space for most polyphenols. The challenge that faces most basic scientists studying polyphenols is not realizing the difficulties they will face in ever seeing their favorite polyphenol being used routinely in the clinic as a chemopreventive or anti-cancer agent. Scientists will need to learn about and become savvy in identifying the various avenues available for creating patent spaces for natural products, including some of the approaches mentioned above such as nanoparticle encapsulation of polyphenols and unique combinations of polyphenols. Such ventures to develop natural product based anti-cancer and chemopreventive agents will require a combined collaborative effort by the scientific community, academic institutions and the pharmaceutical industry.

References

Adachi S, Nagao T, Ingolfsson HI et al (2007) The inhibitory effect of epigallocatechin gallate on activation of the epidermal growth factor receptor is associated with altered lipid order in ht29 colon cancer cells. Cancer Res 13:6493–6501

Adachi S, Nagao T, To S et al (2008) Epigallocatechin gallate causes internalization of the epidermal growth factor receptor in human colon cancer cells. Carcinogenesis 10:1986–1993

Agullo G, Gamet-Payrastre L, Manenti S et al (1997) Relationship between flavonoid structure and inhibition of phosphatidylinositol 3-kinase: a comparison with tyrosine kinase and protein kinase c inhibition. Biochem Pharmacol 11:1649–1657

Ansó E, Zuazo A, Irigoyen M et al (2010) Flavonoids inhibit hypoxia-induced vascular endothelial growth factor expression by a hif-1 independent mechanism. Biochem Pharmacol 11: 1600–1609

Banerjee S, Li Y, Wang Z et al (2008) Multi-targeted therapy of cancer by genistein. Cancer Lett 2:226–242

Bansal SS, Goel M, Aqil F et al (2011) Advanced drug-delivery systems of curcumin for cancer chemoprevention. Cancer Prevent Res 4:1158–1171

Beecher GR (2003) Overview of dietary flavonoids: nomenclature, occurrence and intake. J Nutr 10:3248S–3254S

Benvenuti S, Comoglio PM (2007) The met receptor tyrosine kinase in invasion and metastasis. J Cell Physiol 2:316–325

Bettuzzi S, Brausi M, Rizzi F et al (2006) Chemoprevention of human prostate cancer by oral administration of green tea catechins in volunteers with high-grade prostate intraepithelial neoplasia: a preliminary report from a one-year proof-of-principle study. Cancer Res 2:1234–1240

Bigelow RLH, Cardelli JA (2006) The green tea catechins, (-)-epigallocatechin-3-gallate (egcg) and (-)-epicatechin-3-gallate (ecg), inhibit hgf//met signaling in immortalized and tumorigenic breast epithelial cells. Oncogene 13:1922–1930

Boly R, Gras T, Lamkami T et al (2011) Quercetin inhibits a large panel of kinases implicated in cancer cell biology. Int J Oncol 3:833–842

Brusselmans K, De Schrijver E, Heyns W et al (2003) Epigallocatechin-3-gallate is a potent natural inhibitor of fatty acid synthase in intact cells and selectively induces apoptosis in prostate cancer cells. Int J Cancer 6:856–862

Brusselmans K, Vrolix R, Verhoeven G et al (2005) Induction of cancer cell apoptosis by flavonoids is associated with their ability to inhibit fatty acid synthase activity. J Biol Chem 7:5636–5645

Callahan R, Hurvitz S (2011) Human epidermal growth factor receptor-2-positive breast cancer: Current management of early, advanced, and recurrent disease. Curr Opin Obstet Gynecol 1:37–43

Chen A, Xu J, Johnson AC (2005) Curcumin inhibits human colon cancer cell growth by suppressing gene expression of epidermal growth factor receptor through reducing the activity of the transcription factor egr-1. Oncogene 2:278–287

Chiang C-T, Way T-D, Lin J-K (2007) Sensitizing her2-overexpressing cancer cells to luteolin-induced apoptosis through suppressing p21waf1/cip1 expression with rapamycin. Mol Cancer Ther 7:2127–2138

Choan E, Segal R, Jonker D et al (2005) A prospective clinical trial of green tea for hormone refractory prostate cancer: an evaluation of the complementary/alternative therapy approach. Urologic Oncology: Semin Orig Invest 2:108–113

Chow H-HS, Cai Y, Hakim IA et al (2003) Pharmacokinetics and safety of green tea polyphenols after multiple-dose administration of epigallocatechin gallate and polyphenon e in healthy individuals Clin Cancer Res 9:3312–3319

Chow H-HS, Hakim IA, Vining DR et al (2005) Effects of dosing condition on the oral bioavailability of green tea catechins after single-dose administration of polyphenon e in healthy individuals. Clin Cancer Res 12:4627–4633

Coleman DT, Bigelow R, Cardelli JA (2009) Inhibition of fatty acid synthase by luteolin post-transcriptionally down-regulates c-met expression independent of proteosomal/lysosomal degradation. Mol Cancer Thera 1:214–224

Dashwood W-M, Orner GA, Dashwood RH (2002) Inhibition of [beta]-catenin/tcf activity by white tea, green tea, and epigallocatechin-3-gallate (egcg): minor contribution of h2o2 at physiologically relevant egcg concentrations. Biochem Biophys Res Commun 3:584–588

De Ledinghen V, Monvoisin A, Neaud V et al (2001) Trans-resveratrol, a grapevine-derived polyphenol, blocks hepatocyte growth factor-induced invasion of hepatocellular carcinoma cells. Int J Oncol 1:83–88

Duhon D, Bigelow RLH, Coleman DT et al (2010) The polyphenol epigallocatechin-3-gallate affects lipid rafts to block activation of the c-met receptor in prostate cancer cells. Mol Carcinog 8:739–749

Eddy SF, Kane SE, Sonenshein GE (2007) Trastuzumab-resistant her2-driven breast cancer cells are sensitive to epigallocatechin-3 gallate. Cancer Res 19:9018–9023

Fang J, Zhou Q, Shi X-l et al (2006) Luteolin inhibits insulin-like growth factor 1 receptor signaling in prostate cancer cells. Carcinogenesis 3:713–723

Foley J, Nickerson NK, Nam S et al (2010) Egfr signaling in breast cancer: Bad to the bone. Semin Cell Dev Biol 9:951–960

Fox S, Generali D, Harris A (2007) Breast tumour angiogenesis. Breast Cancer Res 6:216

Fridrich D, Teller N, Esselen M et al (2008) Comparison of delphinidin, quercetin and-epigallocatechin-3-gallate as inhibitors of the egfr and the erbb2 receptor phosphorylation. Mol Nutr Food Res 7:815–822

Fu Y, Chen A (2006) The phyto-chemical (-)-epigallocatechin gallate suppresses gene expression of epidermal growth factor receptor in rat hepatic stellate cells in vitro by reducing the activity of egr-1. Biochem Pharmacol 2:227–238

Fujimura Y, Tachibana H, Kumai R et al (2004) A difference between epigallocatechin-3-gallate and epicatechin-3-gallate on anti-allergic effect is dependent on their distinct distribution to lipid rafts. Biofactors 1–4:133–135

Gao CF, Woude GFV (2005) Hgf/sf-met signaling in tumor progression. Cell Res 1:49–51

Goel A, Jhurani S, Aggarwal BB (2008) Multi-targeted therapy by curcumin: how spicy is it? Mol Nutr Food Res 9:1010–1030

Gu H, Neel BG (2003) The gab' in signal transduction. Trends Cell Biol 3:122–130

Guo Y, Wang S, Hoot DR et al (2007) Suppression of vegf-mediated autocrine and paracrine interactions between prostate cancer cells and vascular endothelial cells by soy isoflavones. The J Nutr Biochem 6:408–417

Gupta S, Kim J, Prasad S et al 2010 Regulation of survival, proliferation, invasion, angiogenesis, and metastasis of tumor cells through modulation of inflammatory pathways by nutraceuticals. Cancer Metastasis Rev 29:405–434

Heber D (2008) Multitargeted therapy of cancer by ellagitannins. Cancer Lett 2:262–268

Hou Z, Sang S, You H et al (2005) Mechanism of action of -epigallocatechin-3-gallate: Auto-oxidation dependent inactivation of epidermal growth factor receptor and direct effects on growth inhibition in human esophageal cancer kyse 150 cells. Cancer Res 17:8049–8056

Huang Y-T, Hwang J-J, Lee P-P et al (1999) Effects of luteolin and quercetin, inhibitors of tyrosine kinase, on cell growth and metastasis-associated properties in a431 cells overexpressing epidermal growth factor receptor. Br J Pharmacol 5:999–1010

Hussain M, Banerjee M, Sarkar FH et al (2003) Soy isoflavones in the treatment of prostate cancer. Nutr Cancer 2:111–117

Jatoi A, Ellison N, Burch PA et al (2003) A phase ii trial of green tea in the treatment of patients with androgen independent metastatic prostate carcinoma. Cancer 6:1442–1446

Jeong J-H, An JY, Kwon YT et al (2008) Quercetin-induced ubiquitination and down-regulation of her-2/neu. J Cell Biochem 2:585–595

Jung JH, Lee JO, Kim JH et al (2010) Quercetin suppresses hela cell viability via ampk-induced hsp70 and egfr down-regulation. J Cell Physiol 2:408–414

Kang NJ, Shin SH, Lee HJ et al (2011) Polyphenols as small molecular inhibitors of signaling cascades in carcinogenesis. Pharmacol Ther 3:310–324

Khan N, Mukhtar H (2008) Multitargeted therapy of cancer by green tea polyphenols. Cancer Lett 2:269–280

Kim EJ, Shin HK, Park JH (2005a) Genistein inhibits insulin-like growth factor-i receptor signaling in ht-29 human colon cancer cells: a possible mechanism of the growth inhibitory effect of genistein. J Med Food 4:431–438

Kim WK, Bang MH, Kim ES et al (2005b) Quercetin decreases the expression of erbb2 and erbb3 proteins in ht-29 human colon cancer cells. J Nutr Biochem 3:155–162

Koch S, Tugues S, Li X et al (2011) Signal transduction by vascular endothelial growth factor receptors. Biochem J 2:169–183

Koh YW, Choi EC, Kang SU et al (2011) Green tea (-)-epigallocatechin-3-gallate inhibits hgf-induced progression in oral cavity cancer through suppression of hgf/c-met. J Nutr Biochem (in press)

Kondo T, Ohta T, Igura K et al (2002) Tea catechins inhibit angiogenesis in vitro, measured by human endothelial cell growth, migration and tube formation, through inhibition of vegf receptor binding. Cancer Lett 2:139–144

Korutla L, Cheung JY, Medelsohn J et al (1995) Inhibition of ligand-induced activation of epidermal growth factor receptor tyrosine phosphorylation by curcumin. Carcinogenesis 8:1741–1745

Kundu JK, Surh Y-J (2008) Cancer chemopreventive and therapeutic potential of resveratrol: mechanistic perspectives. Cancer Lett 2:243–261

Labbe D, Provencal M, Lamy S et al (2009) The flavonols quercetin, kaempferol, and myricetin inhibit hepatocyte growth factor-induced medulloblastoma cell migration. J Nutr 4:646–652

Lamy S, Badard V, Labba D et al (2008) The dietary flavones apigenin and luteolin impair smooth muscle cell migration and vegf expression through inhibition of pdgfr phosphorylation. Cancer Prev Res 6:452–459

Larsen CA, Dashwood RH (2010) (-)-epigallocatechin-3-gallate inhibits met signaling, proliferation, and invasiveness in human colon cancer cells. Arch Biochem Biophys 1:52–57

Larsen CA, Dashwood RH, Bisson WH (2010) Tea catechins as inhibitors of receptor tyrosine kinases: mechanistic insights and human relevance. Pharmacol Res 6:457–464

Lee LT, Huang YT, Hwang JJ et al (2002) Blockade of the epidermal growth factor receptor tyrosine kinase activity by quercetin and luteolin leads to growth inhibition and apoptosis of pancreatic tumor cells. Anticancer Res 3:1615–1627

Lee YK, Bone ND, Strege AK et al (2004) Vegf receptor phosphorylation status and apoptosis is modulated by a green tea component, epigallocatechin-3-gallate (egcg), in b-cell chronic lymphocytic leukemia. Blood 3:788–794

Lee W-J, Wu L-F, Chen W-K et al (2006) Inhibitory effect of luteolin on hepatocyte growth factor/scatter factor-induced hepg2 cell invasion involving both mapk/erks and pi3k-akt pathways. Chemico-Biol Interact 2:123–133

Lee W-J, Chen W-K, Wang C-J et al (2008) Apigenin inhibits hgf-promoted invasive growth and metastasis involving blocking pi3k/akt pathway and [beta]4 integrin function in mda-mb-231 breast cancer cells. Toxicol Appl Pharmacol 2:178–191

Li Y, Bhuiyan M, Sarkar FH (1999) Induction of apoptosis and inhibition of c-erbb-2 in mda-mb-435 cells by genistein. Int J Oncol 3:525–533

Li M, He Z, Ermakova S et al (2007) Direct inhibition of insulin-like growth factor-i receptor kinase activity by epigallocatechin-3-gallate regulates cell transformation. Cancer Epidemiol Biomark Preven 3:598–605

Liang Y-C, Lin-shiau S-Y, Chen C-F et al (1997) Suppression of extracellular signals and cell proliferation through egf receptor binding by -epigallocatechin gallate in human a431 epidermoid carcinoma cells. J Cell Biochem 1:55–65

Lim YC, Park HY, Hwang HS et al (2008) (-)-epigallocatechin-3-gallate (egcg) inhibits hgf-induced invasion and metastasis in hypopharyngeal carcinoma cells. Cancer Lett 1:140–152

Linder ME, Deschenes RJ (2007) Palmitoylation: Policing protein stability and traffic. Nat Rev Mol Cell Biol 1:74–84

Luo H, Jiang BH, King SM et al (2008) Inhibition of cell growth and vegf expression in ovarian cancer cells by flavonoids. Nutr Cancer 6:800–809

Manach C, Williamson G, Morand C et al (2005) Bioavailability and bioefficacy of polyphenols in humans. I. Review of 97 bioavailability studies. Am J Clin Nutr 1:230S–242S

Masuda M, Suzui M, Lim JTE et al (2003) Epigallocatechin-3-gallate inhibits activation of her-2/neu and downstream signaling pathways in human head and neck and breast carcinoma cells. Clin Cancer Res 9:3486–3491

Masuelli L, Marzocchella L, Quaranta A et al (2011) Apigenin induces apoptosis and impairs head and neck carcinomas egfr/erbb2 signaling. Front Biosci 16:1060–1068

McLarty J, Bigelow RLH, Smith M et al (2009) Tea polyphenols decrease serum levels of prostate-specific antigen, hepatocyte growth factor, and vascular endothelial growth factor in prostate cancer patients and inhibit production of hepatocyte growth factor and vascular endothelial growth factor in vitro. Cancer Prev Res 7:673–682

Menendez JA, Lupu R (2007) Fatty acid synthase and the lipogenic phenotype in cancer pathogenesis. Nat Rev Cancer 10:763–777

Menendez JA, Vellon L, Lupu R (2005) Antitumoral actions of the anti-obesity drug orlistat (xenical) in breast cancer cells: Blockade of cell cycle progression, promotion of apoptotic cell death and pea3-mediated transcriptional repression of her2/neu (erbb-2) oncogene. Ann Oncol 8:1253–1267

Merfort I, Heilmann J, Hagedorn-Leweke U et al (1994) In vivo skin penetration studies of camomile flavones. Pharmazie 7:509–511

Milligan SA, Burke P, Coleman DT et al (2009) The green tea polyphenol egcg potentiates the antiproliferative activity of c-met and epidermal growth factor receptor inhibitors in non small cell lung cancer cells. Clin Cancer Rese 15:4885–4894

Miura D, Miura Y, Yagasaki K (2004) Resveratrol inhibits hepatoma cell invasion by suppressing gene expression of hepatocyte growth factor via its reactive oxygen species-scavenging property. Clin Exp Metasta 21:445–451

Moran C (2011) Importance of molecular features of non-small cell lung cancer for choice of treatment. Am J Pathol 5:1940–1948

Nair HB, Sung B, Yadav VR et al (2010) Delivery of antiinflammatory nutraceuticals by nanoparticles for the prevention and treatment of cancer. Biochem Pharmacol 12:1833–1843

Nicolson GL (1982) Cancer metastasis. Organ colonization and the cell-surface properties of malignant cells. Biochim Biophys Acta 2:113–176

Pianetti S, Guo S, Kavanagh KT et al (2002) Green tea polyphenol epigallocatechin-3 gallate inhibits her-2/neu signaling, proliferation, and transformed phenotype of breast cancer cells. Cancer Res 3:652–655

Pike LJ (2009) The challenge of lipid rafts. J Lipid Res Suppl 50:S323–S328

Resh MD (2006) Palmitoylation of ligands, receptors, and intracellular signaling molecules. Science 359:re14

Rosário M, Birchmeier W (2003) How to make tubes: signaling by the met receptor tyrosine kinase. Trends Cell Biol 6:328–335

Sanna V, Pintus G, Roggio AM et al (2011) Targeted biocompatible nanoparticles for the delivery of -epigallocatechin 3-gallate to prostate cancer cells. J Med Chem 5:1321–1332

Sartippour MR, Shao Z-M, Heber D et al (2002) Green tea inhibits vascular endothelial growth factor (vegf) induction in human breast cancer cells. J Nutr 8:2307–2311

Scalbert A, Williamson G (2000) Dietary intake and bioavailability of polyphenols J Nutr 8: 2073S–2085S

Scalbert A, Manach C, Morand C et al (2005) Dietary polyphenols and the prevention of diseases. Crit Rev Food Sci Nutr 4:287–306

Schaeper U, Gehring NH, Fuchs KP et al (2000) Coupling of gab1 to c-met, grb2, and shp2 mediates biological responses. J Cell Biol 7:1419–1432

Sebastian S, Settleman J, Reshkin SJ et al (2006) The complexity of targeting egfr signalling in cancer: from expression to turnover. Biochim Biophys Acta (BBA) 1:120–139

Seol DW, Chen Q, Zarnegar R (2000) Transcriptional activation of the hepatocyte growth factor receptor (c-met) gene by its ligand (hepatocyte growth factor) is mediated through ap-1. Oncogene 9:1132–1137

Shehzad A, Wahid F, Lee YS (2010) Curcumin in cancer chemoprevention: Molecular targets, pharmacokinetics, bioavailability, and clinical trials. Arch Pharm Med Chem 9:489–499

Shimizu M, Shirakami Y, Sakai H et al (2008) Egcg inhibits activation of the insulin-like growth factor (igf)/igf-1 receptor axis in human hepatocellular carcinoma cells. Cancer Lett 1:10–18

Shukla S, Gupta S (2009) Apigenin suppresses insulin-like growth factor i receptor signaling in human prostate cancer: an in vitro and in vivo study. Mol Carcinog 3:243–252

Shutava TG, Balkundi SS, Vangala P et al (2009) Layer-by-layer-coated gelatin nanoparticles as a vehicle for delivery of natural polyphenols. ACS Nano 7:1877–1885

Siddiqui I, Mukhtar H (2010) Nanochemoprevention by bioactive food components: A perspective. Pharma Res 27:1054–1060

Singletary K, Ellington A (2006) Genistein suppresses proliferation and met oncogene expression and induces egr-1 tumor suppressor expression in immortalized human breast epithelial cells. Anticancer Res 2A:1039–1048

Soung YH, Chung J (2011) Curcumin inhibition of the functional interaction between integrin a6b4 and the epidermal growth factor receptor. Mol Cancer Ther 5:883–891

Steffan JJ, Williams BC, Welbourne T et al (2010) Hgf-induced invasion by prostate tumor cells requires anterograde lysosome trafficking and activity of na+-h+ exchangers. J Cell Sci 7: 1151–1159

Stewart JR, O'Brian CA (2004) Resveratrol antagonizes egfr-dependent erk1/2 activation in human androgen-independent prostate cancer cells with associated isozyme-selective pkc inhibition. Invest New Drugs 22:107–117

Suganuma M, Saha A, Fujiki H (2011) New cancer treatment strategy using combination of green tea catechins and anticancer drugs. Cancer Sci 2:317–323

Surh Y-J (2003) Cancer chemoprevention with dietary phytochemicals. Nat Rev Cancer 10: 768–780

Tachibana H, Koga K, Fujimura Y et al (2004) A receptor for green tea polyphenol egcg. Nat Struct Mol Biol 4:380–381

Tang F-Y, Su Y-C, Chen N-C et al (2008) Resveratrol inhibits migration and invasion of human breast-cancer cells. Mol Nutr Food Res 6:683–691

Tanimura S, Kadomoto R, Tanaka T et al (2005) Suppression of tumor cell invasiveness by hydrolyzable tannins (plant polyphenols) via the inhibition of matrix metalloproteinase-2/-9 activity. Biochem Biophys Res Commun 4:1306–1313

Tulasne D, Foveau B (2007) The shadow of death on the met tyrosine kinase receptor. Cell Death Differ 3:427–434

Vazquez-Martin A, Colomer R, Brunet J et al (2008) Overexpression of fatty acid synthase gene activates her1/her2 tyrosine kinase receptors in human breast epithelial cells. Cell Prolife 1:59–85

Walle T (2004) Absorption and metabolism of flavonoids. Free Rad Biol Med 7:829–837

Wang S, DeGroff VL, Clinton SK (2003) Tomato and soy polyphenols reduce insulin-like growth factor-–stimulated rat prostate cancer cell proliferation and apoptotic resistance in vitro via inhibition of intracellular signaling pathways involving tyrosine kinase. J Nutr 7:2367–2376

Wang J, Eltoum I-E, Lamartiniere CA (2004) Genistein alters growth factor signaling in transgenic prostate model (tramp). Mol Cell Endocrinol 1–2:171–180

Way T-D, Kao M-C, Lin J-K (2004) Apigenin induces apoptosis through proteasomal degradation of her2/neu in her2/neu-overexpressing breast cancer cells via the phosphatidylinositol 3-kinase/akt-dependent pathway. J Biol Chem 6:4479–4489

Way T-D, Kao M-C, Lin J-K (2005) Degradation of her2/neu by apigenin induces apoptosis through cytochrome c release and caspase-3 activation in her2/neu-overexpressing breast cancer cells. FEBS Lett 1:145–152

Yu ZJ, He LY, Chen Y et al (2009) Effects of quercetin on the expression of vegf-c and vegfr-3 in human cancer mgc-803 cells. Xi Bao Yu Fen Zi Mian Yi Xue Za Zhi 8:678–680

Yunos NM, Beale P, Yu JQ et al (2011) Synergism from sequenced combinations of curcumin and epigallocatechin-3-gallate with cisplatin in the killing of human ovarian cancer cells. Anticancer Res 4:1131–1140

Zhou Y, Zheng S, Lin J et al (2007) The interruption of the pdgf and egf signaling pathways by curcumin stimulates gene expression of ppar in rat activated hepatic stellate cell in vitro. Lab Invest 5:488–498

Chapter 4
Role of Nutraceuticals on Nrf2 and Its Implication in Cancer Prevention

Constance Lay-Lay Saw and Ah-Ng Tony Kong

Abstract "Nutraceuticals" have recently become a hot topic for the commercial world and the biomedical community. It is postulated that nutraceuticals are relatively non-toxic food supplements with many health benefits including prevention of cancer. Many nutraceuticals are antioxidants by nature; isothiocyanates and polyphenols have been extensively researched in many laboratories including ours. This chapter will cover nutraceuticals from the mechanistic perspectives, and how they would interact with Nuclear factor (erythroid-derived 2)-like 2 (Nrf2), which is the master regulator of the antioxidant response to counteract oxidative stress. Nrf2 deficient (knockout; KO) mice lack response to some nutraceutical cancer chemopreventive agents suggesting the important role of Nrf2 in cancer prevention. Nrf2 is also shown to have protective function against inflammation, a pathological process that is implicated in many diseases including carcinogenesis. Scientific evidence on the role of nutraceuticals on Nrf2 in anti-oxidative stress coupled with anti-inflammatory will also be discussed in this chapter.

Keywords Nutraceuticals · Nrf2 · Antioxidant response element · Oxidative stress · Phase II detoxyfying/antioxidant genes · Anti-inflammatory · NF-κB · Chemoprevention · Carcinogenesis · Epigenetics

Abbreviations

AOM	azoxymethane
ARE	antioxidant response element
BaP	benzo[a]pyrene
COX-2	cyclooxygenase 2
DHA	docosahexaenoic acid
DSS	dextran sulfate sodium
EGCG	epigallocatechin-3-gallate
EPA	eicosapentaenoic acid
ERK2	extracellular signal-regulated protein kinase 2

A.-N.T. Kong (✉)
Department of Pharmaceutics, Ernest-Mario School of Pharmacy, Center for Cancer Prevention Research, Rutgers, The State University of New Jersey, Piscataway, NJ 08854, USA
e-mail: KongT@pharmacy.rutgers.edu

F.H. Sarkar (ed.), *Nutraceuticals and Cancer*, DOI 10.1007/978-94-007-2630-7_4,

GST	glutathione S-transferase
HO-1	heme oxygenase-1
IL-1β	interleukin 1-beta
IL-6	interleukin 6
iNOS	inducible nitric oxide synthase
JNK	c-Jun NH(2)-terminal kinase
Keap1	Kelch-like ECH-associated protein 1
LPS	lipopolysaccharide
Maf	*m*usculo*a*poneurotic *f*ibrosarcoma
MAPKs	mitogen-activated protein kinases
NF-κB	nuclear factor-kappa-B
NQO1	NADP(H):quinone oxidoreductase 1
Nrf2 WT	Nrf2 wild-type
Nrf2	nuclear factor (erythroid-derived 2)-like 2
Nrf2 KO	Nrf2 knockout
PEITC	phenethyl isothiocyanate
PERK	PKR-like endoplasmic reticulum kinase
PI3K	phosphatidylinositol 3-kinase
PKC	protein kinase C
ROS	reactive oxygen species
SFN	sulforaphane
TNF-α	tumor necrosis factor alpha
TRAMP	*tr*ansgenic *a*denocarcinoma of *m*ouse *p*rostate
UGT	UDP-glucuronosyltransferase

4.1 Introduction

4.1.1 Nutraceuticals

"Nutraceuticals" is becoming a hot topic for the commercial world, as well as the biomedical community as it is believed to be relatively non-toxic food supplements and possess nutritional benefits beyond the traditional nutrients of which they are containing. The importance of this term is evidenced by a search in the PubMed database using the term "nutraceuticals" yielded over 33,000 hits, with over 6,400 reviews. The term "nutraceuticals" which was first coined by Stephen DeFelice, MD, founder and chairman of The Foundation for Innovation in Medicine, NJ, in 1989 when he referred to a nutraceutical a food, dietary supplement or medical food that has a medical – health benefit including the prevention and treatment of disease (DeFelice 2011; Kalra 2003). Since then the interest on nutraceuticals is increasing rapidly, not only from the perspective of the healthcare market (Brower 1998), but also from the perspective of general public and patients concern with prevention of diseases including cancer. Although the term "nutraceuticals" were redefined due to its potential overlapping meaning with "functional foods" and "dietary supplements" (Kalra 2003), the following review chapter on "nutraceuticals" focusing on the mechanistic perspectives, and how they would interact and impact on the Nuclear factor (erythroid-derived 2)-like 2 (Nrf2), which is the master regulator of the antioxidant response to counteract oxidative stress (Hu et al. 2010; Nguyen et al. 2009). Oxidative stress appears to the root cause of many diseases such as cardiovascular diseases, neurological diseases, renal diseases, cancer and inflammatory diseases. Because Nrf2 is able to induce antioxidant cellular defense genes to counteract excessive oxidative stress and many nutraceuticals could induce the expression of Nrf2, therefore the role of nutraceuticals on Nrf2 and its implication in cancer prevention will be the major focus in this chapter.

4.1.2 Nrf2, Phase II Detoxifying/Antioxidant Enzymes, Lifestyles and Cancer Prevention

Nrf2 is the key regulator for many phase II detoxifying and antioxidant enzymes. These enzymes are able to scavenge reactive oxygen species (ROS) and metabolize potentially harmful toxic reactive intermediates so as to maintain the homeostatic redox state in the cells. Carcinogens are typically metabolized by phase I drug metabolizing enzymes via oxidation and reduction (Yu and Kong 2007). The resulting products will subsequently undergo phase II conjugations catalyzed by the phase II drug metabolizing enzymes such as glutathione S-transferases (GST) and UDP-glucuronosyltransferases (UGT), resulting in the formation of more water soluble conjugated products that can be excreted easily in the bile or in the urine (Shen and Kong 2009; Yu and Kong 2007). Under normal homeostatic condition, Nrf2 is inhibited in the cytoplasm by the anchor protein Kelch-like ECH-associated protein-1 (Keap1). In the presence of oxidative stress or chemical inducers, Nrf2 is released from Keap1 inhibition, translocates to the nucleus, dimerizes with small *m*usculo*a*poneurotic *f*ibrosarcoma protein (sMaf) and binds the antioxidant response element (ARE) sequence resulting in enhanced expression of the detoxifying and antioxidant enzymes to counteract the stress (Nguyen et al. 2009). Many years of research establish that the signal transduction pathway consisting of the Keap1-Nrf2-sMaf-ARE axis as the primary sensor of the signaling generated by electrophiles and nutraceutical chemopreventive agents, and is essential for eliciting the antioxidant response. Recent evidence suggests that other signaling mechanisms including transcriptional and translational controls mechanisms could also potentially contribute to the overall enhancement of Nrf2-mediated responses (Li and Kong 2009).

Despite the tremendous progress in the early detection and treatment of cancer, the global cancer incidence doubles in the last 30 years of the twentieth century, and it is estimated that the burden will double again between 2000 and 2020 and nearly triple by 2030. However, with the advent of several preventive measures would hopefully reduce the cancer burden, one of which is dietary approach (Boyle and Levin 2008; Jemal et al. 2010a). Thus, cancer prevention research is overwhelming important and much attention would need to be directed to cancer prevention in near term as well as long term.

Epidemiological and population studies have established a close relationship between the incidence of cancer and the consumption of certain types of food (Carter et al. 1990; Tominaga and Kuroishi 1997; Yang et al. 2002). Taking prostate cancer as an example, men in Asia appear to have a lower incidence of prostate cancer than men in North America (Hsing et al. 2000). However, when they migrated to the United States for instance, the incidence of prostate cancer increases substantially (Shimizu et al. 1991). Similarly, non-Western origin immigrants to Europe also show lower cancer risk such as prostate cancer, breast cancer and colorectal cancer, as compared to the native populations of European, this is potentially related to the Western lifestyle (Arnold et al. 2010). Such differences in prostate cancer incidence between different ethnic groups before and after migration to the Western world are believed to be partly due to the different lifestyle and environmental factors (Klassen and Platz 2006). A 30 years follow-up study of men who eat no fish show a two-three-fold higher frequency of prostate cancer than those who eat moderate or high amounts (Terry et al. 2001). The most recent meta-analysis has concluded that the benefit of fish consumption resulted in a 63% reduction of prostate cancer-specific mortality (Szymanski et al. 2010). In addition to dietary factors, lifestyle such as smoking is also implicated in lung cancer (Fielding 1985; Witschi et al. 1997a, b). In this chapter, the different nutraceuticals functioning as Nrf2 inducers and the mechanism of action are discussed in terms of contributing to cancer prevention.

4.2 Different Nutraceuticals, Cancer and Phase II Detoxifying/Antioxidant Genes Regulated by Nrf2

Epidemiological studies indicate that dietary consumption of cruciferous vegetables would reduce various cancer risks (Higdon et al. 2007) including prostate (Chan et al. 2009) and bladder cancers (Tang et al. 2008). Isothiocyanates [sulforaphane (SFN) and phenethyl isothiocyanate (PEITC)] and polyphenols are two major groups of nutraceuticals studied and recognized as detoxifying enzyme inducers via Nrf2 pathways. Dietary isothiocyanates, the naturally sulfur containing compounds, are derived from in vivo hydrolysis of glucosinolates present in cruciferous vegetables such as broccoli, Brussels sprouts, cabbage and cauliflower (Verhoeven et al. 1997). Polyphenols are class of compounds with two or more phenolic rings joined together, and based on their chemical structure, they can be divided into more than ten sub-types (Nichenametla et al. 2006). They are commonly found abundantly in many fruits and vegetables. In addition to their effects on cellular differentiation, proliferation and apoptosis, they were found to be Nrf2 inducers as well. Some examples of polyphenols are curcumin from tumeric, epigallocatechin-3-gallate (EGCG) from green tea, resveratrol from grapes and berries, quercetin from citrus fruits and berries. Our laboratory has been testing these compounds individually in understanding the molecular mechanism particularly related to Nrf2 signaling using in vitro and in vivo systems. In addition, interestingly, some of the combination treatments of these nutraceuticals in cell models reveal that they can also work synergistically by up-regulating the Nrf2 pathways as well as dampening the inflammatory pathway (Cheung et al. 2009; Saw et al. 2010, 2011a).

4.2.1 Isothiocyanates: Sulforaphane (SFN) and Phenethyl Isothiocyanate (PEITC)

More than 120 different glucosinolates have been identified (Fahey et al. 2001). SFN, isolated from broccoli, is one of the isothiocyanates that has received intense attention for its cancer chemopreventive potential possibly due in part to the fact that it is one of the strongest inducers of phase II detoxifying enzymes (Zhang et al. 1994). SFN has been shown to induce ARE in a dose-dependent manner and it was also found that SFN was able to activate c-Jun NH(2)-terminal kinase (JNK) 1/2 in HepG2-C8 cells which is related to apoptosis (Kim et al. 2003). SFN has been found to inhibit carcinogen-induced mammary gland tumorigenesis in the rats (Zhang et al. 1994), azoxymethane (AOM)-induced colonic aberrant crypt foci in rat (Chung et al. 2000), benzo[a]pyrene (BaP)-induced forestomach tumors in mice (Fahey et al. 2002), BaP-induced lung cancer in mice (Hecht et al. 2002; Kalpana Deepa Priya et al. 2011). SFN and PEITC also inhibit the development of adenomatous polypopsis in APCmin/+ mice (Hu et al. 2006; Khor et al. 2008a; Shen et al. 2007) and PEITC can prevent prostate carcinogenesis in transgenic adenocarcinoma of the mouse prostate (TRAMP) mice (Barve et al. 2008) as well as human prostate cancer PC-3 xenograft in nude mice (Khor et al. 2006b). Interestingly, combination of PEITC and curcumin has enhanced potency in lowering the incidence of palpable prostate tumor when compared with PEITC or curcumin alone in the TRAMP mice (Barve et al. 2008). The potential molecular mechanisms responsible for cancer prevention activities by isothiocyanates include the induction of phase II detoxifying/antioxidant enzymes which are regulated by Nrf2, inhibition of phase I cytochrome P450s which in turn inhibit the activation of carcinogens, as well as the induction of anti-proliferative/proapoptotic signaling pathways. Using macrophages collected from Nrf2 knockout (Nrf2 KO) mice and compared to macrophages from Nrf2 wild-type (Nrf2 WT) mice, SFN could also work in part via Nrf2 signaling for its anti-inflammatory activity (Lin et al. 2008). In the same context of Nrf2-mediated anti-inflammatory response, using Nrf2 KO mice, it was found that with UVB-induced skin inflammation model, SFN was able to restore sunburn cells back to basal levels only in the Nrf2 WT and not in Nrf2 KO mice (Saw et al. 2011b).

4.2.2 Polyphenols: Curcumin and Curcmin Analogues

Curcumin, a polyphenol found abundantly in *Curcuma Longa,* family Zingiberaceae, commonly known as turmeric has a long history in herbal Medicine. In addition to inhibiting the key regulator for inflammatory response, nuclear factor-kappa-B (NF-κB), pro-survival kinase Akt and other pathways important to tumor cell survival, curcumin also exerts a cytopreotective effects in non-cancer cells through transcriptional induction of phase II detoxifying enzymes (Hatcher et al. 2008). Our laboratory has used the Nrf2 KO mice and found that curcumin could modulate many Nrf2-mediated genes (Shen et al. 2006). When tested in human islet cells, curcumin and its analogues were found to induce antioxidant enzymes such as NAD(P)H:quinone oxidoreductase 1 (NQO1) (Balamurugan et al. 2009). These studies show that nutraceuticals such as curcumin would dampen oxidative stress by regulating the Nrf2-mediated pathways.

Recently *Curcuma Longa*/curcumin/turmeric have been available over the counter in the United States as dietary supplements. However, the scientific claims and the safety of long-term use of these products may be questionable. Currently there are 61 clinical trials are being conducted on *Curcuma Longa*-related products for various diseases, including prostate and colon cancers and neurodegenerative Alzheimer's disease [listed in http://clinicaltrials.gov/ct2/results?term=curcumin&pg=1; latest accessed website on 1 July 2011]. Some trials are conducted to investigate the effects of the nutraceutical supplememt of curcumin based on its anti-cancer, antioxidant/anti-inflammatory and cognitive activities, turmeric's pharmacokinetics profiles, or combination with chemotherapy such as gemcitabine or combination with other health supplement such as coenzyme Q10. However, the exact mechanisms underlying all these potential human health activities are still unclear. The importance and urgency of further understanding of the mechanism is evidenced by the facts that many *Curcuma Longa* products, curcumin, curcuminoids or turmeric extracts are marketed as capsules or liquids in the US as dietary supplements. Hence, the scientific understanding for these claims would be warranted. Curcumin is the most important bioactive component in *Curcuma Longa*, however, due to its low bioavailability, its effectiveness and the achievable blood levels with human consumption has been questioned (Kidd 2009; Padhye et al. 2010). Many health nutraceutical supplements commercially marketed as curcumin or products have claimed that these products could achieve higher absorption than curcumin itself. However, the actual health benefits of these products are yet to be defined in detail, and the mechanism of such activities remain largely unknown. Several research reports have shown that even at low blood concentrations, curcumin could exhibit cancer chemoprevention activities (Kidd 2009). There are many attempts to synthesize curcumin analogues to circumvent the problem of low bioavailabilities and extensive metabolism (Anand et al. 2007, 2008). In terms of the potential pharmacodynamic effects of curcumin, anti-inflammatory (Tham et al. 2010; Zhao et al. 2010) and antioxidant activities (Dai et al. 2009) are two of the most prominent properties among all others. Interestingly, some analogues have independent anti-inflammatory activities that are not associated with the "antioxidant" activities (Lee et al. 2009).

4.3 Nrf2-Mediated Signaling: Antioxidant/Anti-inflammatory

Current studies have linked chronic inflammation to cancer development (Mantovani et al. 2008). Importantly, many nutraceutical chemopreventive compounds that act on Nrf2 pathway are also having anti-inflammatory activities (Khor et al. 2008c; Kim et al. 2010) and the interplay between Nrf2 signaling pathway and inflammatory pathway has recently been reviewed (Khor et al. 2008c; Kim et al. 2010). Increasing evidence has shown that Nrf2 could play an important role in defense against oxidative stress possibly by activation of cellular antioxidant machinery as well as suppression of pro-inflammatory signaling pathways. In addition, in vitro and in vivo data suggest that many dietary chemopreventive compounds can differentially regulate Nrf2-mediated antioxidant/anti-inflammatory signaling pathways as the first line of defense or induce apoptosis once the cells have been damaged or initiated (Li et al. 2008), and many other pathways can also regulate Nrf2, including a wide variety of kinase signaling pathways such as protein kinase C (PKC) (Huang et al. 2002), mitogen-activated protein kinases (MAPKs) (Yu et al. 2000), phosphatidylinositol 3-kinase (PI3K) (Lee et al. 2001), and PKR-like endoplasmic reticulum kinase (PERK) (Cullinan and Diehl 2004) (Fig. 4.1). Many signaling pathways are involved in the cytokines and inflammatory response, such as NF-κB and MAPKs pathways. We have recently reported the relationship between Nrf2 and NF-κB, a key transcriptional factor involved in inflammatory response using bioinformatic approach (Nair et al. 2008). It was found

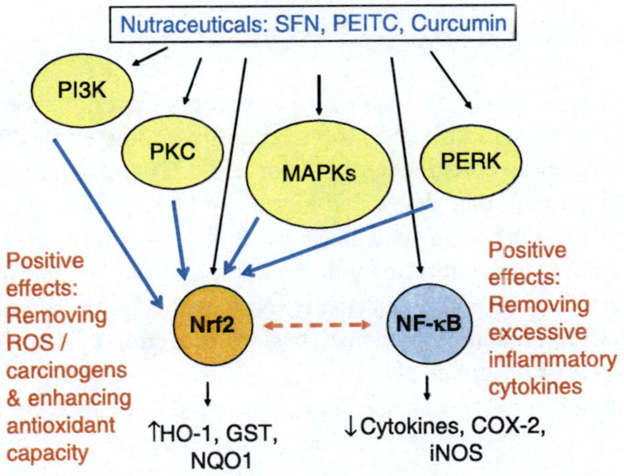

Fig. 4.1 A putative model illustrating the interplay between Nrf2 and NF-κB leading to chemoprevention by nutraceuticals. Nutraceuticals could directly interact with members of upstream kinase signaling pathways such as PI3K, PKC, MAPK and PERK, especially the MAPKs family. The putative cross-talk between Nrf2 and NF-κB is denoted by double head arrows. Nutraceuticals such as SFN, PEITC etc could enhance expression of Nrf2 and related phase II detoxifying and antioxidant genes to remove ROS and carcinogens, as well as to suppress NF-κB mediated excessive inflammatory activities thus confer the cancer preventive activities

that 75% of the members in the regulatory network are MAPKs, which appears to be consistent with the current role of MAPKs in modulation of both Keap1-Nrf2-ARE (Jakubikova et al. 2005; Shen et al. 2004; Svehlikova et al. 2004; Yu et al. 2000; Yuan et al. 2006) and NF-κB signaling pathways (de Sousa et al. 2007; Murakami et al. 2007). As illustrated in Fig. 4.1, a simplified model for the potential concerted modulation of Nrf2 and NF-κB in antioxidation and inflammation via upstream MAPKs pathway; the involvement of the other Nrf2 upstream pathways such as PI3K, PKC and PERK are also incorporated as discussed previously, several nutraceutical/phytochemicals have been shown to interact directly with these kinases.

4.3.1 In Vitro Studies Using Nrf2 KO Macrophages

The potential crosstalk between Nrf2 and NF-κB are also illustrated using Nrf2 KO primary peritoneal macrophages challenged with lipopolysaccharide (LPS) (Lin et al. 2008; Wang et al. 2010). Polyunsaturated fatty acids docosahexaenoic acid (DHA) and eicosapentaenoic acid (EPA) inhibited LPS-induced cyclooxygenase 2 (COX-2), inducible nitric oxide synthase (iNOS), interleukin 1-beta (IL-1β), interleukin 6 (IL-6), or tumor necrosis factor alpha (TNF-α), however, the suppression was attenuated as compared to that in Nrf2 WT macrophages (Wang et al. 2010). Similar observation was seen when the well studied Nrf2 inducer, SFN was tested in the same system (Lin et al. 2008).

4.3.2 In Vivo Studies Using Nrf2 KO Mice

Using Nrf2 KO mice, disruption of Nrf2 gene renders the animals more susceptible to dextran sulfate sodium (DSS)-induced colitis (Khor et al. 2006a) and to AOM-DSS-induced colon carcinogenesis (Khor et al. 2008b). Similar results were seen with Nrf2 KO mice that developed significantly high incidence of colonic tumor in comparison with wild-type mice by Kensler's group when investigating the role of Nrf2 in prevention of inflammation-associated aberrant crypt foci formation (Osburn et al. 2007). Collectively, Nrf2 pathway plays a role in mediating a strong anti-inflammatory response, besides induction of detoxification and antioxidant enzymes as described above.

4.4 Nrf2 in Various Cancers and Chemoprevention by Nutraceuticals

4.4.1 Nutraceuticals and Chemoprevention

Cancer has been reported to be a leading cause of death in the US in persons younger than 85 years old (Jemal et al. 2010b) therefore the importance of cancer prevention cannot be over emphasized. Carcinogenesis is a multi-step process involving initiation, promotion and progression, thus providing numerous opportunities for cancer prevention. The term of chemoprevention was first coined by Michael Sporn in 1976 (Sporn 1976), 13 years before Stephen DeFelice first coined "nutraceuticals" (Kalra 2003). Michael Sporn referred to the prevention of malignancy development by vitamin A and its synthetic analogs (Sporn 1976). Since then, chemoprevention has been adopted as one of the major tactics to modulate the process of carcinogenesis (Hong and Sporn 1997).

Chemoprevention, hence by definition, is the use of pharmacologic or natural agents to inhibit the development of invasive cancer. In this chapter, we have overviewed various nutraceuticals as chemopreventive agents with a cancer preventive activity working via Nrf2 signaling, and some are coupled with anti-inflammatory activities. Current studies have shown that some chemopreventive compounds are not only effective in animal models, but also promising in the ongoing clinical trials (Shu et al. 2010). Generally, chemopreventive compounds may work via multifaceted molecular pathways such as by suppressing inflammation, cell proliferation, invasion, and angiogenesis of tumor cells and by enhancing the antioxidant response (Hu et al. 2010). The "oxidative stress coupled with inflammation hypothesis" has provided compelling evidence that drives initiation, promotion and progression of cancers. A growing body of evidence justifies that targeting the Nrf2 pathway is a viable approach in cancer prevention as oxidative stress is one of the key underlying cause of carcinogenesis (Hu et al. 2010; Slocum and Kensler 2011).

4.4.2 Significant Role of Nrf2 in Chemoprevention

4.4.2.1 Enhanced Susceptibility to Carcinogenesis in Nrf2 KO Mice

The first in vivo evidence showing a critical role of Nrf2 in induction of phase II detoxification enzymes was published in 1997 (Itoh et al. 1997). By using Nrf2 KO mice, Ito et al. found that the magnitude of GST and NQO1 induction was significantly lower in the Nrf2 KO mice than that in Nrf2 heterozygous mice. Such a critical role of Nrf2 in inducing phase II detoxifying and antioxidant enzymes has been further confirmed in many studies using Nrf2 KO mice with and without nutraceutical chemopreventive compounds and have been extensively reviewed (Hu et al. 2010; Saw and Kong 2011; Slocum and Kensler 2011).

Using Nrf2 KO mice, the protective role of Nrf2 has clearly been demonstrated in various carcinogenesis models such as colitis and colon cancer (Khor et al. 2006a, 2008b; Osburn et al. 2007), skin inflammation and cancer (auf dem Keller et al. 2006, Pearson et al. 2008; Saw et al. 2011b; Xu et al. 2006), breast cancer (Becks et al. 2010), bladder cancer (Iida et al. 2004), stomach cancer (Fahey et al. 2002; Ramos-Gomez et al. 2001, 2003), lung diseases and cancer (Aoki et al. 2001, 2007; Iizuka et al. 2005; Rangasamy et al. 2004, 2005; Sussan et al. 2009) and liver cancer (Kitamura et al. 2007).

A general conclusion that can be drawn from these studies is that when Nrf2 is disrupted, induction of cytoprotective phase II detoxifying and antioxidant enzymes would be impaired. Therefore, when Nrf2 KO mice are exposed to oxidative stress or carcinogens, the unchallenged oxidative stress and reactive intermediates generated by carcinogens would damage DNA/cellular macromolecules, potentially induce persistent inflammation, among others, which, in turn would increase genomic instability and enhance neoplastic transformation. In comparison with Nrf2 KO mice, the Nrf2 WT mice would be able to maintain normal induction of phase II detoxifying/antioxidant enzymes, as well as other Nrf2-mediated cellular protective pathways, and hence would limit the cytotoxic effect of carcinogens. As discussed earlier, many chemopreventive compounds have been shown to induce phase II detoxifying and antioxidant enzymes through a mechanism dependent on Keap1-Nrf2-ARE signaling. Given the important role of Nrf2 in protection against carcinogenesis, attempts have been made to develop more effective chemopreventive agents by targeting Nrf2 pathway either from dietary nutraceutical or synthetic sources (Slocum and Kensler 2011).

4.4.2.2 Epigenetic Down-Regulation of Nrf2 in Aging TRAMP Mice Prostate Tumors Correlating to Human Prostate Cancer

The role of Nrf2 in carcinogenesis of prostate cancer in TRAMP mice appears to be implicated with the down-regulation of the expression of Nrf2 and its target genes (Yu et al. 2010), and the prevention of prostate cancer in TRAMP by various nutraceuticals are in part by up-regulating Nrf2 and related genes. The role of Nrf2 in prostate cancer prevention is also clearly demonstrated in TRAMP mice when various nutraceutical chemopreventive compounds were tested such as curcumin, PEITC (Barve et al. 2008), tocopherols (Barve et al. 2009), broccoli sprouts (Keum et al. 2009), dibenzoylmethane (Khor et al. 2009) and tocotrienols (Barve et al. 2010). We have also shown that Nrf2 is epigenetically silenced in prostate cancer in the TRAMP mouse model (Yu et al. 2010). As prostate tumor progresses in TRAMP mice, there appears to be a progressive loss of expression of Nrf2 and its downstream target genes such as UGT, GST and heme oxygenase-1 (HO-1) (Yu et al. 2010), which appears to correlate with human prostate cancer (Frohlich et al. 2008). This leads to a hypothesis that the disruption of the Nrf2-antioxidant axis leads to increased oxidative stress and DNA damage resulting in the initiation of cellular transformation in the prostate gland and drives carcinogenesis. Importantly, nutraceutical compound such as curcumin, which has been shown to be effective in prevention of prostate cancer in TRAMP mice (Barve et al. 2008), would epigenetically demethylate the CpG island found in the promoter of Nrf2 in TRAMP C1 cells, which were derived from TRAMP prostate tumors (Khor et al. 2011).

4.5 Conclusions

Development of effective nutraceuticals in preventing cancer is important and would require conclusive evidence from animal models that emulate human cancers. Excessive oxidative stress and inflammation are implicated in carcinogenesis. Using nutraceutical isothiocyanates and polyphenols as examples, tremendous scientific evidence show that these different nutraceuticals are functioning as Nrf2 inducers, they increase the expression of phase II detoxifying and antioxidant enzymes in cells and animals. When challenged by oxidative stress and carcinogens, these nutraceuticals would dampen and protect against damages. Since there is overlap between antioxidant and anti-inflammatory activities for some nutraceuticals involving Nrf2 and NF-κB pathways, Nrf2 would be one of the very promising target for cancer prevention and other transcription factors can also be targeted for cancer prevention (Colburn and Kensler 2008). The potential of Nrf2 as a chemopreventive target is clearly evident from the findings in Nrf2 KO mice that had increased susceptibility to various carcinogens inducing cancers. Also, the ineffectiveness of nutraceutical chemopreventive compounds to inhibit carcinogenesis in Nrf2 KO mice compared to their Nrf2 WT counterparts further strengthens the Nrf2-dependent susceptibility in Nrf2 KO animals. The studies using Nrf2 KO models have clearly shown the protective role of Nrf2 in cancer prevention particularly during the earlier initiation phase of carcinogenesis.

Acknowledgments Supported in part by Grant NIH R01-CA094828 (A.N.K.). We thank all the members in Dr. Tony Kong's lab for their help in the discussion and preparation of this book chapter.

References

Anand P, Kunnumakkara AB, Newman RA et al (2007) Bioavailability of curcumin: problems and promises. Mol Pharm 4:807–818

Anand P, Thomas SG, Kunnumakkara AB et al (2008) Biological activities of curcumin and its analogues (Congeners) made by man and Mother Nature. Biochem Pharmacol 76:1590–1611

Aoki Y, Sato H, Nishimura N et al (2001) Accelerated DNA adduct formation in the lung of the Nrf2 knockout mouse exposed to diesel exhaust. Toxicol Appl Pharmacol 173:154–160

Aoki Y, Hashimoto AH, Amanuma K et al (2007) Enhanced spontaneous and benzo(a)pyrene-induced mutations in the lung of Nrf2-deficient gpt delta mice. Cancer Res 67:5643–5648

Arnold M, Razum O, Coebergh JW (2010) Cancer risk diversity in non-western migrants to Europe: An overview of the literature. Eur J Cancer 46:2647–2659

auf dem Keller U, Huber M, Beyer TA et al (2006) Nrf transcription factors in keratinocytes are essential for skin tumor prevention but not for wound healing. Mol Cell Biol 26:3773–3784

Balamurugan AN, Akhov L, Selvaraj G et al (2009) Induction of antioxidant enzymes by curcumin and its analogues in human islets: implications in transplantation. Pancreas 38:454–460

Barve A, Khor TO, Hao X et al (2008) Murine prostate cancer inhibition by dietary phytochemicals – curcumin and phenyethylisothiocyanate. Pharm Res 25:2181–2189

Barve A, Khor TO, Nair S et al (2009) Gamma-tocopherol-enriched mixed tocopherol diet inhibits prostate carcinogenesis in TRAMP mice. Int J Cancer 124:1693–1699

Barve A, Khor TO, Reuhl K et al (2010) Mixed tocotrienols inhibit prostate carcinogenesis in TRAMP mice. Nutr Cancer 62:789–794

Becks L, Prince M, Burson H et al (2010) Aggressive mammary carcinoma progression in Nrf2 knockout mice treated with 7,12-dimethylbenz[a]anthracene. BMC Cancer 10:540

Boyle P, Levin B (2008) World Cancer Report 2008: IARC Nonserial Publication, France

Brower V (1998) Nutraceuticals: poised for a healthy slice of the healthcare market? Nat Biotechnol 16:728–731

Carter BS, Carter HB, Isaacs JT (1990) Epidemiologic evidence regarding predisposing factors to prostate cancer. Prostate 16:187–197

Chan R, Lok K, Woo J (2009) Prostate cancer and vegetable consumption. Mol Nutr Food Res 53:201–216

Cheung KL, Khor TO, Kong AN (2009) Synergistic effect of combination of phenethyl isothiocyanate and sulforaphane or curcumin and sulforaphane in the inhibition of inflammation. Pharm Res 26:224–231

Chung FL, Conaway CC, Rao CV et al (2000) Chemoprevention of colonic aberrant crypt foci in Fischer rats by sulforaphane and phenethyl isothiocyanate. Carcinogenesis 21:2287–2291

Colburn NH, Kensler TW (2008) Targeting transcription factors for cancer prevention – the case of Nrf2. Cancer Prev Res (Phila) 1:153–155

Cullinan SB, Diehl JA (2004) PERK-dependent activation of Nrf2 contributes to redox homeostasis and cell survival following endoplasmic reticulum stress. J Biol Chem 279:20108–20117

Dai F, Chen WF, Zhou B et al (2009) Antioxidative effects of curcumin and its analogues against the free-radical-induced peroxidation of linoleic acid in micelles. Phytother Res 23:1220–1228

DeFelice S (2011) The foundation for innovation in medicine. http://www.fimdefelice.org/page.asp?ID=2504. Accessed June 2011

de Sousa RR, Queiroz KC, Souza AC et al (2007) Phosphoprotein levels, MAPK activities and NFkappaB expression are affected by fisetin. J Enzyme Inhib Med Chem 22:439–444

Fahey JW, Zalcmann AT, Talalay P (2001) The chemical diversity and distribution of glucosinolates and isothiocyanates among plants. Phytochemistry 56:5–51

Fahey JW, Haristoy X, Dolan PM et al (2002) Sulforaphane inhibits extracellular, intracellular, and antibiotic-resistant strains of Helicobacter pylori and prevents benzo[a]pyrene-induced stomach tumors. Proc Natl Acad Sci USA 99:7610–7615

Fielding JE (1985) Smoking: health effects and control (1). N Engl J Med 313:491–498

Frohlich DA, McCabe MT, Arnold RS et al (2008) The role of Nrf2 in increased reactive oxygen species and DNA damage in prostate tumorigenesis. Oncogene 27:4353–4362

Hatcher H, Planalp R, Cho J et al (2008) Curcumin: from ancient medicine to current clinical trials. Cell Mol Life Sci 65:1631–1652

Hecht SS, Kenney PM, Wang M et al (2002) Benzyl isothiocyanate: an effective inhibitor of polycyclic aromatic hydrocarbon tumorigenesis in A/J mouse lung. Cancer Lett 187:87–94

Higdon JV, Delage B, Williams DE et al (2007) Cruciferous vegetables and human cancer risk: epidemiologic evidence and mechanistic basis. Pharmacol Res 55:224–236

Hong WK, Sporn MB (1997) Recent advances in chemoprevention of cancer. Science 278:1073–1077

Hsing AW, Tsao L, Devesa SS (2000) International trends and patterns of prostate cancer incidence and mortality. Int J Cancer 85:60–67

Hu R, Khor TO, Shen G et al (2006) Cancer chemoprevention of intestinal polyposis in ApcMin/+ mice by sulforaphane, a natural product derived from cruciferous vegetable. Carcinogenesis 27:2038–2046

Hu R, Saw CL, Yu R et al (2010) Regulation of NF-E2-related factor 2 signaling for cancer chemoprevention: antioxidant coupled with antiinflammatory. Antioxid Redox Signal 13:1679–1698

Huang HC, Nguyen T, Pickett CB (2002) Phosphorylation of Nrf2 at Ser-40 by protein kinase C regulates antioxidant response element-mediated transcription. J Biol Chem 277:42769–42774

Iida K, Itoh K, Kumagai Y et al (2004) Nrf2 is essential for the chemopreventive efficacy of oltipraz against urinary bladder carcinogenesis. Cancer Res 64:6424–6431

Iizuka T, Ishii Y, Itoh K et al (2005) Nrf2-deficient mice are highly susceptible to cigarette smoke-induced emphysema. Genes Cells 10:1113–1125

Itoh K, Chiba T, Takahashi S et al (1997) An Nrf2/small Maf heterodimer mediates the induction of phase II detoxifying enzyme genes through antioxidant response elements. Biochem Biophys Res Commun 236:313–322

Jakubikova J, Sedlak J, Mithen R et al (2005) Role of PI3K/Akt and MEK/ERK signaling pathways in sulforaphane- and erucin-induced phase II enzymes and MRP2 transcription, G2/M arrest and cell death in Caco-2 cells. Biochem Pharmacol 69:1543–1552

Jemal A, Bray F, Center MM et al (2010a) Global cancer statistics. CA Cancer J Clin 60:277–300

Jemal A, Siegel R, Xu J et al (2010b) Cancer statistics, 2010. CA Cancer J Clin 60:277–300

Kalpana Deepa Priya D, Gayathri R, Sakthisekaran D (2011) Role of sulforaphane in the anti-initiating mechanism of lung carcinogenesis in vivo by modulating the metabolic activation and detoxification of benzo(a)pyrene. Biomed Pharmacother 65:9–16

Kalra EK (2003) Nutraceutical – definition and introduction. AAPS PharmSci 5:E25

Keum YS, Khor TO, Lin W et al (2009) Pharmacokinetics and pharmacodynamics of broccoli sprouts on the suppression of prostate cancer in transgenic adenocarcinoma of mouse prostate (TRAMP) mice: implication of induction of Nrf2, HO-1 and apoptosis and the suppression of Akt-dependent kinase pathway. Pharm Res 26:2324–2331

Khor TO, Huang MT, Kwon KH et al (2006a) Nrf2-deficient mice have an increased susceptibility to dextran sulfate sodium-induced colitis. Cancer Res 66:11580–11584

Khor TO, Keum YS, Lin W et al (2006b) Combined inhibitory effects of curcumin and phenethyl isothiocyanate on the growth of human PC-3 prostate xenografts in immunodeficient mice. Cancer Res 66:613–621

Khor TO, Cheung WK, Prawan A et al (2008a) Chemoprevention of familial adenomatous polyposis in Apc(Min/+) mice by phenethyl isothiocyanate (PEITC). Mol Carcinog 47:321–325

Khor TO, Huang MT, Prawan A et al (2008b) Increased susceptibility of Nrf2 knockout mice to colitis-associated colorectal cancer. Cancer Prev Res (Phila Pa) 1:187–191

Khor TO, Yu S, Kong AN (2008c) Dietary cancer chemopreventive agents – targeting inflammation and Nrf2 signaling pathway. Planta Med 74:1540–1547

Khor TO, Yu S, Barve A et al (2009) Dietary feeding of dibenzoylmethane inhibits prostate cancer in transgenic adenocarcinoma of the mouse prostate model. Cancer Res 69:7096–7102

Khor TO, Huang Y, Wu TY et al (2011) Pharmacodynamics of curcumin as DNA hypomethylation agent in restoring the expression of Nrf2 via promoter CpGs demethylation. Biochem Pharmacol 82:1073–1078

Kidd PM (2009) Bioavailability and activity of phytosome complexes from botanical polyphenols: the silymarin, curcumin, green tea, and grape seed extracts. Altern Med Rev 14:226–246

Kim BR, Hu R, Keum YS et al (2003) Effects of glutathione on antioxidant response element-mediated gene expression and apoptosis elicited by sulforaphane. Cancer Res 63:7520–7525

Kim J, Cha YN, Surh YJ (2010) A protective role of nuclear factor-erythroid 2-related factor-2 (Nrf2) in inflammatory disorders. Mutat Res 690:12–23

Kitamura Y, Umemura T, Kanki K et al (2007) Increased susceptibility to hepatocarcinogenicity of Nrf2-deficient mice exposed to 2-amino-3-methylimidazo[4,5-f]quinoline. Cancer Sci 98: 19–24

Klassen AC, Platz EA (2006) What can geography tell us about prostate cancer? Am J Prev Med 30:S7–15

Lee JM, Hanson JM, Chu WA et al (2001) Phosphatidylinositol 3-kinase, not extracellular signal-regulated kinase, regulates activation of the antioxidant-responsive element in IMR-32 human neuroblastoma cells. J Biol Chem 276:20011–20016

Lee KH, Ab Aziz FH, Syahida A et al (2009) Synthesis and biological evaluation of curcumin-like diarylpentanoid analogues for anti-inflammatory, antioxidant and anti-tyrosinase activities. Eur J Med Chem 44:3195–3200

Li W, Kong AN (2009) Molecular mechanisms of Nrf2-mediated antioxidant response. Mol Carcinog 48:91–104

Li W, Khor TO, Xu C et al (2008) Activation of Nrf2-antioxidant signaling attenuates NFkappaB-inflammatory response and elicits apoptosis. Biochem Pharmacol 76:1485–1489

Lin W, Wu RT, Wu T et al (2008) Sulforaphane suppressed LPS-induced inflammation in mouse peritoneal macrophages through Nrf2 dependent pathway. Biochem Pharmacol 76:967–973

Mantovani A, Allavena P, Sica A et al (2008) Cancer-related inflammation. Nature 454:436–444

Murakami A, Song M, Ohigashi H (2007) Phenethyl isothiocyanate suppresses receptor activator of NF-kappaB ligand (RANKL)-induced osteoclastogenesis by blocking activation of ERK1/2 and p38 MAPK in RAW264.7 macrophages. Biofactors 30:1–11

Nair S, Doh ST, Chan JY et al (2008) Regulatory potential for concerted modulation of Nrf2- and Nfkb1-mediated gene expression in inflammation and carcinogenesis. Br J Cancer 99:2070–2082

Nguyen T, Nioi P, Pickett CB (2009) The Nrf2-antioxidant response element signaling pathway and its activation by oxidative stress. J Biol Chem 284:13291–13295

Nichenametla SN, Taruscio TG, Barney DL et al (2006) A review of the effects and mechanisms of polyphenolics in cancer. Crit Rev Food Sci Nutr 46:161–183

Osburn WO, Karim B, Dolan PM et al (2007) Increased colonic inflammatory injury and formation of aberrant crypt foci in Nrf2-deficient mice upon dextran sulfate treatment. Int J Cancer 121:1883–1891

Padhye S, Chavan D, Pandey S et al (2010) Perspectives on chemopreventive and therapeutic potential of curcumin analogs in medicinal chemistry. Mini Rev Med Chem 10:372–387

Pearson KJ, Lewis KN, Price NL et al (2008) Nrf2 mediates cancer protection but not prolongevity induced by caloric restriction. Proc Natl Acad Sci USA 105:2325–2330

Ramos-Gomez M, Kwak MK, Dolan PM et al (2001) Sensitivity to carcinogenesis is increased and chemoprotective efficacy of enzyme inducers is lost in nrf2 transcription factor-deficient mice. Proc Natl Acad Sci USA 98:3410–3415

Ramos-Gomez M, Dolan PM, Itoh K et al (2003) Interactive effects of nrf2 genotype and oltipraz on benzo[a]pyrene-DNA adducts and tumor yield in mice. Carcinogenesis 24:461–467

Rangasamy T, Cho CY, Thimmulappa RK et al (2004) Genetic ablation of Nrf2 enhances susceptibility to cigarette smoke-induced emphysema in mice. J Clin Invest 114:1248–1259

Rangasamy T, Guo J, Mitzner WA et al (2005) Disruption of Nrf2 enhances susceptibility to severe airway inflammation and asthma in mice. J Exp Med 202:47–59

Saw CL, Kong AN (2011) Nuclear factor-erythroid 2-related factor 2 as a chemopreventive target in colorectal cancer. Expert Opin Ther Targets 15:281–295

Saw CL, Huang Y, Kong AN (2010) Synergistic anti-inflammatory effects of low doses of curcumin in combination with polyunsaturated fatty acids: docosahexaenoic acid or eicosapentaenoic acid. Biochem Pharmacol 79:421–430

Saw CL, Cintron M, Wu TY et al (2011a) Pharmacodynamics of dietary phytochemical indoles I3C and DIM: induction of Nrf2-mediated phase II drug metabolizing and antioxidant genes and synergism with isothiocyanates. Biopharm Drug Dispos 32:289–300

Saw CL, Huang MT, Liu Y et al (2011b) Impact of Nrf2 on UVB-induced skin inflammation/photoprotection and photoprotective effect of sulforaphane. Mol Carcinog 50:479–486

Shen G, Kong AN (2009) Nrf2 plays an important role in coordinated regulation of Phase II drug metabolism enzymes and Phase III drug transporters. Biopharm Drug Dispos 30:345–355

Shen G, Hebbar V, Nair S et al (2004) Regulation of Nrf2 transactivation domain activity. The differential effects of mitogen-activated protein kinase cascades and synergistic stimulatory effect of Raf and CREB-binding protein. J Biol Chem 279:23052–23060

Shen G, Xu C, Hu R et al (2006) Modulation of nuclear factor E2-related factor 2-mediated gene expression in mice liver and small intestine by cancer chemopreventive agent curcumin. Mol Cancer Ther 5:39–51

Shen G, Khor TO, Hu R et al (2007) Chemoprevention of familial adenomatous polyposis by natural dietary compounds sulforaphane and dibenzoylmethane alone and in combination in ApcMin/+ mouse. Cancer Res 67:9937–9944

Shimizu H, Ross RK, Bernstein L et al (1991) Cancers of the prostate and breast among Japanese and white immigrants in Los Angeles County. Br J Cancer 63:963–966

Shu L, Cheung KL, Khor TO et al (2010) Phytochemicals: cancer chemoprevention and suppression of tumor onset and metastasis. Cancer Metastasis Rev 29:483–502

Slocum SL, Kensler TW (2011) Nrf2: control of sensitivity to carcinogens. Arch Toxicol 85: 273–284

Sporn MB (1976) Approaches to prevention of epithelial cancer during the preneoplastic period. Cancer Res 36:2699–2702

Sussan TE, Rangasamy T, Blake DJ et al (2009) Targeting Nrf2 with the triterpenoid CDDO-imidazolide attenuates cigarette smoke-induced emphysema and cardiac dysfunction in mice. Proc Natl Acad Sci USA 106:250–255

Svehlikova V, Wang S, Jakubikova J et al (2004) Interactions between sulforaphane and apigenin in the induction of UGT1A1 and GSTA1 in CaCo-2 cells. Carcinogenesis 25:1629–1637

Szymanski KM, Wheeler DC, Mucci LA (2010) Fish consumption and prostate cancer risk: a review and meta-analysis. Am J Clin Nutr 92:1223–1233

Tang L, Zirpoli GR, Guru K et al (2008) Consumption of raw cruciferous vegetables is inversely associated with bladder cancer risk. Cancer Epidemiol Biomarkers Prev 17:938–944

Terry P, Lichtenstein P, Feychting M et al (2001) Fatty fish consumption and risk of prostate cancer. Lancet 357:1764–1766

Tham CL, Liew CY, Lam KW et al (2010) A synthetic curcuminoid derivative inhibits nitric oxide and proinflammatory cytokine synthesis. Eur J Pharmacol 628:247–254

Tominaga S, Kuroishi T (1997) An ecological study on diet/nutrition and cancer in Japan. Int J Cancer Suppl 10:2–6

Verhoeven DT, Verhagen H, Goldbohm RA et al (1997) A review of mechanisms underlying anticarcinogenicity by brassica vegetables. Chem Biol Interact 103:79–129

Wang H, Khor TO, Saw CL et al (2010) Role of nrf2 in suppressing LPS-induced inflammation in mouse peritoneal macrophages by polyunsaturated fatty acids docosahexaenoic acid and eicosapentaenoic acid. Mol Pharm 7:2185–2193

Witschi H, Espiritu I, Maronpot RR et al (1997a) The carcinogenic potential of the gas phase of environmental tobacco smoke. Carcinogenesis 18:2035–2042

Witschi H, Espiritu I, Peake JL et al (1997b) The carcinogenicity of environmental tobacco smoke. Carcinogenesis 18:575–586

Xu C, Huang MT, Shen G et al (2006) Inhibition of 7,12-dimethylbenz(a)anthracene-induced skin tumorigenesis in C57BL/6 mice by sulforaphane is mediated by nuclear factor E2-related factor 2. Cancer Res 66:8293–8296

Yang CX, Kuroishi T, Huang XE et al (2002) Correlation between food consumption and colorectal cancer: An Ecological Analysis in Japan. Asian Pac J Cancer Prev 3:77–83

Yu S, Kong AN (2007) Targeting carcinogen metabolism by dietary cancer preventive compounds. Curr Cancer Drug Targets 7:416–424

Yu R, Chen C, Mo YY et al (2000) Activation of mitogen-activated protein kinase pathways induces antioxidant response element-mediated gene expression via a Nrf2-dependent mechanism. J Biol Chem 275:39907–39913

Yu S, Khor TO, Cheung KL et al (2010) Nrf2 expression is regulated by epigenetic mechanisms in prostate cancer of TRAMP mice. PLoS One 5:e8579

Yuan X, Xu C, Pan Z et al (2006) Butylated hydroxyanisole regulates ARE-mediated gene expression via Nrf2 coupled with ERK and JNK signaling pathway in HepG2 cells. Mol Carcinog 45:841–850

Zhang Y, Kensler TW, Cho CG et al (1994) Anticarcinogenic activities of sulforaphane and structurally related synthetic norbornyl isothiocyanates. Proc Natl Acad Sci USA 91:3147–3150

Zhao C, Cai Y, He X et al (2010) Synthesis and anti-inflammatory evaluation of novel mono-carbonyl analogues of curcumin in LPS-stimulated RAW 264.7 macrophages. Eur J Med Chem 45:5773–5780

Chapter 5
Current Status and Future Prospects of Nutraceuticals in Prostate Cancer

Sanjeev Shukla and Sanjay Gupta

Abstract Nutraceuticals are products derived from food sources that provide health benefits. Several natural dietary agents have been studied for their preventive and/or therapeutic effects against prostate cancer. Although most of the information on nutraceuticals and prostate cancer is drawn from epidemiologic and case-control studies, clinical studies conducted so far have not provided clear-cut results. The lack of evidence-based studies limits the use of nutraceuticals and their clinical recommendations. In spite these limitations, the field of nutraceutical research continues to emerge as many of these nutritional agents are tested for their therapeutic potential in pre-clinical and clinical settings. Nutraceuticals have the potential for significant medical and economic impacts. This chapter highlights the present status of nutraceuticals in prostate cancer and discusses future prospects for nutritional strategies that are safe and clinically beneficial.

Keywords Prostate cancer · Nutraceuticals · Flavonoids · Polyphenols · Dietary agents

Abbreviations

AICR	American Institute for Cancer Research
AKR1C3	aldo-keto reductase family 1 member C3
AR	androgen receptor
CDK	cyclin-dependent kinase
DIM	3,3′-diindolylmethane
HSD3B2	3 beta-hydroxysteroid dehydrogenase type 2
IGF	insulin-like growth factor
IGFBP	insulin-like growth factor binding protein
IL	interleukin
MAPK	mitogen activated protein kinase
mTOR	mammalian target of rapamycin
NCCAM	National Center for Complementary and Alternative Medicine

S. Gupta (✉)
Department of Urology, Case Comprehensive Cancer Center, University Hospitals Case Medical Center, Case Western Reserve University, Cleveland, OH 44106, USA
e-mail: sanjay.gupta@case.edu

F.H. Sarkar (ed.), *Nutraceuticals and Cancer*, DOI 10.1007/978-94-007-2630-7_5,

NEMO	NF-Kappa-B essential modulator
NF-κB	nuclear factor kappa B
NK	natural killer cells
PEITC	phenylethyl isothiocyanate
ppm	parts per million
ProtecT	prostate testing for cancer and treatment
SELECT	selenium and vitamin E cancer prevention trial
SRD5A1	steroid 5alpha reductase type 1
STAT	signal transducer and activator of transcription
TGFβ1	transforming growth factor beta 1
TRAMP	*tr*ansgenic *a*denocarcinoma of the *m*ouse *p*rostate

5.1 Introduction

Prostate cancer is the second leading cause of cancer death, in men, in the United States. Prostate cancer rates are high in North America and northern Europe, intermediate in Mediterranean nations and relatively low in many parts of Asia (Jemal et al. 2011). Epidemiological studies have suggested that diet and nutrition are critical determinants of prostate cancer risk, with dramatic variations in prostate cancer incidence and mortality between different geographic regions (Ross 2010). Prostate cancer incidence is low in Asian countries and this has been attributed to diets and lifestyle factors and diets that are rich in plant-based agents. In contrast, the incidence of prostate cancer is significantly higher in industrialized Western countries where high-calorie diets are commonplace (Parodi 2005). It has been speculated that diets complying with the guidelines by the American Institute for Cancer Research (AICR) would likely reduce the incidence of prostate cancer by at least 60–70%, along with similar reductions in cancers at other sites (Donaldson 2004). It is also apparent from migration studies that Asian men who immigrate to the United States and adopt Western diets have a risk of developing prostate cancer that approaches the average US incidence within one generation (Gann 2002). This information suggests that environmental factors including diet and lifestyle play significant roles in the initiation of prostate cancer, and more importantly, that these factors may also influence the rate of progression of established prostate cancers.

Pharmacological intervention with naturally occurring compounds present in the diet may prevent, inhibit, or reverse carcinogenesis, or suppress the development of invasive cancer. The term 'nutraceutical' arose by combining 'nutrition' and 'pharmaceutical' with intent to categorize natural food or supplement having medical or health benefits (Maddi et al. 2007). Nutraceuticals should possess demonstrable protective action against chronic diseases or should have physiological benefits. Approximately, 40–80% of Americans use alternative remedies, including nutraceuticals, for disease prevention and therapy (Metzger et al. 2009). A large number of macronutrients, micronutrients, and other nutraceuticals have been or are currently being evaluated as potential prostate cancer preventive agents as shown in Table 5.1. These include numerous agents such as carotenoids, vitamins, dietary fiber, selenium, glucosinolates, indoles, isothiocyanates, flavonoids, phenols, protease inhibitors, plant sterols and other complementary agents (Rajasekaran et al. 2008). These nutraceuticals display complementary and overlapping mechanisms of action, including induction of detoxification enzymes, antioxidant effects,

Table 5.1 Current status of nutraceuticals in prostate cancer

Nutraceuticals	**Cell Culture Studies**	**Pre-clinical Studies**	**Clinical**		
			Phase I	**II**	**III**
1.0 Carotenoids					
1.1. β-Carotein	→	→	→	→	→
1.2. Lycopene	→	→	→	→	→
2.0 Vitamins					
2.1. Vitamin A	→	→	→		
2.2. Vitamin C	→	→	→	→	→
2.3. Vitamin D	→	→	→	→	→
2.4. Vitamin E	→	→	→	→	→
3.0 Minerals					
3.1. Selenium	→	→	→	→	→
3.2. Zinc	→	→	→	→	→
4.0 Flavonoids					
4.1. Daidzein	→	→	→		
4.2. Genistein	→	→	→	→	→
4.3. Polyphenols; green tea	→	→	→	→	→
4.4. Resveratrol	→	→			
4.5. Silymarin	→	→			
4.5. Silibinin	→	→	→		
4.6. Grape seed extract	→	→			
4.7. Apigenin	→	→			
4.8. Pomegranate	→	→	→		
4.9. Punic acid	→				
4.10. Delphinidin	→				
5.0 Indoles					
5.1. 3,3'-diindolylmethane	→	→	→		
5.2. Indole -3 -carbinol	→	→			
6.0 Isothiocyanates					
6.1. Phenylethyl isothiocyanate	→	→			
7.0 Phenolic Acids					
7.1. Curcumin	→	→	→		
8.0 Organosulfur Compounds					
8.1. Diallyl disulfide	→				
8.2. Diallyl trisulfide	→	→			
9.0 Terpenes					
9.1. D-Limonene	→				
9.2. Perillyl alcohol	→				
9.3. Betulinic acid	→				
9.4. Ursolic acid	→				
10.0 Other Nutraceuticals					
10.1. PC-SPES	→	→	→		
10.2. Permixon	→	→	→		
10.3. Equiguard	→				

and inhibition of the formation of nitrosamines, binding/dilution of carcinogens in the digestive tract, alteration of hormone metabolism and modulation of epigenetic and carcinogenic events. The long latent period between the initial development of prostate cancer and the onset of clinically relevant prostate cancer affords opportunities for intervention with nutraceuticals to delay disease initiation or progression. This chapter focuses on epidemiologic, clinical and mechanistic studies that have evaluated the anticancer effects of various nutraceuticals in prostate cancer.

5.2 Carotenoids

There has been a remarkable increase in the consumption of dietary supplements in the United States and other developed nations in the past several years (Zambetti 2008). Among the carotenoids, β-carotene and lycopene have been most extensively studied with respect to their possible roles in preventing prostate cancer (Krinsky and Johnson 2005). Reports from epidemiological studies investigating the relationship between β-carotene intake and the risk of prostate cancer have been inconsistent (Cook et al. 2000; Goodman et al. 2003). Prospective cohort studies on intake of α- and β- carotene, vitamins A, C, and E, and lycopene have shown inverse associations for vitamin A and α- and β- carotene in prostate cancer risk (Schuurman et al. 2002). Another case-control study evaluating an association between retinol and various carotenoids has shown a weak protective effect of carotene, particularly β-carotene, on the risk of prostate cancer (Bosetti et al. 2004). Although the results are encouraging, it is difficult to analyze the complex network and the protective role of dietary antioxidants in such clinical settings. Due to the complexity of results, limited preclinical research has been conducted with β-carotene and prostate cancer.

Compelling epidemiological studies have suggested that a diet rich in tomato products is associated with a reduction in prostate cancer risk (Hwang and Bowen 2002). Prospective case-control studies and meta-analysis of observational studies have shown that tomato products may play a role in the prevention of prostate cancer (Jian et al. 2005; Etminan et al. 2004). It is hypothesized that lycopene may be one of the components of tomato that contributes to this association. Lycopene has been shown to be present in the human prostate at significant concentrations, a finding that supports the plausibility of a direct effect on prostate biology (Giovannucci 1999). Studies in cell culture system have shown that lycopene inhibits growth of prostate cancer cells through the pathways that influence expression of gap junction proteins and growth factor signaling (Obermuller-Jevic et al. 2003; Aust et al. 2003). The Carotene and Retinol Efficacy Trial (CARET), a randomized, double-blinded, placebo-controlled trial with a daily dose of 30 mg β-carotene + 25,000 IU of retinyl palmitate in smokers suggested that neither the CARET nor other supplements were associated with total prostate cancer risk (Neuhouser et al. 2009). The conclusion from a recent meta-analysis of randomized controlled trials of β-carotene supplementation, from 13 articles with usable information was that β-carotene supplementation has no substantial effect on prostate cancer risk (Druesne-Pecollo et al. 2010).

A study on a preclinical model of prostate cancer indicates that consumption of tomato powder but not lycopene inhibited prostate carcinogenesis, suggesting that tomato products contain compounds in addition to lycopene that modify the prostate carcinogenic process (Boileau et al. 2003). Recent studies conducted in *tr*ansgenic *a*denocarcinoma of the *m*ouse *p*rostate (TRAMP) mice suggested that the incidence of prostate cancer was significantly decreased in the lycopene beadlet group relative to the control group ($P = 0.0197$) whereas the difference between the tomato paste and control groups was not statistically significant ($P = 0.34$). There was no difference in prostate weights between the groups (Konijeti R et al. 2010). In another study, diet enriched with processed whole tomatoes significantly increased overall survival ($P < 0.01$), delayed progression from prostatic intraepithelial neoplasia to adenocarcinoma, and decreased the incidence of poorly differentiated carcinoma (Pannellini T et al. 2010). These studies are highly encouraging and strongly support further mechanistic studies with lycopene in preclinical models of prostate cancer.

Recent studies on men with prostate cancer supplemented with lycopene-enriched enhancement or tomato products for several weeks prior to radical prostatectomy demonstrated that lycopene concentrations in the prostate could change rapidly in response to dietary intake and induce apoptotic cell death along with modulations in oxidative stress and tumor biology markers (Bowen et al. 2002; Campbell et al. 2004). A phase II randomized clinical trial of 15 mg of lycopene supplementation twice daily for 3 week before radical prostatectomy exhibited a decrease in the plasma insulin-like growth factor (IGF)-1 levels with no significant changes in Bax and Bcl-2 (Kucuk et al. 2001). Another study by this group using tomato oleoresin extract containing the equivalent of 30 mg/day of lycopene extract for 3 week before radical prostatectomy substantially reduced prostate volume in prostate cancer patients (Kucuk et al. 2002). In another study, the efficacy of 10 mg/day supplementation of lycopene to hormone-refractory prostate cancer patients was shown to be effective in reducing serum prostate-specific antigen levels, bone pain, and lower urinary tract symptoms (LUTS) (Ansari and Gupta 2004). Several randomized trials evaluating the potential efficacy of lycopene are still ongoing.

5.3 Vitamins

Much research on dietary influences in prostate cancer has focused on the antioxidant functions of vitamins. Nutritional factors that may influence the disease include total energy intake (as reflected by body mass index), dietary fat, cooked meat, micronutrients and vitamins (carotenoids, retinoids, vitamins A, C, D and E), fruit and vegetable intake, minerals (calcium, selenium), and phytoestrogens (isoflavonoids, flavonoids, lignans). Vitamin A (retinol) and its active metabolites are essential for cell differentiation, visual function, and physiological growth (Blomhoff et al. 1992). The findings in a matched case-control nested study in the United Kingdom population, *viz.* prostate testing for cancer and treatment (ProtecT) study in men ages between 50 and 69 years suggested that circulating B12 and folate were associated with increased risk of prostate cancer (Collin et al. 2010). A recent meta-analysis of fourteen articles supported the notion that vitamins and minerals supplementation may influence cancer incidence in smokers, but neither the use of multivitamin supplementation nor the use of individual vitamin/mineral supplementation affected the overall occurrence of prostate cancer; or the occurrence of advanced/metastatic prostate cancer; or death from prostate cancer (Stratton and Godwin 2011).

Vitamin A and its analogs modulate the growth of cancer cells, presumably by activating gene transcription *via* the nuclear retinoic acid receptors α, β, and γ (Richter et al. 2002). The chemopreventive effects of retinoids are exerted at the tumor promotion phase through inhibition of cell proliferation, induction of apoptosis, cell cycle arrest, and/or a combination of these actions (Igawa et al. 1994; Liang et al. 1999a). All-*trans*-retinoic acids reduce urokinase-type plasminogen-mediated degradation of fibronectin and laminin (Webber and Waghray 1995). Despite numerous studies, no consistent association between vitamin A intake and prostate cancer risk has been established (Schuurman et al. 2002; Bosetti et al. 2004; Giovannucci et al. 1995). Some studies have shown an inverse relationship between serum retinol and the risk of prostate cancer, whereas others indicate a positive association, particularly in men more than 70 years old (Giovannucci et al. 1995; Ohno et al. 1988).

Vitamin C is a potent antioxidant that scavenges reactive oxygen species and other free radicals capable of causing damage to lipids and DNA (Hu and Shih 1997). Vitamin C has shown to inhibit malignant transformation by diminishing cellular chromosomal damage (Menon et al. 1998). Diets that include substantial amounts of fruits and vegetables rich in vitamin C are associated with a low incidence of many forms of cancer (Weisburger 1999). In animal studies, vitamin C has been shown to inhibit prostate tumor growth and viability in athymic nude mice transplanted with both androgen -sensitive and -insensitive human prostate cancer cells (Taper et al. 2001; Agus et al. 1999). Studies have shown that combinations of vitamins C and E inhibit survivin protein, a promoter of prostate cancer cell growth (Gunawardena et al. 2004). However, no individual trial has been conducted with vitamin C alone on prostate cancer.

Vitamin D, and its active form, calcitrol (1α, 25-D3) is produced in the skin through exposure of 7-dehydrocholestrol to ultraviolet light and proximal renal tubules in the kidneys through 1, 25-dihydroxyvitamin D3 hydroxylase (Favus and Langman 1986). Studies have shown that 25-hydroxyvitamin D1α-hydroxylase, the enzyme that synthesizes 1α, 25-dihydroxy D3, is also expressed in cultured prostate cells (Chen et al. 2003). Recent studies have provided evidence that residential sunlight exposure is associated with a decreased risk of prostate cancer that may be linked with vitamin D synthesis (John et al. 2004). Epidemiological studies have further suggested that an increased prostate cancer risk is associated with decreased production of vitamin D (Schwartz et al. 1998; Stewart and Weigel 2004). Studies in cell culture systems and preclinical models of prostate cancer have shown that the biologically active form of vitamin D (1 α, 25-D3) inhibits proliferation of human prostate cancer cells through mechanisms that include cell cycle arrest, induction of apoptosis, and altered activation of growth factor signaling (Blutt et al. 1997; Polek et al. 2003). Consistent with tumor suppressor activity, vitamin D compounds and retinoids have been shown to act synergistically with genistein in inhibiting the growth of human prostate epithelial cells (Rao et al. 2002). Genistein is the component in soy that has been employed in chemoprevention strategies with other putative chemopreventive agents. The combination of vitamin D compounds and retinoids has emerged as an attractive tool for use in controlling prostate cancer progression (Stewart and Weigel 2004). However, hypercalcemia induced by 1 α, 25-D3 in vivo limits its use clinically as a therapeutic agent. Population-based studies with vitamin D as well as plasma 1, 25-dihydroxyvitamin and 25-hydroxyvitamin D levels have not provided any significant data on protective effects in prostate carcinogenesis (Chan and Giovannucci 2001; Platz et al. 2004; Tavani et al. 2005). A recently meta-analysis of 3956 patients with prostate cancer, reported in 11 articles, found no significant association between 25-hydroxyvitamin D and prostate cancer (Gandini et al. 2011).

Vitamin E is a family of naturally occurring; essential, fat-soluble vitamin compounds that constitute at least eight structurally related molecules as four tocopherols and four tocotrienols (Argao and Heubi 1993). Vitamin E functions as the major lipid soluble antioxidant in cell membranes; it is a chain-breaking free-radical scavenger and specifically inhibits lipid peroxidation, a biological activity relevant to carcinogen-induced DNA damage (McCall and Frei 1999). The most active form of vitamin E is α-tocopherol, a compound that is abundant and widely distributed in nature and present in most types of human tissue and plasma (Blatt et al. 2001; Eichholzer et al. 1996). Some epidemiological studies have shown that supplementation of vitamin E in the diet lowers the incidence of prostate carcinoma (Brawley et al. 2001), whereas others did not support the role of vitamin E in prostate cancer prevention (Vlajinac et al. 1997; Rodriguez et al. 2004). In one study, men with lower plasma levels of vitamin E had an increased risk of developing prostate cancer (Eichholzer et al. 1999). Tocopherols have inherent antioxidant affinity for highly reactive and genotoxic electrophiles, such as hydroxyl, superoxide, lipid peroxyl, lipid hydroperoxyl, and nitrogen radicals (Wang and Quinn 1999). Consequently, tocopherols prevent free-radical damage in biological membranes and decrease mutagenesis and carcinogenesis (Wang and Quinn 1999). Animal studies have shown that dietary supplementation of vitamin E slows prostate cancer growth due to its ability to inhibit androgen signaling (Siler et al. 2004). The mechanisms through which tocopherols inhibit cell proliferation include inhibition of protein kinase C activity, induction of NADPH detoxification enzyme, and reduction of arachidonic acid and prostaglandin metabolism (Fazzio et al. 1997). Vitamin E has been shown to inhibit the growth of chemically and hormonally induced prostate cancer cells *via* modulation of cell cycle regulatory machinery and induction of apoptosis (Gunawardena et al. 2000). Other putative mechanisms through which vitamin E may inhibit proliferation of human prostate cancer cells include inhibition of androgen receptor function, inhibition of PSA production, and inhibition of the production of vascular endothelial growth factor (Zhang et al. 2002). The Alpha Tocopherol Beta Carotene (ATBC) cancer prevention trial, in which 29,133 male smokers were studied for prevention of lung cancer using vitamin E (50 mg/day) and/or β-carotene (20 mg/day), demonstrated that, although there was an increase in lung cancer risk, the incidence of prostate cancer was reduced by 32% in men receiving α-tocopherol compared with the control group. Additionally, 41% lower mortality rates were observed in men receiving α-tocopherol. Among subjects receiving β-carotene, the incidence of prostate cancer was 23% higher and mortality rate was up by 15% compared with subjects who did not receive β-carotene supplementation (Heinonen et al. 1998). Studies have shown that α-tocopherol has a stronger association with a lower risk of prostate cancer, and higher circulating levels of major vitamin E fractions α- and γ- tocopherol were similarly associated with lower prostate cancer risk (Weinstein et al. 2005). A recent systemic review and meta-analysis indicates that β-carotene supplementation has no overall effect on the incidence of prostate cancer (Druesne-Pecollo et al. 2010). Although some studies suggest that vitamin E may perhaps be useful in the prevention of prostate cancer, other studies are at odds with this conclusion. For example, the selenium and vitamin E cancer prevention trial (SELECT), a population-based, prospective, randomized clinical trial examined the effect of selenium and vitamin E alone or in combination on prostate cancer risk reduction. The trial was discontinued recently as there was no evidence of a benefit from either agent (Schmid et al. 2011; Ledesma et al. 2011). The totality of results to date suggests that the effects of vitamins on prostate cancer may be limited, and additional studies are required to establish their usefulness as chemopreventive agents for prostate cancer.

5.4 Minerals

Dietary supplement used as multivitamin formulations with or without minerals are typically documented in survey studies (Rock 2007). Minerals that appear to play important roles in the chemoprevention of prostate cancer are selenium and zinc. Selenium is an essential dietary trace element; its concentration in various foods, such as fruits and vegetables, is dependent on the soil content of selenium in the region where these foodstuffs are grown (Ferguson et al. 2004). Selenium appears to exert its cancer chemopreventive effects through induction of cell cycle arrest and apoptosis and reduction of angiogenesis (Jiang et al. 2000). Selenium compounds have been shown to alter the expression and/or activities of a number of cell cycle regulatory proteins, signaling molecules, proteases, mitochondrial associated factors, transcription factors, tumor suppressor genes, polyamines, and glutathione levels (Sinha and El-Bayoumy 2004; Krishnan et al. 2003). Selenium compounds have also been shown to decrease PSA expression by inducing protein degradation and suppressing androgen-stimulated gene transcription (Cho et al. 2004). Combination studies with selenium and vitamin E have shown decreased prostate cancer cell proliferation *via* distinct mechanistic pathways (Siler et al. 2004; Venkateswaran 2004). As a constituent of selenoproteins, selenium has several structural and enzymatic roles (Soriano-Garcia 2004). A number of natural and synthetic organoselenium compounds have been examined as chemopreventive agents in several animal tumor bioassay systems. Selenium in the form of sodium selenite or selenomethionine functions as an essential micronutrient at levels of about 0.1 ppm in the animal diet and acts as a chemopreventive agent at 3–5 ppm and is toxic at levels higher than 5 ppm (Sinha and El-Bayoumy 2004). Most of the selenium chemoprevention studies have used sodium selenite, selenomethionine, or methylseleninic acid as a test agent. Epidemiological studies, preclinical investigations and clinical intervention trials support the role of selenium compounds as potent chemopreventive agents for prostate cancer (Sinha and El-Bayoumy 2004). A randomized trial on selenium supplementation from the National Prevention of Cancer Study in 974 men with 200 μg/day doses of selenium in 0.5 g high-selenium yeast demonstrated a 63% reduction in the incidence of prostate cancer (Clark et al. 1998). However, no significant associations were observed between baseline serum α-tocopherol, dietary vitamin E, or selenium and prostate cancer in the ATBC trial, a randomized, double-blind, placebo-controlled, primary prevention study of lung cancer, upon secondary analysis (Hartman et al. 1998). The compelling findings in the ATBC trial prompted the establishment of a large prospective study, the SELECT trial for prostate cancer chemoprevention (Lippman et al. 2005). The SELECT clinical trial with selenium (200 μg/day from L-selenomethionine) and vitamin E (400 IU/day of all-rac-α- tocopheryl acetate) on 32,400 American men has shown no effects on prostate cancer (Dunn et al. 2010). A 6 month placebo-controlled double-blind clinical trial conducted in 37 men with a combination of silymarin and selenium in radical prostatectomy patients demonstrated that the combination of silymarin and selenium significantly reduced LDL and total cholesterol in the blood of men after surgery, suggesting this may be effective in reducing prostate cancer progression (Vidlar et al. 2010).

Zinc is another essential trace element known to possess antioxidant properties and is present in high concentrations in the prostate (Powell 2011). In cell culture systems, zinc has been shown to inhibit prostate cancer cell growth *via* inhibition of cell cycle and induction of apoptosis through disruption of mitochondrial function (Liang et al. 1999b). Comprehensive prostate needle-biopsy study suggested that the amount of zinc depletion could be used as a measure of the Gleason score of the tumor (Cortesi et al. 2008). Local zinc concentration mapping has the potential to improve patient selection for biopsy, biopsy site selection and local therapy such as cryotherapy and brachytherapy (Cortesi et al. 2008).

Experimental studies suggest that boron may prevent prostate cancer (Gonzalez et al. 2007). A study demonstrated that exposure to pharmacologically-relevant levels of boric acid to human prostate cancer DU145 induces morphological changes consistent with increase in granularity and intracellular vesicle content, enhanced cell spreading and decrease cell volume. Boric acid treatment resulted in increase in β-galactosidase activity suggesting conversion of cancer cells to a senescent-like cellular phenotype. Boric acid also causes a dose-dependent reduction in cyclins

A–E, as well as MAPK proteins, suggesting their contribution to proliferative inhibition. Cells treated with boric acid display reduced adhesion, migration and invasion potential, along with F-actin changes indicative of reduced metastatic potential (Barranco and Eckhert 2006). However, a community based Turkish study in men living and being employed at boron mines in villages with rich boron minerals suggested that exposure to boron might have an implication within the prostatic cellular processes related to hyperplasia and carcinogenesis, even did not find a statistically significant association between prostate cancer and boron exposure (Müezzinoğlu et al. 2002). Further case-control studies are required to substantiate these findings.

5.5 Flavonoids

Flavonoids are polyphenolic compounds that are ubiquitously present in foods of plant origin (Williams and Grayer 2004). The flavonoid family includes about 5,000 compounds that are defined chemically as substances composed of a common phenylchromanone structure (C6–C3–C6), with one or more hydroxyl substituents (Williams and Grayer 2004; Cuyckens and Claeys 2004; Ross and Kasum 2002). These are mainly classified into flavones, flavanols (catechins), isoflavones, flavonols, flavanones, and anthocyanins (Cuyckens and Claeys 2004; Ross and Kasum 2002). The dietary flavonoids possess antioxidant, anti-inflammatory, and possibly anti-carcinogenic properties and are receiving increasing attention (Robak and Gryglewski 1996). The plant flavonoids whose roles in prostate carcinogenesis have been studied are soy isoflavones, catechins from green and black tea, silymarin from milk thistle, resveratrol, apigenin, and proanthocynadins from grape seed, anthocynanins and anthocynadins from various pigmented fruits and vegetables and constituents of pomegranate fruit (Ross and Kasum 2002).

Soy isoflavones have been identified as dietary components that may play an important role in reducing the incidence of prostate cancer (Moyad 1999). The major soy isoflavones include genistein and daidzein. Genistein, the predominant isoflavone found in soy, has been shown to reduce proliferation of prostate cancer cells (Santibanez et al. 1997). The anti-proliferative effects of genistein are attributed to the modulation of genes related to control of cell cycle and apoptosis (Santibanez et al. 1997; Davis et al. 1998). The pathways through which genistein exerts its antiproliferative effects include inhibition of tyrosine kinase, proteasome activity, angiogenesis, metastasis, PI3K/Akt and NF-κB survival signaling pathways, and induction of glutathione peroxidase in human prostate cancer cells (Li and Sarkar 2002a & b). Genistein is also recognized as a phytoestrogen, which targets estrogen- and androgen-mediated signaling pathways in prostate carcinogenesis (Bektic et al. 2004). Administration of a genistein-rich diet to mice has been shown to correlate positively with changes in prostate DNA methylation at CpG islands (Day et al. 2002). This study demonstrates that epigenetic alterations may influence prostate cancer risk. Recent studies have shown that dietary genistein feeding improves survival and reduces expression of osteopontin, which may delay progression of prostate cancer from benign to malignant tumors in a transgenic adenocarcinoma of the mouse prostate (TRAMP) model (Mentor-Marcel et al. 2005). Further studies have shown that dietary genistein feeding inhibits bone metastasis in SCID mice by regulating metastasis-related genes (Li et al. 2004).

Epidemiological and case-control studies are supportive of a chemopreventive action for these compounds; however, clinical studies with soy isoflavones have not been encouraging (Fischer et al. 2004). Various soy isoflavone supplementation regimens in prostate cancer patients have shown no statistically significant changes in serum PSA levels (deVere White et al. 2004). A randomized controlled trial demonstrated that soy isoflavone did not modulate PSA concentration in men between 50 and 80 years of age (Adams et al. 2004). Recently, a double-blind, placebo controlled, randomized clinical trial was conducted in 53 men with prostate cancer enrolled in an active surveillance program, treatment groups were supplement the diet containing 450 mg genistein, 300 mg daidzein, and other isoflavones daily for 6 months. The PSA concentration did not change after 6 months (deVere White et al. 2010). Another pilot study conducted with soy isoflavone supplementation on acute and subacute toxicity ($\leq$6 mo) of external beam radiation therapy in patients with localized prostate cancer. Forty-two patients with prostate cancer were randomly assigned to receive 200 mg soy isoflavone or placebo daily for 6 months beginning with the first day of radiation therapy, which was administered in 1.8–2.5 Gray fractions for a total of 73.8–77.5 Gray. At each time point, urinary, bowel, and sexual adverse symptoms induced by radiation therapy were decreased in the soy isoflavone group compared to placebo group. The results suggested that soy isoflavones taken in conjunction with radiation therapy could reduce the urinary, intestinal, and sexual adverse effects in patients with prostate cancer (Ahmad et al. 2010). Another randomized, double-blind, placebo-controlled was conducted in 33 men undergone androgen deprivation therapy for prostate cancer. Participants were randomly assigned to receive 20 g of soy protein containing 160 mg of total isoflavones versus taste-matched placebo (20 g whole milk protein) for 12 weeks. The results demonstrate that isoflavones did not improve metabolic or inflammatory parameters in androgen-deprived men (Napora et al. 2011). Another double-blind randomized clinical trial was conducted in 85 participants who received combined supplement containing isoflavones and curcumin or placebo daily. Subjects were subdivided by the cut-off of their baseline PSA value at 10 μg/mL. PSA levels decreased in the patients group with PSA less than or equal to 10 μg/mL treated with supplement containing isoflavones and curcumin (Ide et al. 1994). It is possible that soy isoflavones may be more beneficial in preventing prostate cancer when used in combination with other agents. Additional studies are needed to ascertain these findings.

Tea, the most widely consumed beverage in the world, has shown to possess strong antioxidant potential (148). The major catechins present in green tea are (–)-epicatechin, (–)-epicatechin-3-gallate, (–)-epigallocatechin, and (–)-epigallocatechin-3-gallate. Epigallocatechin-3-gallate accounts for approximately 40% of the total polyphenolic mixture in green tea (Saleem et al. 2003). The major constituents of black tea are theaflavins and thearubigins (Saleem et al. 2003; Frei et al.

2003). Epidemiological studies show that, in Asian countries, where tea is very popular, the incidence of all types of cancer, including prostate cancer, is low compared with that in the West (Gupta et al. 2002b). The Japanese and Chinese people, who regularly consume green tea, have the lowest prostate cancer incidence in the world (Gupta et al. 1999 and references therein). Consequently, researchers have developed considerable interest in tea, and especially in green tea polyphenols (GTPs), as a cancer chemopreventive agent. Tea catechins have been shown to modulate a number of cellular signaling pathways that have relevance to prostate cancer (Klein and Fischer 2002; Adhami et al. 2003; Siddiqui et al. 2004; Gupta et al. 2004; Nam et al. 2001). These include proteins related to cell cycle progression, inflammation, angiogenesis, metastasis, tyrosine kinases, PI3K/Akt and NF-κB survival signaling pathways, AR, 5-α reductase, protein kinase C, proteasome inhibition, and apoptosis (Adhami et al. 2003; Siddiqui et al. 2004; Gupta et al. 2004; Nam et al. 2001). We and others have demonstrated that GTPs inhibit DNA methyltransferase and have potential to reactivate methylation-silenced genes in prostate cancer cells (Fang et al. 2003). Recent study with LNCaP cells as well as clinically localized prostate cancer patients represented that prostate cancer cells when incubated with EGCG were able to methylate EGCG to 4"- MeEGCG. Further treatment of LNCaP cells with 4"- MeEGCG resulted in less effective to inhibit proliferation and induce apoptosis compared with EGCG (Wang et al. 2010). Further studies on the TRAMP model have shown that oral infusion of GTPs in drinking water for 24 weeks resulted in approximately 44% reduction in tumor volume and 70% increase in overall survival compared with the control group, which did not receive GTP (Gupta et al. 2001b). More recent studies employing a similar protocol for GTP infusion to TRAMP mice have shown significant reduction in IGF-1 levels with concomitant increase in IGFBP-3 expression in dorsolateral prostate of these mice (Adhami et al. 2004). In addition, GTP infusion has been reported to inhibit protein expression of the S100A4 gene (Mts1) and restored the expression of E-cadherin in TRAMP mice (Saleem et al. 2005). These studies indicate that GTPs may prove useful as chemopreventive agents for prostate cancer. Epidemiological and case-control studies have further supported the chemopreventive properties of green tea; however, clinical studies with green tea have not been encouraging (Jian et al. 2004; Jatoi et al. 2003). A phase II study, in which 6 g/day of tea was administered to 42 patients with asymptomatic, androgen-independent prostate cancer, demonstrated that a single patient achieved a PSA response of >50% that lasted for approximately 1 month (Jatoi et al. 2003). These patients suffered with side effects that include diarrhea, nausea, and fatigue. Another recent clinical study used a 250 mg dose of GTPs twice daily. In this study, 6 of 19 patients had disease control for 3–5 month and only 1 patient whose PSA rise was affected by green tea supplementation. The dose used in this study did not discernibly alter the course of hormone-refractory prostate cancer (Choan et al. 2005). These results suggest that green tea possesses minimal anti-neoplastic activity against advanced-stage prostate cancer. In a clinical case-control trial, Bettuzzi et al. (2006) showed a reduced incidence of prostate cancer in men with prostatic intraepithelial neoplasia after a 1 year green tea supplement intervention compared with a group of men receiving placebo. Likewise, in a single-arm pre-prostatectomy trial of a green tea supplement, McLarty et al. (McLarty et al. 2009) showed a decrease in serum prostate–specific antigen levels, and decreased prostate tissue vascular endothelial growth factor and hepatocyte growth factor concentrations. Well-designed clinical studies are further required to test the validity of GTPs in prevention-based trials.

Resveratrol, a dietary stilbene, is another plant product derivative that has been proposed as a chemopreventive agent based on safety and efficacy studies in cell culture and animal models (Jang et al. 1997). Resveratrol has been shown to possess strong anti-inflammatory, antioxidant, and anticancer properties (Aziz et al. 2003). Resveratrol has shown growth-inhibitory effects on both androgen-sensitive and -insensitive human prostate cancer cells; its effects are mediated through inhibition of the cell cycle and induction of apoptosis (Hsieh and Wu 1999). Interactive gene expression patterns in prostate cancer LNCaP cells exposed to resveratrol have shown alterations in multiple signaling pathways that include p53-responsive genes, the PPAR family, tyrosine kinase family members, Rel/NF-κB family members, heat-shock proteins, cell cycle regulatory genes, and apoptosis-related genes (Narayanan et al. 2003; Narayanan et al. 2002; Shih et al. 2004; Cardile et al. 2003). Resveratrol has also been shown to modulate AR function and inhibits PSA expression in prostate cancer cells (Hsieh and Wu 2000). Based on cell culture studies, further evaluation of resveratrol as a chemopreventive agent in preclinical models of prostate cancer may be warranted.

Silymarin is a plant flavonoid that has been shown to possess exceptionally high anti-inflammatory, antioxidant, and anti-carcinogenic properties (Singh and Agarwal 2002). The major active constituent of silymarin is silibinin; other minor constituents include dehydrosilibinin, silychristin, and silydianin (Chlopcikova et al. 2004). Silymarin and silibinin have shown remarkable anti-proliferative effects on both androgen -responsive and -refractory human prostate cancer cells (Zhu et al. 2001; Zi and Agarwal 1999). The underlying mechanisms of silibinin activity against prostate cancer involve alterations in cell cycle progression and inhibition of mitogenic and cell survival signaling, including modulation of epidermal growth factor receptor, IGF-1, and NF-κB signaling (Singh and Agarwal 2004). Silibinin has been shown to modulate AR function and to inhibit telomerase activity and PSA expression in prostate cancer cells (Singh and Agarwal 2004). Silibinin has been shown to inhibit prostate cancer progression through reduced secretion of pro-angiogenic factors from prostate cancer cells (Thelen et al. 2004). Silibinin has also been shown to synergize the therapeutic effects of doxorubicin in prostate cancer cells and to sensitize it to TNFα-induced apoptosis (Tyagi et al. 2002). Translational studies with silibinin on preclinical models of prostate cancer have demonstrated similar results with reduced tumor proliferation, induction of IGFBP-3 and apoptosis, and inhibition of angiogenesis (Singh et al. 2003). In a recent clinical study, of 12 patients scheduled for radical prostatectomy for cancer, six patients received 13 g of silybin-phytosome daily per-operatively, and 6 patients served as control subjects. There were no significant detectable differences in baseline and post-treatment blood levels of IGF-I and IGFBP-3 (Flaig et al. 2010). These findings raise concern about the bioavailability of silibinin and its constituents in the prostate tissue.

Proanthocyanidins and procynadins are flavonoids that are found in high concentrations in grape seed extract, a popular dietary supplement (Shi et al. 2003). Grape seed extract has been shown to possess significant anti-inflammatory, antioxidant, antiviral, and anti-carcinogenic properties (Zhao et al. 1999). Grape seed extract has been shown to induce apoptosis in prostate cancer cells through activation of caspases and disruption of mitochondrial function (Agarwal et al. 2002). The pathways involved in the chemopreventive activity of grape seed extract on prostate cancer include inhibition of protein tyrosine kinase, matrix metalloproteinases, and Rel/NF-κB family members (Dhanalakshmi et al. 2003; Agarwal et al. 2004). Grape seed extract has recently been shown to inhibit prostate tumor growth and angiogenesis through up-regulation of IGFBP-3 in an athymic nude mouse model (Singh et al. 2004a). More mechanistic studies on cell cultures and in vivo models of prostate cancer are required to assess the possible efficacy of grape seed extract as a chemopreventive agent for prostate cancer.

Apigenin, a widely distributed plant flavonoid abundantly present in fruits and vegetables, is a free-radical scavenger that has been shown to possess anti-inflammatory and anti-carcinogenic effects (O'Prey et al. 2003). Studies have shown that apigenin possesses growth-inhibitory properties against many types of human cancer cells, including prostate cancer (Yin et al. 2001; Gupta et al. 2001a). We have shown that apigenin causes tumor cell growth inhibition cell cycle deregulation and apoptosis in both androgen- sensitive and -insensitive human prostate cancer cells without affecting normal cells (Shukla and Gupta 2004a: Lee et al. 1998). The molecular mechanisms underlying the activities of apigenin include inactivation of tyrosine phosphorylation, inhibition of 17β- hydroxysteroid oxidoreductase, inhibition of AR function, modulation in cell cycle regulatory proteins, disruption of mitochondrial function, and NF-κB inhibition in prostate cancer cells (Lee et al. 1998; Makela et al. 1998; Gupta et al. 2002a). We have shown that apigenin is capable of sensitizing human prostate cancer PC-3 cells to TNFα-induced apoptosis, which correlates with down-regulation of genes relevant for prostate cancer progression (Shukla and Gupta 2004b). Further studies in in vivo TRAMP model have shown that oral intake of apigenin significantly decreased tumor volumes of the prostate, completely abolished distant-site metastases and significantly improved animal overall survival. Furthermore, apigenin resulted in increased levels of E-cadherin with decreased levels of nuclear beta-catenin, c-Myc, and cyclin D1 in the dorsolateral prostates of TRAMP mice (Shukla et al. 2007). Another study with athymic nude mice 22Rv-1 cells tumor xenograft exhibited inhibited tumor growth after apigenin feeding, which was associated with increased accumulation of human IGFBP-3 in mouse serum as well as in xenograft, simultaneous decreased serum IGF-I levels resulting in induction of apoptosis in tumor xenograft (Shukla et al. 2005). Additional mechanistic cell culture studies and in vivo studies with apigenin are required, targeting other signaling pathways that have relevance to prostate cancer development and progression.

Pomegranate has antioxidant, anti-diabetic and anti-atherosclerotic properties. Effects of pomegranate have been extensively studied in prostate cancer cell culture system, animal models, and in a phase II clinical trial in humans. Pomegranate was tested in various forms such as oils, fermented juice polyphenols, and pericarp polyphenols, on human prostate cancer cell growth both in vitro and in vivo (Adhami et al. 2009). In every form it was effective in inhibiting the growth of various human prostate cancer cells, without affecting normal prostate epithelial cells (Khan et al. 2007). Pre-clinical studies with prostate cancer PC-3 cells exhibited inhibited proliferation, induction of apoptosis, which was confirmed by inhibition of tumor growth in athymic nude mice xenograft studies (Khan et al. 2010). Reports suggest the anti-proliferative and pro-apoptotic properties of pomegranate fruit extract (PFE) against human prostate cancer PC-3 cells and CWR22Rν1 in dose-response manner. The induction of apoptosis and cell cycle arrest was associated with upregulation of Bax and Bak and downregulation of Bcl-XL and Bcl-2 (Khan et al. 2010). The reduction in PSA levels was observed in CWR22Rν1 xenograft model which suggested that PFE may have clinical relevance (Adhami et al. 2009). Pomegranate polyphenols inhibited gene expressions, HSD3B2 (3 beta-hydroxysteroid dehydrogenase type 2), AKR1C3 (aldo-keto reductase family 1 member C3) and SRD5A1 (steroid 5alpha reductase type 1) and most consistently AR in the LNCaP-AR cells where androgen receptor was over-expressed (Hong et al. 2008).

Pomgranate extract inhibited NF-κB activity and cell viability of prostate cancer cell lines LAPC4 in a dose-dependent fashion (Rettig et al. 2008). In a phase II clinical trial, Pantuck et al. (2006) recruited patients with rising PSA and provided them 8 ounces of pomegranate juice daily until disease progression. PSA doubling time significantly increased with treatment from a mean of 15 months at baseline to 54 months post-treatment. A major drawback of this study was the absence of a proper placebo control; however, statistically significant prolongation of PSA doubling time suggested a potential role for pomegranate in prostate cancer prevention (Pantuck et al. 2006). Punicic acid, an important fatty acid in pomegranate seeds (70–80% content), was evaluated for its ability to induce intrinsic apoptosis *via* a caspase-dependent pathway and exhibited potent growth inhibitory activities in human prostate cancer LNCaP cells. Further stuies of the constituents of pomegranate appear to be warranted.

Delphinidin, an anthocyanidin, present in many pigmented fruits and vegetables, possesses antioxidant, anti-inflammatory, and anti-angiogenic properties. It has been shown to alter phosphorylation of IκB kinase gamma (NEMO), phosphorylation of NF-κB inhibitory protein and NF-κB/p65 nuclear translocation and its DNA binding activity in a dose-dependent fashion in various prostate cancer cell lines (Soobrattee et al. 2006), suggesting that further studies are warranted.

5.6 Indoles

A diet rich in fruits and vegetables provides a rich source of indoles, which may be responsible for prevention of many types of cancer (Greenwald et al. 2001; Sarkar et al. 2004). Indoles are naturally occurring constituents of Brassica vegetables.

Cruciferous vegetables contain glucobrassicin, which during metabolism yields indole-3-carbinol (I3C) and its in vivo dimeric product 3,3′-diindolylmethane (DIM). These derivatives have been shown to inhibit cell proliferation and induce apoptosis in prostate cancer cells (Nachshon-Kedmi et al. 2003). The mechanisms through which indoles exert their anti-carcinogenic effects include modulations in cell cycle regulatory proteins and inhibition of cell survival pathways (PI3K/Akt) and NF-κB transcription factor (Howells et al. 2002). Gene expression profiles have demonstrated that I3C and DIM affect the expression of a large number of genes that have relevance to cancer, cell survival, and physiological behavior (Li et al. 2003). Recently, DIM alone or in combination with Taxotere, decreased survivin expression as well as androgen receptor and NF-κB DNA-binding activity in LNCaP and C4-2B prostate cancer cells (Rahman et al. 2009). Further, it has been shown that indoles are strong androgen antagonists and that they inhibit PSA production in human prostate cancer cells (Zhang et al. 2003). These findings suggest that dietary indoles may prove useful in the chemoprevention of prostate cancer. Therapeutic studies with plant indoles were performed on preclinical prostate cancer models. DIM fed to TRAMP mice demonstrated inhibition in prostate carcinogenesis. DIM feeding reduced the expression of cyclin A, cyclin-dependent kinase (CDK)2, CDK4, and Bcl-xL, and increased p27 and Bax expression. These results indicated that DIM inhibited prostate carcinogenesis via induction of apoptosis and inhibition of cell cycle progression (Cho et al. 2011). Studies with DIM on C57BL/6 mice injected with TRAMP C2 cells inhibit tumor growth and significantly reduced tumor development in treated animals, compared with untreated controls (Fares et al. 2010; Nachshon-Kedmi et al. 2004). Systemic administration of I3C to Copenhagen rats injected with MAT-LyLu cells has been shown to inhibit prostate tumor growth and metastasis (Garikapaty et al. 2005). More mechanistic in vivo studies are required to assess the potential of indoles in this capacity.

5.7 Isothiocyanates

There is evidence to suggest that thiol conjugates of isothiocyanates present in cruciferous vegetables are effective cancer preventive agents (Chiao et al. 2000). At least two population-based, case-controlled studies have documented reduced risk of prostate cancer in men consuming cruciferous vegetables (Kolonel et al. 2000; Cohen et al. 2000). These salutary effects have been attributed to 2-phenylethyl isothiocyanate, allyl isothiocyanate, and sulforaphane (Wang et al. 2004). These agents exert their anti-carcinogenic activities in cell culture system through mechanisms that include cell cycle inhibition, induction of phase II enzymes, inhibition of extracellular signal-regulated kinases, suppression of NF-κB and its regulated genes, proteasome degradation, caspase activation, and induction of apoptosis (Brooks et al. 2001; Kong et al. 2001; Singh et al. 2004b, c; Xu et al. 2005). Phenylethyl isothiocyanate (PEITC) and allyl isothiocyanate have been shown to inhibit the growth of human prostate cancer PC-3 xenografts through cell cycle perturbation and induction of apoptosis (Singh et al. 2004b). Growth suppression and apoptosis induction was observed in tumor xenografts (PC-3 cells) upon oral administration of PEITC in male athymic mice. Growth factor adapter protein p66 (Shc) was indispensable for PEITC-induced apoptosis which increased in the level of Ser (36)-phosphorylated p66 (Shc) (Xiao and Singh 2010). PEITC significantly inhibited DU145 cell proliferation as well as inhibited both constitutive and IL-6-induced STAT3 activity. IL-6-stimulated phosphorylation of JAK2, an STAT3 upstream kinase, was also attenuated by PEITC (Gong et al. 2009). Further studies with PEITC in TRAMP-derived cells (TRAMP-C1 and TRAMP-C2) demonstrated apoptosis which was associated with a marked increase in the level of proapoptotic protein Bak and/or a decrease in the levels of anti-apoptotic protein Mcl-1 or Bcl-xL and disruption of mitochondrial membrane potential (Xiao et al. 2005).

Epidemiological studies from volunteers were randomly assigned to either a broccoli-rich or a pea-rich diet. After 6 months a significant differences was observed between GSTM1 genotypes on the broccoli-rich diet, associated with transforming growth factor beta 1 (TGFβ1) and epidermal growth factor (EGF) signalling pathways. Sulforaphane (the isothiocyanate derived from 4-methylsuphinylbutyl glucosinolate that accumulates in broccoli) chemically interacts with TGFβ1, EGF and insulin peptides to form thioureas, and enhances TGFβ1/Smad-mediated transcription (Traka et al. 2008). Recent studies with d,l-sulforaphane-treated TRAMP mice exhibited approximately 50% and 63% decrease, in pulmonary metastasis incidence and multiplicity compared with control mice respectively. Additionally, SFN administration enhanced cytotoxicity of co-cultures of natural killer (NK) cells and dendritic cells (DC) against TRAMP-C1 target cells, which correlated with infiltration of T cells in the neoplastic lesions and increased levels of interleukin-12 production by the dendritic cells. This study suggested that sulforaphane administration inhibited prostate cancer progression and pulmonary metastasis by reducing cell proliferation and augmenting NK cell lytic activity in TRAMP mice. More detailed mechanistic studies are required to assess the potential of isothiocyanates in the chemoprevention of prostate cancer.

5.8 Phenolic Acids

Phenolic acids are aromatic secondary plant metabolites, widely present throughout the plant kingdom (Robbins 2003). Phenolic acids are well recognized for their antioxidant potential (Lopez-Velez et al. 2003). Curcumin, a phenolic acid and active component of turmeric, has received a great deal of attention as a possible chemopreventive agent against prostate cancer (Lopez-Velez et al. 2003). Curcumin has been shown to inhibit proliferation of both androgen-sensitive and -insensitive human prostate carcinoma cells via inhibition of the cell cycle and induction of apoptosis (Mukhopadhyay et al. 2002). Recently, curcumin has represented to affect wingless (Wnt)/β-catenin signaling pathway in androgen dependent prostate cancer cells (Teiten et al. 2011; Choi et al. 2010). Other studies explored that curcumin inhibited the phosphorylation of mTOR in DU145 (Beevers et al. 2006) and PC-3 (Li et al. 2007) and also activates the PP2A serine/threonine protein phosphatase and subsequently inhibits the phosphorylation of Akt/PKB, mTOR (Yu et al. 2008). Diets containing 2% curcumin provided to LNCaP tumor xenograft in nude mice for 6 week have shown to induce apoptosis and inhibited proliferation and angiogenesis (Dorai et al. 2001). The molecular pathways that contribute to its anti-carcinogenic activity include tyrosine kinase and protein kinase C inhibition, down-regulation of AR gene expression, inhibition of PI3K/Akt and NF-κB, and modulation of the motility of prostate cancer cells through effects on their microfilament organization (Mukhopadhyay et al. 2002; Gopalakrishna and Gundimeda 2002; Nakamura et al. 2002; Kumar et al. 2003). Curcumin has been shown to enhance tumor necrosis factor-related apoptosis-inducing ligand (TRAIL)–induced apoptosis; it also radiosensitizes prostate carcinoma cells (Sah et al. 2003). Curcumin in combination with radiation showed significant enhancement to radiation-induced clonogenic inhibition and apoptosis in PC-3 cells (Chendil et al. 2004). Eighty-five participants randomized double-blind study of isoflavones and curcumin represented the production of PSA were markedly decreased by the combined treatment (Ide et al. 1994). These findings suggest that curcumin may have some potential as a chemopreventive agent for prostate cancer, and deserves additional study.

5.9 Organosulfur Compounds

Organosulfur compounds are the biologically active components of allium vegetables (Sigounas et al. 1997). The primary sulfur containing constituents in garlic are the gamma-glutamyl-*S*-alk(en)yl-L-cysteines and *S*-alk(en)yl-L-cysteine; the odor of garlic is attributable to allicin and other oil-soluble sulfur components (Amagase et al. 2001; Herman-Antosiewicz and Singh 2004). Once garlic undergoes cutting or crushing, hundreds of organosulfur compounds are released in a short period of time. The transiently formed compound, allicin, comprises 70–80% of the thiosulfinates and quickly decomposes to other compounds, such as diallyl sulfide, diallyl disulfide, diallyl trisulfide, dithiine, and ajoene (Amagase et al. 2001). Many health benefits have been ascribed to organosulfur compounds including inhibition of carcinogenesis. Two studies have shown that *S*-allylmercaptocysteine inhibits prostate cancer cell proliferation (Pinto et al. 2000). Other studies demonstrated that *S*-allylmercaptocysteine suppressed invasion and cell motility in androgen-independent prostate cancer cells via the up-regulation of cell-adhesion molecule E-cadherin (Howard et al. 2007). Diallyl disulfide also inhibited the cell proliferation of prostate cancer PC-3 cells (Arunkumar et al. 2006). Recent studies with diallyl trisulfide (DATS) in prostate cancer cells (LNCaP, C4-2, and TRAMP-C1) suggested that a concentration-dependent decrease in protein level of AR, which was accompanied by suppression of intracellular and secreted levels of PSA. Further DATS treatment inhibited synthetic androgen (R1881)-stimulated nuclear translocation of AR in LNCaP/C4-2 cells and proliferation of LNCaP cells.

Oral administration of DATS (2 mg/day) (three times per week for 13 weeks) markedly suppressed AR protein level in poorly differentiated prostate cancer in TRAMP mice (Stan and Singh 2009). More studies of the potential of organosulfur compounds in prostate cancer chemoprevention appear to be warranted.

5.10 Terpenes

Terpenoids are the most diverse group of plant constituents that play a variety of roles in many different plant species. All terpenes are constructed from isoprenoid units by biochemically unusual pathways involving highly reactive intermediates. They mostly occur as monoterpenoids (essential oils), diterpenoids, triterpenoids, sesquiterpenoids (phytosterols, saponins), and tetraterpenoid carotenoids. All are related by being derived from a common isopentenyl precursor (Zwenger and Basu 2008).

Monoterpenes are oils found in many plants including members of the citrus family. Monoterpenes are commonly used as flavoring agents and food additives and in various fragrances (Grayson 1994). Monoterpenes, especially D-limonene and perillyl alcohol, are recognized as chemopreventive agents through their demonstrated ability to induce phase II carcinogen-metabolizing enzymes, inhibit posttranslational isoprenylation of small G-proteins including *Ras* oncogene, and induce apoptosis in cancer cells (Crowell 1999; Karlson et al. 1996). Only limited efficacy of perillyl alcohol has been observed in clinical studies of patients with advanced prostate cancer (Liu et al. 2003). Other studies have shown that monoterpenes are more effective when used in combination with chemotherapeutic agents (Broitman et al. 1996). Genipin induced apoptosis was observed in PC3 cells which was mediated via activation of ROS-dependent MLK3 (mixed lineage kinase 3), and downstream activation of JNK (Hong and Kim 2007). Another terpene, cannabinoid R+ methanandamide (MET) regulates ceramide metabolism in prostate PC3 cells which resulted in cell death (Olea-Herrero et al. 2009). Treatment of menthol in PC-3 cells resulted in increased c-jun N-terminal kinase (JNK) phosphorylation and cell deaths in supramillimolar concentrations (Kim et al. 2009). It has also been suggested that monoterpenes are capable of radiosensitizing prostate cancer cells (Rajesh and Howard 2003).

Betulinic acid is a pentacyclic triterpene isolated from the stem bark of *Betulin alba,* and the studies show that betulinic acid decreases the expression of VEGF and anti-apoptotic protein survivin in both prostate LNCaP cells and tumors (Chintharlapalli et al. 2007). Betulinic acid exposure to PC-3 cells inhibited DNA binding and reduced nuclear levels of the NF-κB and this reduced expression is due to decreased IKK activity and phosphorylation of IκBα at serine 32/36 followed by its degradation (Rabi et al. 2008).

Ursolic acid is another naturally occurring triterpenoid demonstrated to possess anticancer activity on human prostate cancer cells PC-3 and LNCaP by down-regulation of bcl-2 protein *via* inducing apoptosis. Ursolic acid treatment induced apoptosis in PC-3 cells through activation of c-Jun N-terminal kinase followed by bcl-2 phosphorylation and activation of caspase-9 (Zhang et al. 2010). Additional studies of the potential usefulness of terpenes in the management of prostate cancer are needed.

5.11 Other Potential Nutraceuticals

Several nutraceuticals have been studied in prostate cancer since the year 1994, at which time the Dietary Supplements Health and Education Act opened the market to many herbals, botanicals, and other food ingredients that would have otherwise needed safety testing before being sold; these agents are being used with increasing frequency in men with prostate cancer (Wilkinson and Chodak 2003). Little is known about the efficacy of such agents in cancer. There are limited prospective data supporting the preventive or therapeutic value of such nutraceuticals in prostate cancer.

To date, one of the most studied herbal agents for prostate cancer is PC-SPES (Meyer and Gillatt 2002). PC-SPES is a mixture composed of extracts from eight herbs: *Scutellaria baicalensis*, *Glycyrrhiza glabra*, *Ganoderma lucidium*, *Isatis indigotica*, *Panax pseudo-ginseng*, *Serenoa repens*, *Dendrantherma morifolium*, and *Rabdosia rubescens* (Meyer and Gillatt 2002; Yip et al. 2003). All of these are Chinese herbs except *S. repens*, an extract of the American dwarf palm or saw palmetto. A proprietary herbal blend, PC-SPES has been used since 1996 by thousands of men for 'prostate health' (de la Taille 2001). The clinical effects of PC-SPES appear to be more pronounced in advanced-stage prostate cancer. Additional testing became necessary to identify the active components of PC-SPES and to define its role in the management of patients with prostate cancer. However, these studies identified several synthetic compounds that were present in varying doses in different batches of PC-SPES, including DES, the synthetic estrogens; ethinyl estradiol; warfarin, an anticoagulant; and indomethacin, an anti-inflammatory agent. The presence of these drugs prompted the California Department of Health Services and, subsequently, the Food and Drug Administration to issue warnings describing the adulteration of PC-SPES. The product was recalled, production was subsequently stopped, and studies supported by NCCAM were halted. This incident raised important concern about clinical trials utilizing herbal therapies that must account for issues of purity and consistency (Oh et al. 2004).

Permixon® is another nutraceutical that is an extract from American dwarf palm fruit. *S. repens* is an effective dual inhibitor of 5α-reductase isoenzyme activity in human prostate cancer cells without interfering with PSA expression (Habib et al. 2005). A clinical trial for symptomatic benign prostatic hyperplasia demonstrated significant improvement in peak flow rate and reduction in nocturia, and a five-point reduction in International Prostate Symptom Score in treated patients compared to the outcomes in untreated control subjects (Al-Shukri et al. 2000).

Equiguard is a composite supplement consisting of standardized extracts from nine Chinese herbs, originally formulated to correct physiological decline in kidney functions associated with age. It was fortuitously found to display anti-prostate cancer properties. Ethanol extracts of Equiguard significantly inhibited prostate cancer LNCaP cell growth, induced apoptosis, lowered expression of the AR, decreased intracellular and secreted PSA levels, and completely abolished the colony-forming activities in these cells (Lu et al. 2003).

The number and variety of nutraceuticals on the market are steadily increasing, and now include such entities zyflamend, fish oil and omega-3 fatty acid, Ultraprostate®, flaxseed, pumpkin seed and others need definitive evidence for their preventive or anti-proliferative effects in prostate cancer.

5.12 The Future of Nutraceuticals in Prostate Cancer

Increasing knowledge and awareness of issue related to wellness and health have prompted some individuals to lead presumably healthier lifestyles by exercising more, and consuming a healthy nutritional diet. It is a widely held view that prostate cancer is a preventable disease, since it has a long latency period during which nutraceutical supplementation may provide beneficial effects by delaying or eliminating the onset of clinically relevant prostate cancer. Consequently, the nutraceutical industry has evolved into a highly lucrative market. This may be viewed as both good as well as bad. Although nutraceuticals appear to hold significant promises for the management of prostate cancer, there is an urgent need to move the field forward. Healthcare professional, nutritionists and regulatory toxicologist must strategically work together to plan appropriate regulations to maximize health and therapeutic benefits. *Firstly*, continued efforts are needed to unravel the underlying molecular events through which nutraceuticals may exert their antioxidants and anti-carcinogenic effects. Identification of disease subtypes based on etiological mechanisms may also help to formulate better nutraceutical approaches for individual patients with specific disease susceptibilities. *Secondly*, novel nutraceuticals strategies should be designed that could limit both exposure and adverse health effects from dietary carcinogens and attenuate the incidence of prostate tumorigenesis. *Thirdly*, long-term clinical studies are required to scientifically validate the nutraceuticals in various disease conditions. *Fourthly*, pharmacokinetics and mechanism-based biomarker approaches should be taken to evaluate the efficacy of promising nutraceutical agents. The development of ‘combinations of nutraceuticals’ to study the synergistic effects of interactions between agents will be helpful in explaining epidemiological observations investigating prostate cancer risk and in assessing the interactions between nutraceuticals with food and other drugs.

5.13 Conclusions

Research on nutraceutical research is complex, and it takes huge efforts to consolidate information from cohort studies and generate data on mechanistic effects in pre-clinical settings. Another important aspect of nutraceutical research is the development of surrogate endpoint biomarkers for clinical disease and conduct clinical trials for ascertaining nutraceutical efficacy. Unfortunately, several clinical studies on nutraceutical and prostate cancer were poorly designed, lacking appropriate controls and lacking useful biomarkers; consequently the results of such studies have been inconsistent. Systematic well-designed randomized placebo-controlled trials with adequate power and relevant clinical endpoints are needed. For example, the results generated by the PCPT trial emphasizes that trials with any agents, including nutraceuticals, are not easy to design or interpret and that test agents that appear promising in observational studies may not prove to be as beneficial as expected when evaluated in randomized clinical trials. To ensure that all adverse effects of nutraceuticals are detected, randomized controlled trials need to be carefully monitored for sufficient periods of time. Despite these challenges, nutraceutical research continues to emerge and will offer new and promising nutraceutical agents in the future, with more opportunities for disease prevention, particularly for prostate cancer.

Acknowledgements The original work from author's laboratory outlined in this chapter was supported by United States Public Health Service Grants RO1 CA108512, RO1 CA115491 and RO1 AT002709 and funds from Cancer Research and Prevention Foundation to SG and RO3 CA1376676 to SS.

References

Adams KF, Chen C, Newton KM et al (2004) Soy isoflavones do not modulate prostate-specific antigen concentrations in older men in a randomized controlled trial. Cancer Epidemiol Biomarkers Prev 13:644–648

Adhami VM, Ahmad N, Mukhtar H (2003) Molecular targets for green tea in prostate cancer prevention. J Nutr 133:2417–2424

Adhami VM, Siddiqui IA, Ahmad N et al (2004) Oral consumption of green tea polyphenols inhibits insulin-like growth factor-I-induced signaling in an autochthonous mouse model of prostate cancer. Cancer Res 64:8715–8722

Adhami VM, Khan N, Mukhtar H (2009) Cancer chemoprevention by pomegranate: laboratory and clinical evidence. Nutr Cancer 61:811–815

Agarwal C, Singh RP, Agarwal R (2002) Grape seed extract induces apoptotic death of human prostate carcinoma DU145 cells via caspases activation accompanied by dissipation of mitochondrial membrane potential and cytochrome c release. Carcinogenesis 23:1869–1876

Agarwal C, Singh RP, Dhanalakshmi S et al (2004) Anti-angiogenic efficacy of grape seed extract in endothelial cells. Oncol Rep 11:681–685

Agus DB, Vera JC, Golde DW (1999) Stromal cell oxidation: a mechanism by which tumors obtain vitamin C. Cancer Res 59:4555–4558

Ahmad IU, Forman JD, Sarkar FH et al (2010) Soy isoflavones in conjunction with radiation therapy in patients with prostate cancer. Nutr Cancer 62:996–1000

Al-Shukri SH, Deschaseaux P, Kuzmin IV et al (2000) Early urodynamic effects of the lipido-sterolic extract of Serenoa repens (Permixon®) in patients with lower urinary tract symptoms due to benign prostatic hyperplasia. Prostate Cancer Prostatic Dis 3:195–199

Amagase H, Petesch BL, Matsuura H et al (2001) Intake of garlic and its bioactive components. J Nutr 131:955–962

Ansari MS, Gupta NP (2004) Lycopene: a novel drug therapy in hormone refractory metastatic prostate cancer. Urol Oncol 22:415–420

Argao EA, Heubi JE (1993) Fat-soluble vitamin deficiency in infants and children. Curr Opin Pediatr 5:562–566

Arunkumar A, Vijayababu MR, Srinivasan N (2006) Garlic compound, diallyl disulfide induces cell cycle arrest in prostate cancer cell line PC-3. Mol Cell Biochem 288:107–113

Aust O, Ale-Agha N, Zhang L, Wollersen H et al (2003) Lycopene oxidation product enhances gap junctional communication. Food Chem Toxicol 41:1399–1407

Aziz MH, Kumar R, Ahmad N (2003) Cancer chemoprevention by resveratrol: in vitro and in vivo studies and the underlying mechanisms (review). Int J Oncol 23:17–28

Barranco WT, Eckhert CD (2006) Cellular changes in boric acid-treated DU-145 prostate cancer cells. Br J Cancer 94:884–890

Beevers CS, Li F, Liu L et al (2006) Curcumin inhibits the mammalian target of rapamycin-mediated signaling pathways in cancer cells. Int J Cancer 119:757–764

Bektic J, Berger AP, Pfeil K et al (2004) Androgen receptor regulation by physiological concentrations of the isoflavonoid genistein in androgen-dependent LNCaP cells is mediated by estrogen receptor beta. Eur Urol 45:245–251

Bettuzzi S, Brausi M, Rizzi F et al (2006) Chemoprevention of human prostate cancer by oral administration of green tea catechins in volunteers with high-grade prostate intraepithelial neoplasia: a preliminary report from a one-year proof-of-principle study. Cancer Res 66:1234–1240

Blatt DH, Leonard SW, Traber MG (2001) Vitamin E kinetics and the function of tocopherol regulatory proteins. Nutrition 17:799–805

Blomhoff R, Green MH, Norum KR (1992) Vitamin A: physiological and biochemical processing. Annu Rev Nutr 12:37–57

Blutt SE, Allegretto EA, Pike JW et al (1997) 1,25-Dihydroxyvitamin D3 and 9-cis-retinoic acid act synergistically to inhibit the growth of LNCaP prostate cells and cause accumulation of cells in G1. Endocrinology 138:1491–1497

Boileau TW, Liao Z, Kim S et al (2003) Prostate carcinogenesis in N-methyl-N-nitrosourea (NMU)-testosterone-treated rats fed tomato powder, lycopene, or energy-restricted diets. JNCI 95:1578–1586

Bosetti C, Talamini R, Montella M et al (2004) Retinol, carotenoids and the risk of prostate cancer: a case-control study from Italy. Int J Cancer 112:689–692

Bowen P, Chen L, Stacewicz-Sapuntzakis M et al (2002) Tomato sauce supplementation and prostate cancer: lycopene accumulation and modulation of biomarkers of carcinogenesis. Exp Biol Med 227:886–893

Brawley OW, Barnes S, Parnes H (2001) The future of prostate cancer prevention. Ann NY Acad Sci 952:145–152

Broitman SA, Wilkinson J IV, Cerda S (1996) Effects of monoterpenes and mevinolin on murine colon tumor CT-26 in vitro and its hepatic "metastases" in vivo. Adv Exp Med Biol 401: 111–130

Brooks JD, Paton VG, Vidanes G (2001) Potent induction of phase 2 enzymes in human prostate cells by sulforaphane. Cancer Epidemiol Biomarkers Prev 10:949–954

Campbell JK, Canene-Adams K, Lindshield BL et al (2004) Tomato phytochemicals and prostate cancer risk. J Nutr 134: S3486–S3492

Cardile V, Scifo C, Russo A, Falsaperla M et al (2003) Involvement of HSP70 in resveratrol-induced apoptosis of human prostate cancer. Anticancer Res 23:4921–4926

Chan JM, Giovannucci EL (2001) Dairy products, calcium, and vitamin D and risk of prostate cancer. Epidemiol Rev 23:87–92

Chen TC, Wang L, Whitlatch LW et al (2003) Prostatic 25-hydroxyvitamin D-1alpha-hydroxylase and its implication in prostate cancer. J Cell Biochem 88:315–322

Chendil D, Ranga RS, Meigooni D et al (2004) Curcumin confers radiosensitizing effect in prostate cancer cell line PC-3. Oncogene 23:1599–1607

Chiao JW, Chung F, Krzeminski J et al (2000) Modulation of growth of human prostate cancer cells by the N-acetylcysteine conjugate of phenethyl isothiocyanate. Int J Oncol 16:1215–1219

Chintharlapalli S, Papineni S, Ramaiah SK et al (2007) Betulinic acid inhibits prostate cancer growth through inhibition of specificity protein transcription factors. Cancer Res 67:2816–2823

Chlopcikova S, Psotova J, Miketova P et al (2004) Chemoprotective effect of plant phenolics against anthracycline-induced toxicity on rat cardiomyocytes. I. Silymarin and its flavonolignans. Phytother Res 18:107–110

Cho SD, Jiang C, Malewicz B et al (2004) Methyl selenium metabolites decrease prostate-specific antigen expression by inducing protein degradation and suppressing androgen-stimulated transcription. Mol Cancer Ther 3:605–611

Cho HJ, Park SY, Kim EJ et al (2011) 3,3′-Diindolylmethane inhibits prostate cancer development in the transgenic adenocarcinoma mouse prostate model. Mol Carcinog 50:100–112

Choan E, Segal R, Jonker D et al (2005) A prospective clinical trial of green tea for hormone refractory prostate cancer: an evaluation of the complementary/alternative therapy approach. Urol Oncol 23:108–113

Choi HY, Lim JE, Hong JH (2010) Curcumin interrupts the interaction between the androgen receptor and Wnt/β-catenin signaling pathway in LNCaP prostate cancer cells. Prostate Cancer Prostatic Dis 13:343–349

Clark LC, Dalkin B, Krongrad A et al (1998) Decreased incidence of prostate cancer with selenium supplementation: results of a double-blind cancer prevention trial. Br JUrol 81:730–734

Cohen JH, Kristal AR, Stanford JL (2000) Fruit and vegetable intakes and prostate cancer risk. JNCI 92:61–68

Collin SM, Metcalfe C, Refsum H et al (2010a) Circulating folate, vitamin B12, homocysteine, vitamin B12 transport proteins, and risk of prostate cancer: a case-control study, systematic review, and meta-analysis. Cancer Epidemiol Biomarkers Prev 19:1632–1642

Collin SM, Metcalfe C, Refsum H et al (2010b) Combined inhibitory effects of soy isoflavones and curcumin on the production of prostate-specific antigen. Prostate 70:1127–1133

Cook NR, Le IM, Manson JE et al (2000) Effects of beta-carotene supplementation on cancer incidence by baseline characteristics in the Physicians' Health Study (United States). Cancer Causes Control 11:617–626

Cortesi M, Fridman E, Volkov A et al (1999) Crowell PL: prevention and therapy of cancer by dietary monoterpenes. J Nutr 129: S775–S778

Cortesi M, Fridman E, Volkov A et al (2008) Clinical assessment of the cancer diagnostic value of prostatic zinc: a comprehensive needle-biopsy study. Prostate 68:994–1006

Crowell PL (1999) Prevention and therapy of cancer by dietary monoterpenes. J Nutr 129: 775S–778S

Cuyckens F, Claeys M (2004) Mass spectrometry in the structural analysis of flavonoids. J Mass Spectrom 39:1–15

Davis JN, Singh B, Bhuiyan M et al (1998) Genistein-induced upregulation of p21WAF1, downregulation of cyclin B, and induction of apoptosis in prostate cancer cells. Nutr Cancer 32:123–131

Day JK, Bauer AM, DesBordes C et al (2002) Genistein alters methylation patterns in mice. J Nutr 132: S2419–S2423

de la Taille A (2001) PC SPES in prostatic cancer: critical reviewof the literature. Prog Urol 11:428–432

deVere White RW, Hackman RM et al (2004) Effects of a genistein-rich extract on PSA levels in men with a history of prostate cancer. Urology 63:259–263

deVere White RW, Tsodikov A, Stapp EC et al (2010) Effects of a high dose, aglycone-rich soy extract on prostate-specific antigen and serum isoflavone concentrations in men with localized prostate cancer. Nutr Cancer 62:1036–1043

Dhanalakshmi S, Agarwal R, Agarwal C (2003) Inhibition of NF-kappaB pathway in grape seed extract-induced apoptotic death of human prostate carcinoma DU145 cells. Int J Oncol 23: 721–727

Donaldson MS (2004) Nutrition and cancer: a review of the evidence for an anti-cancer diet. Nutr J 3:1–21

Dorai T, Cao YC, Dorai B et al (2001) Therapeutic potential of curcumin in human prostate cancer. III. Curcumin inhibits proliferation, induces apoptosis, and inhibits angiogenesis of LNCaP prostate cancer cells in vivo. Prostate 47:293–303

Druesne-Pecollo N, Latino-Martel P, Norat T et al (2010) Beta-carotene supplementation and cancer risk: a systematic review and meta-analysis of randomized controlled trials. Int J Cancer 127:172–184

Dunn BK, Richmond ES, Minasian LM et al (2010) A nutrient approach to prostate cancer prevention: the Selenium and Vitamin E Cancer Prevention Trial (SELECT). Nutr Cancer 62:896–918

Eichholzer M, Stahelin HB, Gey KF et al (1996) Prediction of male cancer mortality by plasma levels of interacting vitamins: 17-year follow-up of the prospective Basel study. Int J Cancer 66:145–150

Eichholzer M, Stahelin HB, Ludin E et al (1999) Smoking, plasma vitamins C, E, retinol, and carotene, and fatal prostate cancer: seventeen-year follow-up of the prospective Basal study. Prostate 38:189–198

Etminan M, Takkouche B, Caamano-Isorna F (2004) The role of tomato products and lycopene in the prevention of prostate cancer: a meta-analysis of observational studies. Cancer Epidemiol Biomarkers Prev 13:340–345

Fang MZ, Wang Y, Ai N et al (2003) Tea polyphenol (–)-epigallocatechin-3-gallate inhibits DNA methyltransferase and reactivates methylation-silenced genes in cancer cell lines. Cancer Res 63:7563–7570

Fares F, Azzam N, Appel B et al (2010) The potential efficacy of 3,3′-diindolylmethane in prevention of prostate cancer development. Eur J Cancer Prev 19:199–203

Favus MJ, Langman CB (1986) Evidence for calcium-dependent control of 1,25-dihydroxyvitamin D3 production by rat kidney proximal tubules. J Biol Chem 261:11224–11229

Fazzio A, Marilley D, Azzi A (1997) The effect of alpha-tocopherol and beta-tocopherol on proliferation, protein kinase C activity and gene expression in different cell lines. Biochem Mol Biol Int 41:93–101

Ferguson LR, Philpott M, Karunasinghe N (2004) Dietary cancer and prevention using antimutagens. Toxicology 198:147–159

Fischer L, Mahoney C, Jeffcoat AR et al (2004) Clinical characteristics and pharmacokinetics of purified soy isoflavones: multiple-dose administration to men with prostate neoplasia. Nutr Cancer 48:160–170

Flaig TW, Glodé M, Gustafson D et al (2010) A study of high-dose oral silybin-phytosome followed by prostatectomy in patients with localized prostate cancer. Prostate 70:848–855

Frei B, Higdon JV (2003) Antioxidant activity of tea polyphenols in vivo: evidence from animal studies. J Nutr 133:3275–3284

Gandini S, Boniol M, Haukka J et al (2005) Anti carcinogenic and anti-metastatic properties of indole-3-carbinol in prostate cancer. Oncol Rep 13:89–93

Gandini S, Boniol M, Haukka J et al (2011) Meta-analysis of observational studies of serum 25-hydroxyvitamin D levels and colorectal, breast and prostate cancer and colorectal adenoma. Int J Cancer 128:1414–1424

Gann PH (2002) Risk factors for prostate cancer. Rev Urol 4 Suppl 5:S3–S10

Garikapaty VP, Ashok BT, Chen YG (2005) Anti-carcinogenic and anti-metastatic properties of indole-3-carbinol in prostate cancer. Oncol Rep 13:89–93

Giovannucci E (1999) Tomatoes, tomato-based products, lycopene, and cancer: review of the epidemiologic literature. JNCI 91:317–331

Giovannucci E, Ascherio A, Rimm EB et al (1995) Intake of carotenoids and retinol in relation to risk of prostate cancer. JNCI 87:1767–1776

Gong A, He M, Krishna Vanaja D et al (2009) Phenethyl isothiocyanate inhibits STAT3 activation in prostate cancer cells. Mol Nutr Food Res 53:878–886

Gonzalez A, Peters U, Lampe JW et al (2007) Boron intake and prostate cancer risk. Cancer Causes Contr 18:1131–1140

Goodman GE, Schaffer S, Omenn GS et al (2003) The association between lung and prostate cancer risk, and serum micronutrients: results and lessons learned from beta-carotene and retinol efficacy trial. Cancer Epidemiol Biomarkers Prev 12:518–526
Gopalakrishna R, Gundimeda U (2002) Antioxidant regulation of protein kinase C in cancer prevention. J Nutr 132: S3819–S3823
Grayson DH (1994) Monoterpenoids. Nat Prod Rep 11:225–247
Greenwald P, Clifford CK, Milner JA (2001) Diet and cancer prevention. Eur J Cancer 37:948–965
Gunawardena K, Murray DK, Meikle AW (2000) Vitamin E and other antioxidants inhibit human prostate cancer cells through apoptosis. Prostate 44:287–295
Gunawardena K, Campbell LD, Meikle AW (2004) Combination therapy with vitamins C plus E inhibits survivin and human prostate cancer cell growth. Prostate 59:319–327
Gupta S, Ahmad N, Mukhtar H (1999) Prostate cancer chemoprevention by green tea. Semin Urol Oncol 17:70–76
Gupta S, Afaq F, Mukhtar H (2001a) Selective growth-inhibitory, cell-cycle deregulatory and apoptotic response of apigenin in normal versus human prostate carcinoma cells. Biochem Biophys Res Commun 287:914–920
Gupta S, Hastak K, Ahmad N et al (2001b) Inhibition of prostate carcinogenesis in TRAMP mice by oral infusion of green tea polyphenols. Proc Natl Acad Sci USA 98:10350–10355
Gupta S, Afaq F, Mukhtar H (2002a) Involvement of nuclear factor-kappa B, Bax and Bcl-2 in induction of cell cycle arrest and apoptosis by apigenin in human prostate carcinoma cells. Oncogene 21:3727–3738
Gupta S, Saha B, Giri AK (2002b) Comparative antimutagenic and anticlastogenic effects of green tea and black tea: a review. Mutat Res 512:37–65
Gupta S, Hastak K, Afaq F et al (2004) Essential role of caspases in epigallocatechin-3-gallate-mediated inhibition of nuclear factor kappa B and induction of apoptosis. Oncogene 23: 2507–2522
Habib FK, Ross M, Ho CK et al (2005) Serenoa repens (Permixon) inhibits the 5alpha-reductase activity of human prostate cancer cell lines without interfering with PSA expression. Int J Cancer 114:190–194
Hartman TJ, Albanes D, Pietinen P et al (1998) The association between baseline vitamin E, selenium, and prostate cancer in the alpha-tocopherol, beta-carotene cancer prevention study. Cancer Epidemiol Biomarkers Prev 7:335–340
Heinonen OP, Albanes D, Virtamo J et al (1998) Prostate cancer and supplementation with alpha-tocopherol and beta-carotene: incidence and mortality in a controlled trial. JNCI 90:440–446
Herman-Antosiewicz A, Singh SV (2004) Signal transduction pathways leading to cell cycle arrest and apoptosis induction in cancer cells by Allium vegetable-derived organosulfur compounds: a review. Mutat Res 555:121–131
Hong HY, Kim BC (2007) Mixed lineage kinase 3 connects reactive oxygen species to c-Jun NH2-terminal kinase-induced mitochondrial apoptosis in genipin-treated PC3 human prostate cancer cells. Biochem Biophys Res Commun 362:307–312
Hong MY, Seeram NP, Heber D (2008) Pomegranate polyphenols down-regulate expression of androgen-synthesizing genes in human prostate cancer cells overexpressing the androgen receptor. J Nutr Biochem 19:848–855
Howard EW, Ling MT, Chua CW et al (2007) Garlic-derived S-allylmercaptocysteine is a novel in vivo antimetastatic agent for androgen-independent prostate cancer. Clin Cancer Res 13: 1847–1856
Howells LM, Gallacher-Horley B, Houghton CE (2002) Indole-3-carbinol inhibits protein kinase B/Akt and induces apoptosis in the human breast tumor cell line MDA MB468 but not in the nontumorigenic HBL100 line. Mol Cancer Ther 1:1161–1172
Hsieh TC, Wu JM (1999) Differential effects on growth, cell cycle arrest, and induction of apoptosis by resveratrol in human prostate cancer cell lines. Exp Cell Res 249:109–115

Hsieh TC, Wu JM (2000) Grape-derived chemopreventive agent resveratrol decreases prostate-specific antigen (PSA) expression in LNCaP cells by an androgen receptor (AR)-independent mechanism. Anticancer Res 20:225–228

Hu ML, Shih MK (1997) Ascorbic acid inhibits lipid peroxidation but enhances DNA damage in rat liver nuclei incubated with iron ions. Free Radic Res 26:585–592

Hwang ES, Bowen PE (2002) Can the consumption of tomatoes or lycopene reduce cancer risk? Integr Cancer Ther 1:121–132

Ide H, Tokiwa S, Sakamaki K et al (1994) N-(4-Hydroxyphenyl) retinamide induces cell cycle specific growth inhibition in PC3 cells. Prostate 24:299–305

Igawa M, Tanabe T, Chodak GW (1994) N-(4-hydroxyphenyl) retinamide induces cell cycle specific growth inhibition in PC3 cells. Prostate 24:299–305

Jang M, Cai L, Udeani GO et al (1997) Cancer chemopreventive activity of resveratrol, a natural product derived from grapes. Science 275:218–220

Jatoi A, Ellison N, Burch PA et al (2003) A phase II trial of green tea in the treatment of patients with androgen independent metastatic prostate carcinoma. Cancer 97:1442–1446

Jemal A, Bray F, Center MM et al (2011) Global cancer statistics. CA Cancer J Clin 61:69–90

Jian L, Xie LP, Lee AH et al (2004) Protective effect of green tea against prostate cancer: a case-control study in southeast China. Int J Cancer 108:130–135

Jian L, Du CJ, Lee AH et al (2005) Do dietary lycopene and other carotenoids protect against prostate cancer? Int J Cancer 113:1010–1014

Jiang C, Ganther H, Lu J (2000) Monomethyl selenium-specific inhibition of MMP-2 and VEGF expression: implications for angiogenic switch regulation. Mol Carcinog 29:236–250

John EM, Dreon DM, Koo J et al (2004) Residential sunlight exposure is associated with a decreased risk of prostate cancer. J Steroid Biochem Mol Biol 89–90:549–552

Karlson J, Borg-Karlson AK, Unelius R et al (1996) Inhibition of tumor cell growth by monoterpenes in vitro: evidence of a Ras-independent mechanism of action. Anticancer Drugs 7:422–429

Khan N, Afaq F, Mukhtar H (2007) Apoptosis by dietary factors: the suicide solution for delaying cancer growth. Carcinogenesis 28:233–239

Khan N, Adhami VM, Mukhtar H (2010) Apoptosis by dietary agents for prevention and treatment of prostate cancer. Endocr Relat Cancer 17:R39–R52

Kim SH, Nam JH, Park EJ et al (2009) Menthol regulates TRPM8-independent processes in PC-3 prostate cancer cells. Biochim Biophys Acta 1792:33–38

Klein RD, Fischer SM (2002) Black tea polyphenols inhibit IGF-I-induced signaling through Akt in normal prostate epithelial cells and DU145 prostate carcinoma cells. Carcinogenesis 23: 217–221

Kolonel LN, Hankin JH, Whittemore AS et al (2000) Vegetables, fruits, legumes and prostate cancer: a multiethnic case-control study. Cancer Epidemiol Biomarkers Prev 9:795–804

Kong AN, Yu R, Hebbar V et al (2001) Signal transduction events elicited by cancer prevention compounds. Mutat Res 480–481:231–241

Konijeti R, Henning S, Moro A et al (2010) Chemoprevention of prostate cancer with lycopene in the TRAMP model. Prostate 70:1547–1554

Krinsky NI, Johnson EJ (2005) Carotenoid actions and their relation to health and disease. Mol Aspects Med 26:459–516

Krishnan K, Campbell S, Abdel-Rahman F et al (2003) Cancer chemoprevention drug targets. Curr Drug Targets 4:45–54

Kucuk O, Sarkar FH, SakrW et al (2001) Phase II randomized clinical trial of lycopene supplementation before radical prostatectomy. Cancer Epidemiol Biomarkers Prev 10:861–868

Kucuk O, Sarkar FH, Djuric Z et al (2002) Effects of lycopene supplementation in patients with localized prostate cancer. Exp Biol Med 227:881–885

Kumar AP, Garcia GE, Ghosh R et al (2003) 4-Hydroxy-3-methoxybenzoic acid methyl ester: a curcumin derivative targets Akt/NF kappa B cell survival signaling pathway: potential for prostate cancer management. Neoplasia 5:255–266

Ledesma MC, Jung-Hynes B, Schmit TL et al (2011) Selenium and vitamin E for prostate cancer: post-SELECT (Selenium and Vitamin E Cancer Prevention Trial) status. Mol Med 17:134–143

Lee SC, Kuan CY, Yang CC et al (1998) Bioflavonoids commonly and potently induce tyrosine ephosphorylation/inactivation of oncogenic proline-directed protein kinase FA in human prostate carcinoma cells. Anticancer Res 18:1117–1121

Li Y, Sarkar FH (2002a) Inhibition of nuclear factor kappaB activation in PC3 cells by genistein is mediated via Akt signaling pathway. Clin Cancer Res 8:2369–2377

Li Y, Sarkar FH (2002b) Down-regulation of invasion and angiogenesis-related genes identified by cDNA microarray analysis of PC3 prostate cancer cells treated with genistein. Cancer Lett 186:157–164

Li Y, Li X, Sarkar FH (2003) Gene expression profiles of I3C- and DIM-treated PC3 human prostate cancer cells determined by cDNA microarray analysis. J Nutr 133:1011–1019

Li Y, Che M, Bhagat S et al (2004) Regulation of gene expression and inhibition of experimental prostate cancer bone metastasis by dietary genistein. Neoplasia 6:354–363

Li M, Zhang Z, Hill DL, Wang H et al (2007) Curcumin, a dietary component, has anticancer, chemosensitization, and radiosensitization effects by down-regulating the MDM2 oncogene through the PI3K/mTOR/ETS2 pathway. Cancer Res 67:1988–1996

Liang JY, Fontana JA, Rao JN et al (1999a) Synthetic retinoid CD437 induces S-phase arrest and apoptosis in human prostate cancer cells LNCaP and PC-3. Prostate 38:228–236

Liang JY, Liu YY, Zou J et al (1999b) Inhibitory effect of zinc on human prostatic carcinoma cell growth. Prostate 40:200–207

Lippman SM, Goodman PJ, Klein EA et al (2005) Designing the Selenium and Vitamin E Cancer Prevention Trial (SELECT). JNCI 97, 94–102

Liu G, Oettel K, Bailey H et al (2003) Phase II trial of perillyl alcohol (NSC 641066) administered daily in patients with metastatic androgen independent prostate cancer. Invest NewDrugs 21:367–372

Lopez-Velez M, Martinez-Martinez F, Del Valle-Ribes C (2003) The study of phenolic compounds as natural antioxidants in wine. Crit RevFood Sci Nutr 43:233–244

Lu X, Guo J, Hsieh TC et al (2003) Inhibition of proliferation and expression of AR/PSA by herbal supplement Equiguard in LNCaP cells cultured in androgen-proficient FBS and androgen-deficient charcoal-stripped FBS is correlated with increased serine-15 phosphorylation of the tumor suppressor gene p53. Anticancer Res 23:2489–2498

Maddi VS, Aragade PD, Digge VG et al (2007) Importance of nutraceuticals in health management. Pharmacog Rev 1:377–379

Makela S, Poutanen M, Kostian ML et al (1998) Inhibition of 17beta-hydroxysteroid oxidoreductase by flavonoids in breast and prostate cancer cells. Proc Soc Exp Biol Med 217:310–316

McCall MR, Frei B (1999) Can antioxidant vitamins materially reduce oxidative damage in humans? Free Radic Biol Med 26:1034–1053

McLarty J, Bigelow RL, Smith M et al (2009) Tea polyphenols decrease serum levels of prostate-specific antigen, hepatocyte growth factor, and vascular endothelial growth factor in prostate cancer patients and inhibit production of hepatocyte growth factor and vascular endothelial growth factor in vitro. Cancer Prev Res (Phila) 2:673–682

Menon M, Maramag C, Malhotra RK et al (1998) Effect of vitamin C on androgen independent prostate cancer cells (PC3 and Mat-Ly-Lu) in vitro: involvement of reactive oxygen species-effect on cell number, viability and DNA synthesis. Cancer Biochem Biophys 16:17–30

Mentor-Marcel R, Lamartiniere CA, Eltoum IA et al (2005) Dietary genistein improves survival and reduces expression of osteopontin in the prostate of transgenic mice with prostatic adenocarcinoma (TRAMP). J Nutr 135:989–995

Metzger BT, Barnes DM, Reed JD (2009) A comparison of pectin, polyphenols, and phytosterols, alone or in combination, to lovastatin for reduction of serum lipids in familial hypercholesterolemic swine. J Med Food 12:854–860

Meyer JP, Gillatt DA (2002) PC-SPES: A herbal therapy for the treatment of hormone refractory prostate cancer. Prostate Cancer Prostatic Dis 5:13–15

Moyad MA (1999) Soy, disease prevention, and prostate cancer. Semin UrolOncol 17:97–102

Müezzinoğlu T, Korkmaz M, Neşe N et al (2002) Curcumin induced suppression of cell proliferation correlates with down-regulation of cyclin D1 expression and CDK4-mediated retinoblastoma protein phosphorylation. Oncogene 21:8852–8861

Mukhopadhyay A, Banerjee S, Stafford LJ (2002) Curcumin-induced suppression of cell proliferation correlates with down-regulation of cyclin D1 expression and CDK4-mediated retinoblastoma protein phosphorylation. Oncogene 21:8852–8861

Nachshon-Kedmi M, Yannai S, Haj A et al (2003) Indole-3-carbinol and 3,3′-diindolylmethane induce apoptosis in human prostate cancer cells. Food Chem Toxicol 41:745–752

Nachshon-Kedmi M, Fares FA, Yannai S (2004) Therapeutic activity of 3,3′-diindolylmethane on prostate cancer in an in vivo model. Prostate 61:153–160

Nakamura K, Yasunaga Y, Segawa T, Ko D et al (2002) Curcumin down-regulates AR gene expression and activation in prostate cancer cell lines. Int J Oncol 21:825–830

Nam S, Smith DM, Dou QP (2001) Ester bond-containing tea polyphenols potently inhibit proteasome activity in vitro and in vivo. J Biol Chem 276:13322–13330

Napora JK, Short RG, Muller DC et al (2011) High-dose isoflavones do not improve metabolic and inflammatory parameters in androgen-deprived men with prostate cancer. J Androl 32:40–48

Narayanan BA, Narayanan NK, Stoner GD (2002) Interactive gene expression pattern in prostate cancer cells exposed to phenolic antioxidants. Life Sci 70:1821–1839

Narayanan BA, Narayanan NK, Re GG et al (2003) Differential expression of genes induced by resveratrol in LNCaP cells: P53-mediated molecular targets. Int J Cancer 104:204–212

Neuhouser ML, Barnett MJ, Kristal AR (2009) Dietary supplement use and prostate cancer risk in the Carotene and Retinol Efficacy Trial. Cancer Epidemiol Biomarkers Prev 18:2202–2206

Obermuller-Jevic UC, Olano-Martin E, Corbacho AM (2003) Lycopene inhibits the growth of normal human prostate epithelial cells in vitro. J Nutr 133:3356–3360

Oh WK, Kantoff PW, WeinbergV, Jones G, Rini BI et al (2004) Prospective, multicenter, randomized phase II trial of the herbal supplement, PC-SPES, and diethylstilbestrol in patients with androgen-independent prostate cancer. J Clin Oncol 22:3705–3712

Ohno Y, Yoshida O, Oishi K et al (1988) Dietary beta-carotene and cancer of the prostate: a case-control study in Kyoto, Japan. Cancer Res 48:1331–1336

Olea-Herrero N, Vara D, Malagarie-Cazenave S et al (2009) The cannabinoid R+ methanandamide induces IL-6 secretion by prostate cancer PC3 cells. J Immunotoxicol 6:249–256

O'Prey J, Brown J, Fleming J (2003) Effects of dietary flavonoids on major signal transduction pathways in human epithelial cells. Biochem Pharmacol 66:2075–2088

Pannellini T, Iezzi M, Liberatore M, Sabatini F et al (2010) A dietary tomato supplement prevents prostate cancer in TRAMP mice. Cancer Prev Res (Phila) 3:1284–1291

Pantuck AJ, Leppert JT, Zomorodian N et al (2006) Phase II study of pomegranate juice for men with rising prostate-specific antigen following surgery or radiation for prostate cancer. Clin Cancer Res 12:4018–4026

Parodi PW (2005). Dairy product consumption and the risk of breast cancer. J Am Coll Nutr (6 Suppl):556S–568S

Pinto JT, Qiao C, Xing J et al (2000) Alterations of prostate biomarker expression and testosterone utilization in human LNCaP prostatic carcinoma cells by garlic-derived S-allylmercaptocysteine. Prostate 45:304–314

Platz EA, Leitzmann MF, Hollis BW et al (2004) Plasma 1,25-dihydroxy- and 25-hydroxyvitamin D and subsequent risk of prostate cancer. Cancer Causes Contr 15:255–265

Polek TC, Stewart LV, Ryu EJ et al (2003) p53 is required for 1,25-dihydroxyvitamin D3-induced G0 arrest but is not required for G1 accumulation or apoptosis of LNCaP prostate cancer cells. Endocrinology 144:50–60

Powell SR (2011) The antioxidant properties of zinc. J Nutr 130:S1447–S1454; 2000. Prevalence of prostate cancer in high boron-exposed population: a community-based study. Biol Trace Elem Res Mar 23. [Epub ahead of print]

Rabi T, Shukla S, Gupta S (2008) Betulinic acid suppresses constitutive and TNFalpha-induced NF-kappaB activation and induces apoptosis in human prostate carcinoma PC-3 cells. Mol Carcinog 47:964–973

Rahman KM, Banerjee S, Ali S et al (2009) 3,3′-Diindolylmethane enhances taxotere-induced apoptosis in hormone-refractory prostate cancer cells through survivin down-regulation. Cancer Res 69:4468–4475

Rajasekaran A, Sivagnanam G, Xavier R (2008) Nutraceuticals as therapeutic agents: a review. Res J Pharm Tech 1:328–340

Rajesh D, Howard SP (2003) Perillyl alcohol mediated radiosensitization via augmentation of the Fas pathway in prostate cancer cells. Prostate 57:14–23

Rao A, Woodruff RD, Wade WN et al (2002) Genistein and vitamin D synergistically inhibit human prostatic epithelial cell growth. J Nutr 132:3191–3194

Rettig MB, Heber D, An J et al (2008) Pomegranate extract inhibits androgen-independent prostate cancer growth through a nuclear factor-kappaB-dependent mechanism. Mol Cancer Ther 7:2662–2671

Richter F, Joyce A, Fromowitz F et al (2002) Immunohistochemical localization of the retinoic acid receptors in human prostate. J Androl 23:830–838

Robak J, Gryglewski RJ (1996) Bioactivity of flavonoids. Pol JPharmacol 48:555–564

Robbins RJ (2003) Phenolic acids in foods: an overview of analytical methodology. J Agric Food Chem 51:2866–2887

Rock CL (2007) Multivitamin-multimineral supplements: who uses them? Am J Clin Nutr 85:277S–279S

Rodriguez C, Jacobs EJ, Mondul AM et al (2004) Vitamin E supplements and risk of prostate cancer in U.S. men. Cancer Epidemiol Biomarkers Prev 13:378–382

Ross SA (2010) Evidence for the relationship between diet and cancer. Exp Oncol 32:137–142

Ross JA, Kasum CM (2002) Dietary flavonoids: bioavailability, metabolic effects, and safety. Annu Rev Nutr 22:19–34

Sah NK, Munshi A, Kurland JF et al (2003) Translation inhibitors sensitize prostate cancer cells to apoptosis induced by tumor necrosis factor-related apoptosis-inducing ligand (TRAIL) by activating c-Jun N-terminal kinase. J Biol Chem 278:20593–20602

Saleem M, Adhami VM, Siddiqui IA (2003) Tea beverage in chemoprevention of prostate cancer: a mini-review. Nutr Cancer 47:13–23

Saleem M, Adhami VM, Ahmad N et al (2005) Prognostic significance of metastasis-associated protein S100A4 (Mts1) in prostate cancer progression and chemoprevention regimens in an autochthonous mouse model. Clin Cancer Res 11:147–153

Santibanez JF, Navarro A, Martinez J (1997) Genistein inhibits proliferation and in vitro invasive potential of human prostatic cancer cell lines. Anticancer Res 17:1199–1204

Sarkar FH, Li Y (2004) Cell signaling pathways altered by natural chemopreventive agents. Mutat Res 555:53–64

Schmid HP, Fischer C, Engeler DS et al (2011) Nutritional aspects of primary prostate cancer prevention. Recent Results Cancer Res 188:101–107

Schuurman AG, Goldbohm RA, Brants HA et al (2002) A prospective cohort study on intake of retinol, vitamins C and E, and carotenoids and prostate cancer risk (Netherlands). Cancer Causes Contr 13:573–582

Schwartz GG, Whitlatch LW, Chen TC et al (1998) Human prostate cells synthesize 1,25-dihydroxyvitamin D3 from 25-hydroxyvitamin D3. Cancer Epidemiol Biomarkers Prev 7:391–395

Shi J, Yu J, Pohorly JE et al (2003) Polyphenolics in grape seeds—biochemistry and functionality. J Med Food 4:291–299

Shih A, Zhang S, Cao HJ et al (2004) Inhibitory effect of epidermal growth factor on resveratrol-induced apoptosis in prostate cancer cells is mediated by protein kinase C-alpha. Mol Cancer Ther 3:1355–1364

Shukla S, Gupta S (2004a) Molecular mechanisms for apigenin-induced cell-cycle arrest and apoptosis of hormone refractory human prostate carcinoma DU145 cells. Mol Carcinog 39:114–126

Shukla S, Gupta S (2004b) Suppression of constitutive and tumor necrosis factor alpha-induced nuclear factor (NF)-kappaB activation and induction of apoptosis by apigenin in human prostate carcinoma PC-3 cells: correlation with down-regulation of NF-kappaB-responsive genes. Clin Cancer Res 10:3169–3178

Shukla S, Mishra A, Fu P et al (2005) Up-regulation of insulin-like growth factor binding protein-3 by apigenin leads to growth inhibition and apoptosis of 22Rv1 xenograft in athymic nude mice. FASEB J 19:2042–2044

Shukla S, MacLennan GT, Flask CA et al (2007) Blockade of beta-catenin signaling by plant flavonoid apigenin suppresses prostate carcinogenesis in TRAMP mice. Cancer Res 67: 6925–6935

Siddiqui IA, Adhami VM, Afaq F et al (2004) Modulation of phosphatidylinositol-3-kinase/protein kinase B- and mitogen-activated protein kinase-pathways by tea polyphenols in human prostate cancer cells. J Cell Biochem 91:232–242

Sigounas G, Hooker J, Anagnostou A (1997) S-Allylmercaptocysteine inhibits cell proliferation and reduces the vi-ability of erythroleukemia, breast, and prostate cancer cell lines. Nutr Cancer 27:186–191

Siler U, Barella L, Spitzer V et al (2004) Lycopene and vitamin E interfere with autocrine/paracrine loops in the Dunning prostate cancer model. FASEB J 18:1019–1021

Singh RP, Agarwal R (2002) Flavonoid antioxidant silymarin and skin cancer. Antioxid Redox Signal 4:655–663

Singh RP, Agarwal R (2004) Prostate cancer prevention by silibinin. Curr Cancer Drug Targets 4:1–11

Singh RP, Sharma G, Dhanalakshmi S et al (2003) Suppression of advanced human prostate tumor growth in athymic mice by silibinin feeding is associated with reduced cell proliferation, increased apoptosis, and inhibition of angiogenesis. Cancer Epidemiol Biomarkers Prev 12:933–939

Singh RP, Tyagi AK, Dhanalakshmi S et al (2004a) Grape seed extract inhibits advanced human prostate tumor growth and angiogenesis and upregulates insulin-like growth factor binding protein-3. Int J Cancer 108:733–740

Singh AV, Xiao D, Lew KL et al (2004b) Sulforaphane induces caspase-mediated apoptosis in cultured PC-3 human prostate cancer cells and retards growth of PC-3 xenografts in vivo. Carcinogenesis 25:83–90

Singh SV, Herman-Antosiewicz A, Singh AV et al (2004c) Sulforaphane-induced G2/M phase cell cycle arrest involves checkpoint kinase 2-mediated phosphorylation of cell division cycle 25C. J Biol Chem 279:25813–25822

Sinha R, El-Bayoumy K (2004) Apoptosis is a critical cellular event in cancer chemoprevention and chemotherapy by selenium compounds. Curr Cancer Drug Targets 4:13–28

Soobrattee MA, Bahorun T, Aruoma OI (2006) Chemopreventive actions of polyphenolic compounds in cancer. Biofactors 27:19–35

Soriano-Garcia M (2004) Organoselenium compounds as potential therapeutic and chemopreventive agents: a review. Curr Med Chem 11:1657–1669

Stan SD, Singh SV (2009) Transcriptional repression and inhibition of nuclear translocation of androgen receptor by diallyl trisulfide in human prostate cancer cells. Clin Cancer Res 15:4895–4903

Stewart LV, Weigel NL (2004) Vitamin D and prostate cancer. Exp Biol Med 229:277–284

Stratton J, Godwin M (2011) The effect of supplemental vitamins and minerals on the development of prostate cancer: a systematic review and meta-analysis. Fam Pract 28:243–252

Taper HS, Jamison JM, Gilloteaux J et al (2001) In vivo reactivation of DNases in implanted human prostate tumors after administration of a vitamin C/K(3) combination. J Histochem Cytochem 49:109–120

Tavani A, Bertuccio P, Bosetti C et al (2005) Dietary intake of calcium, vitamin d, phosphorus and the risk of prostate cancer. Eur Urol 48:27–33

Teiten MH, Gaascht F, Cronauer M et al (2011) Anti-proliferative potential of curcumin in androgen-dependent prostate cancer cells occurs through modulation of the Wingless signaling pathway. Int J Oncol 38:603–611

Thelen P, WuttkeW, Jarry H (2004) Inhibition of telomerase activity and secretion of prostate specific antigen by silibinin in prostate cancer cells. J Urol 171:1934–1938

Traka M, Gasper AV, Melchini A et al (2008). Broccoli consumption interacts with GSTM1 to perturb oncogenic signalling pathways in the prostate. PLoS One 3:e2568.

Tyagi AK, Singh RP, Agarwal C et al (2002) Silibinin strongly synergizes human prostate carcinoma DU145 cells to doxorubicin-induced growth inhibition, G2-M arrest, and apoptosis. Clin Cancer Res 8:3512–3519

Venkateswaran V, Fleshner NE, Klotz LH (2004) Synergistic effect of vitamin E and selenium in human prostate cancer cell lines. ProstateCancer Prostatic Dis 7:54–56

Vidlar A, Vostalova J, Ulrichova J et al (1997) Diet and prostate cancer: a case-control study. Eur J Cancer 33:101–107

Vidlar A, Vostalova J, Ulrichova J et al (2010) The safety and efficacy of a silymarin and selenium combination in men after radical prostatectomy – a six month placebo-controlled double-blind clinical trial. Biomed Pap Med Fac Univ Palacky Olomouc Czech Repub 154:239–244

Vlajinac HD, Marinković JM, Ilić MD (1997) Diet and prostate cancer: a case-control study. Eur J Cancer 33:101–107

Wang X, Quinn PJ (1999) Vitamin E and its function in membranes. Prog Lipid Res 38:309–336

Wang L, Liu D, Ahmed T et al (2004) Targeting cell cycle machinery as a molecular mechanism of sulforaphane in prostate cancer prevention. Int J Oncol 24:187–192

Wang P, Aronson WJ, Huang M (2010) Green tea polyphenols and metabolites in prostatectomy tissue: implications for cancer prevention. Cancer Prev Res (Phila) 3:985–993

Webber MM, Waghray A (1995) Urokinase-mediated extracellular matrix degradation by human prostatic carcinoma cells and its inhibition by retinoic acid. Clin Cancer Res 1:755–761

Weinstein SJ, Wright ME, Pietinen P et al (2005) Serum alpha-tocopherol and gamma-tocopherol in relation to prostate cancer risk in a prospective study. JNCI 97:396–399

Weisburger JH (1999) Mechanisms of action of antioxidants as exemplified in vegetables, tomatoes and tea. Food Chem Toxicol 37:943–948

Wilkinson S, Chodak GW (2003) Critical review of complementary therapies for prostate cancer. J Clin Oncol 21:2199–2210

Williams CA, Grayer RJ (2004) Anthocyanins and other flavonoids. Nat Prod Rep 21:539–573

Xiao D, Singh SV (2010) p66Shc is indispensable for phenethyl isothiocyanate-induced apoptosis in human prostate cancer cells. Cancer Res 70:3150–3158

Xiao D, Zeng Y, Choi S et al (2005) Caspase-dependent apoptosis induction by phenethyl isothiocyanate, a cruciferous vegetable-derived cancer chemopreventive agent, is mediated by Bak and Bax. Clin Cancer Res 11:2670–1679

Xu C, Shen G, Chen C et al (2005) Suppression of NF-kappaB and NF-kappaB-regulated gene expression by sulforaphane and PEITC through IkappaBalpha, IKK pathway in human prostate cancer PC-3 cells. Oncogene 24:4486–4495

Yin F, Giuliano AE, Law RE et al (2001) Apigenin inhibits growth and induces G2/M arrest by modulating cyclin-CDK regulators and ERK MAP kinase activation in breast carcinoma cells. Anticancer Res 21:413–420

Yip I, Cudiamat M, Chim D (2003) PC-SPES for treatment of prostate cancer: herbal medicine. Curr Urol Rep 4:253–257

Yu S, Shen G, Khor TO et al (2008) Curcumin inhibits Akt/mammalian target of rapamycin signaling through protein phosphatase-dependent mechanism. Mol Cancer Ther 7:2609–2620

Zambetti P (2008) Global market growth for dietary supplements. www.naturalproductsinsider.com/.../2008/.../global-market-growth-for-dietary-supplements.aspx

Zhang Y, Ni J, Messing EM et al (2002) Vitamin E succinate inhibits the function of androgen receptor and the expression of prostate-specific antigen in prostate cancer cells. Proc Natl Acad Sci USA 99:7408–7413

Zhang J, Hsu JC, Kinseth MA et al (2003) Indole-3-carbinol induces a G1 cell cycle arrest and inhibits prostate-specific antigen production in human LNCaP prostate carcinoma cells. Cancer 98:2511–2520

Zhang Y, Kong C, Zeng Y et al (2010) Ursolic acid induces PC-3 cell apoptosis via activation of JNK and inhibition of Akt pathways in vitro. Mol Carcinog 49:374–385

Zhao J, Wang J, Chen Y (1999) Anti-tumor-promoting activity of a polyphenolic fraction isolated from grape seeds in the mouse skin two-stage initiation-promotion protocol and identification of procyanidin B5–3′-gallate as the most effective antioxidant constituent. Carcinogenesis 20:1737–1745

Zhu W, Zhang JS, Young CY (2001) Silymarin inhibits function of the androgen receptor by reducing nuclear localization of the receptor in the human prostate cancer cell line LNCaP. Carcinogenesis 22:1399–1403

Zi X, Agarwal R (1999) Silibinin decreases prostate-specific antigen with cell growth inhibition via G1 arrest, leading to differentiation of prostate carcinoma cells: implications for prostate cancer intervention. Proc Natl Acad Sci USA 96:7490–7495

Zwenger S, Basu C (2008) Plant terpenoids: applications and future potentials. Biotechnol Mol Biol Rev 3:001–007

Chapter 6
Cellular, Molecular and Biological Insight into Chemopreventive and Therapeutic Potential of 3,3'-Diindolylmethane (DIM)

Sanjeev Banerjee, Mansi A. Parasramka, and Fazlul H. Sarkar

Abstract Emerging evidence suggest that bioactive phytochemical is achievable by consuming moderate amount of cruciferous vegetables, such as broccoli, brussel sprouts, cauliflower and cabbage. Evaluation for chemopreventive effectiveness of these vegetables led to the identification of 3,3'-Diindolylmethane (DIM) which is generated in the acidic environment of the stomach following dimerization of Indole-3-Carbinol (I3C) monomers originating from the aforementioned class of vegetables. This article evaluates the potential targets and biological effects elicited by DIM against tumor cells to ascertain chemopreventive and therapeutic efficacy. We provide mechanistic insight into their pleiotropic action resulting in the induction of cell cycle arrest and apoptosis, and the disruption of intracellular signaling network cascade that are known to regulate angiogenesis, metastasis and invasion. The beneficial effect of DIM has been observed by preclinical in vitro and in vivo studies, suggesting that DIM could be useful as a chemopreventive agent and an adjunct to conventional therapeutics. Moreover, DIM has moved through preclinical development into clinical trials and the outcome of such investigation would likely provide definitive role of DIM in human health and diseases.

Keywords 3,3'-Diindolylmethane · Brassica genus · Prevention · Therapy

6.1 Introduction

In the United States 1,529,560 new cancer cases were diagnosed in 2010, and 569,490 deaths has been estimated (Jemal et al. 2011). These alarming statistics underscore the importance of cancer prevention using novel strategies. Consistent with the history of therapeutic interventions, we present evidence of a natural bioactive phytochemical showing benefit due to its pleiotropic actions, which could be

F.H. Sarkar (✉)
Departments of Pathology and Oncology, Karmanos Cancer Institute, Wayne State University, 740 HWCRC, Detroit, Michigan 48201, USA
e-mail: fsarkar@med.wayne.edu

F.H. Sarkar (ed.), *Nutraceuticals and Cancer*, DOI 10.1007/978-94-007-2630-7_6,

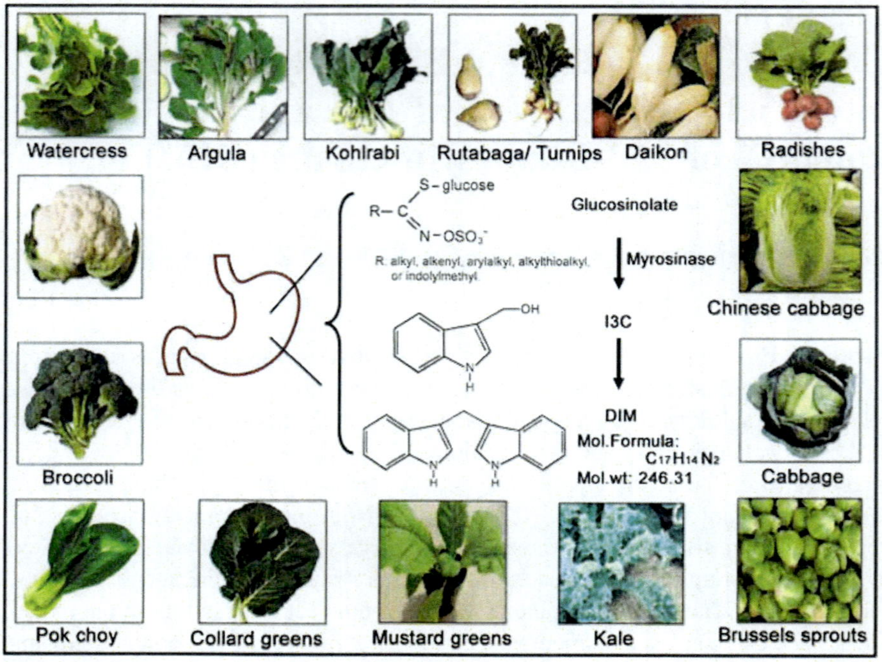

Fig. 6.1 Potential sources, origin and molecular structure of 3,3′-Diindolylmethane (DIM). DIM is dimeric bioactive product of Indole 3-carbinol generated in acid environment of the stomach following consumption of diet rich in cruciferous vegetables. Other relevant information are indicated in the figure

useful for cancer prevention and therapy. This promising agent is found in substantial amounts in vegetables belonging to *Cruciferae* family, particularly the genus *Brassica,* which includes broccoli, cauliflower, kale, cabbage, brussel sprouts, turnips, kohlrabi, bok-choy, and radish (Fig. 6.1). The anticancer properties of cruciferous vegetables were first recognized by the Roman statesman, Cato the Elder (234-149 BC), who in his treatise of medicine wrote: "If a cancerous ulcer appears on the breasts, apply a crushed cabbage leaf and it will make it well." Cruciferous vegetables contain a precursor phytochemical – glucosinolate, that undergoes hydrolysis by the plant enzyme myrosinase, yielding a bioactive compound identified as indole 3-carbinol (I3C). I3C is chemically unstable in aqueous and gastric acidic environment, and is rapidly converted to numerous condensation products. A major in vivo condensation product of I3C is 3,3'-diindolylmethane (DIM; Fig. 6.1). DIM has distinct synchronizing molecular effects on cancer cells, overriding survival signaling, and simultaneously activating multiple death pathways – the two prerequisite of tumor cells to survive and metastasize.

DIM is safe for human consumption and causes no known toxicity. Interestingly, this is the only compound that is detected in the plasma of women ingesting I3C, implying DIM is the predominant bioactive compound that mediates the biological effects of dietary Brassica (Reed et al. 2006). Upon administration of DIM to human volunteers, adequate serum levels were detected and considered to be biologically noteworthy (Crowell et al. 2006; Reed et al. 2006; Reed et al. 2008). Furthermore, when consumed orally, crystalline DIM exhibits poor bioavailability due to its lower aqueous and lipid solubility. To overcome this effect, most pharmacokinetic studies and clinical trials' have now been using Bioresponse-DIM (BR-DIM); a patented, oral formulation containing D-α-tocopheryl acid succinate, phosphatidylcholine, and silica microencapsulated in starch which exhibits 50% higher bioavailability than does crystalline DIM. Consequenently, high concentrations of DIM was detected in the blood samples of humans receiving the same dose of BR-DIM as the crystalline form along with increased net exposure to DIM (Jacobs IC and Zeligs MA 1999; Jacobs IC and Zeligs MA 2000). Furthermore, evaluation for pharmacokinetics, clinical safety, and tolerability of single ascending doses of BR-DIM revealed a linear dose-exposure relationship over the range of 50–300 mg and that a single 200 mg dose of BR-DIM produces a mean C_{max} of 104 ng/ml, and a mean AUC of 553 h* ng/ml (Reed et al. 2008). It has been estimated that consumption of 200 gms of broccoli provides ~12 mg of DIM; with maximum absorption, the blood concentration of DIM would be expected to reach ~10 μM, similar to the effective levels of DIM shown in cultured cells (Chang et al. 2006).

Here, we are summarizing the effect of DIM from an evidence-based perspective for unbiased appraisal of its benefit, as it relates to chemoprevention and by extension, justify the use of DIM in developing oncology therapeutics. A generalized global overview of pleiotropic targets related to DIM action has been summarized in Fig. 6.2. Nevertheless, it is understood that any promising forthcoming effects may also be influenced by individual genetic polymorphism.

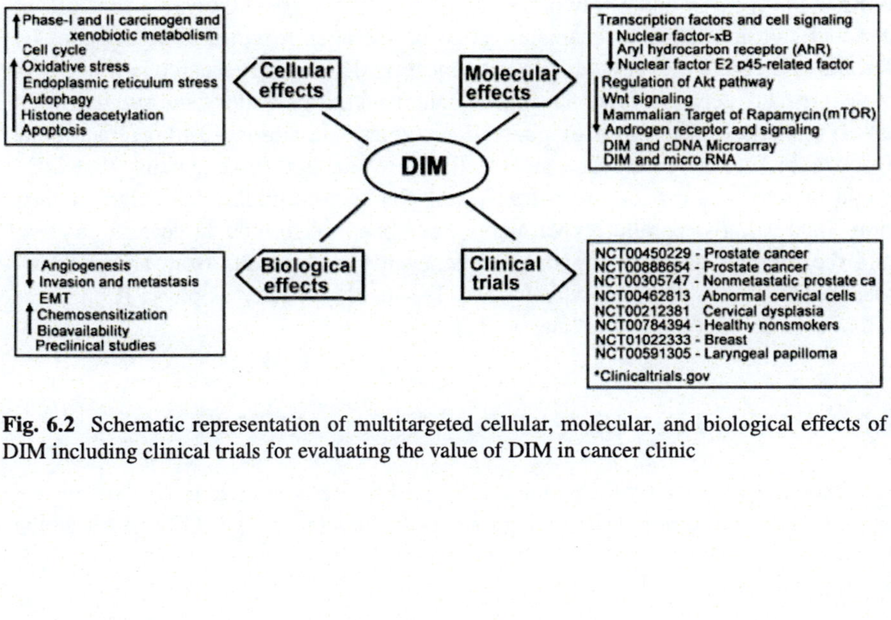

Fig. 6.2 Schematic representation of multitargeted cellular, molecular, and biological effects of DIM including clinical trials for evaluating the value of DIM in cancer clinic

6.2 Cellular Effects of DIM

6.2.1 DIM and Phase-I and II Carcinogen and Xenobiotic Metabolism

The metabolic biotransformation of lipophilic xenobiotics and endogenous hydrophobic substances, including steroids, to inactive hydrophilic waste metabolites, is mediated by the superfamily of heme-containing monooxygenases (cytochrome P450s (CYP) enzymes), and phase-II enzyme systems (GST isoenzymes, UDP-glucuronosyltransferase, sulfotransferase, and catechol O-methyltransferase) (Morse and Stoner 1993; Wattenberg 1985). Several studies point towards DIM's ability to inhibit activities of a range of CYP isoforms, as the basis of its anti-carcinogenic mechanism of action. Using various CYP-specific activity assays, DIM was found to inhibit human CYP1A1 and CYP1A2, and rat CYP2B1 (Stresser et al. 1995). In vitro studies revealed potent inhibition of CYP-mediated metabolism of ubiquitous food contaminant and hepatocarcinogen- aflatoxin B1 by DIM treatment (Stresser et al. 1995). Paradoxically, DIM is reported to interfere with regulation of estrogen-metabolizing CYP enzymes associated with cancer susceptibility. In this context, an interesting observation relates to DIM-mediated inhibition of a CYP complement- CYP3A1/2 activity (catalyzing 4-hydroxylation) that results in enhanced activity of hepatic microsomes to metabolize 17β-estradiol (E2) and estrone (E1) to less estrogenic 2-catechols, estrogenic 4-catechols and the 6-α, 6-β and 16α-hydroxy (OH) derivatives (Parkin and Malejka-Giganti 2004). This interesting finding suggests that DIM contributes to the formation of advanced level of 2-catechol metabolites (good estrogen), provides a crucial logical basis for attempting to prevent the tumorigenic process in estrogen-responsive sites. Contextually, DIM may offer more augmented benefit than currently understood, since estrogen metabolism is important to suppress viral oncogene expression, especially in infections with types 16 and 18, two "high-risk" HPV that are responsible for 70% of cervical cancers. Other mechanisms based on estrogen receptor-β target genes by DIM are emerging (Vivar et al. 2010), suggesting that further research is warranted.

Microarray gene-expression profiling data from our laboratory showed that DIM up-regulates the expression of phase-II enzymes, glutathione-S-transferase theta I and aldo-keto reductase in cancer cells (Li et al. 2003), suggesting that DIM could increase the capacity to detoxify, and thus would inhibit carcinogen activation. Interestingly, parallel experiments have been performed in several cancers, and the findings are well supported concurrently with results from animal models; specifically in rat liver, where DIM elevates the activity of phase-II enzymes (Bonnesen et al. 2001; Wortelboer et al. 1992).

6.2.2 DIM and Cell Cycle

The processes through which tumor cells proliferate is similar to that of normal cells, progressing through the four phases of cell cycle – G1, S, G2 and M, which are regulated by various cyclin-dependent kinases (CDK) and associated CDK inhibitors (CKI). Accumulating evidence suggest that DIM causes a predominant G1 cytostatic cell cycle arrest in breast, ovarian, prostate, colon, thyroid cancer cells, along with HUVEC cells (Chang et al. 2005; Chang et al. 2006; Choi et al. 2009; Tadi et al. 2005). A thorough analyses of G1-acting cell cycle components suggests a potent role of DIM in reducing the activity of cyclin-dependent kinase 2 (CDK2) via up-regulation in the expression of CDK inhibitor-$p21^{Cip1/Waf1}$ (Gong et al. 2006b; Hong et al. 2002b). $p21^{Cip1/Waf1}$ is a well-characterized Cip/Kip family CDK inhibitor, which induces G1-arrest and blocks entry into S-phase by inactivating CDKs or by inhibiting the activity of proliferating cell nuclear antigen, PCNA (Gartel et al. 1996). The cycle-dependent effects of BR-DIM on synchronized cancer cells progressing from G1 to S-phase has been reported previously (Chinnakannu et al. 2009), suggesting that BR-DIM induces $p27^{Kip1}$ – another CDK inhibitor in these cells. Substantial evidence indicates the role of DIM in modulating other crucial G1-acting cell cycle components in human cancer cell lines (Garikapaty et al. 2006; Rajoria et al. 2011). Included among these components are CDK4, CDK6 and cyclin D. It is also noteworthy that DIM diminishes the levels of cyclin A and D1 along with the activity of CDK4, CDC2, and CDC25C phosphatase, causing a "brake" in cell cycle progression (Choi et al. 2009). In human breast cancer cells, DIM is able to halt cell cycle progression, independent of the estrogen-dependence and p53 status of the cells (Choi et al. 2009; Jin et al. 2010; Tadi et al. 2005).

6.2.3 DIM and Oxidative Stress

Oxidative stress is a key trigger in mediating the cellular activity of DIM. Experimental evidence suggests that DIM causes hyperpolarization of mitochondrial inner membrane potential due to noncompetitive inhibition of mitochondrial H^+-ATPase, thus compromising cellular ATP level and thereby leading to generation of mitochondrial reactive oxygen species (ROS) (Gong et al. 2006b) (Fig. 6.3). The ROS production leads to activation of stress-activated pathways involving p38 and c-jun-NH2 terminal kinase with an increasing inhibitory effect on cell proliferation. It is apparent that DIM rapidly induces ROS production in breast and prostate cancer cells, hepatoma cells, leukemia cells, and primary endothelial cells. A related study involving ovarian cancer cells, reported that DIM treatment caused ROS generation, which when blocked by the compound, N-acetyl cysteine, protected the cells from DIM-mediated G2M arrest and apoptosis (Kandala and Srivastava 2010). Intriguingly, another reported revealed that low dose of DIM (1 μmol/L) could stimulate BRCA1 expression and protect normal or non-tumor-derived HMECs cells against oxidative stress, in part, through BRCA1 (Fan et al. 2009), which regulates various DNA repair processes (Gudmundsdottir and Ashworth 2006). Thus, from foregoing account one may infer that DIM like a "double edge sword" executes a protective effect (via increased ability of normal cells to repair oxidative DNA damage by upregulating BRCA1) or mounts an oxidative stress response, based on cell type specificity.

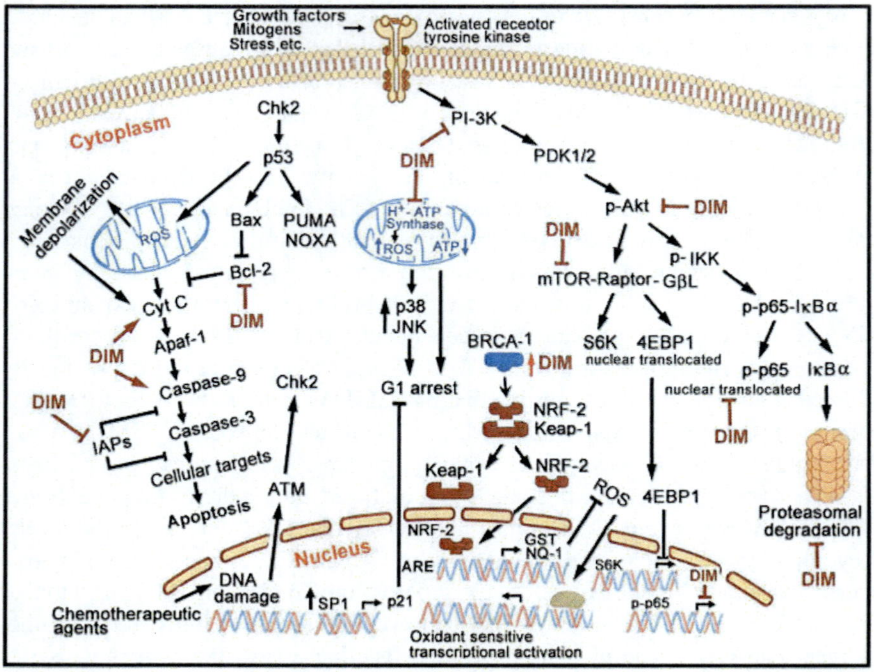

Fig. 6.3 A schematic summary of the molecular targets and cell signaling pathways altered by DIM. DIM is able to stimulate ROS production in mitochondria and downregulates Bcl-2 and IAP protein expression causing activation of the caspase cascade leading to apoptosis. DIM affects MAPK signaling mechanisms; some of the phosphorylated signal transducers translocate to the nucleus to activate transcription factors (such as AP-1) which regulate the expression of select set of genes. Multiple growth factor receptors are activated at the cell surface during cancer. Activation of these receptors activates several downstream signaling pathways. Nrf2 is released from Keap1 by activation of upstream BRCA-1 and translocates into the nucleus, where Nrf2 binds to the ARE with association of small Maf proteins resulting in the transcriptional activation of a battery of detoxification and antioxidant proteins. DIM induced BRCA1 may directly cause the cleavage of disulfide bond between Nrf2 and Keap1. The P13K-Akt, mTOR and NF-κB pathways are of significance and targets of DIM. By dephosphorylating these molecules, DIM modulates downstream signaling pathways impinging on proliferation, angiogenesis and apoptosis. NF-κB pathway is inactive as a result of the binding of p50 and p65 to I-κB. When I-κB is phosphorylated by IKKs and degraded, p50 and p65 are set free and are translocated into the nucleus to activate a specific set of genes. This pathway has been shown to be inhibited both in vitro and in vivo

6.2.4 DIM and ER Stress

There is growing evidence showing that certain pharmacologically active compounds generate stress within the endoplasmic reticulum (ER) of cells by unfolded protein response (UPR) activation, culminating into apoptosis. The induction of stress response genes – GADD153, GADD34 and GADD45A, XBP-1, GRP78, GRP94, and asparagine synthase following exposure to DIM in cervical (C33A), breast (MCF-7) and prostate (DU145) cancer cells is consistent with the activation of more than one stress response pathway coinciding with the onset of apoptosis

(Sun et al. 2004). In pancreatic cancer cells, activation of ER stress by DIM and select methylene-substituted DIMs (C-DIMs) has been hypothesized (Abdelrahim et al. 2006). A related phenomenon involving DIM-mediated alterations in Ca^{2+} homeostasis in ER and promoting apoptosis via mechanisms related to calcium homeostasis, depending on cell types, have also been proposed (Cheng et al. 2011; Savino, III et al. 2006).

6.2.5 DIM and MAP Kinase

There are three distinct, but parallel MAPK cascades identified in mammalian cells such as, extracellular signal-regulated kinase (ERK), c-Jun N-terminal kinase (JNK) and p38 (Cano and Mahadevan 1995; Juge et al. 2007). DIM up-regulates the expression and stimulates secretion of interferon-gamma (IFNγ) in human MCF-7 breast cancer cells via activation of both JNK and p38 pathways (Xue et al. 2005). This novel finding reveals another probable explanation of the anticancer effects of DIM, since it is well known that IFNγ plays an important role in preventing the development of primary and transplanted tumors. DIM activates both JNK and p38 pathways, induces phosphorylation of c-Jun and ATF-2, and increases binding of the homodimer or heterodimer of c-Jun/ATF-2 to the proximal AP-1/CREB-ATF-binding element (Gong et al. 2006b; Xue et al. 2005). An important therapeutic trait of DIM is its ability to disrupt MAPK signaling in vascular endothelial cells by functioning as a negative regulator of VEGF-stimulated MAPK activity that renders these cells insensitive to VEGF. This phenomenon leads to impairment in vasculature involving endothelial cell migration and differentiation, thereby affecting angiogenesis (Chang et al. 2006). DIM-induced activation of all three MAPK pathways in a single cell line has not been reported to date.

6.2.6 DIM and the Inhibition of Histone Deacetylation

Histone deacetylase (HDAC) inhibitors are gaining recognition as novel, therapeutically efficacious anti-tumor agents with multi-target effects including, stimulation of apoptosis. Butyrate, produced naturally in the colon by bacterial fermentation of dietary fibers has been extensively studied in colon cancer prevention and shown to inhibit histone deacetylase. It has been shown that mutations in the adenomatous polyposis coli (APC) gene confer resistance to HDAC inhibitor-induced apoptosis in colon cancer (Huang and Guo 2006). Contextually, it has been found that conventional pre-treatment of cells with DIM augment butyrate-induced apoptosis in colon cancer cells expressing mutant APC (Bhatnagar et al. 2009). Thus, combination of DIM and butyrate could potentially be an effective strategy for the prevention of colon cancer via targeting HDACs. In addition, DIM can selectively induce proteasome-mediated degradation of class I histone deacetylases (HDAC1, HDAC2, HDAC3, and HDAC8) without affecting the class II HDAC proteins in human colon cancer cells in vitro and in vivo as demonstrated using tumor xenograft recently (Li et al. 2010).

6.2.7 DIM and Inhibition of Autophagy

Autophagy is an evolutionary conserved intracellular pathway that sequesters and degrades cytosolic proteins and damaged organelles within autophagosomes, recycling substrates, so as to maintain cellular energy homeostasis under conditions of limited nutrients or stress (Fan et al. 2009). At present, it is difficult to appraise autophagy as a target for DIM-mediated chemoprevention; although limited in vitro experiments using human breast cancer cells treated with H_2O_2 and DIM provided some preliminary evidence showing that autophagy could be one of DIM-mediated mechanisms for cell death (Fan et al. 2009). Further studies are needed to characterize DIM-induced autophagy in other established models and cell lines.

6.2.8 DIM and Apoptosis

Previous studies from our laboratory as well as from others provided ample evidence in support of the anti-cancer effects of DIM in several human cancers. One interesting observation regarding DIM is its apparent selective apoptosis inducing effects in cancer cells but not on normal cells such as human keratinocytes (Chen et al. 2001), CRL2221 human prostate epithelial cells (Li et al. 2005), and human pancreatic ductal epithelial cells (Banerjee et al. 2009). DIM intervenes mechanistically by disrupting mitochondrial membrane potential and cytochrome-c release, followed by activation of caspases 3, 9 and poly(ADP-ribose) polymerase; all of which are mediated through the mitochondrial pathway (Fig. 6.3). In addition, apoptosis is accompanied by down-regulation of anti-apoptotic Bcl-2 protein and increased expression in the pro-apoptotic Bax expression following DIM treatment; supporting the role of DIM as a potential anti-cancer agent, which further underscores the potential clinical importance of DIM as an adjunct to conventional therapeutics.

The induction of apoptosis by DIM has been documented in human colon adenocarcinoma cells, S-174, Caco-2 (Bonnesen et al. 2001), HT-29, and HCT-116 (Kim et al. 2009), human esophageal adenocarcinoma cells (Seg-1 and Bic-1), breast carcinoma cells, including the highly invasive and metastatic breast cancer cells, MDA-MB-231 (Ahmad et al. 2009b; Rahman et al. 2006; Rahman and Sarkar 2005), melanoma cells (Maciejewska et al. 2009), pancreatic carcinoma cells (Ali et al. 2008; Banerjee et al. 2009), hepatoma HepG2 cells (Gong et al. 2006a), thyroid cancer cells representative of papillary (B-CPAP and 8505-C) and follicular carcinoma of the thyroid (CGTH-W-1 and ML-1) (Tadi et al. 2005), numerous human leukemia cell lines (Contractor et al. 2005), and lung cancer cells (Ichite et al. 2009). In androgen-dependent human prostate carcinoma LNCaP cells, DIM-induced apoptosis was associated with stabilization of p53 and down-regulation of NF-κB activity, resulting in decreased expression of the anti-apoptotic protein Bcl-2 (Chen et al. 2001; Nachshon-Kedmi et al. 2003; Nachshon-Kedmi et al. 2004b).

We have previously compared the effect of DIM treatment in breast cancer cell lines harboring different molecular signatures such as, over-expression of Her-2 and activated Akt [BT-20 and BT-474] and cells deficient in estrogen receptor [BT-20].

Upon treatment, DIM induced p27^{KIPI} transcript expression, as well as its nuclear localization in investigated cell lines, independent of Her-2, Akt, or estrogen receptor status, suggesting distinctive role of DIM against breast cancer (Wang et al. 2008). Similarly, another report using estrogen receptor positive (MCF-7) and negative (MDA-MB-231) cells demonstrated DIM-induced apoptosis in both cell lines independent of ER status (Hong et al. 2002a).

In addition to classical targets of apoptosis, other contemporary molecular targets have been identified and reported as being modulated by DIM. These include, p75(NTR), decreased FLICE-like-inhibitory-protein (FLIP), activation and promotion of FasL-mediated apoptosis and Prostate apoptosis response-4 (Par-4). Par-4 is a unique pro-apoptotic protein that selectively induces apoptosis in prostate cancer cells. The influence of DIM in up-regulating Par-4 in a panel of pancreatic cancer cell lines as the basis of apoptosis induction has been reported by our laboratory (Azmi et al. 2008). Additionally, DIM was found to sensitize these cells to cytotoxic action of chemotherapeutic drug such as gemcitabine, through up-regulation of Par-4 (Azmi et al. 2008). Another molecular entity, Nonsteroidal Anti-inflammatory drug-activated Gene-1 (NAG-1), is a TGF-beta super family gene associated with pro-apoptotic and anti-tumorigenic activities. Studies have shown that DIM represses cell proliferation through up-regulation of NAG-1; in addition, activating transcription factor 3 (ATF3) is known to play a pivotal role in DIM-induced NAG-1 expression in human colorectal cancer cells (Lee et al. 2005). These studies provide additional potential molecular basis for the anti-tumorigenenic effects of DIM.

A promising and unique molecular target involving inhibition of DNA topoisomerase (-I and -II alpha) by DIM, affecting mitochondrial F0F1-ATP synthase (which in turn cause depletion of the mitochondrial ATP levels), has been cited (Gong et al. 2006a; Roy et al. 2008). This molecular pathway causes a significant stimulation of mitochondrial ROS production, causing intracellular catastrophe and induction of programmed cell death, and these limited studies suggests that further development of DIM as a potential therapeutic agent is warranted.

6.3 Selective Molecular Effects of DIM

6.3.1 DIM and Transcription Factors

6.3.1.1 Nuclear Transcription Factor-κB

The nuclear transcription factor-κB (NF-κB) signaling plays critical roles in regulating cell proliferation, survival, tumor invasion, metastasis, drug resistance, and stress response. A large number of cancer cells, especially, poorly differentiated cancer cells show activated NF-κB in the nucleus, suggesting that nuclear-localized activated form of NF-κB regulates downstream genes to promote cancer cell growth. Therefore, NF-κB has emerged as a target for prevention and/or treatment of cancer. We found that DIM, or the formulated BR-DIM treatment, could restrict its nuclear localization and inactivate NF-κB DNA-binding activity in prostate (Li et al. 2005), breast (Rahman et al. 2007; Rahman et al. 2009; Wang et al. 2008), head and neck (Ali et al. 2009), and pancreatic cancer cells (Ali et al. 2008; Banerjee et al. 2009), resulting in the inhibition of transcriptional down-regulation of several NF-κB downstream genes (Fig. 6.3) causing inhibition of cell growth and inducing apoptotic cell death.

DIM has also been found to potentiate the anti-tumor activity of chemotherapeutic agents through regulation of NF-κB. It has been reported that some chemotherapeutic agents could result in the activation of NF-κB in cancer cells, and this mechanism might play a pivotal role in inducing drug resistance in cancer cells. We confirmed that NF-κB activity is significantly up-regulated by docetaxel, gemcitabine or oxaliplatin treatment, and that the NF-κB inducing activity of these agents was completely abrogated in cells pre-treated with DIM (Banerjee et al. 2009; Rahman et al. 2009). Collectively, these results clearly suggest that DIM pre-treatment, which inactivates NF-κB activity, along with other cellular effects of DIM, may contribute to enhanced cell growth inhibition and apoptosis with sub-optimal doses of cytotoxic chemotherapeutic agents with minimal side effects.

6.3.1.2 Aryl Hydrocarbon Receptor (AhR)

The AhR is a ligand-dependent transcription factor belonging to the basic helix-loop-helix/Per-ARNT-Sim family of proteins (Hankinson 1995). A variety of structurally diverse xenobiotic and bioactive food compounds can bind to AhR in a ligand-dependent manner as agonists and activate this transcription factor (Degner et al. 2009). In vitro and in vivo studies indicate that AhR ligands can inhibit formation and proliferation of breast tumors, and DIM has been reported to be a selective AhR modulator (Vivar et al. 2010). In estrogen-responsive breast cancer cells, DIM binds to AhR with lower affinity compared to AhR proto-type agonists 2,3,7,8 tetrachlorodibenzo (p) dioxin (TCDD) (Jellinck et al. 1993), and thus, by analogy bear resemblance to selective estrogen receptor modulators (SERM) used in breast cancer treatment. As studied in MCF-7 breast cancer cells, DIM reverses epigenetic activation of cyclooxygenase-2 (COX-2) expression induced by environmental (TCDD) agent, which is known to cause inflammation and tumorigenesis (Degner et al. 2009). Methyl-substituted DIM analogs with preclinical evidence against breast cancer also exhibit selective modulation of the AhR (SAhRMs) signaling in cancer cells (McDougal et al. 2001).

6.3.1.3 Nuclear Factor E2 p45-Related Factor (Nrf-2)

Nuclear factor E2 p45-related factor 2 (Nrf2), is a cap'n'collar basic leucine zipper (Bzip) transcription factor, which after activation, translocates into the nucleus and binds to the "antioxidant response element" (ARE) in conjugation with small Maf proteins and plays a central role in the regulation (basal and/or inducible expression) of several Phase 2 genes (*e.g., GST* and *NQO1*) by binding to the ARE in their promoters (Thimmulappa et al. 2002) (Fig. 6.3). DIM stimulates several Nrf2-regulated promoters, including NQO1 (an oxidoreductase), GSTα1(a glutathione S-transferase), and x-CT (cystine/glutamate transporter) (Fan et al. 2009). Our recent reports suggest a pivotal role of this transcription factor in DIM-stimulated signaling through antioxidant response element in a BRCA1-dependent manner (Fan et al. 2009).

6.3.1.4 Akt Pathway

Most human cancers display reduced expression of the Akt inhibitor, PTEN (the tumor suppressor phosphatase and tensin homologue deleted on chromosome 10). Hence, proteins regulating signaling through the phosphatidylinositol 3-kinase (PI3K)/Akt pathway are frequently activated in tumors because of the loss of PTEN (Fig. 6.3). Inhibition of phosphorylated Akt signaling sensitizes cancer cells to chemotherapy, suggesting the importance of the inhibition of phosphorylated Akt signaling as a vital therapeutic arsenal in cancer therapy. DIM showed to inhibit cancer cell growth and induces apoptosis through the inhibition of the Akt pathway in breast, prostate and pancreatic cancer cells (Banerjee et al. 2009; Bhuiyan et al. 2006; Li et al. 2005; Wang et al. 2008).

A significant finding reported by our laboratory showed the existence of a potential crosstalk between Akt, NF-κB, and androgen receptor (AR) and most interestingly, we reported that B-DIM could interrupt these cross-talks (Bhuiyan et al. 2006). In breast cancer cells with constitutively active Akt, the ability of DIM to induce apoptosis and sensitization to taxotere chemotherapy, highlights the importance of the inhibition of phosphorylated Akt signaling as clinically significant strategy (Rahman et al. 2007). In cholangiocarcinoma cells with increased constitutive phosphorylation of Akt, DIM inhibited phosphorylation of Akt and activation of FLICE-like-inhibitory-protein (FLIP) augmenting Fas-mediated apoptosis (Chen et al. 2006). We reported inhibition of the angiogenic features of human umbilical vein endothelial cells in vitro by DIM, which was correlated with the inactivation of Akt, suppression of vascular endothelial growth factor (VEGF) secretion, and the down-regulation of VEGF receptor 2 protein levels (Kong et al. 2007). In addition, we also reported that DIM inhibits the growth of breast cancer cell lines that over-express Her-2 and activated Akt, via modulation of the PI3K/Akt pathway and $p27^{Kip1}$, independent of estrogen receptor status (Wang et al. 2008), suggesting that DIM is a front runner pleiotropic agent, and thus could be useful for the prevention of tumor progression and/or treatment of cancers that have defects in multiple genes.

6.3.1.5 Mammalian Target of Rapamycin (mTOR) Pathway and DIM

Mammalian target of rapamycin (mTOR) is a serine/threonine kinase pathway that has emerged as an attractive cancer therapeutic target because it is a critical player controlling several key cellular processes e.g., cell growth, proliferation and cell division. Despite limited studies reported to date regarding DIM and the modulation of mTOR pathway, our group, using a newly recognized-Platelet-derived growth factor-D (PDGF-D) over-expressing PC3 cells (referred to as PC3 PDGF-D) provided further insights into probable mechanisms regulating this pathway. These cells exhibits rapid growth rate and enhanced cell invasion associated with the activation of mTOR and reduced Akt activity (Kong et al. 2008). Rapamycin, an inhibitor that function by decreasing mTOR protein levels, repressed mTOR activity in these cells but concomitantly resulted in the activation of Akt, which compromises the overall therapeutic effects of Rapamycin. Interestingly, we reported that B-DIM significantly inhibits both mTOR and Akt in PC3 PDGF-D cells, and this was correlated with decreased cell proliferation and invasion and also elicited other therapeutic effects by inactivation of both mTOR and Akt activity (Kong et al. 2008). In this respect, B-DIM appears to be superior to Rapamycin and other analogs that have otherwise shown some clinical activity as a single agent in a limited number of tumor types (Faivre et al. 2006).

6.3.1.6 Wnt Signaling and DIM

The canonical Wnt signaling pathway operates by stabilizing β-catenin and has emerged as an important mechanism in the regulation of cell proliferation and survival. We previously reported that in hormone-sensitive LNCaP and hormone-insensitive C4-2B prostate cancer cells, BR-DIM causes a significant increase in the phosphorylation of β-catenin, and inhibits β-catenin nuclear translocation, leading to the inhibition of cell growth and induction of apoptosis (Li et al. 2007). The results highlight the existence of a molecular cross-talk between Akt, Wnt and AR signaling in prostate cancer cells and that GSK-3β was found to be the key enzyme bridging these pathways (Li et al. 2007).

6.3.2 Androgen Receptor (AR)

As a member of the steroid receptor super-family of transcription factors, AR and its cognate natural ligand – androgen, have been implicated in the normal prostate development as well as in the growth and maintenance of castrate-resistant prostate cancer (CRPC) (Narayanan et al. 2010). Current treatment modalities for CRPC rely on therapies that target AR, since most CPRC express AR and the androgen inducible, PSA. Studies have shown that DIM function as a novel AR antagonist, represses AR function through competitive binding and employ intracellular signaling pathways to alter AR nuclear accumulation and degradation by the ubiquitin proteasome pathway (Chinnakannu et al. 2009). It has been known that FOXO3a, GSK-3β, and β-catenin are all AR co-regulators which regulate the activity of AR (Li et al. 2007) (Fig. 6.4). We reported that B-DIM inhibits FOXO3a binding to the promoter of *AR* and promotes FOXO3a binding to the $p27^{KIP1}$ promoter, resulting in alteration of AR and $p27^{KIP1}$ expression, thereby inhibiting cell proliferation and inducing apoptosis in both, androgen-sensitive and insensitive prostate cancer cells. Further these results confirmed that B-DIM-induced cell growth inhibition

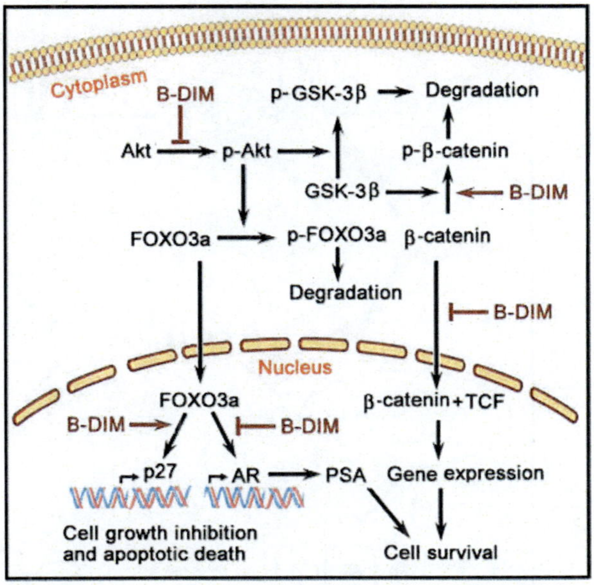

Fig. 6.4 Schematic representation of molecular effect of DIM on Akt/FOXO3a/GSK-3β/β-catenin/AR signaling. DIM acts at multiple level integrating and abrogating cross talks between molecules inhibiting proliferation and induces apoptosis in androgen dependent and independent cancer cells. A similar mechanism may be operational in breast cancer and other malignancies. Adapted from Li et al. (2007)

and apoptosis are mediated through the regulation of Akt/FOXO3a/GSK-3β/β-catenin/AR signaling, attesting that B-DIM is a promising, non-toxic agent for the treatment of not only hormone-sensitive but also metastatic CRPC.

6.3.3 DIM and MicroRNA

A class of endogenous small non-coding RNA molecules of 20–25 nucleotides in length is called microRNAs (miRNAs) that are cleaved from ~70- to 100 nucleotide hairpin pre-miRNAs precursors (Bartel 2009). Increasing evidence reveals deregulation of miRNAs expression consistent with tumorigenesis because they are key regulatory molecules in various biological and pathologic processes. There is also increasing evidence showing that over-expressed miRNAs (such *mir-17-92*), may function as oncogene and promote cancer development by negatively regulating tumor suppressor genes and/or genes that control cell differentiation or apoptosis (Zhang et al. 2007). Many studies have established this concept by discovering the up-regulation or down-regulation of specific miRNAs in various types of cancer and identifying some of their molecular targets (Casalini and Iorio 2009; Iorio et al. 2005; Iorio and Croce 2009). Experimental evidence of diet-specific miRNA biomarker profiles in different cancers is emerging. Relatively few studies have documented the effect of DIM in altering the expression of miRNAs profile. Li et al. from our laboratory assessed the expression profile of miRNAs between gemcitabine-sensitive and gemcitabine-resistant pancreatic cancer cells and showed that the miRNA expression pattern was different between these two cell lines. By

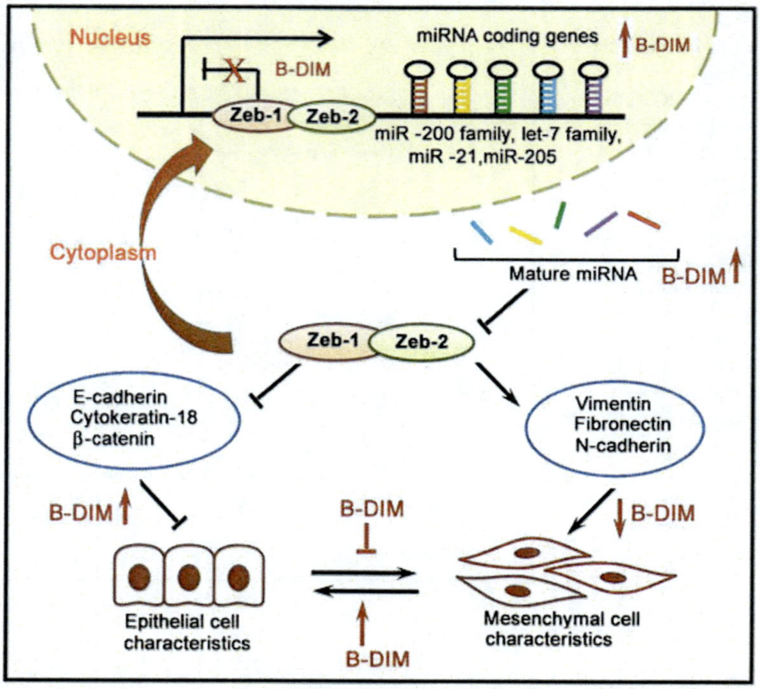

Fig. 6.5 Micro RNA, EMT and the effect of DIM in integrating reversal of EMT as described in the text

miRNA microarray and RT-PCR, we also showed that B-DIM treatments caused alterations in the expression of 28 miRNAs (Li et al. 2009). Further narrowing to miR-200 and let-7 family revealed that miR-200b, miR-200c, let-7b, let-7c, let-7d, and let-7e were all increased by B-DIM treatment in the gemcitabine-resistant cells concomitant with reversal of mesenchymal phenotype to epithelial phenotype (Fig. 6.5).

6.4 Biological Effects of DIM

6.4.1 DIM and Angiogenesis

Accumulating evidence reveals VEGF to be a major mediator of angiogenesis by targeting endothelial cells. Additionally, it is evident that the α-subunit of potent tumorigenic factor, hypoxia inducible factor-1 (HIF-1α) becomes elevated in tumors due to hypoxia, and that HIF-1α transcriptional activity contributes to tumor angiogenesis, invasion and progression. Interestingly, DIM causes a concentration-dependent decrease in proliferation, migration, invasion and capillary tube formation of cultured HUVECs and induce a G1-phase cell cycle arrest in actively proliferating HUVECs (Chang et al. 2005). Additionally, within in vivo Matrigel plug angiogenesis assay, neovascularization was inhibited up to 76% compared to vehicle control following DIM administration, testifying not only anti-angiogenic activity but DIM is active in vivo.

We explored the molecular mechanisms by which DIM inhibits angiogenesis and invasion, by assessing the role of angiogenic factors secreted by cancer cells, and reported that BR-DIM reduces the bioavailability of vascular endothelial growth factor (VEGF), resulting in reduced vascularity (angiogenesis) in vivo (Kong et al. 2007). We also found that BR-DIM treatment inhibited DNA binding activity of nuclear factor-κB (NF-κB), which is known to mediate the expression of many of its downstream target genes, including VEGF, IL-8, uPA, and MMP-9, all of which are involved in angiogenesis, invasion, and metastasis (Kong et al. 2007).

In another study from our laboratory, the tube forming capability of HUVEC cells following exposure to conditioned medium from PC3-PDGF-D cells was found to be abrogated by B-DIM treatment (Kong et al. 2008). These original findings suggested that B-DIM could serve as an efficient chemopreventive and/or therapeutic agent by inhibiting angiogenic factors in cancer cells. Additional evidence in support of anti-angiogenic effect of DIM include the citation that DIM reduces the level of hypoxia-inducible factor (HIF)-1α in hypoxic tumor cell lines, as well as HIF-1 transcriptional activity, resulting in the reduced expression of key hypoxia responsive factors such as VEGF, furin, enolase-1, glucose transporter-1 and phosphofructokinase (Riby et al. 2008). Collectively, these results extend support showing that DIM can decrease the accumulation and activity of the key angiogenesis regulatory factor-HIF-1α in hypoxic tumor cells.

6.4.2 The Role of DIM in Invasion and Metastasis

Cancer metastasis represents the primary reason for morbidity and mortality in the majority of solid tumors. Our knowledge relating to the transcriptional factors that serve as repressors in metastatic and invasion remains obscure. However, closely related to this phenomenon, the expression and activation of uPA contributes to metastasis, and high endogenous levels of uPA and its receptor, uPAR have been found in advanced metastatic cancers. It has been shown that DIM down-regulates uPA-uPAR leading to reduced production of VEGF/MMP-9 which led to the inhibition of cell growth, migration and aggressiveness of prostate and breast cancer cells (Ahmad et al. 2009a, b), suggesting the importance of uPA/uPAR in BR-DIM-mediated regulation of cancer cell growth and migration. Other metastatic regulators, including proteolytic enzymes MMP-2 and MMP-9 have been reported to be inhibited by DIM (Rajoria et al. 2011). DIM has also been reported to be potentially effective in inhibiting growth and invasion of drug resistant human cancer cells from breast, glioma and non-small cell lung cancer expressing EGFR mutant (Rahimi et al. 2010).

A common sequel to progression of breast, prostate and lung cancer is bone metastasis that leads to debilitating complications and pain. We simulated a model of experimental bone metastasis in SCID mice and noted that B-DIM treatment results in the reduction of osteoblastic and osteoclastic reactions. A closely related study reported the influence of DIM in impeding osteoclastogenesis showing reduction in the expression of several inflammatory cytokines, and the expression of RANK L, (Dong et al. 2010). Thus, DIM could additionally be useful in alleviating pain in bone metastasis and associated disorders: however, further in-depth mechanistic studies are required.

6.4.3 DIM and Epithelial Mesenchymal Transition (EMT)

For most epithelial tumors, progression towards malignancy is accompanied by a loss of epithelial differentiation and a shift towards mesenchymal phenotype is defined as "Epithelial-to-Mesenchymal Transition" (EMT) (Fig. 6.5). It has been envisaged that inhibitors of EMT or agents that could either reverse the EMT phenotype or kill EMT-type cells would constitute a novel strategy for the treatment of most cancers. DIM's ability to target major molecular players promoting EMT include increased expression of E-cadherin and decreased expression of transcription factors – ZEB1, slug, and mesenchymal marker – vimentin leading to reversal of the EMT phenotype and augmenting cancer cell death in vitro (Li et al. 2009). Furthermore, it has been reported that the morphology of MiaPaCa-2 cells changed from fibroblastoid to epithelial-like appearance after B-DIM treatment (Li et al. 2009). These limited studies are interesting because we believe that B-DIM could be useful to eradicate tumors by altering or killing the EMT-type cells, which are believed to be the root cause of tumor recurrence.

6.4.4 DIM and Preclinical Studies

DIM has not been established as a direct cause or cure for cancer. With few exceptions, most preclinical studies reported are of a kind involving combination therapy aimed at achieving a superior chemotherapeutic efficacy relative to monotherapy (chemosensitization). Agents so far tested with DIM include Taxotere, Cisplatin, Oxaliplatin, Gemcitabine, Erlotinib and TRAIL (Ali et al. 2008; Ali et al. 2009; Ali et al. 2010; Banerjee et al. 2009; Rahman et al. 2007; Rahman et al. 2009). Current knowledge related to the underlying molecular mechanism of action of DIM conferring sensitivity is limited although apoptotic response appears to be mediated through the down-regulation of NF-κB. In pancreatic cancer, we reported that DIM pretreatment could enhance the apoptotic and therapeutic effectiveness of multiple chemotherapeutic agents (gemcitabine, oxaliplatin and cisplatin) as well as targeted agents such as EGFR inhibitor – Erlotinib in a relevant orthotopic mouse model of pancreatic cancer (Ali et al. 2008; Banerjee et al. 2009). Furthermore, in a mouse xenograft model, gemcitabine and erlotinib in combination with DIM appears to be a promising strategy in future clinical trial (Ali et al. 2010). In HER2/Neu human breast cancer cells, DIM in combination with paclitaxel inhibited cell growth by 74% compared with 42 and 62% by DIM and paclitaxel alone, respectively (McGuire et al. 2006). Other combination studies using DIM have been reported in breast and prostate cancer (Ahmad et al. 2011; Rahman et al. 2007; Rahman et al. 2009). Another study evaluated synergistic effect of DIM following co-treatment with activation of death receptor pathways, suggesting its potential in cancer therapy to overcome TRAIL resistance (Zhang et al. 2005). Mechanistically, DIM sensitizes TRAIL-resistant cancer cells to TRAIL-induced apoptosis via enhancement of c-FLIP ubiquitination and proteasome-dependent degradation.

From a therapeutic viewpoint, DIM has been evaluated as a single agent in xenograft model established with TRAMP-C2, a mouse prostate cancer cell line. Of interest, intraperitoneal injections of DIM significantly diminished tumor growth accompanied by apoptosis and reduced cell proliferation relative to vehicle controls (Nachshon-Kedmi et al. 2004a). In transgenic adenocarcinoma mouse prostate (TRAMP) model, DIM feeding inhibited prostate carcinogenesis accompanied by increase in the number of terminal dUTP nick-end labeling-positive cells in the dorsolateral lobes of the prostate (Cho et al. 2011). In the context of therapeutic response to metastasis, DIM inhibited lung metastasis of 4T1 murine mammary carcinoma cells in the syngenic BALB/c mice along with reduction in the levels of matrix metalloproteinase (MMP-2 and 9), Tissue Inhibitor of Matrix Metalloproteinase-1 (TIMP-1), and the serum concentration of IL-β, IL-6 and TNF-α (Kim et al. 2009). These outcome merits serious consideration since in principle these parameters are relevant to human cancer pathogenesis and chemoprevention. The efficacy of DIM in K14-HPV16 transgenic mouse model of cervical cancer have also been evaluated and reported wherein 2,000 ppm DIM given for 12 weeks either delayed or inhibited the progression from cervical dysplasia to cervical cancer (Sepkovic et al. 2009). To seek an answer for the most effective minimum dose of DIM administration for future human studies to augment the efficacy of preventive and therapeutic HPV vaccines, the dose of 1000 ppm of DIM was extrapolated as the minimum effective and viable dose for future human studies (Sepkovic et al. 2011). This 1000 ppm DIM dose compare favorably to DIM measured in women taking either 200 or 400 mg of DIM twice daily for 4 weeks as reported earlier (Sepkovic et al. 2001).

6.5 Clinical Trials Using DIM for Cancer Therapy

Based on the information available at http//www.clinicaltrials.gov, several clinical trials are under way which mirrors the clinical usefulness of DIM in cancer patients (Table 6.1). Majority of the clinical trials focus on investigating the effects of DIM in the treatment of prostate cancer or cervical dysplasia, and one study is focused on laryngeal papilloma in children. Phase I data support the non-toxic nature of DIM in healthy volunteers (Reed et al. 2008). In Phase-I clinical trials in prostate cancer patients, BR-DIM was well tolerated with serum PSA stabilization, and a recommended B-DIM dose of 225 mg twice daily in prostate cancer was suggested

Table 6.1 Clinical trials elucidating the value of DIM in cancer clinic (Clinicaltrials.gov)

NCT ID	Status	Site/organ	Title of study and end points
NCT00888654	Recruiting	Prostate	DIM in treating patients with Stage I or Stage II prostate cancer undergoing radical prostatectomy.
NCT00450229	Completed	Prostate	Patients undergoing surgery for stage I or stage II prostate cancer.
NCT00305747	Active, not recruiting	Prostate	DIM in treating patients with non-metastatic prostate cancer has not responded to previous hormone therapy.
NCT00462813	Unknown	Cervix	DIM in treating patients with abnormal cervical cells.
NCT00212381	Unknown	Cervix	DIM for the treatment of cervical dysplasia.
NCT00784394	Completed	Healthy	DIM in healthy non-smokers.
NCT01022333	Recruiting	Breast	The potential for oral DIM supplementation to increase the production of the BRCA1 protein in BRCA1 mutation carriers.
NCT00591305	Recruiting	Papilloma	New therapy of laryngeal papilloma in children.

(Heath EI et al. 2009). This dose is being tested currently in a phase II study in our institution in collaboration with Henry Ford Health System.

A pilot study on patients with cervical intraepithelial neoplasia (CIN) grade 2 or 3 lesions has been completed with DIM at dose of 2 mg/kg/day for 12 weeks had improved CIN in 47% cases including reversion to normal stage (Del et al. 2010). Other studies regarding DIM in a clinical setting include its inclusion as an adjunct to conventional therapy for recurrent respiratory papillomatosis (Auborn 2002).

6.6 Conclusions and Perspectives

In conclusion, based on the aforementioned overview, one may conclude from multifaceted and diversified effects of DIM and its broad pharmacologic effects that results in the inhibition and/or progression of cancer development. It is of interest that these anti-proliferative and pro-apoptotic effects of DIM are apparently selective for tumor cells, as normal cells remain unaffected by this compound. The ability of DIM to sensitize tumor cells to chemotherapy may be overwhelmingly beneficial supporting to include DIM as an adjunct to conventional therapies for the treatment of human malignancies in the future. It should be emphasized that the foregoing narrative are "proof-of-principle" that needs to be evaluated in controlled clinical trials and stratify patients who will benefit the most from existing therapy.

Moreover, with emerging technologies including the use of genetically modified mouse models of human diseases and computational analysis, further molecular insights into basic, translational and clinical research will aid in the advancement of our knowledge to prove or disprove whether DIM could fulfill its promise as a chemopreventive and/or therapeutic agent against human cancers. However, the data available in the literature to-date provide strong support in favor of the use of DIM as a cancer preventive and even as therapeutic agent for human malignancies.

Acknowledgement Grant support from National Cancer Institute/NIH grants 5R01CA083695, 5R01CA108535 and 5R01CA101870 is gratefully acknowledged. The authors also express their sincere appreciation to Ms Jacqueline Schaffert for her editorial assistance.

References

Abdelrahim M, Newman K, Vanderlaag K et al (2006) 3,3′-diindolylmethane (DIM) and its derivatives induce apoptosis in pancreatic cancer cells through endoplasmic reticulum stress-dependent upregulation of DR5. Carcinogenesis 27:717–728

Ahmad A, Kong D, Sarkar SH et al (2009a) Inactivation of uPA and its receptor uPAR by 3,3′-diindolylmethane (DIM) leads to the inhibition of prostate cancer cell growth and migration. J Cell Biochem 107:516–527

Ahmad A, Kong D, Wang Z et al (2009b) Down-regulation of uPA and uPAR by 3,3′-diindolylmethane contributes to the inhibition of cell growth and migration of breast cancer cells. J Cell Biochem 108:916–925

Ahmad A, Ali S, Wang Z et al (2011) 3, 3′-diindolylmethane enhances taxotere-induced growth inhibition of breast cancer cells through down-regulation of FoxM1. Int J Cancer 129:1781–1791

Ali S, Banerjee S, Ahmad A et al (2008) Apoptosis-inducing effect of erlotinib is potentiated by 3,3′-diindolylmethane in vitro and in vivo using an orthotopic model of pancreatic cancer. Mol Cancer Ther 7:1708–1719

Ali S, Varghese L, Pereira L et al (2009) Sensitization of squamous cell carcinoma to cisplatin induced killing by natural agents. Cancer Lett 278:201–209

Ali S, Banerjee S, Schaffert JM et al (2010) Concurrent inhibition of NF-kappaB, cyclooxygenase-2, and epidermal growth factor receptor leads to greater anti-tumor activity in pancreatic cancer. J Cell Biochem 110:171–181

Auborn KJ (2002) Therapy for recurrent respiratory papillomatosis. Antivir Ther 7:1–9

Azmi AS, Ahmad A, Banerjee S et al (2008) Chemoprevention of pancreatic cancer: characterization of Par-4 and its modulation by 3,3′ diindolylmethane (DIM). Pharm Res 25:2117–2124

Banerjee S, Wang Z, Kong D et al (2009) 3,3′-Diindolylmethane enhances chemosensitivity of multiple chemotherapeutic agents in pancreatic cancer. Cancer Res 69:5592–5600

Bartel DP (2009) MicroRNAs: target recognition and regulatory functions. Cell 136:215–233

Bhatnagar N, Li X, Chen Y et al (2009) 3,3′-diindolylmethane enhances the efficacy of butyrate in colon cancer prevention through down-regulation of survivin. Cancer Prev Res (Phila Pa) 2:581–589

Bhuiyan MM, Li Y, Banerjee S et al (2006) Down-regulation of androgen receptor by 3,3′-diindolylmethane contributes to inhibition of cell proliferation and induction of apoptosis in both hormone-sensitive LNCaP and insensitive C4-2B prostate cancer cells. Cancer Res 66:10064–10072

Bonnesen C, Eggleston IM, Hayes JD (2001) Dietary indoles and isothiocyanates that are generated from cruciferous vegetables can both stimulate apoptosis and confer protection against DNA damage in human colon cell lines. Cancer Res 61:6120–6130

Cano E, Mahadevan LC (1995) Parallel signal processing among mammalian MAPKs. Trends Biochem Sci 20:117–122

Casalini P, Iorio MV (2009) MicroRNAs and future therapeutic applications in cancer. J BUON 14 Suppl 1:S17–S22

Chang X, Tou JC, Hong C et al (2005) 3,3′-Diindolylmethane inhibits angiogenesis and the growth of transplantable human breast carcinoma in athymic mice. Carcinogenesis 26:771–778

Chang X, Firestone GL, Bjeldanes LF (2006) Inhibition of growth factor-induced Ras signaling in vascular endothelial cells and angiogenesis by 3,3′-diindolylmethane. Carcinogenesis 27: 541–550

Chen DZ, Qi M, Auborn KJ et al (2001) Indole-3-carbinol and diindolylmethane induce apoptosis of human cervical cancer cells and in murine HPV16-transgenic preneoplastic cervical epithelium. J Nutr 131:3294–302

Chen Y, Xu J, Jhala N et al (2006) Fas-mediated apoptosis in cholangiocarcinoma cells is enhanced by 3,3′-diindolylmethane through inhibition of AKT signaling and FLICE-like inhibitory protein. Am J Pathol 169:1833–1842

Cheng JS, Shu SS, Kuo CC et al (2011) Effect of diindolylmethane on Ca(2^{+}) movement and viability in HA59T human hepatoma cells. Arch Toxicol 85:1257–1266

Chinnakannu K, Chen D, Li Y et al (2009) Cell cycle-dependent effects of 3,3′-diindolylmethane on proliferation and apoptosis of prostate cancer cells. J Cell Physiol 219:94–99

Cho HJ, Park SY, Kim EJ et al (2011) 3,3′-Diindolylmethane inhibits prostate cancer development in the transgenic adenocarcinoma mouse prostate model. Mol Carcinog 50:100–112

Choi HJ, Lim dY, Park JH (2009) Induction of G1 and G2/M cell cycle arrests by the dietary compound 3,3′-diindolylmethane in HT-29 human colon cancer cells. BMC Gastroenterol 9:39

Contractor R, Samudio IJ, Estrov Z et al (2005) A novel ring-substituted diindolylmethane,1,1-bis[3′-(5-methoxyindolyl)]-1-(p-t-butylphenyl) methane, inhibits extracellular signal-regulated kinase activation and induces apoptosis in acute myelogenous leukemia. Cancer Res 65: 2890–2898

Crowell JA, Page JG, Levine BS et al (2006) Indole-3-carbinol, but not its major digestive product 3,3′-diindolylmethane, induces reversible hepatocyte hypertrophy and cytochromes P450. Toxicol Appl Pharmacol 211:115–123

Degner SC, Papoutsis AJ, Selmin O et al (2009) Targeting of aryl hydrocarbon receptor-mediated activation of cyclooxygenase-2 expression by the indole-3-carbinol metabolite 3,3′-diindolylmethane in breast cancer cells. J Nutr 139:26–32

Del PG, Gudipudi DK, Montemarano N et al (2010) Oral diindolylmethane (DIM): pilot evaluation of a nonsurgical treatment for cervical dysplasia. Gynecol Oncol 116:464–467

Dong L, Xia S, Gao F et al (2010) 3,3′-Diindolylmethane attenuates experimental arthritis and osteoclastogenesis. Biochem Pharmacol 79:715–721

Faivre S, Kroemer G, Raymond E (2006) Current development of mTOR inhibitors as anticancer agents. Nat Rev Drug Discov 5:671–688

Fan S, Meng Q, Saha T et al (2009) Low concentrations of diindolylmethane, a metabolite of indole-3-carbinol, protect against oxidative stress in a BRCA1-dependent manner. Cancer Res 69:6083–6091

Garikapaty VP, Ashok BT, Tadi K et al (2006) 3,3′-Diindolylmethane downregulates pro-survival pathway in hormone independent prostate cancer. Biochem Biophys Res Commun 340: 718–725

Gartel AL, Serfas MS, Tyner AL (1996) p21 – negative regulator of the cell cycle. Proc Soc Exp Biol Med 213:138–149

Gong Y, Firestone GL, Bjeldanes LF (2006a) 3,3′-diindolylmethane is a novel topoisomerase IIalpha catalytic inhibitor that induces S-phase retardation and mitotic delay in human hepatoma HepG2 cells. Mol Pharmacol 69:1320–1327

Gong Y, Sohn H, Xue L et al (2006b) 3,3′-Diindolylmethane is a novel mitochondrial H(+)-ATP synthase inhibitor that can induce p21(Cip1/Waf1) expression by induction of oxidative stress in human breast cancer cells. Cancer Res 66:4880–4887

Gudmundsdottir K, Ashworth A (2006) The roles of BRCA1 and BRCA2 and associated proteins in the maintenance of genomic stability. Oncogene 25:5864–5874

Hankinson O (1995) The aryl hydrocarbon receptor complex. Annu Rev Pharmacol Toxicol 35:307–340

Heath EI, Heilbrun lk, Vaishampayan UN et al (2009) A phase-I dose escalation study of oral BR-DIM (BioResponse 3,3′-Diindolylmethane) in castrate-resistant, non-metastatic, PSA relapse prostate cancer patients. ASCO Meeting Genitourinary Cancer Symposium, Chicago, IL

Hong C, Firestone GL, Bjeldanes LF (2002a) Bcl-2 family-mediated apoptotic effects of 3,3′-diindolylmethane (DIM) in human breast cancer cells. Biochem Pharmacol 63:1085–1097

Hong C, Kim HA, Firestone GL et al (2002b) 3,3′-Diindolylmethane (DIM) induces a G(1) cell cycle arrest in human breast cancer cells that is accompanied by Sp1-mediated activation of p21(WAF1/CIP1) expression. Carcinogenesis 23:1297–1305

Huang X, Guo B (2006) Adenomatous polyposis coli determines sensitivity to histone deacetylase inhibitor-induced apoptosis in colon cancer cells. Cancer Res 66:9245–9251

Ichite N, Chougule MB, Jackson T et al (2009) Enhancement of docetaxel anticancer activity by a novel diindolylmethane compound in human non-small cell lung cancer. Clin Cancer Res 15:543–552

Iorio MV, Croce CM (2009) MicroRNAs in cancer: small molecules with a huge impact. J Clin Oncol 27:5848–5856

Iorio MV, Ferracin M, Liu CG et al (2005) MicroRNA gene expression deregulation in human breast cancer. Cancer Res 65:7065–7070

Jacobs IC, Zeligs MA (1999) Facilitated absorption of a hydrophobic dietary ingredient. Proc Int Symp Control Rel Bioact Mater 26:958–959

Jacobs IC, Zeligs MA (2000) New formulation strategies for bioavailability enhancement of two poorly absorbed phytonutrient supplements: diindolylmethane and yohimbine bark extract. Proc Int Symp Control Rel Bioact Mater 27:1324–1325

Jellinck PH, Forkert PG, Riddick DS et al (1993) Ah receptor binding properties of indole carbinols and induction of hepatic estradiol hydroxylation. Biochem Pharmacol 45:1129–1136

Jemal A, Bray F, Center MM et al (2011) Global cancer statistics. CA Cancer J Clin 61:69–90

Jin Y, Zou X, Feng X (2010) 3,3′-Diindolylmethane negatively regulates Cdc25A and induces a G2/M arrest by modulation of microRNA 21 in human breast cancer cells. Anticancer Drugs 21:814–822

Juge N, Mithen RF, Traka M (2007) Molecular basis for chemoprevention by sulforaphane: a comprehensive review. Cell Mol Life Sci 64:1105–1127

Kandala PK, Srivastava SK (2010) Activation of checkpoint kinase 2 by 3,3′-diindolylmethane is required for causing G2/M cell cycle arrest in human ovarian cancer cells. Mol Pharmacol 78:297–309

Kim EJ, Shin M, Park H et al (2009) Oral administration of 3,3′-diindolylmethane inhibits lung metastasis of 4T1 murine mammary carcinoma cells in BALB/c mice. J Nutr 139:2373–2379

Kong D, Li Y, Wang Z et al (2007) Inhibition of angiogenesis and invasion by 3,3′-diindolylmethane is mediated by the nuclear factor-kappaB downstream target genes MMP-9 and uPA that regulated bioavailability of vascular endothelial growth factor in prostate cancer. Cancer Res 67:3310–3319

Kong D, Banerjee S, Huang W et al (2008) Mammalian target of rapamycin repression by 3,3′-diindolylmethane inhibits invasion and angiogenesis in platelet-derived growth factor-D-overexpressing PC3 cells. Cancer Res 68:1927–1934

Lee SH, Kim JS, Yamaguchi K et al (2005) Indole-3-carbinol and 3,3′-diindolylmethane induce expression of NAG-1 in a p53-independent manner. Biochem Biophys Res Commun 328:63–69

Li Y, Li X, Sarkar FH (2003) Gene expression profiles of I3C- and DIM-treated PC3 human prostate cancer cells determined by cDNA microarray analysis. J Nutr 133:1011–1019

Li Y, Chinni SR, Sarkar FH (2005) Selective growth regulatory and pro-apoptotic effects of DIM is mediated by AKT and NF-kappaB pathways in prostate cancer cells. Front Biosci 10:236–243

Li Y, Wang Z, Kong D et al (2007) Regulation of FOXO3a/beta-catenin/GSK-3beta signaling by 3,3′-diindolylmethane contributes to inhibition of cell proliferation and induction of apoptosis in prostate cancer cells. J Biol Chem 282:21542–21550

Li Y, VandenBoom TG, Kong D et al (2009) Up-regulation of miR-200 and let-7 by natural agents leads to the reversal of epithelial-to-mesenchymal transition in gemcitabine-resistant pancreatic cancer cells. Cancer Res 69:6704–6712

Li Y, Li X, Guo B (2010) Chemopreventive agent 3,3′-diindolylmethane selectively induces proteasomal degradation of class I histone deacetylases. Cancer Res 70:646–654

Maciejewska D, Rasztawicka M, Wolska I et al (2009) Novel 3,3′-diindolylmethane derivatives: synthesis and cytotoxicity, structural characterization in solid state. Eur J Med Chem 44: 4136–4147

McDougal A, Gupta MS, Morrow D et al (2001) Methyl-substituted diindolylmethanes as inhibitors of estrogen-induced growth of T47D cells and mammary tumors in rats. Breast Cancer Res Treat 66:147–157

McGuire KP, Ngoubilly N, Neavyn M et al (2006) 3,3′-diindolylmethane and paclitaxel act synergistically to promote apoptosis in HER2/Neu human breast cancer cells. J Surg Res 132:208–213

Morse MA, Stoner GD (1993) Cancer chemoprevention: principles and prospects. Carcinogenesis 14:1737–1746

Nachshon-Kedmi M, Yannai S, Haj A et al (2003) Indole-3-carbinol and 3,3′-diindolylmethane induce apoptosis in human prostate cancer cells. Food Chem Toxicol 41:745–752

Nachshon-Kedmi M, Fares FA, Yannai S (2004a) Therapeutic activity of 3,3′-diindolylmethane on prostate cancer in an in vivo model. Prostate 61:153–160

Nachshon-Kedmi M, Yannai S, Fares FA (2004b) Induction of apoptosis in human prostate cancer cell line, PC3, by 3,3′-diindolylmethane through the mitochondrial pathway. Br J Cancer 91:1358–1363

Narayanan R, Yepuru M, Szafran AT et al (2010) Discovery and mechanistic characterization of a novel selective nuclear androgen receptor exporter for the treatment of prostate cancer. Cancer Res 70:842–851

Parkin DR, Malejka-Giganti D (2004) Differences in the hepatic P450-dependent metabolism of estrogen and tamoxifen in response to treatment of rats with 3,3′-diindolylmethane and its parent compound indole-3-carbinol. Cancer Detect Prev 28:72–79

Rahimi M, Huang KL, Tang CK (2010) 3,3′-Diindolylmethane (DIM) inhibits the growth and invasion of drug-resistant human cancer cells expressing EGFR mutants. Cancer Lett 295:59–68

Rahman KW, Sarkar FH (2005) Inhibition of nuclear translocation of nuclear factor-{kappa}B contributes to 3,3′-diindolylmethane-induced apoptosis in breast cancer cells. Cancer Res 65:364–371

Rahman KW, Li Y, Wang Z et al (2006) Gene expression profiling revealed survivin as a target of 3,3′-diindolylmethane-induced cell growth inhibition and apoptosis in breast cancer cells. Cancer Res 66:4952–4960

Rahman KM, Ali S, Aboukameel A et al (2007) Inactivation of NF-kappaB by 3,3′-diindolylmethane contributes to increased apoptosis induced by chemotherapeutic agent in breast cancer cells. Mol Cancer Ther 6:2757–2765

Rahman KM, Banerjee S, Ali S et al (2009) 3,3′-Diindolylmethane enhances taxotere-induced apoptosis in hormone-refractory prostate cancer cells through survivin down-regulation. Cancer Res 69:4468–4475

Rajoria S, Suriano R, George A et al (2011) Estrogen induced metastatic modulators MMP-2 and MMP-9 are targets of 3,3′-diindolylmethane in thyroid cancer. PLoS One 6:e15879

Reed GA, Arneson DW, Putnam WC et al (2006) Single-dose and multiple-dose administration of indole-3-carbinol to women: pharmacokinetics based on 3,3′-diindolylmethane. Cancer Epidemiol Biomarkers Prev 15:2477–2481

Reed GA, Sunega JM, Sullivan DK et al (2008) Single-dose pharmacokinetics and tolerability of absorption-enhanced 3,3′-diindolylmethane in healthy subjects. Cancer Epidemiol Biomarkers Prev 17:2619–2624

Riby JE, Firestone GL, Bjeldanes LF (2008) 3,3′-diindolylmethane reduces levels of HIF-1alpha and HIF-1 activity in hypoxic cultured human cancer cells. Biochem Pharmacol 75:1858–1867

Roy A, Ganguly A, BoseDasgupta S et al (2008) Mitochondria-dependent reactive oxygen species-mediated programmed cell death induced by 3,3′-diindolylmethane through inhibition of F0F1-ATP synthase in unicellular protozoan parasite Leishmania donovani. Mol Pharmacol 74: 1292–1307

Savino JA, III, Evans JF, Rabinowitz D et al (2006) Multiple, disparate roles for calcium signaling in apoptosis of human prostate and cervical cancer cells exposed to diindolylmethane. Mol Cancer Ther 5:556–563

Sepkovic DW, Bradlow HL, Bell M (2001) Quantitative determination of 3,3′-diindolylmethane in urine of individuals receiving indole-3-carbinol. Nutr Cancer 41:57–63

Sepkovic DW, Stein J, Carlisle AD et al (2009) Diindolylmethane inhibits cervical dysplasia, alters estrogen metabolism, and enhances immune response in the K14-HPV16 transgenic mouse model. Cancer Epidemiol Biomarkers Prev 18:2957–2964

Sepkovic DW, Stein J, Carlisle AD et al (2011) Results from a dose response study using 3, 3′-diindolylmethane in the K14-HPV16 transgenic mouse model: Cervical histology. Cancer Prev Res (Phila) 4:890–896

Stresser DM, Bjeldanes LF, Bailey GS et al (1995) The anticarcinogen 3,3′-diindolylmethane is an inhibitor of cytochrome P-450. J Biochem Toxicol 10:191–201

Sun S, Han J, Ralph WM, Jr et al (2004) Endoplasmic reticulum stress as a correlate of cytotoxicity in human tumor cells exposed to diindolylmethane in vitro. Cell Stress Chaperones 9:76–87

Tadi K, Chang Y, Ashok BT et al (2005) 3,3′-Diindolylmethane, a cruciferous vegetable derived synthetic anti-proliferative compound in thyroid disease. Biochem Biophys Res Commun 337:1019–1025

Thimmulappa RK, Mai KH, Srisuma S et al (2002) Identification of Nrf2-regulated genes induced by the chemopreventive agent sulforaphane by oligonucleotide microarray. Cancer Res 62:5196–5203

Vivar OI, Saunier EF, Leitman DC et al (2010) Selective Activation of Estrogen Receptor-{beta} Target Genes by 3,3′-Diindolylmethane. Endocrinology 151:1662–1667

Wang Z, Yu BW, Rahman KM et al (2008) Induction of growth arrest and apoptosis in human breast cancer cells by 3,3-diindolylmethane is associated with induction and nuclear localization of p27kip. Mol Cancer Ther 7:341–349

Wattenberg LW (1985) Chemoprevention of cancer. Cancer Res 45:1–8

Wortelboer HM, de Kruif CA, van Iersel AA et al (1992) Acid reaction products of indole-3-carbinol and their effects on cytochrome P450 and phase II enzymes in rat and monkey hepatocytes. Biochem Pharmacol 43:1439–1447

Xue L, Firestone GL, Bjeldanes LF (2005) DIM stimulates IFNgamma gene expression in human breast cancer cells via the specific activation of JNK and p38 pathways. Oncogene 24: 2343–2353

Zhang S, Shen HM, Ong CN (2005) Down-regulation of c-FLIP contributes to the sensitization effect of 3,3′-diindolylmethane on TRAIL-induced apoptosis in cancer cells. Mol Cancer Ther 4:1972–1981

Zhang B, Pan X, Cobb GP et al (2007) microRNAs as oncogenes and tumor suppressors. Dev Biol 302:1–12

Chapter 7
Mechanism of Action of the Anti-cancer Agent, Triptolide

Veena Sangwan and Ashok K. Saluja

Abstract Triptolide, a dipertene triepoxide isolated from the roots of the Chinese herb *Tripterygium wilfordii* Hook F., is a promising anti-cancer agent. While its role as a promoter of cell death, both in vivo and in vitro, in various cancers is well established, the mechanism by which it induces cell death in cancer cells is not well understood, and has therefore been the subject of intense interest in the past decade. Studies to date have shown that triptolide acts in a pleiotropic fashion, resulting in decrease of HSP70 expression, affecting calcium release, causing lysosomal membrane depolarization, inhibiting NFκB activity, iNOS and Cox-2 expression, as well as acting as a transcription inhibitor and an anti-angiogenesis factor. In this review, we discuss the possible modes of action of triptolide in various cancers, as well as a novel compound derived from triptolide currently being prepared for Phase I clinical trials.

Keywords Triptolide · Cancer · HSP70 · NFκB · Calcium · Lysosome · iNOS · Cox-2

7.1 Introduction

The search for novel efficacious anti-cancer drugs has led to the use of natural plant-derived compounds as anti-proliferative agents causing tumor regression. Triptolide, a dipertene triepoxide isolated from the roots of the Chinese herb *Tripterygium wilfordii* Hook F. (family Celastraceae), is one such compound gaining prominence in the field of anti-cancer therapy. *Tripterygium wilfordii*, native to southern China and Taiwan, has been used as an anti-inflammatory agent for diseases such as rheumatoid arthritis for centuries in China. It was first isolated and structurally characterized in 1972 (Carter et al. 2006) and has been used as an immunosuppressant in patients that have undergone organ and tissue transplantation. Recently, triptolide has been shown to have anti-tumor properties leading to the suppression of growth and induction of apoptosis in a broad range of human tumor cells. Underscoring its efficacy as an anti-tumor agent, triptolide is capable of acting synergistically with

A.K. Saluja (✉)
Department of Surgery, University of Minnesota, Minneapolis, MN, USA
e-mail: asaluja@umn.edu

F.H. Sarkar (ed.), *Nutraceuticals and Cancer*, DOI 10.1007/978-94-007-2630-7_7,

conventional therapeutic drugs by sensitizing cells to Apo2L/TRAIL- and TNF-α-induced cell death (Borja-Cacho et al. 2010; Carter et al. 2008). However, despite evidence supporting the use of triptolide as an anti-cancer agent, our knowledge regarding the mechanism of its action is limited.

7.2 Triptolide as an Anti-cancer Agent in Various Cancers

Recent reports highlighting triptolide as a potent anti-tumor agent come from its ability to act on different cancers. In vivo, triptolide prevents colitis-induced colon cancer, and in vitro, colon cancer cell lines, such as SW480, Caco-2, HT-29 and HCT116, exhibit a decrease in both invasive and migratory potential its presence (Johnson et al. 2011; Ko et al. 2007; Wang et al. 2009). A soluble derivative of triptolide, PG490-88 also causes tumor regression in xenograft mouse models induced by the metastatic COLO205 cell line (Fidler et al. 2003).

In support of its efficacy as a broad spectrum chemotherapeutic agent, triptolide decreases human breast cancer cell line (MDA-435)-induced tumor size in vivo in subcutaneous mouse models, and compares favorably with other known chemotherapeutic agents against breast cancer such as Adriamycin, mitomycin and cisplatin. Interestingly, triptolide is effective in causing cytotoxicity, both in vivo and in vitro, in taxol-resistant cells over-expressing MDR-1, believed to be responsible for the development of drug resistance (Yang et al. 2003). Although breast tumor cell lines showed potent cytotoxicity in a panel of mammalian cell lines, in vivo, triptolide is unable to decrease tumor growth at concentrations of 25 μg/kg body weight injected three times per week (Shamon et al. 1997), suggesting cancer-specific targeting of the compound. Triptolide has also been used as a cytotoxicity-inducing agent in gastric cancer cell lines of varying p53 status, wherein a functional p53 is required for the pro-apoptotic effect of this compound (Jiang et al. 2001). Assessment of triptolide as a potential chemotherapy for acute myeloid leukemia has been tested on patient samples and shown to cause apoptosis in AML-blasts tested, but no substantial loss of viability was observed in normal bone marrow. Triptolide was able to lower the IC_{50} of arabinoside-C- resistant patients, suggesting a potential role for the compound in lowering drug resistance (Carter et al. 2006). A further report by the same group has demonstrated that triptolide sensitizes AML cells to TRAIL-induced apoptosis by abrogation of the anti-apoptotic protein XIAP, and an increase of the death receptor, DR5 (Carter et al. 2008). Efficacy of triptolide in vitro has been demonstrated in the cervical carcinoma cells (Wang et al. 2006; Westerheide et al. 2006), and both in vivo and in vitro in neuroblastoma cell lines, N2a and SKNSH (Antonoff et al. 2009), cholangiocarcinoma (Clawson et al. 2010), as well as osteosarcoma, lung and prostate cancer (unpublished data, Saluja lab). Pancreatic cancer, the fourth leading cause of cancer related deaths in the United States, with a 5-year survival of less than 5%, is also a target for triptolide. Using a pancreatic cancer cell lines of varying metastatic potential, such as Panc-1, MIA Paca-2, and the highly metastatic S2VP-10, it has been shown that triptolide is able to induce cytotoxicity, as well as cause tumor regression (Figs. 7.1 and 7.2) (Aghdassi et al. 2007; Phillips et al. 2007; Wang et al. 2006). Most importantly, triptolide is unable to induce significant cell death in normal pancreatic cells (Phillips et al. 2007), highlighting its specificity as a chemotherapeutic agent (Fig. 7.1).

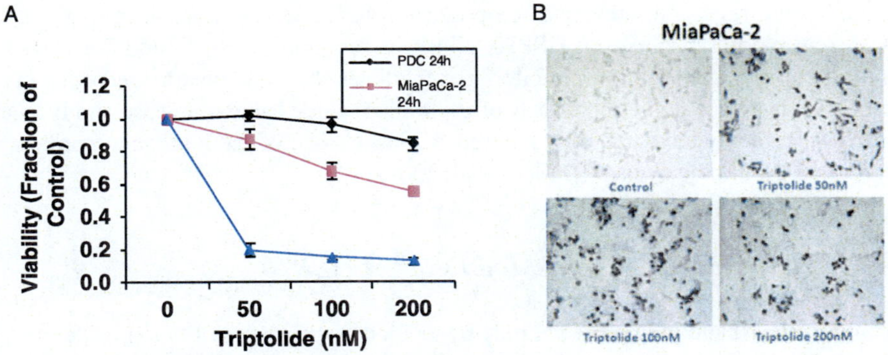

Fig. 7.1 (**a**) Decreased viability (MTT Assay) of MIA PaCa-2 cells after 24 h of treatment with triptolide. Note that triptolide does not affect the viability of normal pancreatic ductal cells (PDC). (**b**) Increased apoptosis of MIA PaCa-2 cells treated with triptolide for 48 h as determined by TUNEL staining

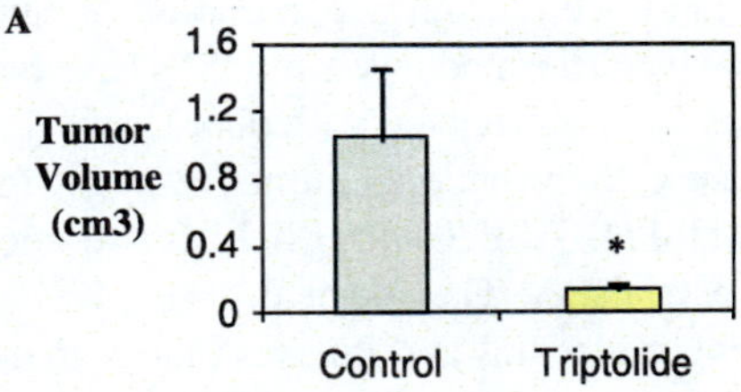

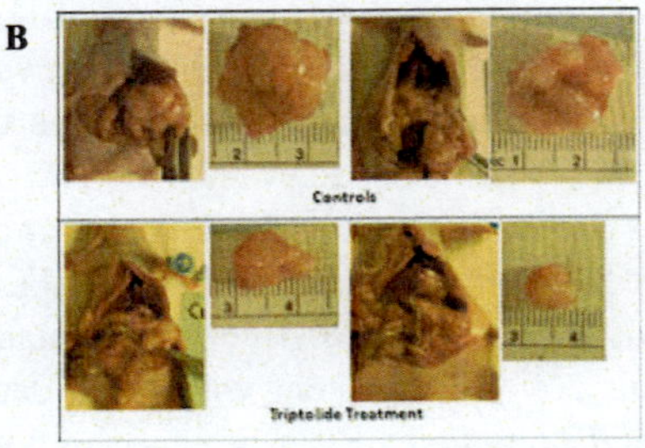

C

Organ	Control	Triptolide
Spleen	4/8	0/8 *
Liver	2/8	1/8
Gall Bladder	1/8	0/8
Kidney	2/8	0/8
Intestine	5/8	0/8 *
Total Number of Organs Invaded	14 *	1

Fig. 7.2 Triptolide decreases in vivo tumor growth in nude mice. (**a**) Mice with orthotopic MIA PaCa-2 tumors were given daily triptolide injections (0.2 mg/kg) for 60 days. Tumor volume was significantly reduced compared with controls injected with vehicle (DMSO) alone (control). In addition, our preliminary macroscopic observations indicate that triptolide also reduces metastases. (**b**) Representative photographs of tumors dissected from the pancreas and corresponding photo of tumors in situ. $*p<0.05$; $n=7$ (**c**) Triptolide markedly reduced the locoregional spread of pancreatic cancer

7.3 Mechanism of Triptolide Action

The potential of triptolide as a chemotherapeutic agent is supported by numerous studies using cell lines representing a wide range of cancers mentioned in the previous section of this review. However, the mechanism by which this compound carries out its pro-apoptotic function in cancer cells is not well understood. A review of the literature reveals a number of proposed mechanisms of action, including, but not exclusive to, an effect on HSP70, NFκB, Cox-2 and iNOS. In addition, triptolide acts as a transcription inhibitor, and mediates the inflammatory response in cancer cells. Other suggested effects of triptolide include calcium release and lysosomal membrane depolarization, assayed by an increase of the lysosomal marker, cathepsin B, into the cytosol (Dudeja et al. 2009).

7.3.1 Triptolide as a Down-Modulator of HSP70

Tumor cells expand in number not only by an increase in their ability to proliferate, but also in a decrease in rate of cell attrition. Acquired resistance towards apoptosis is a hallmark of almost all types of cancer. Early studies show that activation of HSPs via thermal stress led to a decrease in response to subsequent chemotherapeutic treatments. It was only later that a more general role of HSPs as pro-survival proteins upregulated in cancers began to emerge. It is currently believed that an increase in HSPs protects cancer cells from accumulation of misfolded proteins, resulting in increased cell survival. Elevated levels of HSPs have been shown to be a biomarker for various cancers and is correlated with poor survival, therefore, down-modulation of HSPs in cancer cells provide an attractive target for chemotherapy. Among the HSPs, the role of HSP90, HSP70 and HSP27 as anti-apoptotic promoters of cancer cell growth is well established (Garrido et al. 2006). HSPs also regulate the activity of important signaling molecules and kinases that promote cancer including NFκB, p53, Raf1, Akt and steroid aporeceptors. Given the importance of HSPs in cell survival, several cancer strategies have focused on down-regulation of heat shock proteins as a means to cause cell death in cancer cells. Specifically, over-expression of HSP70 in cancer cell lines as compared to normal cells is believed to prevent cell death in cancer cells. This finding is clinically relevant since HSP70 levels in human pancreatic tumor specimens were higher than the adjacent margins (Aghdassi et al. 2007). Similar increase in HSP70 expression has also been observed in hepatocellular carcinoma, and this increase in HSP70 levels correlates with poor outcome (Joo et al. 2005; Li et al. 2007). Consistent with these data, decrease in the levels of HSP70 either by HSP70-targeted siRNA or pharmacological inhibitors like quercetin and triptolide causes cell death in pancreatic cancer cells (Aghdassi et al. 2007; Antonoff et al. 2009; Dudeja et al. 2009; Phillips et al. 2007). Triptolide decreases the levels of both HSP70 mRNA and protein in a time and dose dependent fashion in both pancreatic cancer and neuroblastoma cell lines, but does not affect cell viability in normal cells (Aghdassi et al. 2007; Antonoff et al. 2009; Dudeja et al. 2009; Phillips et al. 2007). Induction of cell death takes place via apoptosis in MIA PaCa-2, Panc-1 and the neuroblastoma cells, N2a and SKNSH, as measured by an increase in Annexin-V positivity, a hallmark of early apoptosis, and caspase 3/9 activation (Aghdassi et al. 2007; Antonoff et al. 2009; Dudeja et al. 2009; Phillips et al. 2007). Similar efficacy of anti-HSP70 therapy has been reported in other tumors. The HSP70 inhibitor, quercetin, decreased tumor growth and angiogenesis in mice with lung, hepatoma and colon cancer (Sherman and Multhoff 2007), and inhibition of HSP70 by anti-sense causes tumor regression in breast, colon and gliomas (Garrido et al. 2006). However, quercetin, although an effective anti-cancer therapy, shows non-specific toxicity and a high efficacious dose (50 mg/kg/day) of this compound precludes its use in the clinic. Making triptolide an even more attractive target is its ability to prevent tumor progression in vivo in several cancers, including the ones reported above, such as osteosarcoma, prostate and lung cancer, at 0.2–0.3 mg/kg concentrations (unpublished data, Saluja group).

Evaluation of the mechanism by which HSP70 induces cell death has shown that its downregulation can inhibit both death receptor-mediated extrinsic and intracellular stress-mediated intrinsic pathways. Recent studies also suggest that HSP70 acts simultaneously at multiple points in the cell, both at the pre-mitochondrial events which result in cytochrome c release, as well as events downstream such as the interaction of cytosolic cytochrome c with apoptosis protease-activating factor-1 (APAF-1) and pro-caspase-9 (Phillips et al. 2007; Li et al. 1997).

7.3.2 Triptolide Causes Calcium Release in Cancer Cells

The calcium ion (Ca^{2+}) regulates various cell processes ranging from cellular proliferation to apoptosis, as well as cancer-relevant pathways such as metastasis, invasion and angiogenesis (Monteith et al. 2007). Increased expression of calcium channels and pumps have been used as biomarkers in cancer, and identified as anti-cancer therapeutic targets, since they show restricted tissue distribution. Sustained increase in cytosolic Ca^{2+} levels can trigger cell death or deregulate potential tumorigenic pathways that are dependent on Ca^{2+}. Therefore, therapies, of which triptolide is one, that result in an increase in levels of cytosolic Ca^{2+} would activate apoptotic events in cancer cells. Treatment with triptolide increases cytosolic Ca^{2+} in the pancreatic cancer cell lines, MIA PaCa-2 and Panc-1. This increase in cytosolic Ca^{2+} is attributed to a decrease in HSP70 levels in cells, as quercetin, a known HSP70 inhibitor, as well as siRNA against HSP70 are able to elicit similar increases in Ca^{2+} levels in the cytosol. The efficacy of triptolide in inducing cytotoxicity is dependent upon Ca^{2+} release since chelation of Ca^{2+} using BAPTA-AM decreases the ability of triptolide to induce apoptosis, as seen by a significant decrease in caspase-3 activation and Annexin V positivity (Dudeja et al. 2009). However, intracellular Ca^{2+} chelation is unable to provide complete protection against cell death, leading to the conclusion that HSP70/triptolide induced cell death by other mechanisms also. In support of this data, triptolide-induced cell-death is delayed in the absence of Ca^{2+} (Leuenroth and Crews 2005).

7.3.3 Triptolide Causes Lysosomal Depolarization

Lysosomes are cytoplasmic membrane enclosed organelles which contain hydrolytic enzymes such as proteases, lipases, nucleases, glycosidases, phospholipases, phosphatases and sulfatases active at low pH (<5) (Luzio et al. 2007). Several degradative pathways, including receptor endocytosis, and bacteria and apoptotic cells converge at the lysosome where they are degraded. Upon release of the hydrolytic enzymes from the lysosome, indiscriminate degradation of cellular components results in cell death. Lysosomal proteases associated with cell death are those that can function at neutral pH, such as cathepsin B, cathepsin D and cathepsin L. Complete permeabilization of the lysosome promotes necrosis, whereas partial depolarization results in apoptosis. Inhibition of HSP70 either using HSP70-specific siRNA, or HSP70 inhibitors, namely triptolide and quercetin, results in lysosomal depolarization, as measured by the release of cathepsin B into the cytosol in pancreatic cancer cells. Inhibition of cathepsin B using the cathepsin B inhibitor CA074me results in protection against cell death. However, similar to calcium chelation, the protection against apoptosis is incomplete. In the presence of inhibitors against both cytosolic increase in calcium and cathepsin release, protection against triptolide-induced cell death is additive, but still not complete as measured by increase in cell viability and decrease in caspase-3 activation (Dudeja et al. 2009). These data show that although both calcium release and cathepsin B activation are important for cell death, both pathways are independent of each other (Dudeja et al. 2009), and suggest several triptolide-induced mechanisms of induction of cell death. In support of the role of triptolide in lysosomal permeabilization, in a recent article, Messina and Halaby hypothesize that triptolide-induced oxidative stress may result in lysosomal permeabilization, leading to caspase activation and cell death in breast cancer cells (Messina and Halaby 2011).

7.3.4 Triptolide as a Modulator of NF-κB Activity

NFκB is a transcription factor comprising of closely related protein dimers that bind to a common sequence motif known as the κB site (Ghosh et al. 1998). NF-κB regulates cell survival by the activation of several anti-apoptotic factors such as cellular inhibitors of apoptosis (cIAP), caspase-8/FADD-like-IL-1β-converting enzyme inhibitory protein (FLIP), and members of the BCL2 family (Karin and Lin 2002). Additionally, constitutive action of NF-κB has been associated with resistance to anti-cancer drugs (Wang et al. 1999), and promotion of angiogenesis (Huang et al. 2000).

Several studies have shown that triptolide inhibits TNF-α and IL-1β-induced transcription at a level after NFκB binding to DNA. It is suggested that triptolide may interfere with p65 modifications or recruitment of a transcriptional cofactor. Using HeLa cells in a transient luciferase assay to detect NFκB activation in the presence of TNF-a, Leuenroth and Crews demonstrated that at concentrations of 25 nM at which triptolide induces cell death at 24 h, no effect on NFκB activity was observed 6 h post-triptolide treatment, whereas at 50 nM, there was a 20% decrease in NFκB activity. However, triptolide effectively inhibits cell growth in a dose-dependent manner in multiple myeloma cell lines exhibiting constitutive activation of NF-κB, and is associated with suppression of NF-κB in these cells (Yinjun et al. 2005). Inhibition of NF-κB activation, either in the presence of its inhibitor, MG132, or by triptolide, is shown to sensitize lung cancer cells to TRAIL-mediated apoptosis (Lee et al. 2002). By its ability to block NF-κB activation, triptolide is able to sensitize TNF-α resistant cell lines to TNF-α induced apoptosis (Lee et al. 1999).

7.3.5 *Triptolide as a Transcriptional Inhibitor*

Cancer cells have defects in regulatory circuits that govern normal cell function and homeostasis. Triptolide is a compound that has been shown to target several transcription factors know to regulate cell signaling and proliferation, including NFκB, c-myc, STAT1, Bcl-2, cyclins and CDK1. Recent data has shown that HSF1, a transcriptional modulator of HSP70 and HSP27, is overexpressed in pancreatic cancer patients when compared to adjacent normal tissue (Dudeja et al. 2011). Treatment with triptolide causes downregulation of HSF1, and knockdown using HSF1-specific siRNA results in cell death of pancreatic cancer cells as well as a decrease in RNA and protein levels of its downstream targets (Dudeja et al. 2011).

Since triptolide downregulates several key transcription factors and affects multiple aspects of cell function, investigation into its role as an overall transcriptional regulator suggest that it is a general transcription blocker of newly formed mRNA (McCallum et al. 2007). Its ability to induce transcriptional arrest was assessed by the rounding of nuclear speckles in HeLa cells, which represented transcriptional arrest. This rounding was associated with a decrease in RNA Polymerase II CTD Ser2 phosphorylation, and was accompanied by calcium-independent changes to nuclear substructure (Leuenroth and Crews 2008). Microarray studies on triptolide-treated A549 cells show that 169 genes are over-expressed and 1,511 genes are under-expressed in response to triptolide. The authors suggest that triptolide primarily affects short-lived mRNA, through its ability to stimulate proteosomal degradation of RNA-polymerase II subunit, RBP1 (Vispe et al. 2009). Microarray data from the same study show that the mode of action of triptolide on the NCI-60 panel of cell lines is different from other known chemotherapeutic compounds (Vispe et al. 2009). However, these data are based on treatment of cells with high doses of triptolide (22.5 fold higher than the EC50 value for this cell line). A recent paper by Titov et al. proposes that triptolide covalently binds XPB, a subunit of transcription factor TFIIH, resulting in the inhibition of RNA Polymerase II. The authors based their conclusions on in vitro experiments carried out at 10–20 μM concentration of triptolide. In vitro studies on cancer cell lines typically use a nanomolar range of triptolide for assaying decrease in cell viability. Phillips et al. have shown that a dose of 200 nM of triptolide exhibits an effect on normal pancreatic cells 48 h post-treatment (Phillips et al. 2007). It is therefore not surprising that high concentrations of triptolide causes transcriptional arrest. A careful study using low doses of triptolide is needed to unequivocally show if triptolide indeed acts by inhibiting general transcription.

7.3.6 Triptolide Mediates Inflammatory Response in Cancer Cells

Free radicals cause DNA damage and protein modifications, leading to the hypothesis that these radicals are involved in carcinogenesis. Nitric oxide ($NO^{\cdot}$) is a short lived free radical synthesized from L-arginine by nitric oxide synthase (NOS) (Alderton et al. 2001; Moncada et al. 1991a, b), the rate limiting enzyme in the synthesis of $NO^{\cdot}$ that exists in both an inducible and a constitutive form. Constitutive NOS is found in normal tissues, whereas inducible nitric oxide synthase (iNOS) produces $NO^{\cdot}$ in response to various inflammatory signals. (Alderton et al. 2001; Liu and Hotchkiss 1995; MacMicking et al. 1997; Moncada et al. 1991b). When activated by inflammatory cytokines or bacterial products including IFN-γ, LPS or TNF-α, macrophages express inducible nitric oxide synthase (iNOS) (Chiou et al. 2001; Nathan and Xie 1994). iNOS, a key molecule in inflammation-mediated cancer, is regulated by nuclear factor (NF-κB) binding, activator protein-1(AP-1), interferon regulatory factor 1(IRF1) and signal transducer and activator of transcription 1 (STAT1) (Marks-Konczalik et al. 1998; Martin et al. 1994; Ohmori and Hamilton 2001; Taylor et al. 1998; Xie et al. 1994). $NO^{\cdot}$ produced by iNOS action diffuses over cells, forming reactive species which are released from inflammatory cells and act upon neighboring dividing epithelial cells, leading to somatic mutations in cancer-causing genes. Free radicals cause structural and functional damage to key signaling proteins and apoptotic modulators, allowing $NO^{\cdot}$ to influence events involved in carcinogenesis such as cell-cycle checkpoints, apoptosis and DNA repair. Using Min/iNOS–/– mice, Ahn and Ohshima have shown that $NO^{\cdot}$ and its derivatives promote colon carcinogenesis in an APC mutant background (Ahn and Ohshima 2001).

Triptolide has been shown to inhibit $NO^{\cdot}$ production and iNOS expression, both at the mRNA and protein levels, in murine primary peritoneal macrophages and RAW 264.7 cells upon stimulation with IFN-γ, LPS or both by preventing NF-κB from binding to the iNOS promoter, as well as by suppressing JNK activation (Kim et al. 2004; Zhou et al. 2006). Inhibition of iNOS by 1400 w (an inducible nitric oxide synthase-specific inhibitor) blocks triptolide-induced apoptosis in macrophages, but not through mitochondria-mediated apoptosis, suggesting that triptolide mediates apoptosis in a caspase-independent manner (Bao et al. 2007).

7.3.7 Triptolide as an Inhibitor of COX-2

It is well established that chronic inflammation promotes tumor formation, and developing tumors promote a pro-inflammatory environment (Balkwill and

Mantovani 2001). Since inflammation also promotes innate immune responses, the tumor is required to overcome immune surveillance by a process known as "immune editing" (Dunn et al. 2002). Cyclooxygenase-2 (Cox-2) is an enzyme that affects several processes relevant to tumorigenesis including inflammation/immunosuppression, apoptosis and angiogenesis, and is overexpressed in many tumor types such as breast, colon, gastric and non-small cell lung carcinomas (NSCLCs) (Pereg and Lishner 2005). Cox-2 activity, which is regulated by iNOS, is a key step in the conversion of arachidonic acid to prostaglandins (Muller and Scherle 2006). Clinical studies using inhibitors against cox-2 in patients with breast, pancreatic, NSCLC and colorectal cancers, have shown additional advantage over chemotherapy alone (Csiki et al. 2005; Ferrari et al. 2006; Gasparini et al. 2005a, b; Nugent et al. 2005). Triptolide is an anti-cancer agent that decreases cox-2 expression by abolishing TNF-α and IL-1β, and protects dopaminergic neurons from inflammation-mediated damage induced by LPS (Zhou et al. 2005). It also suppresses COX-2 expression in LPS stimulated U937 cells and TNF-α stimulated synovial fibroblasts from rheumatoid arthritis patients (Tao et al. 1998; Yao et al. 2005), as well as interferon-γ or LPS induced production of IL-12 in THP-1 cells (Liu et al. 2005). It has also been shown to inhibit COX-2 expression via NF-κB pathway in astrocytes (Dai et al. 2006).

7.4 Mode of Triptolide-Mediated Cell Death Is Cell-Type Dependent

The cytotoxic effect of triptolide in cell lines representing different types of cancers is well documented. However, very little has been done to elucidate the type of cell death initiated by triptolide. Using different pancreatic cancer cell lines representing varying metastatic potential, it has recently been shown that while MIA PaCa-2 and Panc-1 cells undergo apoptosis in response to triptolide, as evidenced by an increase in caspase-3 activation and Annexin V positivity in the presence of triptolide, S2-VP10 and S2-013, two highly metastatic cell lines, showed a decrease in cell viability in the presence of triptolide, but there was no activation of caspase-3 or Annexin V positivity (Fig. 7.3). Upon further investigation, it was determined that triptolide does not lead to a change in cell cycle distribution, suggesting an alternative pathway of cell death.

An increasing number of studies have shown that cancer cells can undergo autophagy in response to various anti-cancer therapies (Bursch et al. 2000). Autophagy is an evolutionary conserved process required to maintain cellular homeostasis by removal and breakdown of cellular materials. (Klionsky and Emr 2000). Autophagic cells show the presence of double membrane vesicles in the cytoplasm known as autophagic vacuoles. Autophagy is caspase-independent, and the nucleus remains intact until the late stage of cell death. We therefore examined whether S2 cells that do not die via triptolide mediated apoptosis use autophagy as a mechanism of cell death. Induction of autophagy can be monitored by

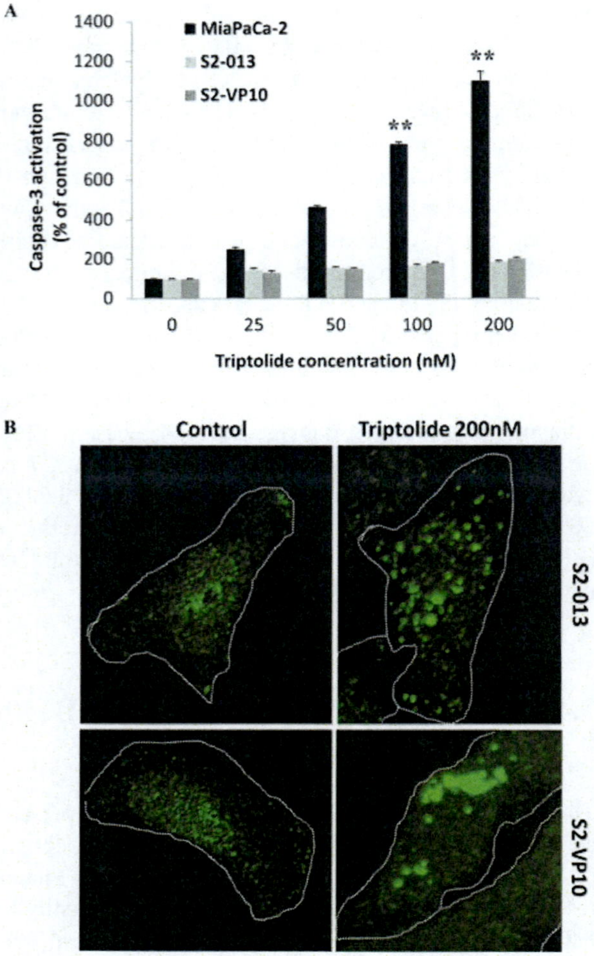

Fig. 7.3 MIA PaCa-2 cells undergo apoptosis, but S2-VP10 and S2-013 cells undergo autophagy (**a**) MIA PaCa-2 shows a significant time- and dose-dependent increase in caspase-3 activity after triptolide treatment which is absent in S2-013 and S2-VP10. (**b**) The formation of LC3 II after exposure of S2-013 and S2-VP10 cells to 200 nM of triptolide for 24 h was monitored by immunofluorescence. There is a significant increase in the LC3 II punctate staining pattern (*green*) on triptolide treatment when compared with untreated cells. The *white dotted line* indicates the outline of the cells. Results shown are representative of four independent experiments

studying LC3I, a cytosolic autophagosome specific protein that upon binding to phosphatidylethanolamine leads to the formation of LC3II, a protein that is localized to the membrane of the autophagosome. Using both immunoblotting and immunofluorescence microscopy, it was established that the S2 cell lines undergo autophagy-induced cell death (Fig. 7.3). The importance of this mechanism of cell death was investigated by blocking autophagy using siRNA against the autophagy-essential genes Atg5 and Beclin3. Intriguingly, inhibition of autophagy did not prevent triptolide-mediated cell death. Instead, upon blocking autophagy, S2 cells underwent apoptosis-mediated cell death, as evidenced by an increase in caspase activation, providing evidence for cross talk between these two mechanisms of cell death. However, preventing apoptosis by using caspase-3 mediated siRNA in MIA PaCa-2 cells prevented triptolide-mediated cell death, suggesting that the autophagy-mediated cell death pathway is not functional in these cells (Mujumdar et al. 2010). These data demonstrate that triptolide-mediated cell death in different cell lines follows a non-uniform pattern, underscoring the pleiotropic mechanism of action of triptolide.

7.5 Triptolide as a Combination Therapy in Cancer

Induction of apoptosis is believed to be the most promising molecular mechanisms for chemotherapeutic drugs. It is not surprising, therefore, that the TNF superfamily, which includes the TNF-a and Fas ligands, were used to target malignant cells. However, promising in vitro results were followed by disappointing in vivo results in which both ligands resulted in systemic shock response induced by death of both malignant and normal cells. Further research led to the identification of TNF-related apoptosis-inducing ligand (TRAIL) which only targets malignant cells proved to be an effective chemotherapy in several in vivo models. Additionally, early results in human patients have shown that this therapy is effective in humans. However, not all cancers respond to TRAIL therapy, and the mechanisms that confer resistance to apoptosis vary among different tumor types. Monotherapy eventually lead to chemoresistance, making the identification of novel combinatorial therapies an important area of investigation. TRAIL is a ligand for Death Receptor 4/5, a therapy which not been successful in pancreatic cancer, and in vitro data has demonstrated that pancreatic cancer cells are resistant to TRAIL therapy. However, a combination of TRAIL and triptolide results in cell death of TRAIL-resistant pancreatic cancer, at low concentrations of both TRAIL and triptolide. Cell death is mediated via apoptosis, as evidenced by an increase in caspase activation (Garcia-Becerra et al. 2006). In another study, Yang et al. have shown that triptolide can be combined with hydrocamptothecin, a topoisomerase inhibitor derived from *Camptotheca accuminata* to inhibit proliferation and induce cell death in Panc-1 pancreatic cancer cells (Yang et al. 2011). These data allow us to conclude that triptolide can be used at very low doses in combination with other known therapies.

7.6 Conclusion

Triptolide is a compound that induces cell death in cancer cells through a multifaceted approach (Figs. 7.3 and 7.4). Although it shows great potential as an anti-cancer agent, its progression into the clinic has been slow due to its insolubility in water, requiring the presence of organic solvents. We have recently synthesized a water-soluble pro-drug of triptolide, named Minnelide which shows chemotherapeutic effects similar to those seen for the parent compound. We are currently in the process of entering Phase I clinical trials with this drug.

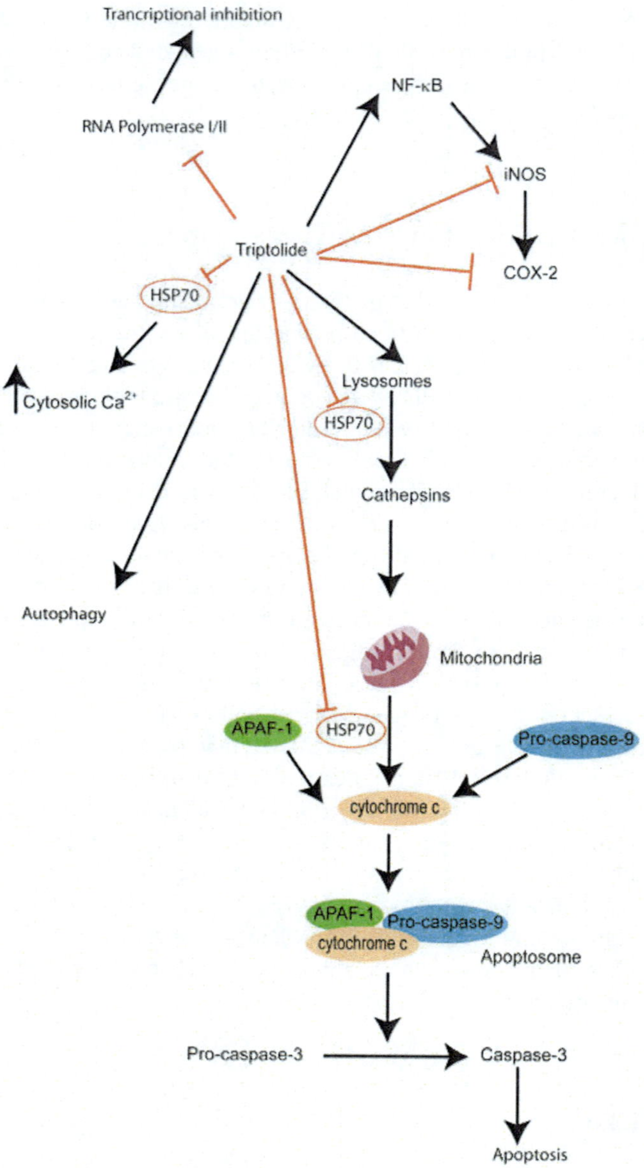

Fig. 7.4 An overview of the known mechanisms of action of triptolide

References

Aghdassi A, Phillips P, Dudeja V, Dhaulakhandi D, Sharif R, Dawra R, Lerch MM, Saluja A (2007) Heat shock protein 70 increases tumorigenicity and inhibits apoptosis in pancreatic adenocarcinoma. Cancer Res 67(2):616–625

Ahn B, Ohshima H (2001) Suppression of intestinal polyposis in Apc(Min/+) mice by inhibiting nitric oxide production. Cancer Res 61(23):8357–8360

Alderton WK, Cooper CE, Knowles RG (2001) Nitric oxide synthases: structure, function and inhibition. Biochem J 357(Pt 3):593–615

Antonoff MB, Chugh R, Borja-Cacho D, Dudeja V, Clawson KA, Skube SJ, Sorenson BS, Saltzman DA, Vickers SM, Saluja AK (2009) Triptolide therapy for neuroblastoma decreases cell viability in vitro and inhibits tumor growth in vivo. Surgery 146(2):282–290

Balkwill F, Mantovani A (2001) Inflammation and cancer: back to Virchow? Lancet 357(9255):539–545

Bao X, Cui J, Wu Y, Han X, Gao C, Hua Z, Shen P (2007) The roles of endogenous reactive oxygen species and nitric oxide in triptolide-induced apoptotic cell death in macrophages. J Mol Med 85(1):85–98

Borja-Cacho D, Yokoyama Y, Chugh RK, Mujumdar NR, Dudeja V, Clawson KA, Dawra RK, Saluja AK, Vickers SM (2010) TRAIL and triptolide: an effective combination that induces apoptosis in pancreatic cancer cells. J Gastrointest Surg 14(2):252–260

Bursch W, Ellinger A, Gerner C, Frohwein U, Schulte-Hermann R (2000) Programmed cell death (PCD). Apoptosis, autophagic PCD, or others? Ann N Y Acad Sci 926:1–12

Carter BZ, Mak DH, Schober WD, McQueen T, Harris D, Estrov Z, Evans RL, Andreeff M (2006) Triptolide induces caspase-dependent cell death mediated via the mitochondrial pathway in leukemic cells. Blood 108(2):630–637

Carter BZ, Mak DH, Schober WD, Dietrich MF, Pinilla C, Vassilev LT, Reed JC, Andreeff M (2008) Triptolide sensitizes AML cells to TRAIL-induced apoptosis via decrease of XIAP and p53-mediated increase of DR5. Blood 111(7):3742–3750

Chiou WF, Chou CJ, Chen CF (2001) Camptothecin suppresses nitric oxide biosynthesis in RAW 264.7 macrophages. Life Sci 69(6):625–635

Clawson KA, Borja-Cacho D, Antonoff MB, Saluja AK, Vickers SM (2010) Triptolide and TRAIL combination enhances apoptosis in cholangiocarcinoma. J Surg Res 163(2):244–249

Csiki I, Morrow JD, Sandler A, Shyr Y, Oates J, Williams MK, Dang T, Carbone DP, Johnson DH (2005) Targeting cyclooxygenase-2 in recurrent non-small cell lung cancer: a phase II trial of celecoxib and docetaxel. Clin Cancer Res 11(18):6634–6640

Dai YQ, Jin DZ, Zhu XZ, Lei DL (2006) Triptolide inhibits COX-2 expression via NF-kappa B pathway in astrocytes. Neurosci Res 55(2):154–160

Dudeja V, Mujumdar N, Phillips P, Chugh R, Borja-Cacho D, Dawra RK, Vickers SM, Saluja AK (2009) Heat shock protein70 inhibits apoptosis in cancer cells through simultaneous and independent mechanisms. Gastroenterology 136(5):1772–1782

Dudeja V, Chugh RK, Sangwan V, Skube SJ, Mujumdar NR, Antonoff MB, Dawra RK, Vickers SM, Saluja AK (2011) Prosurvival role of heat shock factor 1 in the pathogenesis of pancreatobiliary tumors. Am J Physiol Gastrointest Liver Physiol 300(6):G948–955

Dunn GP, Bruce AT, Ikeda H, Old LJ, Schreiber RD (2002) Cancer immunoediting: from immunosurveillance to tumor escape. Nat Immunol 3(11):991–998

Ferrari V, Valcamonico F, Amoroso V, Simoncini E, Vassalli L, Marpicati P, Rangoni G, Grisanti S, Tiberio GA, Nodari F, Strina C, Marini G (2006) Gemcitabine plus celecoxib (GECO) in advanced pancreatic cancer: a phase II trial. Cancer Chemother Pharmacol 57(2):185–190

Fidler JM, Li K, Chung C, Wei K, Ross JA, Gao M, Rosen GD (2003) PG490-88, a derivative of triptolide, causes tumor regression and sensitizes tumors to chemotherapy. Mol Cancer Ther 2(9):855–862

Garcia-Becerra R, Borja-Cacho E, Cooney AJ, Smith CL, Lemus AE, Perez-Palacios G, Larrea F (2006) Synthetic 19-nortestosterone derivatives as estrogen receptor alpha subtype-selective ligands induce similar receptor conformational changes and steroid receptor coactivator recruitment than natural estrogens. J Steroid Biochem Mol Biol 99(2–3):108–114

Garrido C, Brunet M, Didelot C, Zermati Y, Schmitt E, Kroemer G (2006) Heat shock proteins 27 and 70: anti-apoptotic proteins with tumorigenic properties. Cell Cycle 5(22):2592–2601

Gasparini G, Gattuso D, Morabito A, Longo R, Torino F, Sarmiento R, Vitale S, Gamucci T, Mariani L (2005a) Combined therapy with weekly irinotecan, infusional 5-fluorouracil and the selective COX-2 inhibitor rofecoxib is a safe and effective second-line treatment in metastatic colorectal cancer. Oncologist 10(9):710–717

Gasparini G, Meo S, Comella G, Stani SC, Mariani L, Gamucci T, Avallone A, Lo Vullo S, Mansueto G, Bonginelli P, Gattuso D, Gion M (2005b) The combination of the selective cyclooxygenase-2 inhibitor celecoxib with weekly paclitaxel is a safe and active second-line therapy for non-small cell lung cancer: A phase II study with biological correlates. Cancer J 11(3):209–216

Ghosh S, May MJ, Kopp EB (1998) NF-kappa B and Rel proteins: evolutionarily conserved mediators of immune responses. Annu Rev Immunol 16:225–260

Huang S, Robinson JB, Deguzman A, Bucana CD, Fidler IJ (2000) Blockade of nuclear factor-kappaB signaling inhibits angiogenesis and tumorigenicity of human ovarian cancer cells by suppressing expression of vascular endothelial growth factor and interleukin 8. Cancer Res 60(19):5334–5339

Jiang XH, Wong BC, Lin MC, Zhu GH, Kung HF, Jiang SH, Yang D, Lam SK (2001) Functional p53 is required for triptolide-induced apoptosis and AP-1 and nuclear factor-kappaB activation in gastric cancer cells. Oncogene 20(55):8009–8018

Johnson SM, Wang X, Mark Evers B (2011) Triptolide inhibits proliferation and migration of colon cancer cells by inhibition of cell cycle regulators and cytokine receptors. J Surg Res 168(2):197–205

Joo M, Chi JG, Lee H (2005) Expressions of HSP70 and HSP27 in hepatocellular carcinoma. J Korean Med Sci 20(5):829–834

Karin M, Lin A (2002) NF-kappaB at the crossroads of life and death. Nat Immunol 3(3):221–227

Kim YH, Lee SH, Lee JY, Choi SW, Park JW, Kwon TK (2004) Triptolide inhibits murine-inducible nitric oxide synthase expression by down-regulating lipopolysaccharide-induced activity of nuclear factor-kappa B and c-Jun NH2-terminal kinase. Eur J Pharmacol 494(1):1–9

Klionsky DJ, Emr SD (2000) Autophagy as a regulated pathway of cellular degradation. Science 290(5497):1717–1721

Ko JK, Leung WC, Ho WK, Chiu P (2007) Herbal diterpenoids induce growth arrest and apoptosis in colon cancer cells with increased expression of the nonsteroidal anti-inflammatory drug-activated gene. Eur J Pharmacol 559(1):1–13

Lee KY, Chang W, Qiu D, Kao PN, Rosen GD (1999) PG490 (triptolide) cooperates with tumor necrosis factor-alpha to induce apoptosis in tumor cells. J Biol Chem 274(19):13451–13455

Lee KY, Park JS, Jee YK, Rosen GD (2002) Triptolide sensitizes lung cancer cells to TNF-related apoptosis-inducing ligand (TRAIL)-induced apoptosis by inhibition of NF-kappaB activation. Exp Mol Med 34(6):462–468

Leuenroth SJ, Crews CM (2005) Studies on calcium dependence reveal multiple modes of action for triptolide. Chem Biol 12(12):1259–1268

Leuenroth SJ, Crews CM (2008) Triptolide-induced transcriptional arrest is associated with changes in nuclear substructure. Cancer Res 68(13):5257–5266

Li H, Sui C, Kong F, Zhang H, Liu J, Dong M (2007) Expression of HSP70 and JNK-related proteins in human liver cancer: Potential effects on clinical outcome. Dig Liver Dis 39(7): 663–670

Li P, Nijhawan D, Budihardjo I, Srinivasula SM, Ahmad M, Alnemri ES, Wang X (1997) Cytochrome c and dATP-dependent formation of Apaf-1/caspase-9 complex initiates an apoptotic protease cascade. Cell 91:479–489

Liu RH, Hotchkiss JH (1995) Potential genotoxicity of chronically elevated nitric oxide: a review. Mutat Res 339(2):73–89

Liu J, Wu QL, Feng YH, Wang YF, Li XY, Zuo JP (2005) Triptolide suppresses CD80 and CD86 expressions and IL-12 production in THP-1 cells. Acta Pharmacol Sin 26(2):223–227

Luzio JP, Pryor PR, Bright NA (2007) Lysosomes: fusion and function. Nat Rev Mol Cell Biol 8(8):622–632

MacMicking J, Xie QW, Nathan C (1997) Nitric oxide and macrophage function. Annu Rev Immunol 15:323–350

Marks-Konczalik J, Chu SC, Moss J (1998) Cytokine-mediated transcriptional induction of the human inducible nitric oxide synthase gene requires both activator protein 1 and nuclear factor kappaB-binding sites. J Biol Chem 273(35):22201–22208

Martin E, Nathan C, Xie QW (1994) Role of interferon regulatory factor 1 in induction of nitric oxide synthase. J Exp Med 180(3):977–984

McCallum C, Kwon S, Leavitt P, Shen DM, Liu W, Gurnett A (2007) Triptolide binds covalently to a 90 kDa nuclear protein. Role of epoxides in binding and activity. Immunobiology 212(7): 549–556

Messina ME, Jr., Halaby R (2011) Does triptolide induce lysosomal-mediated apoptosis in human breast cancer cells? Med Hypotheses 77(1):91–93

Moncada C, Arvin B, Le Peillet E, Meldrum BS (1991a) Non-NMDA antagonists protect against kainate more than AMPA toxicity in the rat hippocampus. Neurosci Lett 133(2):287–290

Moncada S, Palmer RM, Higgs EA (1991b) Nitric oxide: physiology, pathophysiology, and pharmacology. Pharmacol Rev 43(2):109–142

Monteith GR, McAndrew D, Faddy HM, Roberts-Thomson SJ (2007) Calcium and cancer: targeting Ca2+ transport. Nat Rev Cancer 7(7):519–530

Mujumdar N, Mackenzie T, Dudeja V, Chugh R, Antonoff M, Borja-Cacho D, Sangwan V, Dawra R, Vickers SM, Saluja AK (2010) Triptolide induces cell death in pancreatic cancer cells by apoptotic and autophagic pathways. Gastroenterology 139(2):598–608

Muller AJ, Scherle PA (2006) Targeting the mechanisms of tumoral immune tolerance with small-molecule inhibitors. Nat Rev Cancer 6(8):613–625

Nathan C, Xie QW (1994) Regulation of biosynthesis of nitric oxide. J Biol Chem 269(19): 13725–13728

Nugent FW, Mertens WC, Graziano S, Levitan N, Collea R, Gajra A, Marshall J, McCann J (2005) Docetaxel and cyclooxygenase-2 inhibition with celecoxib for advanced non-small cell lung cancer progressing after platinum-based chemotherapy: a multicenter phase II trial. Lung Cancer 48(2):267–273

Ohmori Y, Hamilton TA (2001) Requirement for STAT1 in LPS-induced gene expression in macrophages. J Leukoc Biol 69(4):598–604

Pereg D, Lishner M (2005) Non-steroidal anti-inflammatory drugs for the prevention and treatment of cancer. J Intern Med 258(2):115–123

Phillips PA, Dudeja V, McCarroll JA, Borja-Cacho D, Dawra RK, Grizzle WE, Vickers SM, Saluja AK (2007) Triptolide induces pancreatic cancer cell death via inhibition of heat shock protein 70. Cancer Res 67(19):9407–9416

Shamon LA, Pezzuto JM, Graves JM, Mehta RR, Wangcharoentrakul S, Sangsuwan R, Chaichana S, Tuchinda P, Cleason P, Reutrakul V (1997) Evaluation of the mutagenic, cytotoxic, and antitumor potential of triptolide, a highly oxygenated diterpene isolated from Tripterygium wilfordii. Cancer Lett 112(1):113–117

Sherman M, Multhoff G (2007) Heat shock proteins in cancer. Ann N Y Acad Sci 1113:192–201

Tao X, Schulze-Koops H, Ma L, Cai J, Mao Y, Lipsky PE (1998) Effects of Tripterygium wilfordii hook F extracts on induction of cyclooxygenase 2 activity and prostaglandin E2 production. Arthritis Rheum 41(1):130–138

Taylor BS, Alarcon LH, Billiar TR (1998) Inducible nitric oxide synthase in the liver: regulation and function. Biochemistry (Mosc) 63(7):766–781

Vispe S, DeVries L, Creancier L, Besse J, Breand S, Hobson DJ, Svejstrup JQ, Annereau JP, Cussac D, Dumontet C, Guilbaud N, Barret JM, Bailly C (2009) Triptolide is an inhibitor of RNA polymerase I and II-dependent transcription leading predominantly to down-regulation of short-lived mRNA. Mol Cancer Ther 8(10):2780–2790

Wang CY, Cusack JC, Jr., Liu R, Baldwin AS, Jr (1999) Control of inducible chemoresistance: enhanced anti-tumor therapy through increased apoptosis by inhibition of NF-kappaB. Nat Med 5(4):412–417

Wang X, Matta R, Shen G, Nelin LD, Pei D, Liu Y (2006) Mechanism of triptolide-induced apoptosis: Effect on caspase activation and Bid cleavage and essentiality of the hydroxyl group of triptolide. J Mol Med 84(5):405–415

Wang Z, Jin H, Xu R, Mei Q, Fan D (2009) Triptolide downregulates Rac1 and the JAK/STAT3 pathway and inhibits colitis-related colon cancer progression. Exp Mol Med 41(10):717–727

Westerheide SD, Kawahara TL, Orton K, Morimoto RI (2006) Triptolide, an inhibitor of the human heat shock response that enhances stress-induced cell death. J Biol Chem 281(14):9616–9622

Xie QW, Kashiwabara Y, Nathan C (1994) Role of transcription factor NF-kappa B/Rel in induction of nitric oxide synthase. J Biol Chem 269(7):4705–4708

Yang S, Chen J, Guo Z, Xu XM, Wang L, Pei XF, Yang J, Underhill CB, Zhang L (2003) Triptolide inhibits the growth and metastasis of solid tumors. Mol Cancer Ther 2(1):65–72

Yang SW, Wang W, Xie XY, Zhu WP, Li FQ (2011) In vitro synergistic cytotoxic effect of triptolide combined with hydroxycamptothecin on pancreatic cancer cells. Am J Chin Med 39(1): 121–134

Yao H, Zhou J, Li D, Wu N, Bader A, Hoxtermann S, Altmeyer P, Brockmeyer NH (2005) FK506 enhances triptolide-induced down-regulation of cyclooxygenase-2, inducible nitric oxide synthase as well as their products PGE2 and NO in TNF-alpha-stimulated synovial fibroblasts from rheumatoid arthritic patients. Eur J Med Res 10(3):110–116

Yinjun L, Jie J, Yungui W (2005) Triptolide inhibits transcription factor NF-kappaB and induces apoptosis of multiple myeloma cells. Leuk Res 29(1):99–105

Zhou HF, Liu XY, Niu DB, Li FQ, He QH, Wang XM (2005) Triptolide protects dopaminergic neurons from inflammation-mediated damage induced by lipopolysaccharide intranigral injection. Neurobiol Dis 18(3):441–449

Zhou R, Zheng SX, Tang W, He PL, Li XY, Yang YF, Li YC, Geng JG, Zuo JP (2006) Inhibition of inducible nitric-oxide synthase expression by (5R)-5-hydroxytriptolide in interferon-gamma- and bacterial lipopolysaccharide-stimulated macrophages. J Pharmacol Exp Ther 316(1): 121–128

Chapter 8
Nutraceuticals in Human Urinary Bladder Cancer Prevention and Treatment

Xiaolin Zi and Christopher Blair

Abstract Bladder cancer is a major public health burden. Tumor resection with possible intravesical treatments for superficial disease, and cystectomy or chemotherapy with radiation protocols for invasive bladder cancer have associated limitations and large costs. In addition, exposure to carcinogens contributes to the majority of bladder cancer risk. All of these represent profound opportunities to use nutraceuticals for improvement of current bladder cancer prevention and treatment. We discuss the clinical opportunities for use of nutraceuticals in bladder cancer prevention and treatment, including preventing the first occurrence of bladder cancer in high risk populations, delaying progression of the disease, use in combination with existing intravesical agents, and delaying or preventing radical cystectomy. We review randomized controlled trials of nutraceuticals in bladder cancer, current promising chemopreventive agents under preclinical development for bladder cancer prevention, and future directions of bladder cancer chemoprevention, including the concept of individualized bladder cancer chemoprevention.

Abbreviations

4HRP	N-4-hydroxyphenylretinamide
5-ALA	5-aminolevulinic acid
ATBC	alpha-Tocopherol Beta-Carotene
CIS	carcinoma in situ
CPS-II	cancer prevention study II
EMT	epithelial-to-mesenchymal transformation
NMIBC	non-muscle-invasive bladder cancers
RDA	recommended daily allowance
RTK	the receptor tyrosine kinases
TCC	transitional cell carcinoma
TURBT	transurethral resection of bladder tumor
UC	urothelial carcinoma
UVB	ultraviolet B

X. Zi (✉)
Departments of Urology and Pharmaceutical Sciences, Chao Family Comprehensive Cancer Center, University of California, Irvine, Orange, CA 92868, USA
e-mail: xzi@uci.edu

F.H. Sarkar (ed.), *Nutraceuticals and Cancer*, DOI 10.1007/978-94-007-2630-7_8,

8.1 Bladder Cancer Represents a Major Public Health Burden

Bladder cancer is the fourth most common cancer in men and eighth most common in women in the United States. There will be an estimated 69,250 new cases of bladder cancer and 14,990 related deaths during 2011 (Siegel et al. 2011). In addition, the estimated prevalence is over 500,000 with recurrence rate up to 85% (Patton et al. 2002). The cost per patient with bladder cancer from diagnosis to death is the highest among all cancers ($96,000 to $187,000 per patient in the US) (Avritscher et al. 2006). It is estimated that approximately $3.5 billion is spent in the United States each year on bladder cancer treatment (Noyes et al. 2008). Because of the high frequency of tumor recurrence, the lifetime need for surveillance, the treatment of recurrent tumors, and the high cost of complications associated with treatments, the psychological and economic burdens of the management of human bladder cancer on the health care system are substantial. Therefore, the reduction of bladder cancer occurrence and recurrence would be a definitive approach to easing the burden of bladder cancer.

The reduction of bladder cancer burden can be achieved through (1) preventing cancer occurrence by avoiding exposure to cancer risk factors or preventing their carcinogenic effects in healthy individuals, and (2) preventing or delaying recurrence and progression in those who have been diagnosed with and treated for cancer and are currently free of disease. Current approaches for preventing bladder cancer occurrence and recurrence can be summarized as Fig. 8.1.

8.2 Bladder Cancer Prevention Through Modification of Risk Factors

Cigarette smoking and occupational exposure to aromatic amines are major modifiable risk factors for bladder cancer (Yu et al. 2004). Cigarette smoking has been estimated to be a contributing factor in over 50% of all bladder cancer cases in the USA (Yu et al. 2004). The cessation of smoking has demonstrated a reduction in the incidence of bladder cancer (Barnoya and Glantz 2004). The less common or less potent risk factors include disinfection byproducts, artificial sweeteners, arsenic (particularly in Argentina, Chile and Taiwan), urinary tract infection (patients with spinal cord injuries and schistosomiasis in East Africa and the Middle East), hair dyes, a Chinese herbal weight-reduction supplement *Aristolochia fangchi*, and treatments with radiation, phenacetin, or cyclophosphamide (Johansson and Cohen 1997; Yang et al. 2005). Therefore, primary prevention to reduce the incidence of bladder cancer should primarily be focused on cessation of smoking and avoiding exposures to industrial and other risk factors.

As bladder carcinogens are excreted and concentrated in urine, high fluid intake may reduce the concentration and the duration of exposure and therefore influence the risk of bladder cancer. In the largest Health Professionals Follow-up Study, 48,000 men were followed for a period of 10 years; Michaud et al. (1999)

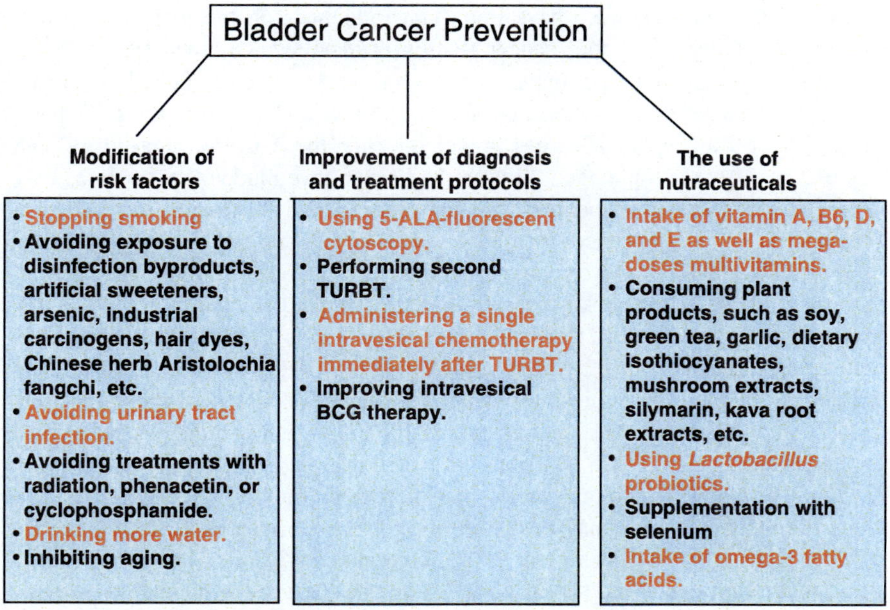

Fig. 8.1 Current approaches for preventing bladder cancer occurrence and recurrence. Currently the following methods are studied for preventing bladder cancer occurrence and recurrence: (**1**) Modification of bladder cancer risk factors can be achieved by stopping smoking, carrying out sensitive education programs on the cessation of tobacco usage in adolescence, avoiding exposure to bladder-related carcinogens, avoiding urinary tract infections, drinking more water to decrease concentrations of carcinogens in the bladder, inhibiting aging and avoiding treatments that may cause bladder cancer. In addition, research on sex differences in bladder cancer may provide new strategies/approaches for bladder cancer prevention. (**2**) Improvement in bladder cancer diagnosis and treatment protocols can reduce bladder cancer recurrence and progression. The use of 5-ALA–fluorescent cystoscopy and single-dose intravesical chemotherapy administered immediately after transurethral resection of bladder tumor (TURBT), performing second TURBT, and improvement of intravesical BCG therapy would reduce residual disease, leading to an increase in recurrence-free survival and a lower residual tumor rate. (**3**) The use of nutraceuticals for bladder cancer prevention has the advantages of non-invasiveness, fewer side effects, and prevention of tumor recurrence at sites that are inaccessible to intravesical therapy

demonstrated that fluid intake was inversely associated with the risk of bladder cancer. Men who drank an estimated fluid of more than 2,531 ml/day exhibited approximately 50% lower risk of developing bladder cancer than those with the lowest fluid consumption (1,290 ml/day). A meta-analysis of ten case-controlled studies also suggested a weak positive relationship between high total fluid consumption and reduced bladder cancer risk (Zeegers et al. 2004). However, other studies failed to show any connection between total fluid consumption and bladder cancer risk (Villanueva et al. 2006). The link between total and different types of fluid intakes and bladder cancer remains inconclusive (Villanueva et al. 2006).

Age, gender, and race also have important influences on the incidence, prognosis and mortality of bladder cancer (Patton et al. 2002; Fajkovic et al. 2011). Over 71% of first diagnoses of bladder cancer and 85.5% of related deaths occur in patients after 65 years of age (Patton et al. 2002). Bladder cancer rates for people aged 55–69 are up to 20 times higher than for those in the range of 30–54 (Siegel et al. 2011). People aged 70 years and older have bladder cancer rates two to three times higher than people aged between 55 and 69 (Siegel et al. 2011). Relative risks of bladder cancer incidence were 4.6, 5.3, and 5.7 for the age groups 70–74, 75–79, and 80 or more years, respectively, compared with those aged 50–54 years after adjusting for pack-years of cigarettes smoked (Siegel et al. 2011). As the population ages, one can expect an increasing burden of bladder cancer in the coming years. Interventions that slow down aging may delay bladder cancer. When considering all possible aging interventions evaluated to date, caloric restriction is the most robust and consistent approach for anti-aging. Studies in numerous species including nonhuman primates have demonstrated that reduction of calories 30–50% below ad libitum levels of a nutritious diet can increase lifespan, reduce the incidence and delay the onset of age-related diseases including cancer (Colman et al. 2009; Blagosklonny 2008). Experiments in mice have shown that caloric restriction decreased serum IGF1 levels and the growth of bladder tumors in mice (Dunn et al. 1997). The protective effect of caloric restriction on bladder carcinogenesis was reversed by restoring serum IGF-1 levels via the administration of exogenous human IGF-1 (Dunn et al. 1997). However, given the degree and length of caloric restriction required for its antitumor effect in animals, its application in humans would not be practical. Therefore, new strategies that can mimic the effects of caloric restriction may be developed for bladder cancer prevention in the elderly.

Men are nearly 3–4 times more likely to develop bladder cancer than women (Fajkovic et al. 2011). The difference between genders cannot be attributed to environmental or lifestyle factors alone. Genetic, anatomical, hormonal, and societal factors may play a role in sex differences in bladder cancer risk. In addition, Whites are about twice as likely to develop bladder cancer as African Americans and Hispanics. Asians have the lowest incidence of bladder cancer. The reason for the differences between genders and races in bladder cancer remains largely unknown.

8.3 Improved Diagnosis and Treatment for Decreasing Bladder Cancer Recurrence and Progression

Transitional cell carcinomas (TCCs) are the most common bladder cancer in Western countries and constitute approximately 95% of all cases (Patton et al. 2002). TCC or urothelial carcinoma (UC) of the bladder is not a single disease, but occurs in distinct forms with diversified morphology, natural history, and prognosis. TCC has been categorized into non-muscle-invasive (pTa, pT1, and carcinoma in situ) and muscle invasive (pT2-4) cancer depending on whether or not tumor infiltration extends to the muscular bladder wall (Villanueva et al. 2006; Fajkovic et al. 2011; Colman et al. 2009). The clinical treatment of bladder cancer greatly varies from non-muscle to muscle invasive or metastatic disease, which provides a second opportunity for bladder cancer prevention in Non-muscle-invasive bladder cancers (NMIBC). NMIBC can be subdivided into several sub-types with varying risk factors for recurrence and progression.

NMIBC are initially treated by transurethral resection of bladder tumor (TURBT) (Snyder et al. 2003). TURBT frequently fails to completely eradicate tumors, even when performed by skilled urologists (Adiyat et al. 2010; Herr 2011). After TURBT, many patients will still have residual disease. Recurrence of NMIBC may be due to new tumor development at other regions of the urothelium, implantation of tumor cells that may occur spontaneously and be caused by urothelial injuries during cystoscopy or TURBT, and failure to resect the original tumors. The use of 5-aminolevulinic acid (5-ALA)-fluorescent cytoscopy may improve the effectiveness of the initial TURBT, leading to a reduction of tumor recurrence in NMIBC. Several single-center studies have shown that the use of 5-ALA-fluorescent cytoscopy exhibited an overall improvement in bladder cancer diagnosis, a lower residual tumor rate and an increase in recurrence-free survival (Denzinger et al. 2007). However, a multiple center, randomized study with 370 patients followed up to 12 months did not show an increase in recurrence-free and progression-free survival rates (Stenzl et al. 2011). Further multiple center randomized studies are needed to better define the nature of fluorescent cytoscopy's role.

In addition, a nonrandomized retrospective study suggested that a second TURBT may also improve local obliteration of tumor (Herr. 2005), specifically for stage T1 bladder cancer and achieved better response to subsequent BCG intravesical therapy (Herr 2005). Reduction of bladder cancer recurrence can also be achieved by decreasing procedure-facilitated tumor implantation and by treating incompletely resected tumors using a single intravesical instillation of chemotherapy administered immediately after TURBT. Several prospective, randomized clinical trials have shown that immediate post-TURBT instillation therapy reduces recurrence by 17–44% (Dalbagni and Herr 2000; Duque and Loughlin 2000; Sylvester et al. 2002, 2004). Despite this fact, Madeb et al. (2009) reported that only 49 (0.33%) of 14,677 newly diagnosed bladder cancer patients received same-day intravesical instillation of chemotherapy. A single intravesical instillation of chemotherapeutic drugs immediately after TURBT is estimated to result in a 3-year savings of nearly $700 in medical expenses per year over TURBT alone.

Carcinoma in situ (CIS) of the bladder can occur as a primary urothelial lesion or in combination with another form of TCC either concomitantly or secondarily. CIS, when left untreated, may lead to progression to muscle-invasive disease in approximately 50% of patients and to disease recurrence in up to 90% of patients (Siegel et al. 2011; Patton et al. 2002). Intravesical BCG therapy is currently the most effective agent for treatment and prevention of recurrence of CIS, but it has the highest rate of side effects and a debatable impact on progression and overall survival rates of bladder cancer (Crawford 2002, Crawford et al. 2003). Moreover, some patients are refractory to BCG therapy (Crawford et al. 2003). Because of a considerable risk of recurrence anywhere in the urinary tract, CIS often requires life-long fellow-up. In addition, a group of patients with BCG failure will undergo early cystectomy. Muscle-invasive TCC also requires a radical cystectomy or chemotherapy with radiation protocols (Snyder et al. 2003; Crawford 2002, Crawford et al. 2003). Treatment options for metastatic bladder cancers are extremely limited, with 6% 5-year survival rate and median survival time of 12–20 months (Crawford 2002; Lobel et al. 1998).

Therefore, because the high recurrence of NMIBC requires repeated cytoscopies and resections, and development of metastatic disease is fatal, efforts focused on preventing recurrence and progression to invasive and metastatic bladder cancer in those with NMIBC are highly desirable and feasible.

8.4 Bladder Cancer Prevention by the Use of Nutraceuticals

Chemoprevention is an approach to impede, arrest, or reverse carcinogenesis by administration of natural or synthetic agents before a complex series of genetic and epigenetic events leads to invasive and metastatic malignancy (Sporn and Suh 2002). Bladder cancer represents an unique opportunity for chemoprevention to reduce the risk of developing new or recurrent cancers because of: (1) the long history of this disease in the majority of patients (Cookson et al. 1997; Siegel et al. 2011), (2) the ready accessibility of the bladder to repeated cytoscopic examinations and biopsies (Kelloff et al. 1992; Gee et al. 2002), (3) agents with a systematic effect that have the advantage of potentially reducing the risk of tumors inaccessible to intravesical therapy, and (4) preclinical and limited clinical data demonstrating that bladder cancer is responsive to preventive efforts (Barnoya and Glantz 2004; Tang and Zhang 2004; Becci et al. 1978; Grubbs et al. 2000; Zhou et al. 1998). More importantly, the high incidence and prevalence of bladder cancer in aging people suggests that agents that even moderately inhibit or delay disease development and progression could yield significant reductions in cancer morbidity and mortality.

Most epidemiological studies report an inverse relationship between fruit and vegetable intake and bladder cancer risk (Go et al. 2001; Reddy 1996; Riboli and Norat 2003; Steinmaus et al. 2000). In a prospective study of atomic bomb survivors (Nagano et al. 2000), high consumption of vegetables and fruit was a protective factor for bladder cancer with the relative risk of 0.6 and 0.5, respectively. However, due to inaccuracy in dietary questionnaires, poorly defined dietary composition and difficulty in conducting mechanistic studies on populations, available data from epidemiological studies are inadequate to provide indications for prevention.

Nutraceutical, a term combining the words "nutrition" and "pharmaceutical", refers to a food or food product that provides health and medical benefits, including the prevention and treatment of disease. A nutraceutical is demonstrated to have a physiological benefit or provide protection against chronic disease. Such products may range from isolated nutrients, dietary supplements and specific diets to genetically engineered foods, herbal products, and processed foods such as cereals, soups, and beverages. Many nutraceuticals have shown promising anticancer results with little or no toxicity to normal cells (Gupta et al. 2001). In addition, most nutraceuticals are excreted through the urinary tract and are therefore concentrated in urine, which leads to prolonged and direct exposure to the mucosal lining. Furthermore, nutraceuticals working systematically could potentially reduce the risk of developing tumors on the sites that are normally inaccessible to intravesical therapy. Thus, investigation of these nutraceuticals for prevention and therapeutic intervention against urinary bladder cancer is plausible. Moreover, prevention and therapeutic intervention by using well-studied, effective nutraceuticals could be a newer approach with potentially fewer side effects and, if targeted correctly, more efficacy as compared with current chemotherapeutic agents in cancer management. Therefore, we summarize current evidence regarding the potential usefulness of nutraceuticals in bladder cancer prevention and treatment.

8.4.1 Vitamins

Vitamin A and its related natural and synthetic retinoids have been widely studied in bladder cancer in cell culture systems, animal models and clinical trials. Although existing evidence showed that retinoids induced apoptosis in bladder cancer cell lines and inhibited carcinogen induced tumors in animal models, results from epidemiological studies have been conflicting. A case-control study of 1,592 bladder cancer patients and neighborhood controls showed that the high intake of carotenoids in current or former smokers was associated with reduced risk for bladder cancer (Castelao et al. 2004). However, two large-scale epidemiological studies, the Netherlands Cohort Study (Zeegers et al. 2001) and the Alpha-Tocopherol Beta-Carotene (ATBC) Cancer Prevention Study (Michaud et al. 2002) failed to show an association between higher intake of vitamin A or carotenoids and reduced risk of bladder cancer. Excessive consumption of vitamin A can lead to acute and chronic toxicities and cause the Retinoid syndrome. The syndrome includes a steady fever, hypotension, respiratory dysfunction, conjunctivitis, cheilosis, and arthralgia. The symptoms can disappear when the intake of vitamin A stops. In addition, synthetic forms of vitamin A analogs have reduced toxicity, with only infrequent episodes of grade 3 and 4 toxicity reported, and higher therapeutic index. A prospective, randomized, double-blind phase II trial (Studer et al. 1995) demonstrated that etretinate, an aromatic retinoid, extended the time to second recurrence of stage Ta-T1 papillary bladder cancer by an average of about 7 months without affecting time to the first recurrence, and therefore resulted in a decrease in the annual TURBT rate from 2.1 to 0.92 ($p<0.001$). These results suggested that etretinate decreased new tumor development rather than eradicated existing tumors. However, Sabichi et al. (2008) reported in a phase III, multiple center trial that fenretinide (N-4-hydroxyphenylretinamide, 4HRP) did not increase the time to first recurrence in patients with NMIBC compared to placebo controls.

Vitamin C supplements are available in caplets, tablets, capsules, drink mix packets, in multi-vitamin formulations, in multiple antioxidant formulations with bioflavonoids such as quercetin, hesperidin, and rutin, and as crystalline powder. Vitamin C acts as a potent antioxidant by protecting the body against oxidative stress and preventing free radical induced DNA damage and the formation of carcinogens (e. g. N-nitroso compounds), as well as by decreasing the concentration of bladder carcinogen 3-hydro xanthranilic acid. Results regarding the relationship between vitamin C intake and bladder cancer have been inconsistent. Nomura et al. (1991) reported that high intake of vitamin C was associated with a relative risk of 0.4 in women and 0.6 in men for bladder cancer. In the prospective Health Professionals Follow-Up Study (Michaud et al. 2000), the intake of vitamin C was also inversely associated with bladder cancer risk but only in those who used vitamin C supplementation. The association was no longer statistically significant after controlling for smoking history. However, in the ATBC Cancer Prevention Study following up 27,111 male smokers aged 50–69 years (Michaud et al. 2002), dietary intake of vitamin C was not associated with risk of bladder cancer. In the Cancer Prevention Study II (CPS-II) cohort examining the association between vitamin C supplements and bladder cancer mortality among 991,522 US adults, vitamin C supplementation was also not associated with bladder cancer mortality (Jacobs et al. 2002).

Vitamin E is an important lipid-soluble antioxidant, consisting of tocopherols and tocotrienols. Vitamin E protects cell membranes and metabolic enzymes from oxidation damage by reacting with lipid radicals produced in the lipid peroxidation chain reaction and by playing a role in glutathione peroxidase pathway. In addition, vitamin E inhibits carcinogenic nitrosamine formation and resulted in 30 to 60% inhibition of nitroso compound induced carcinogenesis in most experiments (Mirvish 1986; Tamano et al. 1987). Several epidemiological studies showed an inverse relationship between the intake of vitamin E and bladder cancer risk (Liang et al. 2008; Jacobs et al. 2002). However, in a meta- analysis of 19 clinical trials testing vitamin E alone and vitamin E plus other vitamins or minerals, Miller et al. (2005) reported that high-dosage vitamin E was associated with increased risk of all-cause mortality.

Vitamin B6 is a water-soluble vitamin. Vitamin B6 plays an important role in tryptophan metabolism. Metabolites of tryptophan may interact with nitrite to become mutagenic nitrosamines that cause bladder cancer. Therefore, vitamin B6 supplementation for bladder cancer prevention is plausible. In a prospective clinical trial of 121 patients with Stage I bladder cancer randomized to placebo, pyridoxine (vitamin B6), or intravesical thiotepa, Byar and Blackard (1977) reported that pyridoxine significantly reduced bladder cancer recurrence in those patients with more than 10 months of follow-up and that its efficacy is similar to thiotepa. A prospective, randomized phase III study carried out by the European Organisation for Research and Treatment Cancer genitourinary group failed to replicate this result, in which vitamin B6 showed no difference with respect to time to first recurrence or recurrence rate compared to placebo control (Newling et al. 1995).

Vitamin D is one nutritional factor that is thought to protect against cancer at many sites. 25(OH)D is converted to its active form, 1-25-dihydroxyvitamin D (1,25(OH)2D), by 1-α-hydroxylase. Epidemiological studies showed that ultraviolet B irradiance (UVB) and intake of vitamin D were inversely associated with bladder cancer incidence and mortality (Boscoe and Schymura 2006; Chen et al. 2010; Grant 2002). In an ecological study of UVB irradiance and incidence rates of bladder cancer in 174 countries worldwide, bladder cancer incidences were independently and inversely related with solar UVB radiation after controlling for per capita cigarette consumption (Mohr et al. 2010). Furthermore, in a nested case-control study of male smokers from the ATBC cohort, lower serum 25(OH)D was shown to be significantly associated with an increased risk of bladder cancer (Mondul et al. 2010). These results suggest that vitamin D deserves further investigation in bladder cancer chemoprevention.

Vitamin megadoses and combinations: Epidemiological studies provided inconsistent evidence for a benefit from multivitamin intake for bladder cancer prevention (Neuhouser et al. 2009; Bruemmer et al. 1996). However, in a prospective, randomized, double-blinded, small clinical trial (Lamm et al. 1994), 65 bladder cancer patients treated with BCG were supplemented with the recommended daily allowance (RDA) of individual vitamins plus 40,000 IU of vitamin A, 100 mg of vitamin B6, 2000 mg of vitamin C, 400 IU of vitamin E, and 90 mg zinc or the RDA of individual vitamins alone. Mega-dose multivitamin supplementation demonstrated significantly decreased recurrence rates by 50% compared to the RDA of individual vitamins.

8.4.2 Minerals

Selenium is also an antioxidant. A meta-analysis for summarization of seven published epidemiological studies before 2010 showed that levels of selenium measured in serum and toenails were inversely associated with risk of bladder cancer (Amaral et al. 2010). A more significant protective effect of selenium against bladder cancer was observed in women. However, in the VITamins and Lifestyle study following-up 77,050 eligible VITAL participants for 6 years, mineral and vitamin supplementation has been shown not to be associated with the risk of urothelial cancers (Hotaling et al. 2011).

8.4.3 Lactobacillus Probiotics

Probiotics are live microbial food supplements beneficial to the host when administered in adequate amounts. Probiotics have been used in urology for preventing urogenital infections and recurrent bladder cancer since the early part of the 20th century. *Lactobacillus casei* strain Shirota is commercially available in Japan since 1935 as the fermented milk drink Yakult. Preclinical studies have shown that *Lactobacillus casei* strain Shirota inhibited N-butyl-N-(4-hydroxybutyl)nitrosamine induced rat bladder cancer and reduced tumor growth in a murine orthotopic bladder tumor MBT-2 model when administrated by intravesicular instillation (Tomita et al. 1994; Takahashi et al. 2001; Seow et al. 2010). In a clinical trial with 52 Japanese patients, an oral preparation of *Lactobacillus casei* strain Shirota increased superficial bladder cancer recurrence-free survival time by 1.8 fold compared to the placebo control arm (350 versus 195 days) (Aso and Akazan 1992). In a double-blinded placebo-controlled randomized trial, 138 patients were stratified into three subgroups with: A, primary multiple tumors, B, recurrent single tumors, or C, recurrent multiple tumors (Aso et al. 1995). Compared to placebo control patients, the intake of *Lactobacillus casei* strain Shirota resulted in a decreased tumor recurrence in group A and B patients, but not in group C patients. A case-control study performed in 7 Japanese cities (Ohashi et al. 2002) also showed that the habitual intake of *Lactobacillus casei* strain Shirota was associated with lower risk of bladder cancer. Mechanisms of *Lactobacillus casei* strain Shirota's action remain largely unknown. It is plausible that *Lactobacillus casei* strain Shirota changes the flora of various tissue sites allowing these organisms to detoxify carcinogens. In addition, *Lactobacillus* has been shown to secrete a tumor antigen and cytokines to activate neutrophils, dendritic cells and cytotoxic T lymphocytes against bladder cancer cells (Kandasamy et al. 2011).

8.4.4 Omega-3

Omega-3 fatty acids are essential to normal growth and health. Epidemiological studies have suggested that the intake of diets high in omega-3 fatty acids was associated with lower risk of several cancers. Therefore, a number of omega-3 fatty acid containing dietary supplements that claim to have health promoting and anti-cancer activity has become popular on the market. Studies on the relationship between consumption of omega-3 fatty acid and bladder cancer risk are very limited. Chyou et al. (1993) reported that men consuming fish (rich in omega-3) 5 times per week or more were associated with a non-significant reduction of bladder cancer risk than those who eat 1 time per week or less (the RR, 0.67; 95% CI, 0.26–1.67). In a rat multi-organ carcinogenesis model, Toriyama-Baba et al. (2001) reported that n-3 unsaturated fatty acids did not affect preneoplastic and neoplastic lesion development in the urinary bladder.

8.4.5 Plant Products and Phytochemicals

Soy is rich in isoflavones including genistein, daidzein and biochanin. Singh et al. (2006) has shown that genistein and an isoflavone-rich soy phytochemical concentrate inhibited the in vivo tumor growth of bladder cancer cells by 56 and 52%, respectively. The isoflavone-rich soy phytochemical concentrate, but not genistein, also inhibited lung metastasis by 95%. On the contrary, an epidemiology study in China demonstrated that consumption of soy products 3 to more than 7 times was associated with a significantly increased risk of bladder cancer (the relative risk: 4.61, 95% CI: 1.57–13.51) (Sun et al. 2004).

Green tea is one of the most commonly consumed beverages worldwide and contains potent antioxidants: polyphenol and catechins. Lubet et al. (2007) demonstrated that Polyphenon E, a standardized mixture of green tea polyphenols, significantly inhibited 4-hydroxybutyl(butyl) nitrosamine induced palpable urinary bladder tumors in rats in a dose-dependent manner. However, epidemiological studies failed to demonstrate a benefit of drinking green tea in reducing bladder cancer risk (Hemelt et al. 2010; Wakai et al. 2004) Wakai et al. (2004) even reported that moderate drinkers of green tea exhibited an increased risk for bladder cancer.

Garlic (*Allium sativum*) and garlic supplements contains numerous chemical compounds that exhibit antibiotic, lipid-lowering, detoxification, immune stimulation and antitumor activity against a variety of cancers. In the MBT2 murine bladder carcinoma model, intralesional and oral administration of aged garlic extracts was demonstrated to be more efficacious than BCG or Keyhole limpet hemocyanin immunotherapy (Marsh et al. 1987). However, it was also noted in these studies that garlic extract caused severe toxicity to mice. Currently, there are no or limited epidemiological or clinical studies on the relationship between the use of garlic supplements and bladder cancer risk.

Dietary isothiocyanates are derived from glucosinolate breakdown products of cruciferous vegetables. Most isothiocyanates are shown to be inhibitors of carcinogenesis when administered before, or concurrently with carcinogens. This mechanism of isothiocyanates' action is mostly likely due to inhibition of cytochrome-P450 isoenzymes for carcinogen activation and induction of phase 2 enzymes involved in carcinogen detoxification. However, existing epidemiological studies on the relationship between cruciferous vegetable intake and bladder cancer risk have been inconsistent. In the ATBC Cancer Prevention Study following up 27,111 male smokers aged 50–69 years, consumption of cruciferous vegetables was shown to be not associated with bladder cancer risk (Michaud et al. 2002). On the contrary, a recent hospital-based, case-control study showed that raw cruciferous vegetable intake (adjusted OR for highest versus lowest category = 0.64; 95% CI, 0.42–0.97) was inversely associated with bladder cancer risk (Tang et al. 2008a).

Mushroom extracts have long been used as folk medicine for treating cancer in Asia. Mushroom extracts play important roles in immunomodulating activities. Several mushroom extracts, such as cordyceps militaris, maitake (Grifola frondosa), ganoderma lucidum, meshimakobu, *antrodia camphorata*, *coriolus versicolor* and *Lentinus edode,* have shown their anti-bladder cancer activities either in cell culture systems, carcinogenesis models or in clinics (Yang et al. 1999; Peng et al. 2007; Yuen et al. 2008; Park et al. 2009; Rajamahanty et al. 2009). Yang et al. (1999) reported that bladder cancer patients, who were treated with BCG or the Chinese herbal medicine Zhuling mushroom (Grifola umbellata pilat) and followed up for 2–15 years after TURBT or partial cystectomy, had a similar recurrence rate, which was significantly lower than those patients who were treated with mitomycin C or thiotepa or received no treatment. However, a study also showed that the methanol extract of fresh *Agaricus bisporus* mushrooms and an active compound Agaritine existing in these mushrooms were carcinogenic to the mouse bladder epithelium

(Hashida et al. 1990). These studies suggested that different types of mushrooms may have different effects on bladder carcinogenesis.

Silymarin is a mixture of flavonoid antioxidants isolated from milk thistle seeds. Silymarin is being used clinically in Europe and Asia for the treatment of alcoholic liver diseases without any toxicity. In several preclinical studies, silymarin has been shown to inhibit tumor growth in bladder cancer xenograft models and bladder carcinogenesis in the carcinogen OH-BBN induced bladder cancer model (Vinh et al. 2002; Tyagi et al. 2007; Singh et al. 2008). Silymarin also has been shown to inhibit the erbB1 mediated cell growth pathway in cancer cells (Zi et al. 1998). Therefore, silymarin could be a promising chemopreventive agent for bladder cancer.

Kava root extracts have been part of the Pacific Islanders' culture for thousands of years, serving as a beverage and medication and used during socioreligious functions. Consumption of the traditional kava preparation was reported to correlate with low and uncustomary gender ratios (more cancer in women than men) of cancer incidences in three kava-drinking countries: Fiji, Vanuatu, and Western Samoa despite the high prevalence of smoking in their populations (Henderson et al. 1985; Steiner 2000). We have identified flavokawain A, B, and C, but not the major kavalactone, kawain, in kava extracts as causing strong antiproliferative and apoptotic effects in human bladder cancer cells (Zi and Simoneau 2005). We also found that flavokawain A more effectively inhibited the growth of p53 mutant versus wild type bladder cancer and inhibited tumor growth in a bladder cancer xenograft model (Tang et al. 2008b). These results suggest that flavokawain A deserves further investigation in bladder cancer chemoprevention.

8.5 Conclusion and Future Directions

In view of the demographic trend toward an aging population, and the absence of effective preventive strategies, bladder cancer incidence is expected to increase in the coming years. In addition, bladder cancer patients can survive for a long time, but have a very high recurrence rate in a short period of time after their first diagnosis and treatment. Bladder cancer will represent an increasing public health burden in the coming years. One important strategy to address this public health concern is to prevent the occurrence, recurrence and progression of the disease. Therefore, there is a specific need to emphasize bladder cancer prevention in public policy, and for the development of effective preventive approaches.

The ability of nutraceuticals to reduce the risk of bladder cancer is not yet well known. Results from chemoprevention trials of vitamin C supplements, retinoids (e.g. 13cRA and etretinate) and Vitamin B6 in bladder cancer patients have been conflicting, and implementation of these agents for cancer prevention in the clinical community is debated. Other clinical trials of potential chemopreventive agents for bladder cancer including fenretinide and green tea polyphenols are currently either ongoing or have been completed but have not yet released their results. Dietary fat, soy protein, garlic, isothiocyanates, silymarin, kava root extracts, mushroom extracts and selenium have shown anticancer properties in animal experiments, but remain largely unstudied in humans. Probiotics, such as Lactobacillus casei strain Shirota (Yakult) have demonstrated their potential ability to prevent urogenital infection and recurrent bladder cancer in several clinical trials on a small scale. Production according to the Good Manufacturing Practices guidelines and guaranteed survival over a long storage time would be essential for the use of the bacteria for bladder cancer prevention on a large scale in the population. Therefore, currently there is no sufficient evidence to make a routine recommendation of any nutraceuticals for bladder cancer chemoprevention.

The future of cancer chemoprevention depends on innovative agents, molecular targets and trials. The development of chemopreventive agents is greatly hindered by the fact that chemoprevention trials require a large sample size, the difficulty recruiting patients due to potential toxicity, and tissue sampling issues in relatively healthy people. However, recent successes in the targeted therapy of advanced cancers suggest that molecularly targeted approaches for risk assessment, drug development and outcome evaluation may be the future of cancer chemoprevention. Since molecularly targeted approaches can (1) define populations who are most likely to benefit, (2) increase event rates, (3) develop rational, effective and safe preventive drugs with the ability to treat both early and advanced disease, and (4) effectively evaluate outcomes, molecularly targeted approaches represent a promising future for bladder cancer chemoprevention.

Bladder cancer is a suitable candidate disease for molecularly targeted approaches. Bladder cancer arises via two distinct but somewhat overlapping pathways (Fig. 8.2). Seventy to 80% of bladder TCCs progress from urothelial hyperplasia to low-grade, superficial papillary tumors, whereas the remaining 20 to 30% either have muscle-invasive tumors at diagnosis or arise from flat, high-grade CIS and progress to invasive tumors (Wu 2005; Spruck 3rd et al. 1994). Invasive TCCs often progress to the metastatic stage. After transurethral resection, papillary TCCs have about a 70% rate of recurrence, but the risk of progression to muscle invasive TCC is much lower (Wu 2005). In contrast, 50% of those with CIS ultimately progress to invasive TCC (Wu 2005). Genetic analyses of bladder cancer specimens have correlated these two bladder tumorigenesis pathways with different molecular events. Loss of a chromosome 9 sequence has been considered an early event for both superficial and invasive bladder tumors (Hartmann et al. 2002). Activation of the receptor tyrosine kinases (RTK)-Ras pathway through mutations in the H-Ras (30–40%) and FGFR genes (about 70%), as well as overexpression of H-Ras, ERBB3 and 4 have been frequently found in superficial bladder tumors, whereas inactivation of the p53 and pRB tumor suppressors (over 50%) are often detected in muscle invasive TCC (Wu 2005). Inactivation of p53 and pRB tumor suppressors is believed to initiate a progressive genetic instability and accumulation of genetic defects, leading to muscle invasive TCC. These molecular characteristics of bladder cancer provide an important foundation for future molecularly targeted approaches of bladder cancer chemoprevention.

In addition, trials of single agents may not be the most favorable approach for bladder cancer prevention; rather, future chemoprevention trials for bladder cancer should include novel combinations of different agents.

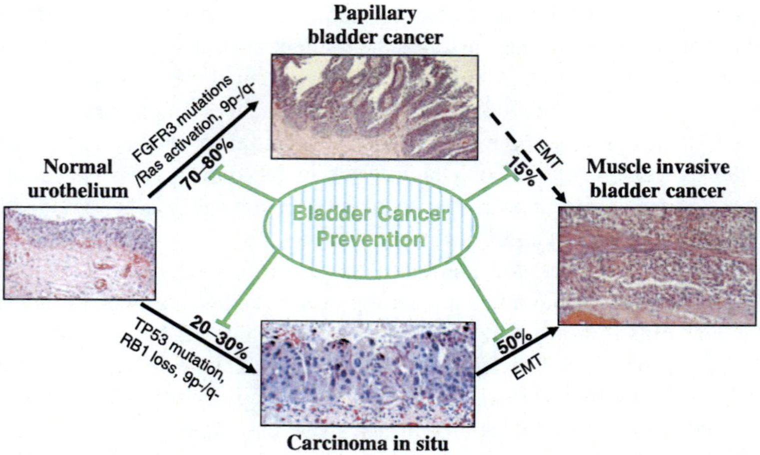

Fig. 8.2 Two distinctive molecular pathways for papillary TCC and CIS, respectively, and strategies of bladder cancer prevention. TCCs typically progress from urothelial hyperplasia to low-grade, superficial papillary tumors, whereas the remaining 20–30% of patients either have muscle-invasive tumors at diagnosis or arise from flat, high-grade CIS and progress to invasive tumors. Invasive TCCs often progress to the metastatic stage. After transurethral resection, papillary TCCs have about a 70% rate of recurrence, but the risk of progression to muscle invasive TCC is much lower. In contrast, 50% of those with CIS ultimately progress to invasive TCC. Genetic analyses of bladder cancer specimens have correlated these two bladder tumorigenesis pathways with different molecular events. Loss of a chromosome 9 sequence has been identified as an early event for both superficial and invasive bladder tumors. Activation of the RTK-Ras pathway through mutations in the H-Ras (30–40%) and FGFR genes (about 70%), as well as overexpression of H-Ras, ERBB3 and 4 have been frequently found in superficial bladder tumors, whereas inactivation of p53 and pRB tumor suppressors (over 50%) are often detected in muscle invasive TCC. Inactivation of p53 and pRB tumor suppressors is believed to initiate a progressive genetic instability and an accumulation of genetic defects, leading to muscle invasive TCC. In addition, bladder cancer may develop a gene expression profile characteristic of epithelial-to-mesenchymal transformation (EMT) but microscopically retain a full epithelial/urothelial phenotype, or partially or completely lose the epithelial phenotype and change into mesenchymal sarcoma-like tumors during its progression to muscle invasive TCC. The hallmark feature of EMT is a loss of the homotypic adhesion markers, E-cadherin. The role of EMT in bladder cancer progression remains largely unknown. Molecularly targeted approaches for bladder cancer prevention could benefit from these well-characterized molecular pathways in bladder carcinogenesis

Acknowledgments Work cited from our laboratory was supported by NIH award 5R01CA122558-03 and 1R21CA152804-01A1 (to X. Z.).

References

Adiyat KT, Katkoori D, Soloway CT et al (2010) "Complete transurethral resection of bladder tumor": are the guidelines being followed? Urology 75:365–367

Amaral AF, Cantor KP, Silverman DT et al (2010) Selenium and bladder cancer risk: a meta-analysis. Cancer Epidemiol Biomarkers Prev 19:2407–2415

Aso Y, Akazan H (1992) Prophylactic effect of a Lactobacillus casei preparation on the recurrence of superficial bladder cancer. BLP Study Group. Urol Int 49:125–129

Aso Y, Akaza H, Kotake T (1995) Preventive effect of a Lactobacillus casei preparation on the recurrence of superficial bladder cancer in a double-blind trial. The BLP Study Group. Eur Urol 27:104–109

Avritscher EB, Cooksley CD, Grossman HB et al (2006) Clinical model of lifetime cost of treating bladder cancer and associated complications. Urology 68:549–553

Barnoya J, Glantz S (2004) Association of the California tobacco control program with declines in lung cancer incidence. Cancer Causes Control 15:689–695

Becci PJ, Thompson HJ, Grubbs CJ et al (1978) Inhibitory effect of 13-cis-retinoic acid on urinary bladder carcinogenesis induced in C57BL/6 mice by N-butyl-N-(4-hydroxybutyl)-nitrosamine. Cancer Res 38:4463–4466

Blagosklonny MV (2008) Prevention of cancer by inhibiting aging. Cancer Biol Ther 7:1520–1524

Boscoe FP, Schymura MJ (2006) Solar ultraviolet-B exposure and cancer incidence and mortality in the United States, 1993–2002. BMC Cancer 6:264

Bruemmer B, White E, Vaughan TL (1996) Nutrient intake in relation to bladder cancer among middle-aged men and women. Am J Epidemiol 144:485–495

Byar D, Blackard C (1977) Comparisons of placebo, pyridoxine, and topical thiotepa in preventing recurrence of stage I bladder cancer. Urology 10:556–561

Castelao JE, Yuan JM, Gago-Dominguez M et al (2004) Carotenoids/vitamin C and smoking-related bladder cancer. Int J Cancer 110:417–423

Chen W, Clements M, Rahman B et al (2010) Relationship between cancer mortality/incidence and ambient ultraviolet B irradiance in China. Cancer Causes Control 21:1701–1709

Chyou PH, Nomura AM, Stemmermann GN (1993) A prospective study of diet, smoking, and lower urinary tract cancer. Ann Epidemiol 3:211–216

Colman RJ, Anderson RM, Johnson SC et al (2009) Caloric restriction delays disease onset and mortality in rhesus monkeys. Science 325:201–204

Cookson MS, Herr HW, Zhang ZF et al (1997) The treated natural history of high risk superficial bladder cancer: 15-year outcome. J Urol 158:62–67

Crawford ED (2002). Intravesical therapy for superficial cancer: need for more options. J Clin Oncol 20:3185–3186

Crawford ED, Wood DP, Petrylak DP et al (2003) Southwest Oncology Group studies in bladder cancer. Cancer 97(8 Suppl):2099–2108

Dalbagni G, Herr HW (2000) Current use and questions concerning intravesical bladder cancer group for superficial bladder cancer. Urol Clin North Am 27:137

Denzinger S, Burger M, Walter B (2007) Clinically relevant reduction in risk of recurrence of superficial bladder cancer using 5-aminolevulinic acid-induced fluorescence diagnosis: 8-year results of prospective randomized study. Urology 69:675–679

Dunn SE, Kari FW, French J et al (1997) Dietary restriction reduces insulin-like growth factor I levels, which modulates apoptosis, cell proliferation, and tumor progression in p53-deficient mice. Cancer Res 57:4667–4672

Duque JL, Loughlin KR (2000) An overview of the treatment of superficial bladder cancer. Intravesical chemotherapy. Urol Clin North Am 27:125

Fajkovic H, Halpern JA, Cha EK et al (2011) Impact of gender on bladder cancer incidence, staging, and prognosis. World J Urol (Epub ahead of print)

Gee J, Sabichi AL, Grossman HB (2002) Chemoprevention of superficial bladder cancer. Crit Rev Oncol Hematol 43:277–286

Go VL, Wong DA, Butrum R (2001) Diet, nutrition and cancer prevention: where are we going from here? J Nutr 131(11 Suppl):3121S–2126S

Grant WB (2002) an estimate of premature cancer mortality in the U.S. due to inadequate doses of solar ultraviolet-B radiation. Cancer 94:1867–1875

Grubbs CJ, Lubet RA, Koki AT (2000) Celecoxib inhibits N-butyl-N-(4-hydroxybutyl)-nitrosamine-induced urinary bladder cancers in male B6D2F1 mice and female Fischer-344 rats. Cancer Res 60:5599–5602

Gupta S, Afaq F, Mukhtar H (2001) Selective growth-inhibitory, cell-cycle deregulatory and apoptotic response of apigenin in normal versus human prostate carcinoma cells. Biochem Biophys Res Commun 287:914–920

Hartmann A, Schlake G, Zaak D et al (2002) Occurrence of chromosome 9 and p53 alterations in multifocal dysplasia and carcinoma in situ of human urinary bladder. Cancer Res 62:809–818

Hashida C, Hayashi K, Jie L et al (1990) Quantities of agaritine in mushrooms (Agaricus bisporus) and the carcinogenicity of mushroom methanol extracts on the mouse bladder epithelium). Nippon Koshu Eisei Zasshi 37:400–405

Hemelt M, Hu Z, Zhong Z et al (2010) Fluid intake and the risk of bladder cancer: results from the South and East China case-control study on bladder cancer. Int J Cancer 127:638–645

Henderson BE, Kolonel LN, Dworsky R et al (1985) Cancer incidence in the islands of the Pacific. Natl Cancer Inst Monogr 69:73–81

Herr H (2005) Restaging transurethral resection of high risk superWcial bladder cancer improves the initial response to bacillus Calmette-Guerin therapy. J Urol 174:2134

Herr HW (2011) Role of re-resection in non-muscle-invasive bladder cancer. Sci World J 11: 283–288

Hotaling JM, Wright JL, Pocobelli G et al (2011) Long-term use of supplemental vitamins and minerals does not reduce the risk of urothelial cell carcinoma of the bladder in the VITamins and Lifestyle study. J Urol 185:1210–1215

Jacobs EJ, Henion AK, Briggs PJ et al (2002) Vitamin C and vitamin E supplement use and bladder cancer mortality in a large cohort of US men and women. Am J Epidemiol 156:1002–1010

Johansson SL and Cohen SM (1997) Epidemiology and etiology of bladder cancer. Semin Surg Oncol 13:291–298

Kamat AM, Lamm DL (2000) Diet and nutrition in urologic cancer. W V Med J 96:449–454

Kandasamy M, Bay BH, Lee YK et al (2011) Lactobacilli secreting a tumor antigen and IL15 activates neutrophils and dendritic cells and generates cytotoxic T lymphocytes against cancer cells. Cell Immunol (Epub ahead of print)

Kelloff GJ, Boone CW, Malone WF (1992) Development of chemopreventive agents for bladder cancer. J Cell Biochem Suppl 16I:1–12

Lamm DL, Riggs DR, Shriver JS et al (1994) Megadose vitamins in bladder cancer: a double-blind clinical trial. J Urol 151:21–26

Liang D, Lin J, Grossman HB (2008) Plasma vitamins E and A and risk of bladder cancer: a case-control analysis. Cancer Causes Control 19:981–992

Lobel B, Abou CC, Brausi MA et al (1998) Guidelines for diagnosis, treatment, and follow-up of bladder cancer: the influence of prognostic factors and the significance of random biopsies. Urol Oncol 4:94

Lubet RA, Yang CS, Lee MJ et al (2007) Preventive effects of polyphenon E on urinary bladder and mammary cancers in rats and correlations with serum and urine levels of tea polyphenols. Mol Cancer Ther 6:2022–2028

Madeb R, Golijanin D, Noyes K et al (2009) Treatment of nonmuscle invading bladder cancer: do physicians in the United States practice evidence based medicine? The use and economic implications of intravesical chemotherapy after transurethral resection of bladder tumors. Cancer 115:2660–2670

Marsh CL, Torrey RR, Woolley JL et al (1987) Superiority of intravesical immunotherapy with Corynebacterium parvum and Allium sativum in control of murine bladder cancer. J Urol 137:359–362

Michaud DS, Spiegelman D, Clinton SK et al (1999) Fluid intake and the risk of bladder cancer in men. N Engl J Med 340:1390–1397

Michaud DS, Spiegelman D, Clinton SK et al (2000) Prospective study of dietary supplements, macronutrients, micronutrients, and risk of bladder cancer in US men. Am J Epidemiol 152:1145–1153

Michaud DS, Pietinen P, Taylor PR et al (2002) Intakes of fruits and vegetables, carotenoids and vitamins A, E, C in relation to the risk of bladder cancer in the ATBC cohort study. Br J Cancer 87:960–965

Miller ER 3rd, Pastor-Barriuso R, Dalal D et al (2005) Meta-analysis: high-dosage vitamin E supplementation may increase all-cause mortality. Ann Intern Med 142:37–46

Mirvish SS. (1986) Effects of vitamins C and E on N-nitroso compound formation, carcinogenesis, and cancer. Cancer 58(8 Suppl):1842–1850

Mohr SB, Garland CF, Gorham ED et al (2010) Ultraviolet B irradiance and incidence rates of bladder cancer in 174 countries. Am J Prev Med 38:296–302

Mondul AM, Weinstein SJ, Männistö S et al (2010) Serum vitamin D and risk of bladder cancer. Cancer Res 70:9218–9223

Nagano J, Kono S, Preston DL et al (2000) Bladder-cancer incidence in relation to vegetable and fruit consumption: a prospective study of atomic-bomb survivors. Int J Cancer 86:132–138

Neuhouser ML, Wassertheil-Smoller S, Thomson C et al (2009) Multivitamin use and risk of cancer and cardiovascular disease in the Women's Health Initiative cohorts. Arch Intern Med 169:294–304

Newling DW, Robinson MR, Smith PH et al (1995) Tryptophan metabolites, pyridoxine (vitamin B6) and their influence on the recurrence rate of superficial bladder cancer. Results of a prospective, randomised phase III study performed by the EORTC GU Group. EORTC Genito-Urinary Tract Cancer Cooperative Group. Eur Urol 27:110–116

Nomura AM, Kolonel LN, Hankin JH et al (1991) Dietary factors in cancer of the lower urinary tract. Int J Cancer 48:199–205

Noyes K, Singer EA, Messing EM (2008) Healthcare economics of bladder cancer: cost-enhancing and cost-reducing factors. Curr Opin Urol 18:533–539

Ohashi Y, Nakai S, Tsukamoto T et al (2002) Habitual intake of lactic acid bacteria and risk reduction of bladder cancer. Urol Int 68:273–280

Park BT, Na KH, Jung EC et al (2009) Antifungal and Anticancer Activities of a Protein from the Mushroom Cordyceps militaris. Korean J Physiol Pharmacol 2009 Feb;13(1):49–54

Patton SE, Hall C, Ozen H (2002) Bladder cancer. Curr Opin Oncol 14:265:272

Peng CC, Chen KC, Peng RY et al (2007) Antrodia camphorata extract induces replicative senescence in superficial TCC, and inhibits the absolute migration capability in invasive bladder carcinoma cells. J Ethnopharmacol 109:93–103

Rajamahanty S, Louie B, O'Neill C et al (2009) Possible disease remission in patient with invasive bladder cancer with D-fraction regimen. Int J Gen Med 2:15–17

Reddy BS (1996) Micronutrients as chemopreventive agents. IARC Sci Publ 139:221–235

Riboli E, Norat T (2003) Epidemiologic evidence of the protective effect of fruit and vegetables on cancer risk. Am J Clin Nutr 78(3 Suppl):559S–569S

Sabichi AL, Lerner SP, Grossman HB (1998) Retinoids in the chemoprevention of bladder cancer. Curr Opin Oncol 10:479–484

Sabichi AL, Lerner SP, Atkinson EN et al (2008) Phase III prevention trial of fenretinide in patients with resected non-muscle-invasive bladder cancer. Clin Cancer Res 14:224–229

Seow SW, Cai S, Rahmat JN et al (2010) Lactobacillus rhamnosus GG induces tumor regression in mice bearing orthotopic bladder tumors. Cancer Sci 101:751–758

Siegel R, Ward E, Brawley O et al (2011) Cancer statistics, 2011: the impact of eliminating socioeconomic and racial disparities on premature cancer deaths. CA Cancer J Clin 61:212–236

Singh AV, Franke AA, Blackburn GL et al (2006) Soy phytochemicals prevent orthotopic growth and metastasis of bladder cancer in mice by alterations of cancer cell proliferation and apoptosis and tumor angiogenesis. Cancer Res 66:1851–1858

Singh RP, Tyagi A, Sharma G et al (2008) Oral silibinin inhibits in vivo human bladder tumor xenograft growth involving down-regulation of survivin. Clin Cancer Res 14:300–308

Snyder C Harlan L, Knopf K et al (2003) Patterns of care for the treatment of bladder cancer. J Urol 169:1697–1701
Sporn MB, Suh N (2002) Chemoprevention: an essential approach to controlling cancer. Nat Rev Cancer 2:537–543
Spruck CH 3rd, Ohneseit PF, Gonzalez-Zulueta M et al (1994) Two molecular pathways to transitional cell carcinoma of the bladder. Cancer Res 54:784–788
Steiner GG (2000) The correlation between cancer incidence and kava consumption. Hawaii Med J 59:420–422
Steinmaus CM, Nunez S, Smith AH (2000) Diet and bladder cancer: a meta-analysis of six dietary variables. Am J Epidemiol 151:693–702
Stenzl A, Penkoff H, Dajc-Sommerer E et al (2011) Detection and clinical outcome of urinary bladder cancer with 5-aminolevulinic acid-induced fluorescence cystoscopy: a multicenter randomized, double-blind, placebo-controlled trial. Cancer 117:938–947
Studer UE, Jenzer S, Biedermann C et al (1995) Adjuvant treatment with a vitamin A analogue (etretinate) after transurethral resection of superficial bladder tumors. Final analysis of a prospective, randomized multicenter trial in Switzerland. Eur Urol 28:284–290
Sun CL, Yuan JM, Wang XL (2004) Dietary soy and increased risk of bladder cancer: a prospective cohort study of men in Shanghai, China. Int J Cancer 112:319–23
Sylvester RJ, van der Meijden AP, Lamm DL (2002) Intravesical bacillus Calmette-Guerin reduces the risk of progression in patients with superficial bladder cancer: a meta-analysis of the published results of randomized clinical trials. J Urol 168:1964
Sylvester RJ, Oosterlinck W, van der Meijden AP (2004) A single immediate postoperative instillation of chemotherapy decreases the risk of recurrence in patients with stage Ta T1 bladder cancer: a meta-analysis of published results of randomized clinical trials. J Urol 171:2186
Takahashi T, Kushiro A, Nomoto K et al (2001) Antitumor effects of the intravesical instillation of heat killed cells of the Lactobacillus casei strain Shirota on the murine orthotopic bladder tumor MBT-2. J Urol 166:2506–2511
Tamaño S, Fukushima S, Shirai T et al (1987) Modification by alpha-tocopherol, propyl gallate and tertiary butylhydroquinone of urinary bladder carcinogenesis in Fischer 344 rats pretreated with N-butyl-N-(4-hydroxybutyl) nitrosamine. Cancer Lett 35:39–46
Tang L, Zhang Y (2004) Isothiocyanates in the chemoprevention of bladder cancer. Curr Drug Metab 5:193–201
Tang L, Zirpoli GR, Guru K et al (2008a) Consumption of raw cruciferous vegetables is inversely associated with bladder cancer risk. Cancer Epidemiol Biomarkers Prev 17:938–944
Tang Y, Simoneau AR, Xie J et al (2008b) Effects of the kava chalcone flavokawain A differ in bladder cancer cells with wild-type versus mutant p53. Cancer Prev Res (Phila) 1:439–451
Tomita K, Akaza H, Nomoto K et al (1994) Influence of Lactobacillus casei on rat bladder carcinogenesis Nippon Hinyokika Gakkai Zasshi 85:655–663
Toriyama-Baba H, Iigo M, Asamoto M et al (2001) Organotropic chemopreventive effects of n-3 unsaturated fatty acids in a rat multi-organ carcinogenesis model. Jpn J Cancer Res 92: 1175–1183
Tyagi A, Raina K, Singh RP et al (2007) Chemopreventive effects of silymarin and silibinin on N-butyl-N-(4-hydroxybutyl) nitrosamine induced urinary bladder carcinogenesis in male ICR mice. Mol Cancer Ther 6:3248–3255
Villanueva CM, Cantor KP, King WD et al (2006) Total and specific fluid consumption as determinants of bladder cancer risk 118:2040–2047
Vinh PQ, Sugie S, Tanaka T, Hara A, Yamada Y, Katayama M, Deguchi T, Mori H (2002) Chemopreventive effects of a flavonoid antioxidant silymarin on N-butyl-N-(4-hydroxybutyl) nitrosamine-induced urinary bladder carcinogenesis in male ICR mice. Jpn J Cancer Res 93:42–49
Wakai K, Hirose K, Takezaki T (2004) Foods and beverages in relation to urothelial cancer: case-control study in Japan. Int J Urol 11:11–19
Wu XR (2005) Urothelial tumorigenesis: a tale of divergent pathways. Nat Rev Cancer 5:713–725

Yang D, Li S, Wang H et al (1999) Prevention of postoperative recurrence of bladder cancer: a clinical study. Zhonghua Wai Ke Za Zhi 37:464–465

Yang CY, Chiu HF, Chang CC et al (2005) Bladder cancer mortality reduction after installation of a tap-water supply system in an arsenious-endemic area in southwestern Taiwan. Environ Res 98:127–132

Yu MC, Skipper PL, Tannenbaum SR, Chan KK, Ross RK (2004) Arylamine exposures and bladder cancer risk. Mutation Res 506–507:21–28

Yuen JW, Gohel MD, Au DW (2008) Telomerase-associated apoptotic events by mushroom ganoderma lucidum on premalignant human urothelial cells. Nutr Cancer 60:109–119

Zeegers MP, Goldbohm RA, van den Brandt PA (2001) Are retinol, vitamin C, vitamin E, folate and carotenoids intake associated with bladder cancer risk? Results from the Netherlands Cohort Study. Br J Cancer 85:977–983

Zeegers MP, Kellen E, Buntinx F (2004) The association between smoking, beverage consumption, diet and bladder cancer: a systematic literature review. World J Urol 21:392–401

Zhou JR, Mukherjee P, Gugger ET et al (1998) Inhibition of murine bladder tumorigenesis by soy isoflavones via alterations in the cell cycle, apoptosis, and angiogenesis. Cancer Res 58: 5231–5238

Zi X, Simoneau AR (2005) Flavokawain A, a novel chalcone from kava extract, induces apoptosis in bladder cancer cells by involvement of Bax protein-dependent and mitochondria-dependent apoptotic pathway and suppresses tumor growth in mice. Cancer Res 65:3479–3486

Zi X, Grasso AW, Kung HJ et al (1998) A flavonoid antioxidant, silymarin, inhibits activation of erbB1 signaling and induces cyclin-dependent kinase inhibitors, G1 arrest, and anticarcinogenic effects in human prostate carcinoma DU145 cells. Cancer Res 58:1920–1929

Chapter 9
Exploiting Resveratrol for the Treatment of Cancer

Simone Fulda

Abstract Resveratrol is a naturally occurring polyphenolic phytoalexin that is widely consumed with the diet. Its multitude of health beneficial effects has been attributed to the modulation of various signaling pathways. For example, the cancer chemopreventive and antitumor activities of resveratrol have been shown to involve the regulation of cell death and survival signaling cascades by resveratrol. In most circumstances, resveratrol suppresses signaling events that are critical to maintain tumor growth and survival, while it promotes pathways that lead to cell death. A better understanding of the molecular processes that are under the control of resveratrol in cancer cells will optimize the opportunities to exploit resveratrol for the treatment of cancer.

Keywords Resveratrol · Apoptosis · Signal transduction · Cancer

9.1 Resveratrol

Resveratrol (3,4′,5-trihydroxystilbene) is a naturally occurring polyphenolic compound that is well known for its multiple beneficial effects on human health (Pervaiz 2003). It is a constituent of red wine and considered to be responsible for the so-called "French Paradox", i.e. the observation that people from Southern France suffer a relatively low incidence of ischemic heart disease, although they eat a diet that is rich in saturated fats (Ferrieres 2004). Besides these cardiovascular effects, resveratrol has been well characterized for its chemopreventive or antitumor activities (Pervaiz 2003).

Studies that aimed at identifying the structural basis for the anticancer properties of resveratrol have highlighted the importance of the 4-hydroxy group in the trans-conformation on positions 4 and 4′ of the stilbenic backbone (Stivala et al. 2001). The fact that the stilbene-like structure of resveratrol resembles the structure of the synthetic estrogen derivative diethylstilbestrol has led to the classification of resveratrol as phytoestrogene (Pervaiz 2003).

S. Fulda (✉)
Institute for Experimental Cancer Research in Pediatrics, Goethe-University Frankfurt, 60528 Frankfurt, Germany
e-mail: simone.fulda@kgu.de

F.H. Sarkar (ed.), *Nutraceuticals and Cancer*, DOI 10.1007/978-94-007-2630-7_9,

The biological activities of resveratrol are mediated by its effect on various signal transduction pathways that are involved in the regulation of tumor initiation as well as tumor progression and treatment resistance. For example, resveratrol interferes with cell survival cascades while simultaneously promoting cell death (Cal et al. 2003; Gusman et al. 2001; Pervaiz and Holme 2009). As a net result, resveratrol causes tumor growth inhibition and/or tumor regression in a large variety of cancer models (Gusman et al. 2001; Pervaiz and Holme 2009).

9.2 Regulation of Apoptotic Pathways by Resveratrol

One of the prominent characteristics of resveratrol is its apoptosis-promoting activity. Apoptosis is the best characterized form of programmed cell death that is tightly regulated in order to sustain tissue homeostasis (Degterev et al. 2008; Lockshin and Zakeri 2007; Lowe et al. 2004). Two key signaling pathways of apoptosis can be distinguished: (1) the death receptor (extrinsic) pathway and (2) the mitochondrial (intrinsic) pathway (Taylor et al. 2008). However, it has also to be pointed out that apoptosis is not the only mode of cell death. A variety of additional cell death forms have been delineated, including necrosis, necroptosis, autophagy or lysosomal cell death, just to name a few (Festjens et al. 2006; Kirkegaard and Jaattela 2009; Maiuri et al. 2007; Okada and Mak 2004; Vandenabeele et al. 2010).

One hallmark of human cancers is their ability to evade apoptosis (Hanahan and Weinberg 2011). This characteristic of cancer cells facilitates tumor formation as well as various facets of tumor progression, including treatment resistance. Importantly, resveratrol has been shown to be able to antagonize those mechanisms that prevent apoptosis in cancer cells by various means, thereby lowering the threshold for cell death induction (Fig. 9.1). For example, resveratrol has been demonstrated to suppress survivin, an anti-apoptotic protein of the "Inhibitor of Apoptosis" (IAP) family of proteins, in various models of cancer including hematological malignancies as well as solid cancers (Bhardwaj et al. 2007; Fulda and Debatin 2004; Harikumar et al. 2010; Hayashibara et al. 2002; Ling et al. 2009; Singh et al. 2007; Wang et al. 2008; Yu et al. 2008; Zhao et al. 2010). Mechanistically, this resveratrol-triggered suppression of survivin has been attributed to p21-mediated cell cycle arrest, leading to cell cycle-dependent depletion of the survivin via transcriptional and posttranscriptional mechanisms (Fulda and Debatin 2004). In addition, activation of Sirt1 upon exposure to resveratrol has been implicated to contribute to transcriptional downregulation of survivin expression (Wang et al. 2008). Furthermore, resveratrol has been reported to negatively regulate survivin expression by counteracting the transcription factor Signal Transducer and Activator of Transcription 3 (STAT3) that is known to stimulate survivin expression as one of its target genes (Yu et al. 2008). Thus, various molecular mechanisms may be responsible for resveratrol-imposed suppression of survivin in cancers, likely in a context-dependent manner.

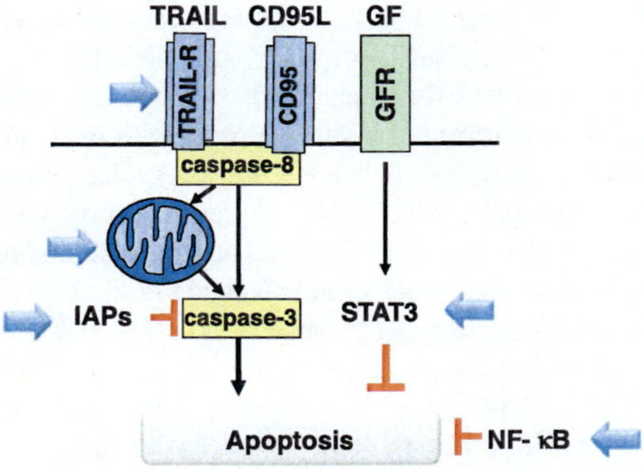

Fig. 9.1 Modulation of signaling pathways by resveratrol. Resveratrol has been shown to interfere with various signaling pathways, e.g. by inhibiting anti-apoptotic proteins such as the Inhibitor of Apoptosis (IAP) protein, by triggering pro-apoptotic proteins such as death receptors or by blocking survival mechanisms, i.e. transcription factors such as STAT3 and NF-κB. See text for more details

It is important to note that not only the anticancer activity of resveratrol, but also its chemopreventive potential has been linked to downregulation of survivin. In a classical mouse model of skin carcinogenesis initiated by ultraviolet (UV) light exposure in hairless mice, the topical application of resveratrol prevented the UV-stimulated upregulation of survivin expression in the skin, thereby counteracting tumor development (Aziz et al. 2005). Similarly, when dimethyl benz(a)anthracene (DMBA) was used as carcinogen in mouse models of skin tumorigenesis, the addition of resveratrol interfered with tumor formation at several points by postponing tumor onset and by reducing the cumulative number of tumors as well as tumor volume (Roy et al. 2009).

Additional anti-apoptotic proteins that are downregulated in expression by resveratrol comprise Bcl-X_L and Mcl-1, for example via resveratrol-mediated inhibition of extracellular signal-regulated kinase 1/2 (ERK1/2) or activator protein-1-dependent pathways (Jazirehi and Bonavida 2004) or via blockade of STAT3 signaling (Kotha et al. 2006). Furthermore, downregulation of Bcl-X_L and cFLIP by resveratrol has been identified as a mechanism conferring sensitivity to TRAIL-induced apoptosis by resveratrol in melanoma cells (Ivanov et al. 2008). Moreover, reduced expression of various anti-apoptotic proteins by resveratrol including Bcl-2, Bcl-X_L, survivin and XIAP has been associated with sensitization of prostate cancer cells that were resistant to TRAIL-induced apoptosis (Shankar et al. 2007).

Moreover, resveratrol can promote apoptosis by directly engaging pro-apoptotic signaling pathways (Fig. 9.1). For example, Reis-Sobreiro et al. reported that treatment with resveratrol triggers the recruitment of the Fas/CD95 receptor into lipid rafts in multiple myeloma and leukemia cells, thereby engaging the death receptor pathway of apoptosis (Reis-Sobreiro et al. 2009). Along these lines, the synergistic induction of apoptosis by resveratrol and death receptor ligands such as

CD95 ligand or TRAIL has been linked to the resveratrol-mediated redistribution of death receptors, i.e. CD95, TRAIL-R1 and TRAIL-R2, into lipid rafts (Delmas et al. 2003, 2004). Also, increased surface expression of Fas/CD95 associated with apoptosis induction was documented upon treatment with resveratrol in anaplastic large-cell lymphoma cells (Ko et al. 2011). Recently, resveratrol was shown to cause translocation of Bax to mitochondria in a XIAP-dependent manner, leading to Bax oligomerization on mitochondria, mitochondrial outer membrane permeabilization, cytochrome c release and caspase activation (Gogada et al. 2011). The resveratrol derivative 4-(6-hydroxy-2-naphthyl)-1,3-benzenediol (HS-1793) can bypass Bcl-2-mediated apoptosis resistance by reducing the expression of 14-3-3, a scaffold protein that binds to and inhibits various client proteins including pro-apoptotic proteins such as Bax and Bad (Jeong et al. 2009). F_1-ATPase, a component of the mitochondrial respiratory complex that is responsible for mitochondrial ATP synthesis, has been identified as another target of resveratrol, leading to a blockade of ATP production and subsequently to cell death (Gledhill et al. 2007).

9.3 Inhibition of the STAT3 Axis by Resveratrol

The antitumor cell activity of resveratrol has at least in part been attributed to the blockade of the STAT3 axis, a transcription factor that is involved in many aspects of oncogenesis. Inhibition of STAT3 signaling results in downregulating of STAT3-regulated target genes such as cyclin D1, Bcl-X_L and Mcl-1, providing a mechanistic basis for the anti-proliferative and apoptosis-promoting effects of resveratrol in tumors with activated STAT3 signaling (Kotha et al. 2006). In glioblastoma tumor-initiating cells, resveratrol suppressed tumor growth and enhanced radiosensitivity by interfering with STAT3 signaling (Yang et al. 2011). Also, the anti-leukemia effect of resveratrol in vitro and in vivo has been attributed to its ability to block STAT3 phosphorylation and STAT3-dependent signaling events, including reduction of Bcl-2 expression (Li et al. 2010). The antitumor activity of a trimeric derivative of resveratrol, i.e. 6-methyl-2-propylimino-6, 7-dihydro-5H-benzo [1, 3]-oxathiol- 4-one (LYR71) has been linked to the inhibition of migration/invasion by blocking the STAT3-mediated expression of matrix metalloproteinase 9 (MMP-9) (Kim et al. 2008). Furthermore, resveratrol induced apoptosis and inhibited proliferation in multiple myeloma cell lines and CD138-positive plasma cells from patients with multiple myeloma by decreasing STAT3-regulated anti-apoptotic and cell survival genes (Bhardwaj et al. 2007).

9.4 Inhibition of NF-κB Signaling by Resveratrol

NF-κB is one of the key transcriptional factors that is a target of resveratrol. NF-κB controls many different facets of cancer biology, including proliferation, invasion, metastasis, apoptosis and treatment resistance (Karin et al. 2002). In unstimulated cells, NF-κB is sequestered in the cytoplasm and held in check by IκB proteins that bind to NF-κB subunits (Hayden and Ghosh 2008). Upon stimulation, the proteasomal degradation of IκB proteins releases NF-κB to translocate to the nucleus to stimulate target gene expression (Hayden and Ghosh 2008). Resveratrol has been shown to interfere with several steps of the NF-κB signaling cascade, including inhibition of IκB kinase activity, nuclear translocation of NFκ-B and NF-κB-dependent transcriptional activation of target genes (Holmes-McNary and Baldwin 2000; Manna et al. 2000). Alternatively, resveratrol can indirectly interfere with NF-κB activation by modifying histone deacetylase activity and chromatin remodeling, which has been associated with its sirtuin-like activity (Howitz et al. 2003; Yeung et al. 2004). Since the NF-κB target genes comprise among others pro-angiogenic factors such as VEGF, the anti-angiogenic properties of resveratrol have been linked to its inhibitory effects on NF-κB (Yu et al. 2011). As hematological malignancies frequently harbor constitutively active NF-κB signaling, the antitumor activity of resveratrol against these malignancies may involve inhibition of NF-κB, leading to downregulation of NF-κB-dependent genes that promote tumor growth, e.g. in acute myeloid leukemic (AML) or multiple myeloma (Estrov et al. 2003; Pervaiz and Holme 2009; Rambaldi et al. 1991). Of note, resveratrol has also been reported to activate NF-κB signaling under certain circumstances, for example in medulloblastoma cells, leading to increased expression of the NF-κB target gene Bcl-2 and suppression of apoptosis (Wen et al. 2011).

9.5 Translational Perspective

A phase I study showed that resveratrol could be safely administered orally and that measurable plasma levels of resveratrol and its metabolites could be achieved (Boocock et al. 2007). Preclinical studies indicate that the potential of resveratrol may especially reside in enhancing the potency of other cytotoxic compounds in combination protocols. Just to give one example, resveratrol has been reported in vitro and in an orthotopic mouse model to augment the antitumor effects of gemcitabine, the first line chemotherapeutic drug in the treatment of pancreatic cancer (Harikumar et al. 2010). Resveratrol is currently evaluated in phase I/II clinical trials as single agent or in combination with e.g. the proteasome inhibitor bortezomib in colon cancer and multiple myeloma (http://clinicaltrials.gov).

9.6 Conclusions

Resveratrol presents a natural compound with promising properties that can be exploited for cancer chemoprevention as well as for cancer therapy. Investigations into the molecular mechanisms of action of resveratrol over the last decades have revealed many signal transduction pathways that are regulated by resveratrol and that account for its pleiotropic activities. Further investigation of the molecular network that is under the control of resveratrol may lead to the identification of novel targets, possibly also in a cancer- or stimulus-specific manner. Another key area for future research includes the development of biomarkers that allow the selection of patients that will benefit the most from resveratrol-based protocols. This approach may pave the avenue to personalized cancer medicine using resveratrol alone or in combination for the prevention or treatment of cancer.

Acknowledgements Work in the author's laboratory is supported by grants from the Deutsche Forschungsgemeinschaft, the Deutsche Krebshilfe, the Bundesministerium für Bildung und Forschung, the European Union (ApopTrain, APO-SYS) and IAP6/18.

References

Aziz MH, Afaq F, Ahmad N (2005) Prevention of ultraviolet-B radiation damage by resveratrol in mouse skin is mediated via modulation in survivin. Photochem Photobiol 81:25–31

Bhardwaj A, Sethi G, Vadhan-Raj S, Bueso-Ramos C, Takada Y, Gaur U et al (2007) Resveratrol inhibits proliferation, induces apoptosis, and overcomes chemoresistance through down-regulation of STAT3 and nuclear factor-kappaB-regulated antiapoptotic and cell survival gene products in human multiple myeloma cells. Blood 109:2293–2302

Boocock DJ, Faust GE, Patel KR, Schinas AM, Brown VA, Ducharme MP et al (2007) Phase I dose escalation pharmacokinetic study in healthy volunteers of resveratrol, a potential cancer chemopreventive agent. Cancer Epidemiol Biomark Prev 16:1246–1252

Cal C, Garban H, Jazirehi A, Yeh C, Mizutani Y, Bonavida B (2003) Resveratrol and cancer: chemoprevention, apoptosis, and chemo-immunosensitizing activities. Curr Med Chem Anti-Cancer Agents 3:77–93

Degterev A, Hitomi J, Germscheid M, Ch'en IL, Korkina O, Teng X et al (2008) Identification of RIP1 kinase as a specific cellular target of necrostatins. Nat Chem Biol 4:313–321

Delmas D, Rebe C, Lacour S, Filomenko R, Athias A, Gambert P et al (2003) Resveratrol-induced apoptosis is associated with Fas redistribution in the rafts and the formation of a death-inducing signaling complex in colon cancer cells. J Biol Chem 278:41482–41490

Delmas D, Rebe C, Micheau O, Athias A, Gambert P, Grazide S et al (2004) Redistribution of CD95, DR4 and DR5 in rafts accounts for the synergistic toxicity of resveratrol and death receptor ligands in colon carcinoma cells. Oncogene 23:8979–8986

Estrov Z, Shishodia S, Faderl S, Harris D, Van Q, Kantarjian HM et al (2003) Resveratrol blocks interleukin-1beta-induced activation of the nuclear transcription factor NF-kappaB, inhibits proliferation, causes S-phase arrest, and induces apoptosis of acute myeloid leukemia cells. Blood 102:987–995

Ferrieres J (2004) The French paradox: lessons for other countries. Heart 90:107–111

Festjens N, Vanden Berghe T, Vandenabeele P (2006) Necrosis, a well-orchestrated form of cell demise: signalling cascades, important mediators and concomitant immune response. Biochim Biophys Acta 1757:1371–1387

Fulda S, Debatin KM (2004) Sensitization for tumor necrosis factor-related apoptosis-inducing ligand-induced apoptosis by the chemopreventive agent resveratrol. Cancer Res 64:337–346

Gledhill JR, Montgomery MG, Leslie AG, Walker JE (2007) Mechanism of inhibition of bovine F1-ATPase by resveratrol and related polyphenols. Proc Natl Acad Sci USA 104:13632–13637

Gogada R, Prabhu V, Amadori M, Scott R, Hashmi S, Chandra D (2011) Resveratrol Induces p53-Independent, XIAP-Mediated Bax oligomerization on mitochondria to initiate cytochrome c release and caspase activation. J Biol Chem 286:28749–28760

Gusman J, Malonne H, Atassi G (2001) A reappraisal of the potential chemopreventive and chemotherapeutic properties of resveratrol. Carcinogenesis 22:1111–1117

Hanahan D, Weinberg RA (2011) Hallmarks of cancer: the next generation. Cell 144:646–674

Harikumar KB, Kunnumakkara AB, Sethi G, Diagaradjane P, Anand P, Pandey MK et al (2010) Resveratrol, a multitargeted agent, can enhance antitumor activity of gemcitabine in vitro and in orthotopic mouse model of human pancreatic cancer. Int J Cancer 127:257–268

Hayashibara T, Yamada Y, Nakayama S, Harasawa H, Tsuruda K, Sugahara K et al (2002) Resveratrol induces downregulation in survivin expression and apoptosis in HTLV-1-infected cell lines: a prospective agent for adult T cell leukemia chemotherapy. Nutr Cancer 44:193–201

Hayden MS, Ghosh S (2008) Shared principles in NF-kappaB signaling. Cell 132:344–362

Holmes-McNary M, Baldwin AS Jr (2000) Chemopreventive properties of trans-resveratrol are associated with inhibition of activation of the IkappaB kinase. Cancer Res 60:3477–3483

Howitz KT, Bitterman KJ, Cohen HY, Lamming DW, Lavu S, Wood JG et al (2003) Small molecule activators of sirtuins extend Saccharomyces cerevisiae lifespan. Nature 425:191–196

Ivanov VN, Partridge MA, Johnson GE, Huang SX, Zhou H, Hei TK (2008) Resveratrol sensitizes melanomas to TRAIL through modulation of antiapoptotic gene expression. Exp Cell Res 314:1163–1176

Jazirehi AR, Bonavida B (2004) Resveratrol modifies the expression of apoptotic regulatory proteins and sensitizes non-Hodgkin's lymphoma and multiple myeloma cell lines to paclitaxel-induced apoptosis. Mol Cancer Ther 3:71–84

Jeong SH, Jo WS, Song S, Suh H, Seol SY, Leem SH et al (2009) A novel resveratrol derivative, HS1793, overcomes the resistance conferred by Bcl-2 in human leukemic U937 cells. Biochem Pharmacol 77:1337–1347

Karin M, Cao Y, Greten FR, Li ZW (2002) NF-kappaB in cancer: from innocent bystander to major culprit. Nat Rev Cancer 2:301–310

Kim JE, Kim HS, Shin YJ, Lee CS, Won C, Lee SA et al (2008) LYR71, a derivative of trimeric resveratrol, inhibits tumorigenesis by blocking STAT3-mediated matrix metalloproteinase 9 expression. Exp Mol Med 40:514–522

Kirkegaard T, Jaattela M (2009) Lysosomal involvement in cell death and cancer. Biochim Biophys Acta 1793:746–754

Ko YC, Chang CL, Chien HF, Wu CH, Lin LI (2011) Resveratrol enhances the expression of death receptor Fas/CD95 and induces differentiation and apoptosis in anaplastic large-cell lymphoma cells. Cancer Lett 309:46–53

Kotha A, Sekharam M, Cilenti L, Siddiquee K, Khaled A, Zervos AS et al (2006) Resveratrol inhibits Src and Stat3 signaling and induces the apoptosis of malignant cells containing activated Stat3 protein. Mol Cancer Ther 5:621–629

Li T, Wang W, Chen H, Ye L (2010) Evaluation of anti-leukemia effect of resveratrol by modulating STAT3 signaling. Int Immunopharmacol 10:18–25

Ling X, He X, Apontes P, Cao F, Azrak RG, Li F (2009) Enhancing effectiveness of the MDR-sensitive compound T138067 using advanced treatment with negative modulators of the drug-resistant protein survivin. Am J Transl Res 1:393–405

Lockshin RA, Zakeri Z (2007) Cell death in health and disease. J Cell Mol Med 11:1214–1224

Lowe SW, Cepero E, Evan G (2004) Intrinsic tumour suppression. Nature 432:307–315

Maiuri MC, Zalckvar E, Kimchi A, Kroemer G (2007) Self-eating and self-killing: crosstalk between autophagy and apoptosis. Nat Rev Mol Cell Biol 8:741–752

Manna SK, Mukhopadhyay A, Aggarwal BB (2000) Resveratrol suppresses TNF-induced activation of nuclear transcription factors NF-kappa B, activator protein-1, and apoptosis: potential role of reactive oxygen intermediates and lipid peroxidation. J Immunol 164:6509–6519

Okada H, Mak TW (2004) Pathways of apoptotic and non-apoptotic death in tumour cells. Nat Rev Cancer 4:592–603

Pervaiz S (2003) Resveratrol: from grapevines to mammalian biology. FASEB J 17:1975–1985

Pervaiz S, Holme AL (2009) Resveratrol: its biologic targets and functional activity. Antioxid Redox Signal 11:2851–2897

Rambaldi A, Torcia M, Bettoni S, Vannier E, Barbui T, Shaw AR et al (1991) Modulation of cell proliferation and cytokine production in acute myeloblastic leukemia by interleukin-1 receptor antagonist and lack of its expression by leukemic cells. Blood 78:3248–3253

Reis-Sobreiro M, Gajate C, Mollinedo F (2009) Involvement of mitochondria and recruitment of Fas/CD95 signaling in lipid rafts in resveratrol-mediated antimyeloma and antileukemia actions. Oncogene 28:3221–3234

Roy P, Kalra N, Prasad S, George J, Shukla Y (2009) Chemopreventive potential of resveratrol in mouse skin tumors through regulation of mitochondrial and PI3K/AKT signaling pathways. Pharm Res 26:211–217

Shankar S, Chen Q, Siddiqui I, Sarva K, Srivastava RK (2007) Sensitization of TRAIL-resistant LNCaP cells by resveratrol (3, 4′, 5 tri-hydroxystilbene): molecular mechanisms and therapeutic potential. J Mol Signal 2:7

Singh SK, Moretta D, Almaguel F, Wall NR, De Leon M, De Leon D (2007) Differential effect of proIGF-II and IGF-II on resveratrol induced cell death by regulating survivin cellular localization and mitochondrial depolarization in breast cancer cells. Growth Factors 25:363–372

Stivala LA, Savio M, Carafoli F, Perucca P, Bianchi L, Maga G et al (2001) Specific structural determinants are responsible for the antioxidant activity and the cell cycle effects of resveratrol. J Biol Chem 276:22586–22594

Taylor RC, Cullen SP, Martin SJ (2008) Apoptosis: controlled demolition at the cellular level. Nat Rev Mol Cell Biol 9:231–241

Vandenabeele P, Galluzzi L, Vanden Berghe T, Kroemer G (2010) Molecular mechanisms of necroptosis: an ordered cellular explosion. Nat Rev Mol Cell Biol 11:700–714

Wang RH, Zheng Y, Kim HS, Xu X, Cao L, Luhasen T et al (2008) Interplay among BRCA1, SIRT1, and Survivin during BRCA1-associated tumorigenesis. Mol Cell 32:11–20

Wen S, Li H, Wu ML, Fan SH, Wang Q, Shu XH et al (2011) Inhibition of NF-kappaB signaling commits resveratrol-treated medulloblastoma cells to apoptosis without neuronal differentiation. J Neurooncol 104:169–177

Yang YP, Chang YL, Huang PI, Chiou GY, Tseng LM, Chiou SH et al (2011) Resveratrol suppresses tumorigenicity and enhances radiosensitivity in primary glioblastoma tumor initiating cells by inhibiting the STAT3 axis. J Cell Physiol [Apr 18, E-pub ahead of print]

Yeung F, Hoberg JE, Ramsey CS, Keller MD, Jones DR, Frye RA et al (2004) Modulation of NF-kappaB-dependent transcription and cell survival by the SIRT1 deacetylase. Embo J 23:2369–2380

Yu LJ, Wu ML, Li H, Chen XY, Wang Q, Sun Y et al (2008) Inhibition of STAT3 expression and signaling in resveratrol-differentiated medulloblastoma cells. Neoplasia (New York) 10:736–744

Yu HB, Zhang HF, Zhang X, Li DY, Xue HZ, Pan CE et al (2011) Resveratrol inhibits VEGF expression of human hepatocellular carcinoma cells through a NF-kappa B-mediated mechanism. Hepatogastroenterology 57:1241–126

Zhao W, Bao P, Qi H, You H (2010) Resveratrol down-regulates survivin and induces apoptosis in human multidrug-resistant SPC-A-1/CDDP cells. Oncol Rep 23:279–286

Chapter 10
Role of Novel Nutraceuticals Garcinol, Plumbagin and Mangiferin in the Prevention and Therapy of Human Malignancies: Mechanisms of Anticancer Activity

Aamir Ahmad, Subhash Padhye, and Fazlul H. Sarkar

Abstract Nutraceuticals from natural sources have been investigated for their putative chemopreventive and cancer therapeutic properties for the last few decades. The interest in these compounds is in part due to their pleiotropic effects and relatively non-toxic nature. A large number of such nutraceuticals are under detailed investigations worldwide but most of them suffer from the lack of sufficient bioavailability in humans. The identification and characterization of novel natural compounds with sufficient anticancer potential is therefore an ongoing process. This article is a summary of anticancer activity of three such novel nutraceuticals, namely garcinol, plumbagin and mangiferin. These compounds have shown promising biological activity in preliminary studies by targeting multiple signaling pathways. In particular, it seems that the inhibition of NF-κB pathway is one of the major mechanism through which these compounds exhibit their anticancer and apoptosis-inducing effects. The data on their anticancer activity is just emerging and the information on their bioavailability is still insufficient to predict their future application in the clinical settings. In this article, we have surveyed the available literature to summarize the mechanisms of anticancer activity of these three novel nutraceuticals. We also discuss the challenges and possible solutions to realize the dream on the translational potential of these compounds into clinical practice for the prevention and/or treatment of human malignancies.

10.1 Introduction

Cancer is a major public health problem worldwide. In the United States, cancer-related deaths are second only to deaths caused by heart diseases and account for close to a quarter of all deaths (Jemal et al. 2011; Siegel et al. 2011). With

---

F.H. Sarkar (✉)
Departments of Pathology and Oncology, Karmanos Cancer Institute, Wayne State University, 740 HWCRC, Detroit, Michigan 48201, USA
e-mail: fsarkar@med.wayne.edu

F.H. Sarkar (ed.), *Nutraceuticals and Cancer*, DOI 10.1007/978-94-007-2630-7_10,

the advancement in our understanding, it is now well accepted that cancer represents a highly heterogeneous disease. Accordingly, various therapeutic regimes are available for specific cancer subtypes, largely determined by the presence and absence of molecular targets. According to the information available on National Cancer Institute's website (http://www.cancer.gov/cancertopics/factsheet/Therapy/targeted), many molecularly targeted therapies are available for the treatment of a number of human cancers. For example, drugs that interfere with estrogen binding to the estrogen receptor (ER), such as tamoxifen, have been approved by the Food and Drug Administration (FDA) for the treatment of ER-positive breast cancers. The enzyme aromatase is necessary to produce estrogen in the body and, therefore, aromatase inhibitors are targeted drugs that interfere with estrogen's ability to promote the growth of ER-positive breast cancers. Other FDA-approved targeted therapies include tyrosine kinase inhibitors, serine/threonine kinase inhibitors, proteasome inhibitors, DNA synthesis inhibitors, angiogenesis inhibitors and monoclonal antibodies against Her-2 and EGFR.

The targeted therapies are clinically quite effective in blocking the proliferation of cancer cells through an effective check-point control of cell proliferation pathway by targeting cell-cycle molecules. However, it is well-known that cancer cells eventually develop resistance to these targeted therapies by activating alternative pathways thereby reducing their dependence on the pathway being targeted by the molecularly targeting agent. To overcome this, the idea of combinational therapy has been developed wherein multiple agents, that target mutually exclusive molecular pathways, are combined in an attempt to block multiple pathways. Such blockage of multiple cell signaling pathways indeed is much effective in ensuring a better check on the progression of malignancies but comes with the undesired side-effect of increased toxicity. Thus, it emerges that in addition to simultaneous targeting of multiple signaling pathways, the therapeutic regime/agent(s) should be associated with no or minimum toxicity.

To that end, the use of naturally occurring compounds has been suggested for many years because of the non-toxic nature of these agents. These compounds are known to be pleiotropic i.e. they possess the ability to deregulate multiple signaling pathways. Also, these compounds, obtained from plants, are part of normal diet and, therefore, they are well tolerated. A number of these agents such as isoflavones, indole-3-carbinol (I3C), 3,3′-diindolylmethane (DIM), curcumin, (-)-epigallocatechin-3-gallate (EGCG), resveratrol, lycopene, etc. have been investigated in considerable detail (Sarkar et al. 2009). These, and many other natural compounds, are being tested in clinical trials for their putative anticancer properties. In addition to the well established natural anticancer agents mentioned above, there are some other compounds that have not been well-investigated in such details or their anticancer potential has been suggested only in last few years. A few examples that fit this description are garcinol, plumbagin and mangiferin. The chemistry of these three natural compounds is relatively well understood. Their anticancer potential has been suggested; however, they have not been thoroughly investigated. This article summarizes our present knowledge on these three promising anticancer agents.

10.2 Occurrence and Chemistry

10.2.1 Garcinol

Garcinol (Fig. 10.1) is isolated from 'Kokum' plant. The kokum plant, *Garcinia indica*, grows extensively on the western coast of India and is known by various names across India including Bindin, Biran, Bhirand, Bhinda, Katambi, Panarpuli, Ratamba or Amsool. It is also known by names such as Mangosteen, wild Mangosteen, or Red Mango. The genus Garcinia includes some 200 species found in the tropics, especially Asia and Africa. Out of 35 species found in India, 17 are endemic. Of these, seven are endemic to the region of Western Ghats including the state of Goa, six in the Andaman and Nicobar Islands and four in the North-Eastern region of India.

Garcinia indica extracts, especially from its rind, are rich in polyisoprenylated benzophenone derivatives, including garcinol. The rind also contains isogarcinol, hydroxycitric acid, hydroxycitric acid lactone, citric acid and oxalic acid. The fruit contains compounds such as malic acid, polyphenols, carbohydrates, anthocyanin, pigments and ascorbic acid. The major organic acid in leaves and rinds of *Garcinia indica* is reported to be (-)-hydroxycitric acid, present to the extent of 4.1–4.6 and 10.3–12.7%, respectively (Jayaprakasha and Sakariah 2002; Jena et al. 2002). Chemically, garcinol is a tri-isoprenylated chalcone (Hamed et al. 2006; Masullo et al. 2008).

10.2.2 Plumbagin

Plumbagin (Fig. 10.1) belongs to the naphthoquinone family of chemical compounds and is the active principle found in *Plumbagenaeace*, *Droseraceae* and *Ebenceae* families. Chemically, it is a hydroxy-naphthoquinone which is generally extracted from the roots of Plumbago species. The oldest reference to this plant is found in the ancient Indian Ayurvedic texts of Charaka (2nd century B.C.) where the plant was known as 'Chitraka' whose roots were credited with therapeutic properties

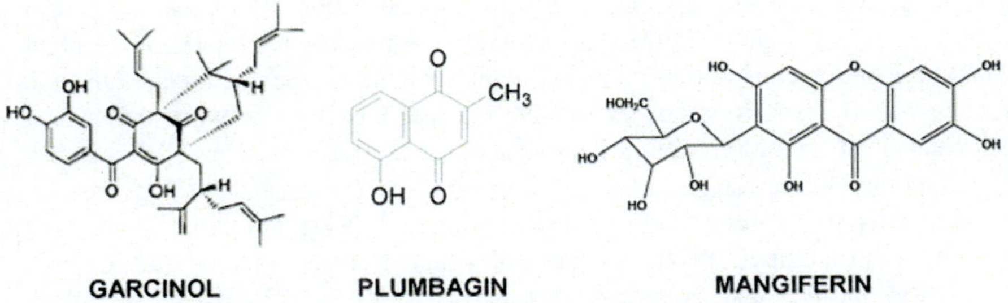

GARCINOL PLUMBAGIN MANGIFERIN

Fig. 10.1 Chemical structures of garcinol, plumbagin and mangiferin against dyspepsia, piles, diarrhea and skin diseases (Chopra et al. 1956; Dutt 1877; Nadkarni 1954). The plant extract was also found to be useful in treating tuberculosis and leprosy. *Plumbaginaceae* is a family of 10 genera and about 300 families mostly found in semi-arid regions of mediterranean and central Asia. In United States, it is represented by a single polymorphic species of Armeria (*A. maritima*) and polymorphic species of *Limonium,* both of which are found on the pacific coasts. Another species, *Plumbago scandens* is native of Florida and is grown from Texas to Arizona. Three species found in India are *Plumbago rosea*, *Plumbago zeylanica* and *Plumbago capensis*. These can be differentiated visually from the color of their flowers which are red, white and blue, respectively (Padhye et al. 2010b).

Isolation of plumbagin from the plant material is usually carried out by solvent extraction of the coarsely powdered roots by solvents of increasing polarity using cold percolation method (de et al. 2003), and it has been reported (Aryanathan 2009) that plumbagin content in *Plumbago rosea* is highest, corresponding to 0.17%, while in *Plumbago capensis* and *Plumbago zeylenica*, it is 0.04 and 0.01%, respectively. In general, the root parts are the rich sources of plumbagin. Interestingly, *Plumbago rosea* has been found to accumulate maximum plumbagin in the roots while, *Plumbago auriculata* and *Plumbago zeylanica* are high yielding species for the leaf and stem parts, respectively (Mallavadhani et al. 2002).

10.2.3 Mangiferin

The compound mangiferin (Fig. 10.1) is found in a variety of plant families in varying concentrations and it usually occurs as a glycoside. Some of the plant sources for Mangiferin include: *Anemmarhena asphodeloides*, *Aphloia theiformis*, *Arrabidaea patellifera*, *Arrabidaea samydoides*, *Bersama abyssinica*, *Bombax ceiba*, *Bombax malabaricum*, *Cratoxylum cochinchinense*, *Cyclopia genistoides*, *Cyclopia subternata*, *Folium mangiferae*, *Folium pyrrosiae*, *Gentiana lutea*, *Gentianella nitida*, *Gnidia involucrata*, *Hypericum perforatum*, *Mahkota Dewa*, *Mangifera indica*, *Mangifera odorata*, *Phaleria cumingii*, *Phaleria macrocarpa*, *Mangifera Persiciformis*, *Polygala hongkongensis*, *Pyrrosia gralla*, *Rhizoma anemarrhenae*, *Rhizoma belamcandae*, *Salacia hainanensis*, *Salacia oblonga*, *Salacia reticulate*, *Swertia macrosperma*, *Swertia chirata*, *Swertia mussotii*, *Swertia punicea*, *Trichomanes reniforme*, *Zizyphus cambodiana*. The easiest source of mangiferin, however, is the mango plant (*Mangifera indica*), especially the leaves of the plant. The tree is indigenous to the Indian sub-continent and has been cultivated in India for over 4000 years. It is thought to have reached East Asia between the 4th and 5th century BC and cultivated in East Africa and thereafter in Brazil, West Indies, China, United States, Carribean and Mexico.

Mangiferin is a natural C-glucoside xanthone [2-C-β-Dgluco-pyranosyl-1,3,6,7-tetrahydroxyxanthone]. It is detected at high concentrations in young mango leaves (172 g/kg) and it is also present in moderate amounts in bark (107 g/kg) and old leaves (Itamaraka) (94 g/kg), respectively (Barreto et al. 2008). Mangiferin has also been found in the mango fruits.

10.3 Antioxidant Activity

Oxidative stress has long been regarded as a factor that contributes to cancer development. More recent research has shown that reactive oxygen species (ROS), produced at elevated levels within tumor tissue, may function as signaling molecules that initiate and/or modulate different regulatory pathways that are involved in tumorigenesis and metastasis (Tertil et al. 2010). Elevated ROS have been detected in almost all cancers and high concentrations of ROS can damage many biomolecules, including lipids, proteins and nucleic acids. To counter the harmful effects of ROS, tumor cells typically express elevated levels of antioxidant proteins, which suggests that a delicate balance of intracellular ROS levels is required for cancer cell function (Liou and Storz 2010). Despite the presence of the cell's antioxidant system, oxidative damage accumulates during the life cycle and plays an important role in the development of many disease conditions, including cancer (Balsano and Alisi 2009). Since oxidative stress plays a crucial role in the development of cancer, a desirable property of any potential anticancer agent is its ability to reverse or minimize cellular damage by oxidative stress, more simply known as its antioxidant potential. This is one of the earliest parameter to judge the efficacy of a novel compound for its anticancer activity. Most of the compounds that are eventually tested for their anticancer activity usually start out as potent antioxidants. It is therefore not surprising that the antioxidant potential of garcinol, plumbagin as well as mangiferin has been suggested as the mode of action of these compounds.

10.3.1 Garcinol

A strong antioxidant activity of garcinol has been documented which is primarily because of the presence of phenolic hydroxyl groups as well as a β-diketone moiety in garcinol. In this respect, it resembles the well-known antioxidant of plant origin, curcumin (Pan et al. 2001). As a proof of its potent antioxidant activity, garcinol has been documented to scavenge DPPH free radicals (3 times more effectively than DL-R-tocopherol), hydroxyl radicals (more effectively than DL-R-tocopherol), methyl radicals and superoxide anions (Yamaguchi et al. 2000). Garcinol reacts with peroxyl radicals by a single electron transfer followed by deprotonation of the hydroxyl group from the enolized 1, 3-diketone to form a resonance pair. Depending on the position of hydroxyl group (C-3 or C-5) which initiates the reaction, different compounds are formed (Sang et al. 2001, 2002). The antioxidant activity of garcinol in the context of its neuroprotective effects has been studied, and it was found that garcinol prevented nitric oxide (NO) radical accumulation in lipopolysaccharide (LPS) – treated astrocytes. In phenazine methosulfate/NADH-nitro blue tetrazolium system, garcinol has been shown to exhibit superoxide anion scavenging activity (Yamaguchi et al. 2000).

10.3.2 Plumbagin

In an earlier study for evaluating the antioxidant effects of plumbagin, plumbago roots was used in medicinal preparations, and a potent antioxidant activity was reported with significant inhibition of lipid peroxidation (Tilak et al. 2004). In the comet assay, using mouse lymphoma L5178Y cells (Demma et al. 2009), plumbagin was able to reduce the catechol-induced DNA damage, suggesting its role as an antioxidant at low concentrations. Plumbagin has also been reported to inhibit ascorbate and NADPH-dependent lipid peroxidation in rats that were fed plumbagin (Sankar et al. 1987). Interestingly, most of the studies on antioxidant ability of plumbagin also seem to suggest its prooxidant activity. This is not very surprising since many naturally occurring compounds are known to possess antioxidant as well as prooxidant properties (Hadi et al. 2000; Khan et al. 2000; Singh et al. 2001), which may function in a context-dependent manner.

10.3.3 Mangiferin

A study to compare five varieties of *Mangifera indica* for their phenolic contents and antioxidant potential of the fruit pulp revealed that the mango variety, Ataulfo has the highest phenolic content and exhibited superior DPPH radical scavenging activity compared to other varieties (Manthey and Perkins-Veazie 2009). The ability of mangiferin to ameliorate glutamate receptors-mediated oxidative stress, neuronal death and mitochondrial depolarization has also been demonstrated (Lemus-Molina et al. 2009). It has also been shown that mangiferin suppresses generation of ROS by triggering enzymatic antioxidant system and rejuvenating mitochondrial membrane potential (Campos-Esparza et al. 2009). A similar antioxidant activity of mangiferin through modulation of mitochondrial membrane potential and lipid peroxidation has been shown in benzo (a) pyrene-induced lung carcinogenesis in mice (Rajendran et al. 2008c). A number of reports have demonstrated the ability of mangiferin to scavenge ROS (Amazzal et al. 2007; Barreto et al. 2008; Bertolini et al. 2007; Hsu et al. 1997; Martinez et al. 2001; Pauletti et al. 2003; Yoshikawa et al. 2002). These studies indicate that one of the mechanisms through which mangiferin affords antioxidant effects is through quenching of reactive oxygen intermediates. In addition, the effects of mangiferin on other oxidation pathways leading to an antioxidant effect have also been reported (Dar et al. 2005; Pardo-Andreu et al. 2008a, b; Prabhu et al. 2006; Rodeiro et al. 2008).

The available literature on the antioxidant potential of garcinol, plumbagin and mangiferin indicates that these compounds are good regulators of cellular oxidative stress. While the reports on garcinol and mangiferin support the ability of these compounds to quench ROS leading to antioxidant effects, the available evidence for plumbagin suggests that this compound can act as a quencher as well as generator of ROS. This property of plumbagin has been suggested to be concentration-dependent but can also be cell type-dependent or cellular microenvironment-dependent. In support of the latter, it has been suggested that many anticancer natural compounds can actually generate ROS in cancer cells through mobilization and redox cycling of chromatin-bound transition metal ion copper (Hadi et al. 2000; Ullah et al. 2011). Such a generation of ROS in copper-rich cancer cells leads to an efficient induction of apoptotic cell death which further underlines the anticancer activity of such compounds.

10.4 Anticancer Activity

With the establishment of a potent antioxidant activity, garcinol, plumbagin and mangiferin have further been evaluated for their anticancer potential in models representing different human cancers. In the next few paragraphs we have discussed a cancer-specific breakdown of reported anticancer activity of these compounds. Named subsections have only been provided for those cancers where there are reports on anticancer effects of all the three compounds, or a minimum of two compounds. The cancers, in which only one of these compounds has been characterized, are listed under 'other cancers'.

10.4.1 Breast Cancer

The first evidence for an anticancer effect of garcinol against breast cancer cells was provided by us (Ahmad et al. 2010). In this study we found that garcinol inhibits proliferation of ER-positive MCF-7 as well as ER-negative MDA-MB-231 breast cancer cells with a concomitant induction of apoptosis, but has no effect on non-tumorigenic MCF-10A cells. Down-regulation of NF-κB signaling pathway was observed to be the mechanism of apoptosis-induction by garcinol. More recently, it has been shown that garcinol can inhibit nicotinic acetylcholine receptor (nAChR) and cyclin D3 expression in human breast cancer cells (Chen et al. 2011). Since nAChRs have been shown to be involved in smoking-induced cancer formation in multiple types of human cancer cells (Wu et al. 2011), their inhibition by garcinol has implications for anticancer activity of garcinol against a number of different cancers.

In an earlier report demonstrating the ability of plumbagin to inhibit proliferation of human breast cancer cells, an involvement of autophagic cell death was suggested (Kuo et al. 2006). It was shown that plumbagin inhibits Akt, and thus plays a crucial role in plumbagin-induced induction of autophagy and cell cycle arrest. In our investigations with plumbagin, we observed that this compound significantly inhibits the growth of MCF-7 and MDA-MB-231 cells, with no effect on MCF-10A cells, (Ahmad et al. 2008). As a mechanism, we found that plumbagin down-regulates Bcl-2 expression and NF-κB activity and that ectopic expression of Bcl-2 was able to attenuate plumbagin-induced effects. Plumbagin has also been shown to inhibit proliferation, and induce apoptosis in Her2/neu-overexpressing SKBR3 breast cancer cells (Nazeem et al. 2009).

The first evidence for an anticancer effect of mangiferin against breast cancer cells was reported few years back when it was shown that mangiferin can inhibit tumor necrosis factor (TNF)-induced activation of NF-κB in MCF-7 cells (Sarkar et al. 2004). More recently, *Mangifera indica* extract has been shown to inhibit proliferation of MDA-MB-231 cells through inhibition of NF-κB pathway (Garcia-Rivera et al. 2011).

10.4.2 Prostate Cancer

Similar to its anticancer action against breast cancer cells (Ahmad et al. 2010), our laboratory was the first one to suggest such an action of garcinol against prostate cancer cells (Ahmad et al. 2011b). In this study, we investigated the mechanism of apoptosis-inducing effect of garcinol in multiple prostate cancer cells – androgen receptor (AR)-positive and responsive LNCaP cells, AR-positive but unresponsive C4-2B cells and AR-negative PC3 cells. We found that garcinol inhibited cell growth of all the cell lines and induced apoptosis in a dose-dependent manner. Garcinol inhibited constitutive levels of NF-κB activity, which was consistent with down-regulation of NF-κB-regulated genes. We also observed a significant decrease in the colony forming ability of prostate cancer cells which suggested the possible use of this compound against metastatic disease.

Regarding the anticancer activity of plumbagin in prostate cancer model, it was first reported that exposure to plumbagin significantly reduces the viability of multiple prostate cancer cells (Powolny and Singh 2008). Plumbagin was found to induce apoptosis which was accompanied by generation of ROS. Later, it was shown that plumbagin can selectively kill prostate cancer cells without affecting non-tumorigenic prostate epithelial RWPE-1 cells (Aziz et al. 2008). Plumbagin was also found to delay tumor growth in mice and the tumor weight was reduced by 90%. This study, thus, established in vitro as well as in vivo activity of plumbagin against prostate cancer.

10.4.3 Pancreatic Cancer

As part of our comprehensive study investigating the anticancer activity of garcinol against prostate as well as pancreatic cancer cells, we showed that garcinol was effective in inducing apoptotic cell death in BxPC-3 pancreatic cancer cells through inhibition of constitutive NF-κB activity (Ahmad et al. 2011b). Another recent study has further confirmed our results (Parasramka and Gupta 2011). In this study two human pancreatic cell lines, BxPC-3 and Panc-1, with wild and mutant k-ras, respectively, were used. Garcinol was found to significantly inhibit cell growth and induce apoptosis and caused G0-G1 phase cell cycle arrest in both the cell lines although the effects were more pronounced in Panc-1 cells.

Plumbagin has also been shown to inhibit the growth of Panc-1 and BxPC-3 pancreatic cancer cells (Chen et al. 2009). It was observed that plumbagin causes an up-regulation of bax and a rapid decline in mitochondrial trans-membrane potential. Activation of caspase-9 and caspase-3, but not caspase-8, was observed. As an in vivo proof, plumbagin was found to significantly inhibit the growth of Panc-1 xenograft tumor. Down-regulation of phosphoinositide 3-kinase (PI3K) activity by plumbagin through a negative feedback mechanism was also suggested, and it was concluded that plumbagin can induce apoptosis through caspase-dependent and caspase-independent cascades.

10.4.4 Lung Cancer

There is evidence to suggest anticancer action of plumbagin in lung cancer models. It has been reported that plumbagin significantly inhibits the growth of H460 cells compared to A549 cells (Gomathinayagam et al. 2008) through down-regulation of EGFR signaling. Plumbagin was also found to induce cell cycle arrest and caspase-3-mediated apoptosis. Another study has actually demonstrated the ability of plumbagin to inhibit cell growth and induce cell cycle arrest and apoptosis in A549 cells as well (Hsu et al. 2006). The ability of plumbagin to inhibit 12-O-tetradecanoylphorbol-13-acetate (TPA)-induced invasion and migration of A549 cancer cells has also been reported (Shieh et al. 2010). Such effect of plumbagin has been attributed to its ability to inhibit matrix metalloproteinases and urokinase-type plasminogen activator.

There is evidence to suggest chemopreventive effect of mangiferin against benzopyrene-induced lung carcinogenesis. In a series of publications, the research group led by Rajendran has investigated such biological effects of mangiferin (Rajendran et al. 2008a–c). Firstly, supplementation of mangiferin was found to enhance detoxification enzymes (glutathione transferase, quinone reductase and uridin 5′-diphosphate-glucuronosyl transferase) and reduce DNA damage in the lung cancer bearing animals (Rajendran et al. 2008a). Thereafter, mangiferin was found to prevent decreased activities of electron transport chain complexes and tricarboxylic acid cycle key enzymes (isocitrate dehydrogenase, succinate dehydrogenase, malate dehydrogenase and alpha-ketoglutarate dehydrogenase), in lung cancer bearing animals (Rajendran et al. 2008b). Lastly, the levels of glutathione and the activities of antioxidant enzymes (superoxide dismutase, catalase, glutathione peroxidase and glutathione reductase) in the mangiferin + benzo(a)pyrene-treated animals were found to be improved, compared with benzo(a)pyrene-treated animals (Rajendran et al. 2008c).

10.4.5 Colon Cancer

In colon cancer models, the effects of garcinol and its oxidative derivatives have been investigated on the growth of HT-29 and HCT-116 colon cancer cells, as well as the normal immortalized intestinal cells IEC-6 and INT-407 (Hong et al. 2007). Garcinol and its derivatives showed potent growth-inhibitory effects on all intestinal cells and was found to be more effective in inhibiting growth of cancer cells than that of normal immortalized cells. These results indicate that garcinol and its derivatives can inhibit intestinal cancer cell growth without affecting normal cells. In another study on HT-29 cells (Liao et al. 2005), it was shown that garcinol can inhibit cell invasion through suppression of Src, MAPK/ERK, PI3K/Akt and FAK signaling pathways. In a study to investigate the effects of mangiferin on azoxymethane-induced tumorigenesis, it was observed that mangiferin significantly inhibits the aberrant crypt foci development in rats treated with azoxymethane (Yoshimi et al. 2001).

10.4.6 Leukemia

In human leukemia HL-60 cells, garcinol has been reported to inhibit cell growth through induction of caspase-3 and caspase-2 activity, but not caspase-1 activity, in a dose- and time-dependent manner (Pan et al. 2001). Treatment with garcinol was found to result in a rapid loss of mitochondrial transmembrane potential, release of mitochondrial cytochrome c into cytosol, and increased procaspase-9 processing. In a study comprising four human leukemia cells lines, loss of mitochondrial membrane potential was observed during garcinol-induced apoptosis (Matsumoto et al. 2003).

In human promyelocytic leukemia cells, NB4, an involvement of mitochondrial pathway during plumbagin-induced apoptosis has been suggested (Xu and Lu 2010). This study also identified generation of ROS as a critical mediator of plumbagin-induced apoptosis. In vivo, the results were confirmed through NB4 tumor xenograft in NOD/SCID mice. Daily plumbagin treatment for 3 weeks resulted in 64.49% reduction of tumor volume. A dose-dependent inhibitory action of plumbagin on proliferation of NB4 cells has also been shown (Zhao and Lu 2006). Plumbagin blocked the G2/M transition of cell cycle and induced apoptosis, as evident by DNA fragmentation.

There is evidence to suggest an anticancer action of mangiferin as well, against leukemia cells. In K562 cells, mangiferin has been found to inhibit telomerase activity and induce apoptosis (Cheng et al. 2007). Earlier studies in the same model also observed an in vitro antiproliferative effect of mangiferin leading to efficient induction of apoptosis (Peng et al. 2004). In HL-60 cells, *Mangifera indica* extract has been shown to inhibit cell cycle in the G0/G1 phase (Percival et al. 2006). Also, the whole mango juice was found to be effective in reducing the number of transformed foci in the neoplastic transformation assay in a dose-dependent manner.

10.4.7 Other Cancers

In a study to evaluate the differential ability of selected compounds to inhibit cell growth in relation to BRCA1 (breast cancer 1, early onset) status in ER-positive ovarian cancer cells (Thasni et al. 2008), plumbagin was found to be the most effective inducer of apoptosis through its binding to and modulation of ER-alpha in BRCA1 silenced cells. In an earlier study, the effect of tamoxifen, emodin, and plumbagin was analyzed in BRCA1-silenced ovarian cancer cells that express ER (Srinivas et al. 2004a). It was observed that the induction of apoptosis was greater in BRCA1-blocked cells and the efficacy was in the order of plumbagin > tamoxifen > emodin.

In a myeloma model (Bringmann et al. 2008), it was first reported that plumbagin has no effect on proliferation of human multiple myeloma cells lines RPMI8226 and INA-6, as evaluated by Annexin V-FITC/PI staining. However, in a later study in myeloma cell lines U266 and MM.1S, it was shown that plumbagin can inhibit both constitutive and interleukin (IL-6)-inducible STAT-3 phosphorylation, leading to the induction of apoptosis (Sandur et al. 2010). These contrasting results suggest that plumbagin might have a cell-line specific effect in myeloma models.

In human melanoma 375.S2 cells, plumbagin has been reported to induce apoptosis and S-G2/M cell cycle arrest leading to cell growth inhibition (Wang et al. 2008). The anticancer effect of plumbagin was also verified in vivo. Plumbagin treatment resulted in elevated p21 levels and reduced levels of cyclin B1, cyclin A, Cdc2, and Cdc25C. It also induced a change in Bax/Bcl-2 ratios and activation of caspase-9 resulting in apoptotic cell death. In A-431 cells, it has been reported that the biological action of plumbagin is mediated through a mechanism that involves redox recycling of transition metal ion copper (Nazeem et al. 2009). There are some other reports on the anticancer ability of plumbagin against melanoma cells as well (Mandala Rayabandla et al. 2010; Prasad et al. 1996).

The effect of plumbagin on liver cancer HepG2 cells has been investigated and it was observed that plumbagin can inhibit the migration and invasion of liver cancer cells through down-regulation of MMP-2 and uPA (Shih et al. 2009). In another study (Parimala and Sachdanandam 1993), administration of plumbagin (4 mg/kg body weight) was found to significantly induce regression of tumor in 3-methyl-4-dimethyl aminoazobenzene (3MeDAB)-induced hepatoma in Wistar male rats. There is also a report on cytotoxic action of plumbagin against HEPA-3B hepatoma cells (Kuo et al. 1997). An anticancer action of plumbagin has been suggested against human embryonic kidney 293 (HEK293) cells (Ding et al. 2005) through inhibition of Nox-4, a renal NAD(P)H oxidase, activity.

Kuo et al. (1997) first demonstrated the anticancer effects of plumbagin against cervical carcinoma HeLa cells. In a later study, Srinivas et al. evaluated the anti-cancer effect of plumbagin against another human cervical cancer cell line, ME-180 (Srinivas et al. 2004b). These studies indicated that plumbagin is an effective inhibitor of cervical cancer cell growth. Plumbagin induced apoptosis through a caspase-dependent pathway. As a further confirmation, another study has also demonstrated a cytotoxic action of plumbagin against HeLa cells (Montoya et al. 2004) through induction of apoptosis. Apoptosis-inducing effect of plumbagin in C33A cells has also been reported (Nair et al. 2008) which, in combination with low doses of radiation, potently inhibited cell growth, and thus suggesting a radio-sensitizing effect of plumbagin against cervical cancer.

The potent cytotoxic activity for the methanol extract of the fruit rinds of *Garcinia indica* against three human cancer cell lines, Colo-320-DM colon, MCF-7 breast and WRL-68 liver has been reported (Kumar et al. 2007). Fractionation of the methanol extract into hexane-, chloroform- and ethyl acetate-soluble portions was performed and their cytotoxic activity was evaluated. The ethyl acetate fraction was found to be the most effective as compared to the two other fractions. In a study that compared the anticancer potential of polyphenolic extracts from several mango varieties (Francis, Kent, Ataulfo, Tommy Atkins and Haden) in multiple cancer cell lines, including Molt-4 leukemia, A-549 lung, MDA-MB-231 breast, LNCaP prostate, and SW-480 colon cancer cells (Noratto et al. 2010), it was found that the extracts exerted anticancer effects against these cancer cells of different origin with great efficacy.

Collectively, these studies suggest a potent anticancer action of garcinol, plumbagin and mangiferin against a number of different cancer cells via modulation of distinct cellular signaling pathways (Table 10.1). It is interesting to note that, of the three compounds, plumbagin stands out as the one that has been shown to be chemopreventive against almost all the human cancer models. The anticancer properties of garcinol are just beginning to be realized and the reports on its action in breast, prostate and pancreatic cancer have only emerged in last 1 year or so. Mangiferin has not been investigated in-detail so far but its potent antioxidant activity and the

Table 10.1 Targets for anticancer activity of garcinol, plumbagin and mangiferin

Target	Agent	Cancer model	Study
Cyclin D3	Garcinol	Breast	Chen et al. (2011)
Caspases	Garcinol	Leukemia	Pan et al. (2001)
FAK	Garcinol	Colon	Liao et al. (2005)
NF-κB	Garcinol	Breast	Ahmad et al. (2010)
NF-κB	Garcinol	Prostate	Ahmad et al. (2011b)
NF-κB	Garcinol	Pancreas	Ahmad et al. (2011b), Parasramka and Gupta (2011)
Akt	Plumbagin	Breast	Kuo et al. (2006)
Bcl-2	Plumbagin	Breast	Ahmad et al. (2008)
Cell cycle	Plumbagin	Leukemia	Zhao and Lu (2006)
Cell cycle	Plumbagin	Myeloma	Wang et al. (2008)
EGFR	Plumbagin	Lung	Gomathinayagam et al. (2008)
ER	Plumbagin	Ovarian	Srinivas et al. (2004a), Thasni et al. (2008)
MMP-uPA	Plumbagin	Liver	Shih et al. (2009)
NF-κB	Plumbagin	Breast	Ahmad et al. (2008)
PI3K	Plumbagin	Pancreas	Chen et al. (2009)
STAT-3	Plumbagin	Myeloma	Sandur et al. (2010)
Cell cycle	Mangiferin	Leukemia	Percival et al. (2006)
NF-κB	Mangiferin	Breast	Sarkar et al. (2004), Garcia-Rivera et al. (2011)
Telomerase	Mangiferin	Leukemia	Cheng et al. (2007)

available information in breast, leukemia, lung and colon cancer models suggests that the compound merits further investigations in other cancer models as well. Moreover, although a number of signaling pathways have been implicated in the anticancer action of these compounds, the one that clearly stands out is the NF-κB pathway. Studies using garcinol in breast, prostate and pancreatic cancer cells have clearly indicated a central role of NF-κB pathway (Ahmad et al. 2011b; Ahmad et al. 2010; Parasramka and Gupta 2011), and all three compounds have been shown to affect signaling mediated through NF-κB pathway leading to anticancer action against breast cancer cells (Ahmad et al. 2008, 2010; Garcia-Rivera et al. 2011; Sarkar et al. 2004). This is not surprising considering the central role of NF-κB signaling in human cancers (Karin 2006). It is therefore only logical that suppression of NF-κB signaling pathway is one of the important mechanism(s) through which natural agents likely exert their anticancer effects (Ahmad et al. 2011a). Next we will briefly discuss the role of NF-κB signaling in human cancers and its modulation by garcinol, plumbagin and mangiferin.

10.5 NF-κB Signaling

Nuclear factor-kappa B (NF-κB) is a molecular target that has gained recognition for its crucial role in the development and progression of human cancers as well as in the acquisition of drug-resistant phenotype in highly aggressive malignancies (Ahmad et al. 2009; Karin et al. 2002; Karin 2006; Sarkar et al. 2009). NF-κB pathway includes several important molecules such as NF-κB, IκB, IKK, etc., however; NF-κB is the key protein in the pathway that has been described as a major culprit and a critical target for therapy of human malignancies (Sarkar et al. 2009; Staudt 2010).

As mentioned above, garcinol has been shown to be a potent inhibitor of NF-κB signaling pathway. Evidence from our own laboratory (Ahmad et al. 2010, 2011b) as well as from others (Parasramka and Gupta 2011) clearly establishes a potent action of this compound against NF-κB signaling. In a direct relevance to human malignancies which are characterized by induced NF-κB signaling, these results showed that garcinol was effective in blocking the constitutive NF-κB activity in various human cancer cells. In addition to a direct inhibition of NF-κB, the downstream targets of NF-κB were also found to be down-regulated, suggesting an efficient blocking of NF-κB signaling pathway.

Plumbagin is also an efficient inhibitor of NF-κB activation (Sandur et al. 2006). It is able to suppress constitutive NF-κB activity, ultimately leading to the suppression of down-stream NF-κB-regulated gene products (Sandur et al. 2006). These observations may explain plumbagin-mediated cell growth modulatory, anti-carcinogenic, and radio-sensitizing effects. Our studies (Ahmad et al. 2008) have revealed that plumbagin induces a dose-dependent inactivation of endogenous NF-κB activity in ER-negative MDA-MB-231 as well as ER-positive MCF-7 breast cancer cells. We also established that the induction of apoptosis in breast cancer cells by plumbagin was mechanistically linked with the inactivation of NF-κB/Bcl-2 pathway. Our results could have greater clinical implications because the activation of NF-κB and expression of Bcl-2 serves as a mechanism of resistance of breast cancer patients to chemotherapy (Buchholz et al. 2005) and, therefore, inhibition of NF-κB/Bcl-2 pathway by plumbagin might be relevant to conventional chemotherapy of advanced and refractory breast cancers.

The ability of mangiferin to inhibit NF-κB signaling pathway was recently investigated and it was shown that mangiferin inhibits classical NF-κB activation by IKK kinases in MDA-MB-231 breast cancer cells, resulting in impaired IκB degradation, NF-κB translocation and NF-κB-DNA binding activity (Garcia-Rivera et al. 2011). Gallic acid, present in *Mangifera indica* extract was found to be a more potent inhibitor of NF-κB in this study, compared to mangiferin. This preliminary report is indicative of NF-κB-modulating activity of mangiferin although more detailed studies are needed to further characterize the anticancer activity of mangiferin.

10.6 Safety and Bioavailability Considerations

As suggested earlier, the interest in natural compounds as anticancer therapeutics stems from the realization that most chemotherapeutic agents used in the clinic are associated with some levels of toxicity which particularly adds-up to alarming levels during combination therapies. It is therefore imperative to evaluate the safety of novel anticancer agents, including the natural agents. In the case of garcinol, it has been shown that garcinol-containing diets do not cause retardation of body weight gain and pathological alterations in liver and other organs including kidney, lung, heart, and esophagus, which is indicative of the low toxicity of the compound (Padhye et al. 2009a).

There are some concerns that have been raised about the safety of plumbagin (Padhye et al. 2010b). Some toxic side effects of plumbagin have been identified in humans which include skin rashes, diarrhea, increases in white blood cell and neutrophil counts, increases in serum phosphatase and acid phosphatase levels and hepatic toxicity (Singh and Udupa 1997). However, there is no report to suggest occupational exposure to plumbagin during its production or processing. Also, there is no report or epidemiological study that can suggest a link between exposure to plumbagin and risk of human cancer (Padhye et al. 2010b).

Studies have been carried out to assess the bioavailability of plumbagin. In an early study on the topic (Chandrasekaran and Nagarajan 1981), it was reported that plumbagin is not detected in blood up to 24 h when administered to rats while in urine it is detectable as early as 4 h after administration. A major portion of the drug was found to be excreted in urine after 24 h and traces of the drug were observed in the urine even after 48 h. Pharmacokinetics of plumbagin in rats have indicated oral bioavailability of plumbagin to be $38.7 \pm 5\%$ (Hsieh et al. 2006), and 49% plumbagin was excreted through feces and it achieved the maximum serum concentration (Cmax) of 0.35 mg/mL at 1 h, after which its serum concentration declined rapidly. The AUC was estimated as 271.9 mg/kg, p.o. with Tmax (min) of 150.

The bioavailability of mangiferin has also been investigated using an ultra-performance liquid chromatography tandem mass spectrometry (UPLC-MS/MS) method employing electrospray ionization (ESI) (Han et al. 2010). The recoveries of mangiferin from rat plasma were 75.0 $\pm$ 7.2%, 86.5 $\pm$ 6.4% and 78.9% $\pm$ 2.3% at concentrations of 0.04, 0.4 and 4.0 μg/ml, respectively while the values were 71.0 $\pm$ 3.8%, 84.6 $\pm$ 9.7% and 81.4% $\pm$ 9.1% at concentrations of 0.8, 8.0 and 80 μg/mL, respectively. The stability experiments demonstrated that mangiferin was stable up to 5.0 h at room temperature (relative error $\leq$ 9.8). Oral bioavailability of mangiferin was found to be 1.2% and it was suggested that novel chemical and pharmaceutical methods should be planned to improve the oral bioavailability of mangiferin.

10.7 Conclusions and Perspectives

Natural compounds garcinol, plumbagin and mangiferin are potent antioxidant and anti-cancer agents (Fig. 10.2). In addition to these effects, there are reports on numerous other biological effects of these agents. For a detailed overview of these activities, we suggest our comprehensive reviews on garcinol (Padhye et al. 2009a) and plumbagin (Padhye et al. 2010b) to our readers. For cancer researchers, an interesting observation is the ability of these compounds to modulate NF-κB especially because NF-κB is known to be a key player in the progression of many human cancers (Sarkar et al. 2008; Sarkar and Li 2008). Interestingly, there is evidence to suggest that these compounds have a selective cytotoxic effect against cancer cells and that they exhibit minimal or no activity against normal cells. For example, our study with breast cancer cells clearly demonstrated that whereas garcinol or plumbagin inhibit the cell growth of MDA-MB-231 and MCF-7 breast cancer cells with effective induction of apoptosis, they do not have any significant effect on MCF-10A cells, the non-tumorigenic 'normal' breast epithelial cells (Ahmad et al. 2008). In a similar study on prostate cancer cells, Aziz et al. (2008) reported an efficient induction of apoptosis by plumbagin in prostate cancer cells (DU145, CWR22rv1, and LNCaP) but no significant effect was observed in non-tumorigenic immortalized prostate epithelial RWPE-1 cells. Garcinol is also known to exhibit a cancer cell-specific action in colon cancer models where it inhibits the growth of

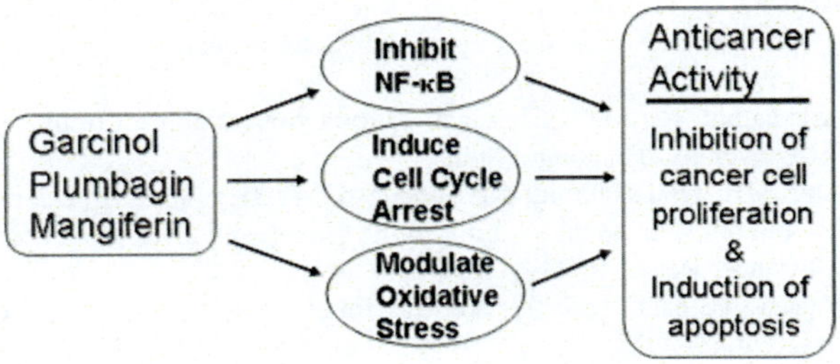

Fig. 10.2 An overview of anticancer activity of garcinol, plumbagin and mangiferin

HT-29 and HCT-116 colon cancer cells without any effect on normal immortalized intestinal IEC-6 and INT-407 cells (Hong et al. 2007). Such a cancer cell-specific action of these novel anticancer agents is very attractive and good indicator of their therapeutic potential although further in-depth studies are warranted.

An important issue that is crucial to the successful translation of these potential compounds into clinically relevant therapeutic agents is that of the bioavailability. The bioavailability of garcinol has not been investigated in detail and there are only a handful reports on bioavailability of plumbagin and mangiferin. Most of the natural compounds fail in the clinic because of their poor bioavailability. It has been suggested that novel synthetic derivatives of natural compounds can significantly enhance their bioavailability and efficacy. A good example is novel analog of curcumin developed by us recently (Padhye et al. 2009b, c). On a similar note, we have recently characterized novel analogs of garcinol (Padhye et al. 2010a) and these compounds have shown promising results against breast and pancreatic cancer cells; however, their bioavailability has not yet been investigated. Efforts are also underway towards the design of novel analogues as well as 'hybrid drug molecules' of plumbagin which can potentially exhibit pleiotropic action and act on multiple pathways leading to an enhanced anticancer activity and reduced toxicity. The emerging data on anticancer activity of garcinol, plumbagin and mangiferin is encouraging. It is envisioned that design of novel synthetic analogs and novel nano-formulation of these compounds can substantially improve their anticancer activity as well as bioavailability, which will lead to their application as lead compounds in human health and diseases.

References

Ahmad A, Banerjee S, Wang Z, et al (2008) Plumbagin-induced apoptosis of human breast cancer cells is mediated by inactivation of NF-kappaB and Bcl-2. J Cell Biochem 105:1461–1471

Ahmad A, Banerjee S, Wang Z et al (2009) Aging and inflammation: etiological culprits of cancer. Curr Aging Sci 2:174–186

Ahmad A, Wang Z, Ali R et al (2010) Apoptosis-inducing effect of garcinol is mediated by NF-kappaB signaling in breast cancer cells. J Cell Biochem 109:1134–1141

Ahmad A, Sakr WA, Rahman KMW (2011a) Role of nuclear factor-kappa B signaling in anticancer properties of indole compounds. J Exp Clin Med 3:55–62

Ahmad A, Wang Z, Wojewoda C et al (2011b) Garcinol-induced apoptosis in prostate and pancreatic cancer cells is mediated by NF- KappaB signaling. Front Biosci (Elite Ed) 3:1483–1492

Amazzal L, Lapotre A, Quignon F et al (2007) Mangiferin protects against 1-methyl-4-phenylpyridinium toxicity mediated by oxidative stress in N2A cells. Neurosci Lett 418: 159–164

Aryanathan S (2009) Chemical examination of three Plumbago species. Ph.D. Thesis, Sastra University, Thanjavur, India

Aziz MH, Dreckschmidt NE, Verma AK (2008) Plumbagin, a medicinal plant-derived naphthoquinone, is a novel inhibitor of the growth and invasion of hormone-refractory prostate cancer. Cancer Res 68:9024–9032

Balsano C, Alisi A (2009) Antioxidant effects of natural bioactive compounds. Curr Pharm Des 15:3063–3073

Barreto JC, Trevisan MT, Hull WE et al (2008) Characterization and quantitation of polyphenolic compounds in bark, kernel, leaves, and peel of mango (Mangifera indica L.). J Agric Food Chem 56:5599–5610

Bertolini F, Novaroli L, Carrupt PA et al (2007) Novel screening assay for antioxidant protection against peroxyl radical-induced loss of protein function. J Pharm Sci 96:2931–2944

Bringmann G, Rudenauer S, Irmer A et al (2008) Antitumoral and antileishmanial dioncoquinones and ancistroquinones from cell cultures of Triphyophyllum peltatum (Dioncophyllaceae) and Ancistrocladus abbreviatus (Ancistrocladaceae). Phytochemistry 69:2501–2509

Buchholz TA, Garg AK, Chakravarti N et al (2005) The nuclear transcription factor kappaB/bcl-2 pathway correlates with pathologic complete response to doxorubicin-based neoadjuvant chemotherapy in human breast cancer. Clin Cancer Res 11:8398–8402

Campos-Esparza MR, Sanchez-Gomez MV, Matute C (2009) Molecular mechanisms of neuroprotection by two natural antioxidant polyphenols. Cell Calcium 45:358–368

Chandrasekaran B, Nagarajan B (1981) Metabolism of echitamine and plumbagin in rats. J Biosci 3:395–400

Chen CA, Chang HH, Kao CY et al (2009) Plumbagin, isolated from Plumbago zeylanica, induces cell death through apoptosis in human pancreatic cancer cells. Pancreatology 9:797–809

Chen CS, Lee CH, Hsieh CD et al (2011) Nicotine-induced human breast cancer cell proliferation attenuated by garcinol through down-regulation of the nicotinic receptor and cyclin D3 proteins. Breast Cancer Res Treat 125:73–87

Cheng P, Peng ZG, Yang J et al (2007) [The effect of mangiferin on telomerase activity and apoptosis in leukemic K562 cells]. Zhong Yao Cai 30:306–309

Chopra RN, Nayar SL, Chopra IC (1956) Glossary of Indian medicinal plants. CSIR, New Delhi, India

Dar A, Faizi S, Naqvi S et al (2005) Analgesic and antioxidant activity of mangiferin and its derivatives: the structure activity relationship. Biol Pharm Bull 28:596–600

de P, Sr., Figueiredo MR, Aragao TV et al (2003) Antimicrobial activity in vitro of plumbagin isolated from Plumbago species. Mem Inst Oswaldo Cruz 98:959–961

Demma J, Hallberg K, Hellman B (2009) Genotoxicity of plumbagin and its effects on catechol and NQNO-induced DNA damage in mouse lymphoma cells. Toxicol In Vitro 23:266–271

Ding Y, Chen ZJ, Liu S et al (2005) Inhibition of Nox-4 activity by plumbagin, a plant-derived bioactive naphthoquinone. J Pharm Pharmacol 57:111–116

Dutt UC (1877) The materia medica of the Hindus. Thacker, Spink & Co., Calcutta, India

Garcia-Rivera D, Delgado R, Bougarne N et al (2011) Gallic acid indanone and mangiferin xanthone are strong determinants of immunosuppressive anti-tumour effects of Mangifera indica L. bark in MDA-MB231 breast cancer cells. Cancer Lett 305:21–31

Gomathinayagam R, Sowmyalakshmi S, Mardhatillah F et al (2008) Anticancer mechanism of plumbagin, a natural compound, on non-small cell lung cancer cells. Anticancer Res 28: 785–792

Hadi SM, Asad SF, Singh S et al (2000) Putative mechanism for anticancer and apoptosis-inducing properties of plant-derived polyphenolic compounds. IUBMB Life 50:167–171

Hamed W, Brajeul S, Mahuteau-Betzer F et al (2006) Oblongifolins A-D, Polyprenylated Benzoylphloroglucinol Derivatives from Garcinia oblongifolia. J Nat Products 69:774–777

Han D, Chen C, Zhang C et al (2010) Determination of mangiferin in rat plasma by liquid-liquid extraction with UPLC-MS/MS. J Pharm Biomed Anal 51:260–263

Hong J, Kwon SJ, Sang S et al (2007) Effects of garcinol and its derivatives on intestinal cell growth: inhibitory effects and autoxidation-dependent growth-stimulatory effects. Free Radic Biol Med 42:1211–1221

Hsieh YJ, Lin LC, Tsai TH (2006) Measurement and pharmacokinetic study of plumbagin in a conscious freely moving rat using liquid chromatography/tandem mass spectrometry. J Chromatogr B Analyt Technol Biomed Life Sci 844:1–5

Hsu MF, Raung SL, Tsao LT et al (1997) Examination of the inhibitory effect of norathyriol in formylmethionyl-leucyl-phenylalanine-induced respiratory burst in rat neutrophils. Free Radic Biol Med 23:1035–1045

Hsu YL, Cho CY, Kuo PL et al (2006) Plumbagin (5-hydroxy-2-methyl-1,4-naphthoquinone) induces apoptosis and cell cycle arrest in A549 cells through p53 accumulation via c-Jun NH2-terminal kinase-mediated phosphorylation at serine 15 in vitro and in vivo. J Pharmacol Exp Ther 318:484–494

Jayaprakasha GK, Sakariah KK (2002) Determination of organic acids in leaves and rinds of Garcinia indica (Desr.) by LC. J Pharm Biomed Anal 28:379–384

Jemal A, Bray F, Center MM et al (2011) Global cancer statistics. CA Cancer J Clin 61:69–90

Jena BS, Jayaprakasha GK, Singh RP et al (2002) Chemistry and biochemistry of (-)-hydroxycitric acid from Garcinia. J Agric Food Chem 50:10–22

Karin M (2006) Nuclear factor-kappaB in cancer development and progression. Nature 441: 431–436

Karin M, Cao Y, Greten FR et al (2002) NF-kappaB in cancer: from innocent bystander to major culprit. Nat Rev Cancer 2:301–310

Khan NS, Ahmad A, Hadi SM (2000) Anti-oxidant, pro-oxidant properties of tannic acid and its binding to DNA. Chem Biol Interact 125:177–189

Kumar S, Chattopadhyay SK, Darokar MP et al (2007) Cytotoxic activities of xanthochymol and isoxanthochymol substantiated by LC-MS/MS. Planta Med 73:1452–1456

Kuo YH, Chang CI, Li SY et al (1997) Cytotoxic constituents from the stems of Diospyros maritima. Planta Med 63:363–365

Kuo PL, Hsu YL, Cho CY (2006) Plumbagin induces G2-M arrest and autophagy by inhibiting the AKT/mammalian target of rapamycin pathway in breast cancer cells. Mol Cancer Ther 5:3209–3221

Lemus-Molina Y, Sanchez-Gomez MV, gado-Hernandez R et al (2009) Mangifera indica L. extract attenuates glutamate-induced neurotoxicity on rat cortical neurons. Neurotoxicology 30: 1053–1058

Liao CH, Sang S, Ho CT et al (2005) Garcinol modulates tyrosine phosphorylation of FAK and subsequently induces apoptosis through down-regulation of Src, ERK, and Akt survival signaling in human colon cancer cells. J Cell Biochem 96:155–169

Liou GY, Storz P (2010) Reactive oxygen species in cancer. Free Radic Res 44:479–496

Mallavadhani UV, Sahu G, Muralidhar J (2002) Screening of Plumbago Species for the Bio-active Marker Plumbagin. Pharmaceut Biol 40:508–511

Mandala Rayabandla SK, Aithal K, Anandam A et al (2010) Preparation, in vitro characterization, pharmacokinetic, and pharmacodynamic evaluation of chitosan-based plumbagin microspheres in mice bearing B16F1 melanoma. Drug Deliv 17:103–113

Manthey JA, Perkins-Veazie P (2009) Influences of harvest date and location on the levels of beta-carotene, ascorbic acid, total phenols, the in vitro antioxidant capacity, and phenolic profiles of five commercial varieties of mango (Mangifera indica L.). J Agric Food Chem 57:10825–10830

Martinez G, Giuliani A, Leon OS et al (2001) Effect of Mangifera indica L. extract (QF808) on protein and hepatic microsome peroxidation. Phytother Res 15:581–585

Masullo M, Bassarello C, Suzuki H et al (2008) Polyisoprenylated benzophenones and an unusual polyisoprenylated tetracyclic xanthone from the fruits of Garcinia cambogia. J Agric Food Chem 56:5205–5210

Matsumoto K, Akao Y, Kobayashi E et al (2003) Cytotoxic benzophenone derivatives from Garcinia species display a strong apoptosis-inducing effect against human leukemia cell lines. Biol Pharm Bull 26:569–571

Montoya J, Varela-Ramirez A, Estrada A et al (2004) A fluorescence-based rapid screening assay for cytotoxic compounds. Biochem Biophys Res Commun 325:1517–1523

Nadkarni KM (1954) Indian materia medica. Popular Book Depot., Bombay

Nair S, Nair RR, Srinivas P et al (2008) Radiosensitizing effects of plumbagin in cervical cancer cells is through modulation of apoptotic pathway. Mol Carcinog 47:22–33

Nazeem S, Azmi AS, Hanif S et al (2009) Plumbagin induces cell death through a copper-redox cycle mechanism in human cancer cells. Mutagenesis 24:413–418

Noratto GD, Bertoldi MC, Krenek K et al (2010) Anticarcinogenic effects of polyphenolics from mango (Mangifera indica) varieties. J Agric Food Chem 58:4104–4112

Padhye S, Ahmad A, Oswal N et al (2009a) Emerging role of Garcinol, the antioxidant chalcone from Garcinia indica Choisy and its synthetic analogs. J Hematol Oncol 2:38

Padhye S, Banerjee S, Chavan D et al (2009b) Fluorocurcumins as cyclooxygenase-2 inhibitor: molecular docking, pharmacokinetics and tissue distribution in mice. Pharm Res 26:2438–2445

Padhye S, Yang H, Jamadar A et al (2009c) New difluoro Knoevenagel condensates of curcumin, their Schiff bases and copper complexes as proteasome inhibitors and apoptosis inducers in cancer cells. Pharm Res 26:1874–1880

Padhye S, Ahmad A, Oswal N et al (2010a) Fluorinated 2′-hydroxychalcones as garcinol analogs with enhanced antioxidant and anticancer activities. Bioorg Med Chem Lett 20:5818–5821

Padhye S, Dandawate P, Yusufi M et al (2010b) Perspectives on medicinal properties of plumbagin and its analogs. Med Res Rev. doi:10.1002/med.20235

Pan MH, Chang WL, Lin-Shiau SY et al (2001) Induction of apoptosis by garcinol and curcumin through cytochrome c release and activation of caspases in human leukemia HL-60 cells. J Agric Food Chem 49:1464–1474

Parasramka MA, Gupta SV (2011) Garcinol inhibits cell proliferation and promotes apoptosis in pancreatic adenocarcinoma cells. Nutr Cancer 63:456–465

Pardo-Andreu GL, Barrios MF, Curti C et al (2008a) Protective effects of Mangifera indica L extract (Vimang), and its major component mangiferin, on iron-induced oxidative damage to rat serum and liver. Pharmacol Res 57:79–86

Pardo-Andreu GL, Paim BA, Castilho RF et al (2008b) Mangifera indica L. extract (Vimang) and its main polyphenol mangiferin prevent mitochondrial oxidative stress in atherosclerosis-prone hypercholesterolemic mouse. Pharmacol Res 57:332–338

Parimala R, Sachdanandam P (1993) Effect of Plumbagin on some glucose metabolising enzymes studied in rats in experimental hepatoma. Mol Cell Biochem 125:59–63

Pauletti PM, Castro-Gamboa I, Siqueira Silva DH et al (2003) New antioxidant C-glucosylxanthones from the stems of Arrabidaea samydoides. J Nat Prod 66:1384–1387

Peng ZG, Luo J, Xia LH et al (2004) [CML cell line K562 cell apoptosis induced by mangiferin]. Zhongguo Shi Yan Xue Ye Xue Za Zhi 12:590–594

Percival SS, Talcott ST, Chin ST et al (2006) Neoplastic transformation of BALB/3T3 cells and cell cycle of HL-60 cells are inhibited by mango (Mangifera indica L.) juice and mango juice extracts. J Nutr 136:1300–1304

Powolny AA, Singh SV (2008) Plumbagin-induced apoptosis in human prostate cancer cells is associated with modulation of cellular redox status and generation of reactive oxygen species. Pharm Res 25:2171–2180

Prabhu S, Jainu M, Sabitha KE et al (2006) Role of mangiferin on biochemical alterations and antioxidant status in isoproterenol-induced myocardial infarction in rats. J Ethnopharmacol 107:126–133

Prasad VS, Devi PU, Rao BS et al (1996) Radiosensitizing effect of plumbagin on mouse melanoma cells grown in vitro. Indian J Exp Biol 34:857–858

Rajendran P, Ekambaram G, Sakthisekaran D (2008a) Protective role of mangiferin against Benzo(a)pyrene induced lung carcinogenesis in experimental animals. Biol Pharm Bull 31:1053–1058

Rajendran P, Ekambaram G, Sakthisekaran D (2008b) Effect of mangiferin on benzo(a)pyrene induced lung carcinogenesis in experimental Swiss albino mice. Nat Prod Res 22:672–680

Rajendran P, Ekambaram G, Sakthisekaran D (2008c) Cytoprotective effect of mangiferin on benzo(a)pyrene-induced lung carcinogenesis in swiss albino mice. Basic Clin Pharmacol Toxicol 103:137–142

Rodeiro I, Donato MT, Martinez I et al (2008) Potential hepatoprotective effects of new Cuban natural products in rat hepatocytes culture. Toxicol In Vitro 22:1242–1249

Sandur SK, Ichikawa H, Sethi G et al (2006) Plumbagin (5-hydroxy-2-methyl-1, 4-naphthoquinone) suppresses NF-kappaB activation and NF-kappaB-regulated gene products through modulation of p65 and IkappaBalpha kinase activation, leading to potentiation of apoptosis induced by cytokine and chemotherapeutic agents. J Biol Chem 281:17023–17033

Sandur SK, Pandey MK, Sung B et al (2010) 5-hydroxy-2-methyl-1,4-naphthoquinone, a vitamin K3 analogue, suppresses STAT3 activation pathway through induction of protein tyrosine phosphatase, SHP-1: potential role in chemosensitization. Mol Cancer Res 8:107–118

Sang S, Pan MH, Cheng X et al (2001) Chemical studies on antioxidant mechanism of garcinol: analysis of radical reaction products of garcinol and their antitumor activities. Tetrahedron 57:9931–9938

Sang S, Liao CH, Pan MH et al (2002) Chemical studies on antioxidant mechanism of garcinol: analysis of radical reaction products of garcinol with peroxyl radicals and their antitumor activities. Tetrahedron 58:10095–10102

Sankar R, Devamanoharan P, Raghupathi G et al (1987) Lipid peroxidation in plumbagin administered rats. J Biosci 12:267–271

Sarkar FH, Li Y (2008) NF-kappaB: a potential target for cancer chemoprevention and therapy. Front Biosci 13:2950–2959

Sarkar A, Sreenivasan Y, Ramesh GT et al (2004) beta-D-Glucoside suppresses tumor necrosis factor-induced activation of nuclear transcription factor kappaB but potentiates apoptosis. J Biol Chem 279:33768–33781

Sarkar FH, Li Y, Wang Z et al (2008) NF-kappaB signaling pathway and its therapeutic implications in human diseases. Int Rev Immunol 27:293–319

Sarkar FH, Li Y, Wang Z et al (2009) Cellular signaling perturbation by natural products. Cell Signal 21:1541–1547

Shieh JM, Chiang TA, Chang WT et al (2010) Plumbagin inhibits TPA-induced MMP-2 and u-PA expressions by reducing binding activities of NF-kappaB and AP-1 via ERK signaling pathway in A549 human lung cancer cells. Mol Cell Biochem 335:181–193

Shih YW, Lee YC, Wu PF et al (2009) Plumbagin inhibits invasion and migration of liver cancer HepG2 cells by decreasing productions of matrix metalloproteinase-2 and urokinase-plasminogen activator. Hepatol Res 39:998–1009

Siegel R, Ward E, Brawley O et al (2011) Cancer statistics, 2011: The impact of eliminating socioeconomic and racial disparities on premature cancer deaths. CA Cancer J Clin

Singh UV, Udupa N (1997) Reduced toxicity and enhanced antitumor efficacy of betacyclodextrin plumbagin inclusion complex in mice bearing Ehrlich ascites carcinoma. Indian J Physiol Pharmacol 41:171–175

Singh S, Asad SF, Ahmad A et al (2001) Oxidative DNA damage by capsaicin and dihydrocapsaicin in the presence of Cu(II). Cancer Lett 169:139–146

Srinivas G, Annab LA, Gopinath G et al (2004a) Antisense blocking of BRCA1 enhances sensitivity to plumbagin but not tamoxifen in BG-1 ovarian cancer cells. Mol Carcinog 39:15–25

Srinivas P, Gopinath G, Banerji A et al (2004b) Plumbagin induces reactive oxygen species, which mediate apoptosis in human cervical cancer cells. Mol Carcinog 40:201–211

Staudt LM (2010) Oncogenic activation of NF-kappaB. Cold Spring Harb Perspect Biol 2:a000109

Tertil M, Jozkowicz A, Dulak J (2010) Oxidative stress in tumor angiogenesis- therapeutic targets. Curr Pharm Des 16:3877–3894

Thasni KA, Rakesh S, Rojini G et al (2008) Estrogen-dependent cell signaling and apoptosis in BRCA1-blocked BG1 ovarian cancer cells in response to plumbagin and other chemotherapeutic agents. Ann Oncol 19:696–705

Tilak JC, Adhikari S, Devasagayam TP (2004) Antioxidant properties of Plumbago zeylanica, an Indian medicinal plant and its active ingredient, plumbagin. Redox Rep 9:219–227

Ullah MF, Ahmad A, Zubair H et al (2011) Soy isoflavone genistein induces cell death in breast cancer cells through mobilization of endogenous copper ions and generation of reactive oxygen species. Mol Nutr Food Res 55:553–559

Wang CC, Chiang YM, Sung SC et al (2008) Plumbagin induces cell cycle arrest and apoptosis through reactive oxygen species/c-Jun N-terminal kinase pathways in human melanoma A375.S2 cells. Cancer Lett 259:82–98

Wu CH, Lee CH, Ho YS (2011) Nicotinic acetylcholine receptor-based blockade: applications of molecular targets for cancer therapy. Clin Cancer Res 17:3533–3541

Xu KH, Lu DP (2010) Plumbagin induces ROS-mediated apoptosis in human promyelocytic leukemia cells in vivo. Leuk Res 34:658–665

Yamaguchi F, Ariga T, Yoshimura Y et al (2000) Antioxidative and anti-glycation activity of garcinol from Garcinia indica fruit rind. J Agric Food Chem 48:180–185

Yoshikawa M, Ninomiya K, Shimoda H et al (2002) Hepatoprotective and antioxidative properties of Salacia reticulata: preventive effects of phenolic constituents on CCl4-induced liver injury in mice. Biol Pharm Bull 25:72–76

Yoshimi N, Matsunaga K, Katayama M et al (2001) The inhibitory effects of mangiferin, a naturally occurring glucosylxanthone, in bowel carcinogenesis of male F344 rats. Cancer Lett 163:163–170

Zhao YL, Lu DP (2006) [Effects of plumbagin on the human acute promyelocytic leukemia cells in vitro]. Zhongguo Shi Yan Xue Ye Xue Za Zhi 14:208–211

Chapter 11
Anthocyanins and Cancer Prevention

Li-Shu Wang, Steven Carmella, Robert Keyes, Chieh-Ti Kuo, Yi-Wen Huang, Stephen S. Hecht, and Gary D. Stoner

Abstract Anthocyanins are members of a class of flavonoid compounds commonly known as plant polyphenols. They are responsible for the blue, purple, red and intermediate colors of many flowers, leaves, vegetables and fruits, especially berries. The daily intake of anthocyanins in the United States diet is estimated to be about 200 mg or about 9-fold higher than that of other dietary flavonoids. Anthocyanins have been evaluated for chemopreventive potential, both in cell cultures and in animal model tumor systems. Limited information on their chemopreventive effects is also available from epidemiological studies. This chapter summarizes the chemistry, synthesis and bioavailability of anthocyanins and the latest developments regarding their anti-carcinogenic effects in cell cultures and in animal model systems. The chemopreventive activity of protocatechuic acid (PCA), one of the most abundant metabolites of anthocyanins, is also discussed due to its prominent role in the overall inhibitory effects of anthocyanins. We suggest that PCA be further evaluated for chemoprevention in animal model systems and in humans in view of its relatively low toxicity and commercial availability.

Keywords Anthocyanins · Chemoprevention · Cell culture · Animals · Humans · Metabolism · Bioavailability

Abbreviations

4-NQO	4-nitroquinoline 1-oxide
8-Iso-PGF2	8-epi-prostaglandin F2α
AgNORs	silver-stained nuclear organizer regions
AOM	azoxymethane
BBN	N-butyl-N-(4-hydroxybutyl)nitrosamine
BOP	N-nitrosobis(2-oxopropyl)amine
BRBs	black raspberries
BrdU	bromodeoxyuridine
CHI	chalcone isomerase
CHS	chalcone synthase

G.D. Stoner (✉)
Division of Hematology and Oncology, Department of Medicine, Medical College of Wisconsin, Milwaukee, WI 53220, USA
e-mail: gstoner@mcw.edu

F.H. Sarkar (ed.), *Nutraceuticals and Cancer*, DOI 10.1007/978-94-007-2630-7_11,

CyG	cyandin-glucoside
DEN	diethylnitrosamine
DFR	dihydroflavonol-4-reductase
DMBA	7,12-dimethylbenz[a]anthracene
DNMT	DNA methyltransferase
F3H	flavonoid 3′ hydroxylase
FHT	flavanone hydroxylase
H_2O_2	hydrogen peroxide
ICAM-1	intercellular adhesion molecule-1
IL	interleukin
MAPK	mitogen-activated protein kinase
MNNG	N-methyl-N′-nitro-N-nitrosoguanidine
NF-kB	nuclear factor-kappa B
NMBA	*N*-nitrosomethylbenzylamine
NNK	4-(methylnitrosamino)-1-(3-pyridyl)-1-butanone
ODC	ornithine decarboxylase
PCA	protocatechuic acid
PhIP	2-amino-1-methyl-6-phenylimidazo[4,5-b]pyridine
PKCe	protein kinase Ce
RB	retinoblastoma
RVS	*Rhus verniciflua* Stokes
TPA	12-O-tetradecanoylphorbol-13-acetate

11.1 Introduction

Anthocyanins are a ubiquitous group of water-soluble plant metabolites of the flavonoid family. They are "nature's colors", responsible for the blue, purple, red and intermediate colors of leaves, flowers, vegetables and fruits, especially berries. Anthocyanins serve as least three functions in plant physiology (Sullivan 1998; Gould 2004). First, they assist in propagating plant species because their bright colors serve as an attractant for insects for pollination and for animals resulting in seed dispersion. Second, they help prevent predation by imparting a bitter taste to plants. Third, through their free radical scavenging activities, they protect the plant photosynthetic apparatus from ultraviolet (UV) irradiation and photo-oxidative stress. Indeed, factors that elicit stress in plants such as UV irradiation, cold, drought, leaf wounding and osmotic stress are known to trigger the formation of anthocyanins (Wheldale 1916; Field et al. 2001; Gould and Lee 2002; Gould et al. 2002; Steyn et al. 2002; Hoch et al. 2003; Gould 2004; Keskitalo et al. 2005).

Of the edible plants, berries are one of the most popular food sources of anthocyanins (Clifford 2000; Scalbert and Williamson 2000). Berries are consumed not only as fresh fruit but also in frozen, canned, jelly and jam, yogurt and beverage forms. Table 11.1 lists examples of commonly eaten sources of anthocyanins and the amounts present in milligrams per 1000 g of foods and beverages (Clifford 2000).

Table 11.1 Amounts of anthocyanins found in representative foods and beverages (Clifford 2000)

Food type	Anthocyanin content (mg/1000 g)	Reference
Blackberry	1150	Wilska-Jeszka et al. (1992)
Blueberry	825–4200	Timberlake (1988) Wilska-Jeszka et al. (1992) Skrede et al. (1992)
Boysenberry	1609	Torre and Barritt (1977)
Cherry	20–4500	Timberlake (1988) Gao and Mazza (1995)
Chokeberry	5060–10,000	Bridle and Timberlake (1997) Wilska-Jeszka et al. (1992)
Cranberry	600–2000	Timberlake (1988)
Cowberry	1000	Timberlake (1988)
Currant (black)	1300–4000	Timberlake (1988)
Elderberry	2000–10,000	Bridle and Timberlake (1997) Wilska-Jeszka et al. (1992)
Grape (red)	300–7500	Bridle and Timberlake (1997) Timberlake (1988)
Loganberry	774	Torre and Barritt (1977)
Orange, blood (juice)	2000	Bridle and Timberlake (1997)
Plum	20–250	Timberlake (1988)
Raspberry (black)	1700–4277	Timberlake (1988) Torre and Barritt (1977) Herrmann (1992)
Raspberry (red)	100–600	Timberlake (1988) Torre and Barritt (1977) Herrmann (1992)
Raspberry (red) single strength juice	4–1101	Boyles and Wrolstad (1993)
Sloe	1600	Casado-Redin et al. (1992)
Strawberry	150–350	Timberlake (1988)
Cabbage (red)	250	Timberlake (1988)
Eggplant	7500	Bajaj et al. (1990)
Onion	up to 250	Timberlake (1988)
Rhubarb	up to 2000	Timberlake (1988)
Wines (port)	140–1100	Timberlake (1988)
Wines (red)	240–350	Bakker and Timberlake (1985) Frankel et al. (1995)

The anthocyanin contents depicted in the table can vary however, as concentrations are affected by factors such as growing conditions, maturity at harvest time, species and cultivar (Siriwoharn et al. 2004; Jing and Giusti 2011). Typically, the color of a plant's fruit and its antioxidant potential is a function of anthocyanin concentration with higher concentrations resulting in intensified colors and increased antioxidant activity (Jing and Giusti 2011).

The daily intake of anthocyanins by residents in the United States is estimated to be about 200 mg or about 9-fold higher than that of other dietary flavonoids.

Epidemiological studies suggest that the consumption of anthocyanins lowers the risk for diabetes, arthritis, cardiovascular disease and cancer due, at least in part, to their anti-inflammatory and anti-oxidant activities (Seeram 2008). In this chapter, we highlight recent studies on the cancer preventive activities of the anthocyanins, including results from in vitro cell culture systems, in vivo animal model systems, and human epidemiological studies. We also discuss the chemopreventive effects of one of their more prevalent metabolites, protocatechuic acid (PCA). Additional in vitro and in vivo studies of the potential preventative effects of PCA in animal model and human systems appear to be warranted. This chapter updates our previous review of the role of anthocyanins in cancer prevention in 2008 (Wang, and Stoner 2008).

11.2 Chemistry of Anthocyanins

Anthocyanins belong to the class of flavonoid compounds commonly known as plant polyphenols. They occur naturally in fruits and vegetables as glycosides, having different sugars bound to an aglycone nucleus (Harborne 1979; Clifford 2000; Giusti and Wrolsted 2003). Anthocyanins are water-soluble and, depending upon pH and the presence of chelating metal ions, are intensely colored in blue, purple and red. The de-glycosylated or aglycone forms of anthocyanins are known as anthocyanidins (Fig. 11.1) (Kong et al. 2003). Anthocyanidins rarely occur in their aglycone form in nature because of their high reactivity (Harborne 1979; Clifford 2000; Giusti and Wrolsted 2003). There are 27 known anthocyanidins in nature (Andersenand and Jordheim 2005), and 6 (cyanidin, peonidin, pelargonidin, delphinidin, petunidin and malvidin) are found in berries (Giusti and Jing 2007). Structurally, the anthocyanidins are glycosylated predominately at the 3-position of the C-ring; however, glycosylation can also occur on the A-ring at positions 5 and 7. Glycosylation is also observed at the 3′, 4′, and 5′ positions on the B ring, but this is extremely rare (Mazza and Miniati 1993). The most common glycosyl units are glucose, arabinose, rhamnose, xylose and galactose; either as monosaccharides or linked in a di- or tri-saccharide manner. The glycosyl moieties can also be acylated with various aliphatic, aromatic and cinnamic acid analogs. The A and B rings are highly oxygenated with hydroxyl and methoxy groups varying in position and number. Broad structural variability results in compounds with molecular weights ranging from 400 to 1200 g/mol. As of 2003, more than 400 anthocyanins had been isolated (Kong et al. 2003). Importantly, in aqueous media, the chemical structure of anthocyanins is pH dependent (Fig. 11.2). In general, they are more stabile in the lower pH range. At low pH (pH 0–2), the C-ring of the anthocyanins has cyclized and aromatized to a red flavylium cation. At higher pHs (pH 2–6), the anthocyanins exist as the colorless hemiacetal with small amounts of yellow ring-opened chalcones (Clifford 2000). The structural variability of anthocyanins as a function of varying pH levels plays a major role in their absorption, distribution, metabolism and excretion.

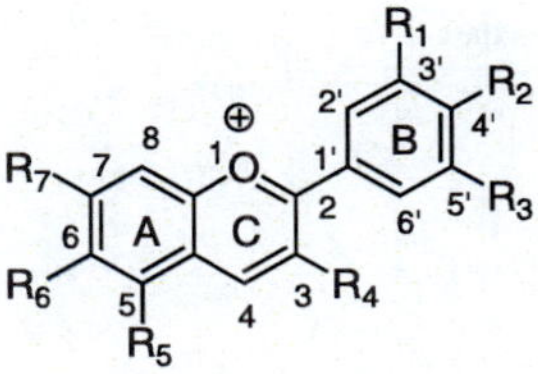

anthocyanidin

anthocyanidin	R_1	R_2	R_3	R_4	R_5	R_6	R_7
cyanidin	OH	OH	H	OH	OH	H	OH
pelargondin	H	OH	H	OH	OH	H	OH
delphinidin	OH	OH	OH	OH	OH	H	OH
aurantinidin	H	OH	H	OH	OH	OH	OH
malvidin	OCH_3	OH	OCH_3	OH	OH	H	OH
peonidin	OCH_3	OH	H	OH	OH	H	OH
petunidin	OCH_3	OH	H	OH	OH	H	OH
europhinidin	OCH_3	OH	OH	OH	OCH_3	H	OH
luteolinidin	OH	OH	H	H	OH	H	OH
rosinidin	OCH_3	OH	H	OH	OH	H	OCH_3

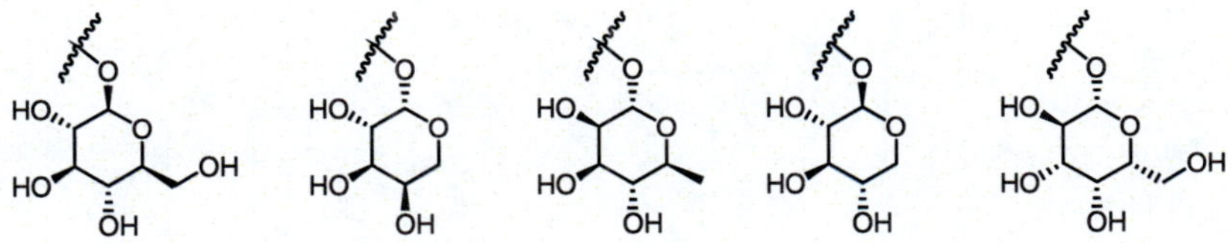

glucose arabinose rhamnose xylose galactose

Fig. 11.1 Chemical structures of some common anthocyanins and their sugar substituents (Kong et al. 2003)

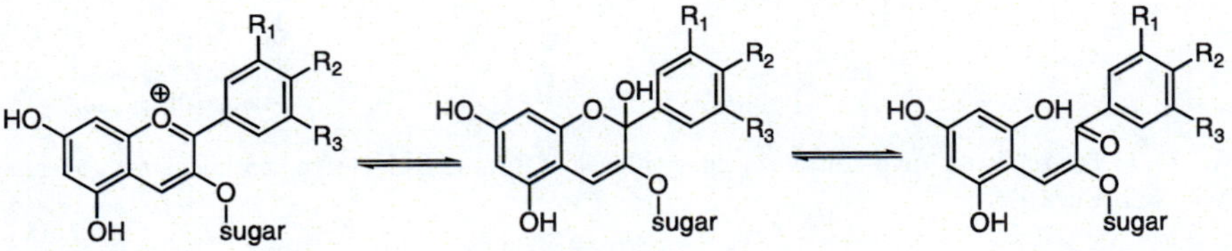

Flavilium at pH = 0–2

Hemiacetal at pH = 2–6

Chalcone

Fig. 11.2 Equilibrium structures of anthocyanins at various pH levels (Clifford 2000)

11.3 Biosynthesis of Anthocyanins

The biosynthesis of anthocyanins (Fig. 11.3) results from the convergence of phenylalanine and three molecules of malonyl CoA (Mann 1987; Sullivan 1998). Phenylalanine arises from the shikimate pathway and is the precursor of the

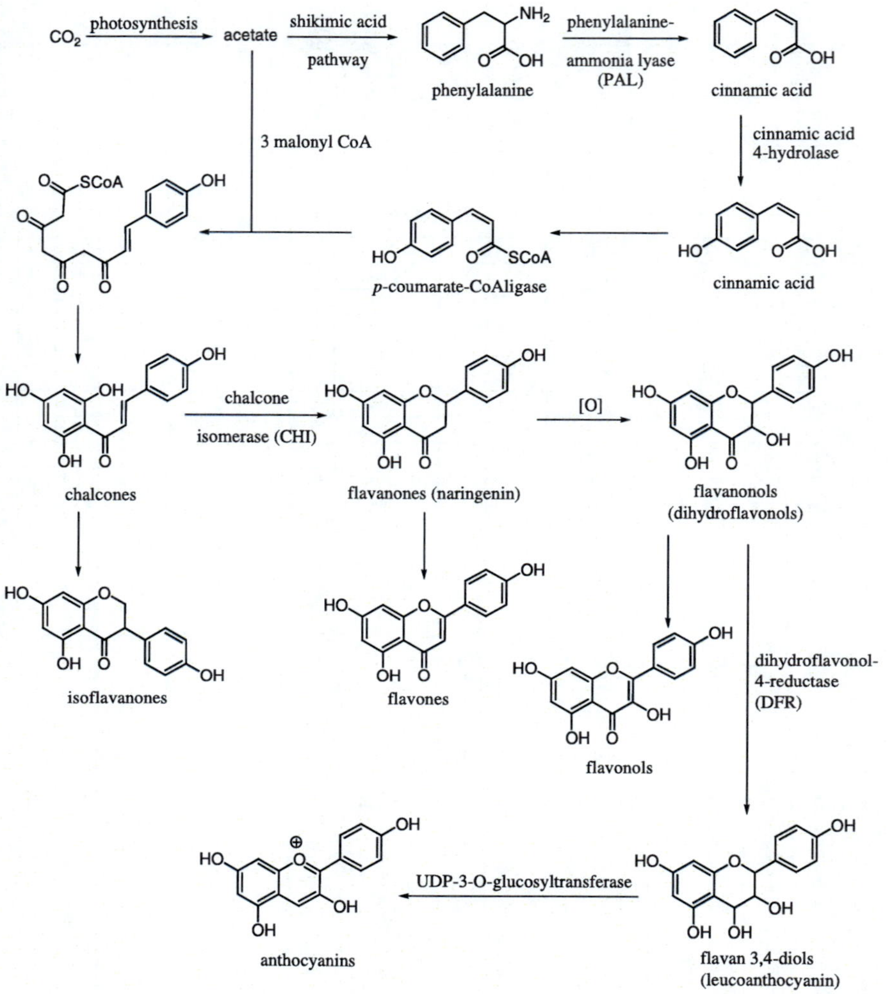

Fig. 11.3 The biosynthetic pathway for the synthesis of flavanoids including anthocyanins (Mann 1987; Sullivan 1998)

p-coumaryl subunit. Malonyl CoA arises from the acetate pathway. *p*-Coumaryl-SCoA and the malonyl CoA units are coupled via chalcone synthase (CHS) to give, after cyclization and aromatization via a polyketide folding mechanism, a chalcone. The hydroxylation pattern of the A-ring is set at the cyclization stage. The B-ring's hydroxylation pattern, on the other hand, is set later in the biosynthetic pathway. Anthocyanin's chalcones are a diverging point in the synthetic pathway giving rise to other flavanoid-like flavanones, isoflavanones, flavones, flavonols, and catechins. Once the chalcone has been produced, it is isomerized by chalcone isomerase (CHI) to the flavanone, naringenin. Naringenin is then oxidized by enzymes such as flavanone hydroxylase (FHT) or flavonoid 3′ hydroxylase (F3H) and flavonoid

3′ 5′-hydroxylase to yield flavanonols (i.e., dihydroxyflavonols). Next, naringenin is reacted with the enzyme dihydroflavonol-4-reductase (DFR) to give leucoanthocyanins (i.e., flavan 3,4-diols) (Nakajima et al. 2001) that are enzymatically dehydrated and aromatized to the anthocyanidins. Next, glycosylation occurs via UDP-3-O-glucosyltransferase to produce the anthocyanins (Kovinich et al. 2010). All enzymes involved in the biosynthetic pathway are bound to the cell membrane. The building blocks, malonyl CoA and phenylalanine, are located in the cytoplasm. Once formed and transported to vacuoles located on the opposite side of the membrane's epidermal cell layer (Sullivan 1998), anthocyanins perform their valuable biological roles.

11.4 Bioavailability of Anthocyanins

The bioavailability of anthocyanins has been discussed in detail by Jing and Giusti (2011). In general, the bioavailability of anthocyanins is low, with very low absorption into plasma and low levels detected in urine after large oral intake of anthocyanin-enriched extracts or berries. In a phase I clinical trial, we reported the uptake of black raspberry anthocyanins and ellagic acid into the plasma of human volunteers who consumed 45 g/day of black raspberry powder for 7 days. The uptake was less than 1% of the administered dose of both anthocyanins and ellagic acid (Stoner et al. 2005). McGhie et al. (2003) studied the bioabsorption of anthocyanins from blueberry, boysenberry, black raspberry and black currant in rats and humans and found that the total amount excreted as a percentage of the amount consumed was less than 0.1% for all anthocyanins. Similar results were reported for the uptake of anthocyanins from strawberries, blackberries, and chokeberries (Felgines et al. 2003; Felgines et al. 2005; Kay et al. 2004). Felgines et al. (2009) studied the distribution of anthocyanins to the bladder, prostate, testes and adipose tissue in rats after an enriched blackberry diet for 12 days and detected anthocyanin metabolites in all organs, among which the bladder contained the highest levels.

The bioavailability of anthocyanins is influenced by the nature of the glycoside and also by the structure of the aglycone. Anthocyanins can be absorbed as glycosides in rats and humans (Miyazawa et al. 1999; Tsuda et al. 1999; Cao et al. 2001; Felgines et al. 2002) with absorption occurring in the stomach and intestines (Passamonti et al. 2003; Talavéra et al. 2003; Talavéra et al. 2004). They can also pass into the gastrointestinal tract where they are metabolized by bacterial enzymes or they degrade due to their instability at neutral and alkaline pH (Fig. 11.4) (Keppler 2005). The anthocyanins are metabolized via methylation, glucuronidation and sulfoconjugation, and anthocyanin metabolites recovered in the urine are glucuronides, sulfoconjugates and methylated derivatives (Jing and Giusti 2011). Microbial metabolism of the anthocyanins involves hydrolysis and ring scission whereas chemical decomposition is due to hydrolysis. When pigs were fed freeze-dried black raspberry powder and the small intestines, cecum and colon analyzed for phenolic acids, the most abundant metabolites detected were protocatechuic acid

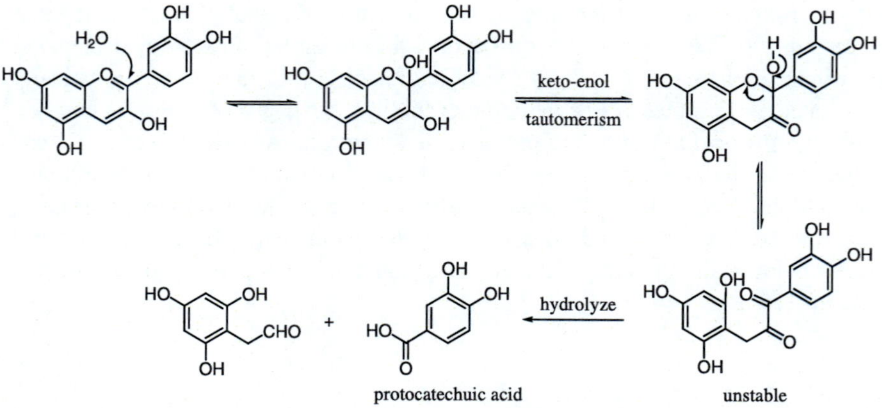

Fig. 11.4 Proposed chemical degradation pathway giving protocatechuic acid (Keppler and Humpf 2005)

and homoprotocatechuic acid (Keppler 2005; Wu et al. 2009). These two phenolic acids and some of the other less abundant metabolites appear to play a pivotal role in the chemopreventive effects of black raspberry.

The reason(s) for the poor absorption of the anthocyanins is/are not clear. It has been speculated that many anthocyanin chemical structures are not efficiently hydrolyzed by β-glucuronidase in the GI tract, resulting in low absorption into the bloodstream (Nemeth et al. 2003; Jing and Giusti 2011). In addition, as stated above, the anthocyanins may be rapidly degraded due to the neutral and mild alkaline conditions of the intestine. Dreiseitel et al. (2009) found that berry anthocyanins and anthocyanidins were bound to efflux transporters such as the multidrug resistance protein 1 (MDR1). Therefore, they may be actively transported out of the intestine, resulting in low levels in plasma. Additional studies are required to fully explain the low bioavailability of the anthocyanins.

11.5 Biological Effects of Anthocyanins and Protocatechuic Acid (PCA)

Due, at least in part, to their anti-oxidant and anti-inflammatory activities, anthocyanins may play important roles in promoting cardiovascular health, vision and eye health, reducing obesity, and preventing cancer (Wang and Stoner 2008). In addition, they appear to promote normal brain function because supplementation of the diet with blueberries has been shown to improve memory in older adults (Krikorian et al. 2010). As described above, PCA is the major metabolite of cyanidin, and it is present naturally in plants and fruits. Studies have shown that PCA has anti-oxidant and anti-carcinogenic effects in various cell culture and animal models. In the remaining portion of this chapter, we summarize the chemopreventive effects of anthocyanins and PCA.

11.5.1 Mechanisms of Chemoprotection by Anthocyanins

11.5.1.1 In Vitro Studies

Most in vitro studies of the anti-carcinogenic effects of the anthocyanidins/anthocyanins have been conducted with human tumor cell lines. These studies have been summarized in detail in our recent review articles (Wang and Stoner 2008, 2009) and the reader is referred to these articles for more detailed information. In vitro studies have used either pure anthocyanidins/anthocyanins for study, or they have employed extract fractions of these compounds from various natural sources. As illustrated in Table 11.2, the anthocyanidins/anthocyanins, and the different extracts enriched in these compounds, elicit multiple anti-carcinogenic effects in vitro including anti-oxidation (Bagchi et al. 2004; Singletary et al. 2007), activation of phase II metabolizing enzymes (Singletary et al. 2007), inhibition of cell proliferation (Zhang et al. 2005), induction of apoptosis (Chen et al. 2005; Mukhtar et al. 2008) and cell differentiation (Fimognari et al. 2004; Rodrigo et al. 2006), and anti-inflammatory (Afaq et al. 2005b; Reddy et al. 2005) anti-angiogenic (Favot et al. 2003; Rodrigo et al. 2006) and anti-invasive effects (Chen et al. 2006a, b). The expression levels of relevant genes associated with these cellular processes are also influenced by these compounds/mixtures (Fig. 11.5). The anti-carcinogenic effects of the anthocyanidins are related to their structure, and are due principally to the presence of hydroxyl groups in position 3 of ring C, and in the 3′, 4′ and 5′ positions of ring B in the molecule. For example, the anti-cancer effects of delphinidin, with three hydroxyl groups on the B-ring, are superior to those of malvidin and peonidin which have only one hydroxyl group on the B-ring (Fig. 11.1). The anthocyanidins appear to be more potent inhibitors of carcinogenesis in vitro than the anthocyanins (Zhang et al. 2005), suggesting that the sugars attached to the anthocyanidin nucleus interfere with its anti-carcinogenic effects. Several investigations have compared the antiproliferative effects of anthocyanidins/anthocyanins on normal vs. cancer cells in vitro and found that these compounds selectively inhibit the growth of cancer cells (Galvano et al. 2004; Hakimuddin et al. 2004). Our laboratory reported that an ethanol extract from black raspberries selectively inhibited the growth and induced apoptosis in a highly tumorigenic rat esophageal epithelial cell line (RE-149 DHD) but not in a weakly tumorigenic line (RE-149). The uptake of the anthocyanins from the extract into RE-149 DHD cells far exceeded their uptake into RE-149 cells, which may have accounted for the selective effects of the extract on growth and apoptosis of RE-149 DHD cells (Zikri et al. 2009).

The concentrations of anthocyanins/anthocyanidins or extract fractions required to elicit anti-carcinogenic effects in vitro are much higher (~10–200 μM) than the levels of these compounds observed in the blood of animals administered anthocyanin-containing diets or juices (~2–25 nM). This may be due, in part, to the instability of the anthocyanins at physiological pH. The half-life of most anthocyanins in culture medium at pH 7.0 is less than 5 h (Duthie et al. 2006). The results of in vitro studies with the anthocyanidins are also difficult to extrapolate to the in vivo situation because the anthocyanidins in vivo are unstable and are

Table 11.2 Anti-carcinogenic effects of anthocyanidin/anthocyanin and anthocyanin-rich extract in vitro

Anti-cancer effect	Anthocyanidin/anthocyanin source	Concentration	Cells	Reference
Anti-oxidation				
↑ ORAC value	6 types of berry extracts	50 μg/ml	Human endothelial cells	Bagchi et al. (2004)
↓ Reactive oxygen species	Concord grape extract	10–20 μg/ml	Normal human breast cells	Singletary et al. (2007)
Phase II enzyme activation				
↑ Glutathione-related enzymes ↑ NAD(P)H: quinone reductase	Concord grape extract	10–20 μg/ml	Normal human breast cells	Singletary et al. (2007)
Anti-cell proliferation				
↓ Cell proliferation	5 anthocyanidins and 5 anthocyanins	12.5–200 μg/ml	Human stomach, colon, breast and lung cancer cells	Zhang et al. (2005)
↓ Cell proliferation	Black raspberry extract, cyanidin-3-O-glucoside and cyanidin-3-Orutinoside	10–100 μg/ml	Rat esophageal highly and weakly tumorigenic epithelial cells	Zikri et al. (2009)
Induction of apoptosis				
↑ Caspase-3 and PARP activity	Cyanidin 3-glucoside and peonidin 3-glucoside	10–100 μM	Human breast, stomach, liver, cervical, and lung cancer cells	Chen et al. (2005)
↑ Cytochrome *c* release ↑ Caspases-3, -6, -8, and -9	Delphinidin	30–180 μM	Human prostate cancer cells	Mukhtar et al. (2008)
Induction of differentiation				
↑ Activation of transglutaminase enzymes involved in keratin production	Black raspberry extract	100 μg/ml	Human oral SCC cells	Rodrigo et al. (2006)
↑ Granulocyte differentiation	cyanidin-3-O-beta-glucopyranoside	25–225 μg/ml	Human leukemic cells	Fimognari et al. (2004)

Table 11.2 (continued)

Anti-cancer effect	Anthocyanidin/anthocyanin source	Concentration	Cells	Reference
Anti-inflammation				
↓ COX-1 and COX-2	Cyanidin-3-O-glucoside	12.5–200 μg/ml	Human breast, colon, stomach, central nervous system and lung cancer cells	Reddy et al. (2005)
↓ NF-κB activation	Pomegranate extract	10–40 μg/ml	Normal human epidermal keratinocytes	Afaq et al. (2005a)
Anti-angiogenesis				
↓ VEGF	Black raspberry extract	1–100 μg/ml	Human oral SCC cells and mouse epidermal cells	Rodrigo et al. (2006)
↓ Matrigel endothelial cell tube formation	6 anthocyanidins and 1 anthocyanin	1–25 μM	Human umbilical vein endothelial cells	Favot et al. (2003)
Anti-invasiveness				
↓ MMP-9 and u-PA ↓ Cell invasion and motility (Matrigel)	Extract from black rice, peonidin 3-glucoside and cyanidin 3-glucoside	50–200 μg/ml (extract), 25–100 μM (anthocyanin)	Human liver and cervical cancer cells	Chen et al. (2006a, b)
Promoter demethylation				
↓ Promoter demethylation of tumor suppressor genes, e.g., p16, SFRP2, SFRP5, WIF1 ↓ DNMT1 and DNMT3B activities	Black raspberry extract	5–25 μg/ml	Human colon cancer cells	Data not published

ORAC oxygen-radical absorbing capacity, *AP-1* activator protein 1, *PARP* Poly (ADP-ribose) polymerase, *COX* cyclooxygenase, *NF-κB* nuclear factor kappa B, *PGE_2* prostaglandin E_2, *VEGF* vascular endothelial growth factor, *SCC* squamous cell carcinoma, *MMP* matrix metalloproteinases, *uPA* urokinase plasminogen activator

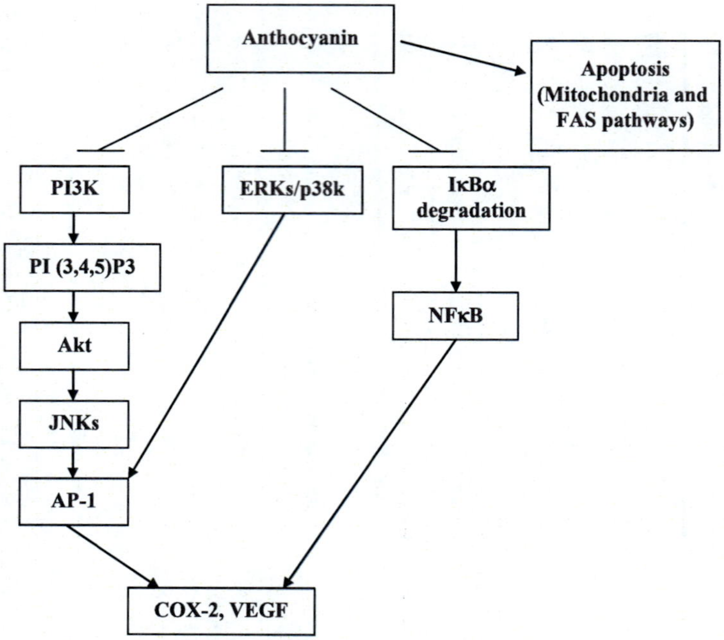

Fig. 11.5 Schematic illustration of known molecular mechanisms that may be involved in the chemopreventive mechanisms of anthocyanidin/anthocyanin (Wang and Stoner 2008)

generally not found in plasma, urine or in tissues (Francis 1989). Thus, perhaps the most appropriate use of the in vitro data in Table 11.2 is that of identifying possible mechanistic biomarkers for clinical investigations with the anthocyanins or anthocyanin-containing foodstuffs.

In addition to the chemopreventive effects mentioned above, we recently observed that black raspberry-derived anthocyanins are capable of causing promoter demethylation of tumor suppressor genes, e.g., p16, in human colon cancer cell lines through suppressing the activities of DNA methyltransferase 3B (DNMT3B) (Fig. 11.6). The co-localization of black raspberry-derived anthocyanins with DNMT3B suggested the possible direct binding of anthocyanins to these enzymes (Fig. 11.7). Similar staining pattern was observed in DNMT1 co-localization with anthocyanins (data not shown).

11.5.1.2 Animal Studies

Anthocyanidins/anthocyanins and fruit extracts enriched in these compounds have been shown to inhibit the development of multiple cancer types in carcinogen-treated animals and in animals with a hereditary predisposition to cancer. Table 11.3 presents results of some of the published studies; the reader is referred to our review articles (Wang and Stoner 2008, 2009) for more extensive discussions. An update

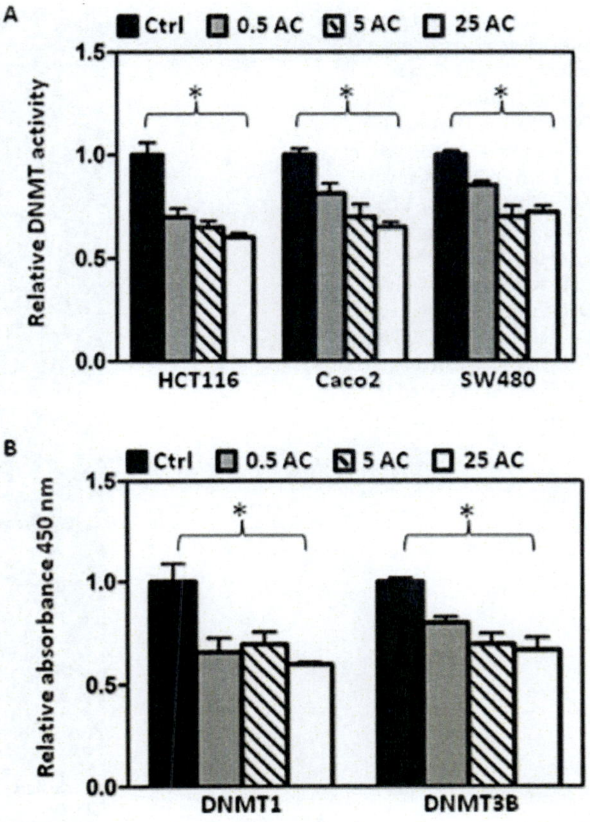

Fig. 11.6 Black raspberry-derived anthocyanins (AC) suppressed DNMT1 and DNMT3B. (**a**) Total DNMT activity in nuclear extracts from human colon cancer cells, HCT116, Caco2 and SW480, treated with AC at 0.5–25 μg/ml for 3 days was decreased. In a cell free in vitro inhibition assay, AC inhibited DNMT1 and DNMT3B (**b**). * $p < 0.05$

of the chemopreventive effects of anthocyanidins/anthocyanins in animals since our last review in 2008 follows.

Using the rat model of esophageal squamous cell carcinoma in which esophageal tumors are induced by the carcinogen, *N*-nitrosomethylbenzylamine (NMBA), an anthocyanin-enriched fraction of black raspberries (BRBs) was tested for its ability to inhibit esophageal cancer (Wang et al. 2009). The anthocyanin-rich fraction, containing the same amount of anthocyanins (~3.8 μmol/g diet) as are present in a diet containing 5% BRBs, was compared along with the 5% BRB diet itself for their ability to inhibit esophageal tumorigenesis . The anthocyanin-rich fraction was equally as effective as the 5% BRB diet in reducing esophageal tumorigenesis, suggesting that the anthocyanins in BRBs are important for chemoprevention (Wang et al. 2009). In molecular studies, we reported the modulation of NMBA-induced gene expression in rat esophagus by the 5% BRB diet and the anthocyanin-enriched fraction (Wang et al. 2009). Using quantitative immunohistochemistry and Western blot analysis, we found that BRB anthocyanins produced similar modulatory effects on protein expression of genes associated with cell proliferation (Ki-67, Erk1/2), inflammation [COX-2 and PGE_2, NFκB, CD45 (leukocyte common antigen)] and

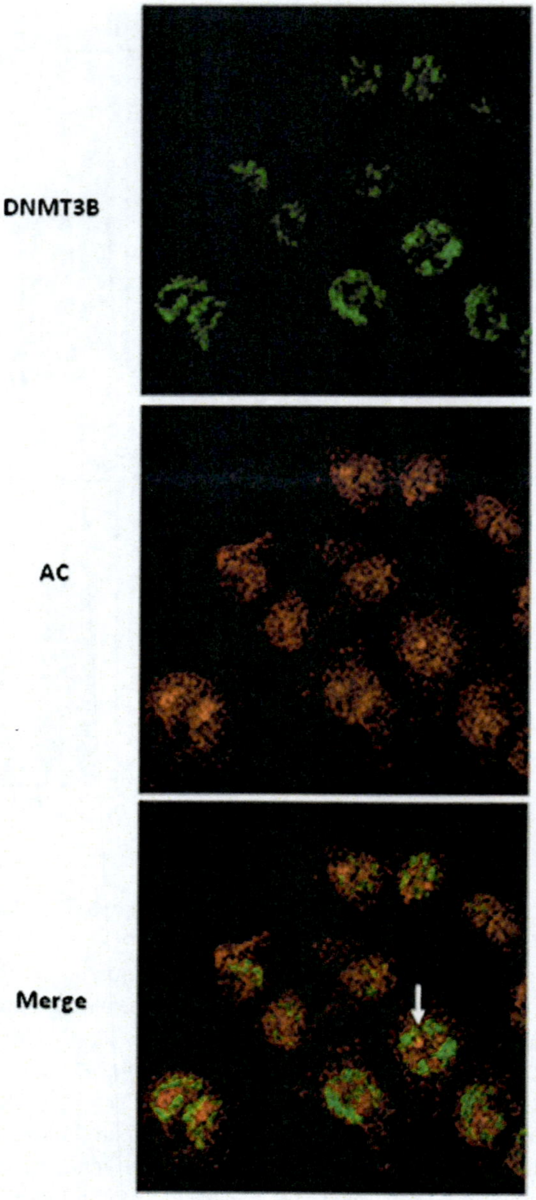

Fig. 11.7 Cellular uptake of black raspberry-derived anthocyanins (AC) and co-localization of AC with DNMT3B in HCT116 cells. AC uptake was observed in HCT116 cells treated with AC at 25 μg/ml for 1 day. AC in *red* presented in both cytoplasm and nuclei. Same cells were stained with DNMT3B shown in *green*. Co-localization of AC with DNMT3B appeared in *yellowish* as indicated by *arrowhead*

angiogenesis (VEGF, HIF1α, CD34) in preneoplastic esophagus and in esophageal papillomas as were observed with the 5% BRB diet. Both diets were also found to induce apoptosis as demonstrated by increased TUNEL staining and modulation of proteins that regulate apoptosis such as Bcl-2 and Bax in NMBA-treated esophagus (Wang et al. 2009).

Table 11.3 Anti-carcinogenic effects of anthocyanidin/anthocyanin and anthocyanin-rich extract in vivo

Cancer types	Anthocyanidin/anthocyanin source	Concentration	Mechanisms	Reference
Esophagus	Anthocyanin-rich extract from black raspberries	3.5 μmole/g diet	↓ Cell proliferation ↑ Apoptosis ↓ Inflammation ↓ Angiogenesis	Wang et al. (2009)
	Black raspberries, red raspberries, strawberries, and blueberries	5% in diet	↓ Interleukin 5 (IL-5) and GRO/KC ↑ Serum antioxidant capacity	Stoner et al. (2010)
	Black raspberries	5% in diet	↓ PGE_2 ↓ LTB_4 ↓ Matrix metalloproteinase 10	Wang et al. (2011a)
Colon	Anthocyanin-rich extract from bilberry, chokeberry and grape	3.85 g/kg diet	↓ Cell proliferation ↓ COX-2 expression	Lala et al. (2006)
Skin	Delphinidin	1 mg/topical application	Inhibition of UVB-mediated apoptosis and DNA damage	Afaq et al. (2005a)
	Anthocyanin- and hydrolysable-tannin- rich pomegranate extracts	2 mg/topical application	Modulation of MAPK and NF-κB pathways	Afaq et al. (2005b)
Lung	Cyanidin-3-glucoside	9.5 mg/kg i.p. injection	ND	Ding et al. (2006)
	Anthocyanins from black rice	0.5% (wt/wt) by oral gavage	ND	Ding et al. (2006)
Mammary	Black raspberries and blueberries	2.5% in diet	↓ Cell proliferation	Ravoori et al. (2008)
	Black raspberries and blueberries	2.5% in diet	Modulating enzymes that metabolitze estrogen	Aiyer and Gupta (2010)
Prostate	Fruit juice from blueberries, red grapes, raspberries and elderberries	10% in drinking water	↓ Cell proliferation	Singh et al. (2008)
	Delphinidin	2 mgKg i.p. injection	↓ NF-κB/p65, Bcl2, Ki67, and PCNA	Hafeez et al. (2008)

MAPK mitogen-activated protein kinases, *i.p.* intraperitoneal, *ND* not determined

Using the same animal model, we compared the ability of BRBs, red raspberries, strawberries and blueberries to suppress tumorigenesis in the rat esophagus, and determined the effects of these berry types on levels of inflammatory cytokines in the serum of NMBA-treated rats (Stoner et al. 2010). All berry types were about equally effective in inhibiting NMBA-induced tumorigenesis in spite of known differences in levels and types of anthocyanins. They also reduced the levels of the serum cytokines, interleukin 5 (IL-5) and GRO/KC, the rat homologue for human interleukin-8 (IL-8), and this was associated with increased serum antioxidant capacity. Serum levels of IL-5 and GRO/KC (IL-8) may be predictive of the inhibitory effect of chemopreventive agents in rat esophageal carcinogenesis. Using cDNA microarray, we studied the mechanistic basis for the chemopreventive effects of BRBs at a late stage of NMBA-induced rat esophageal carcinogenesis (Wang et al. 2011a). Treatment with 5% BRBs reduced the number of dysplastic lesions and the number and size of esophageal papillomas in NMBA-treated rats. When compared to esophagi from control rats, NMBA treatment led to the differential expression of 4807 genes in preneoplastic esophagus (PE) and 17,846 genes in esophageal papillomas. Dietary BRBs modulated 626 of the 4807 differentially expressed genes in PE and 625 of the 17,846 differentially expressed genes in esophageal papillomas towards normal levels of expression. In both PE and in papillomas, BRBs modulated the mRNA expression of genes associated with carbohydrate and lipid metabolism, cell proliferation and death, and inflammation. In these same tissues, BRBs modulated the expression of proteins associated with proliferation, apoptosis, inflammation, angiogenesis, and both cyclooxygenase and lipoxygenase pathways of arachidonic acid metabolism. Interestingly, matrix metalloproteinases involved in tissue invasion and metastasis, and proteins associated with cell-cell adhesion, were also modulated by BRBs. This is the first report of the effects of berries on the expression of genes associated with the late stages of rat esophageal carcinogenesis.

Lala et al. (2006), using the azoxymethane (AOM)-induced colon cancer model in rats, showed that an anthocyanin-rich extract from bilberry, chokeberry and grape administered in the diet significantly reduced AOM-induced aberrant crypt foci. This reduction was associated with decreased cell proliferation and COX-2 gene expression. In the mouse skin cancer model, delphinidin and pomegranate extracts enriched in anthocyanins and tannins were shown to inhibit UVB- or TPA (12-O-tetradecanoylphorbol-13-acetate)-induced skin cancer development when applied topically to the skin. Delphinidin inhibited UVB-mediated DNA damage and the pomegranate extracts modulated the mitogen-activated protein kinase (MAPK) and nuclear factor-kappa B (NF-κB) pathways (Afaq et al. 2005a, b). Using the nude mouse xenotransplant model, cyanidin-3-glucoside and anthocyanins from black rice (Ding et al. 2006) were shown to inhibit the development of tumors produced by subcutaneous injection of lung tumor cells. The mechanism(s) of this inhibition was not investigated. In the rat mammary carcinogenesis model, diets containing 5% blueberry or black raspberry powders reduced the proliferation index in mammary tissues from estrogen-treated animals compared with control rats (Ravoori et al. 2008). The protective effects of berries on estrogen-induced mammary tumors are possibly through their abilities to modulate enzymes that metabolize estrogen

(Aiyer and Gupta 2010). A juice prepared from blueberries, red grapes, raspberries and elderberries reduced the size and cyclin D1 expression of tumors in nude mice produced after subcutaneous injection of human prostate cancer cells (Singh et al. 2008). Delphinidin administration to athymic nude mice implanted with human prostate cancer PC3 cells resulted in a significant inhibition of tumor growth. Analysis of tumors from delphinidin-treated mice showed significant decreases in the expression of NF-κB/p65, Bcl2, Ki67, and PCNA (Hafeez et al. 2008). The positive inhibitory effects of these anthocyanin-rich preparations in the gastrointestinal tract and on the skin are probably mediated by localized absorption of the anthocyanins into the target tissues. However, the observations that whole berries or berry anthocyanins protect against estrogen-induced breast cancer, and against lung and prostate cancer cell growth in xenotransplant models, suggests that berry compounds are absorbed in sufficient quantities to be protective in internal organs and in skin when administered orally.

11.5.1.3 Human Studies

Epidemiological studies in humans have not provided convincing evidence of the anti-cancer effects of anthocyanins (Wang and Stoner 2008). For example, a case-control study involving 805 subjects with oral and pharyngeal cancer and 2081 hospital controls without neoplasia in Italy, showed no significant association between anthocyanidin intake and risk for oral or pharyngeal cancer (Rossi et al. 2007). Also in Italy, the role of six principal classes of flavonoids, including the anthocyanidins, on prostate cancer risk was studied using data from a multicentric case-control study (Bosetti et al. 2006). The results did not support a protective effect of flavonoids, including anthocyanidins, on prostate cancer in this population (Bosetti et al. 2006). Supplementation of anthocyanins in the diet of cancer patients receiving chemotherapy did not result in increased inhibition of tumor development when compared to chemotherapy alone (Bode et al. 1999).

Although epidemiological studies have not shown that anthocyanin intake reduces cancer risk in humans, they suggest that anthocyanin intake may reduce certain parameters of oxidative stress. A study in Germany showed that individuals who consumed an anthocyanin/polyphenolic-rich fruit juice had reduced oxidative DNA damage and a significant increase in reduced glutathione when compared to controls (Weisel et al. 2006). In addition, in an investigation involving Barrett's esophagus patients, the oral administration of freeze-dried black raspberry powder (which contains about 4–6% anthocyanins) in a slurry of water daily for 6 months reduced levels of 8-epi-prostaglandin F2α (8-Iso-PGF2) and 8-OHdG in urine (Kresty et al. 2006). In contrast, a study conducted in the United Kingdom indicated that dietary anthocyanins from cranberry juice had no effect on basal or induced oxidative DNA damage or cellular antioxidant status in leukocytes taken from treated individuals (Duthie et al. 2006).

In a pre-surgical model, we evaluated the effects of BRBs on biomarkers of tumor development in the human colon and rectum including methylation of relevant tumor suppressor genes, cell proliferation, apoptosis, angiogenesis, and expression of Wnt pathway genes (Wang et al. 2011b). Biopsies of adjacent normal tissues and colorectal adenocarcinomas were taken from 20 patients before and after oral consumption of BRB powder (60 g/d) for 1–9 weeks. Methylation status of promoter regions of five tumor suppressor genes was quantified. Protein expression of DNMT1, genes associated with cell proliferation, apoptosis, angiogenesis, and Wnt signaling were measured. The methylation of three Wnt inhibitors, SFRP2, SFRP5, and WIF1, upstream genes in Wnt pathway, and PAX6a, a developmental regulator, was modulated in a protective direction by BRBs in normal tissues and in colorectal tumors only in patients who received BRB treatment for an average of 4 weeks, but not in all 20 patients with 1–9 weeks of BRB treatment. The demethylation effects were associated with decreased expression of the enzyme, DNMT1. BRBs modulated expression of genes associated with Wnt signaling, proliferation, apoptosis, and angiogenesis in a protective direction. These data provide evidence of the ability of BRBs to demethylate tumor suppressor genes and to modulate other biomarkers of tumor development in the human colon and rectum. While demethylation of genes did not occur in colorectal tissues from all treated patients, the positive results with the secondary endpoints suggest that additional studies of BRBs for the prevention of colorectal cancer in humans now appear warranted.

11.5.2 Mechanisms of Chemoprotection by Protocatechuic Acid

Unless otherwise stated, the protective effects of PCA discussed below are not limited to its role as a metabolite of cyanidin because PCA also occurs naturally in fruit. In addition, other polyphenols, such as quercetin, are metabolized to PCA (Boulton et al. 1999). Therefore, when crude extracts or whole fruits were used in the studies described below, the PCA was derived from multiple sources.

11.5.2.1 In Vitro Studies

PCA, and extracts enriched in PCA, have been shown to elicit multiple anti-carcinogenic effects in vitro including anti-oxidation, reduced cell proliferation, induction of apoptosis and anti-invasiveness (Table 11.4). With respect to its anti-oxidant activities, in human colon cancer cell lines HT-29 and HCT-116, PCA did not cause significant changes in COX-1 and COX-2 activities but reduced liposome oxidation (Seeram et al. 2001). Grape seed extracts containing PCA were found to increase oxidative defense and ROS-induced damage by increasing catalase and glutathione *S*-transferase activities in human lymphocytes (Stanković et al. 2008). PCA isolated from the kernels of *Alpinia oxyphylla*, protected against -induced apoptosis, and H_2O_2- and Fe^{2+}-induced cell damage in rat PC12 cells by increasing catalase activity and glutathione levels in the cells (Guan et al. 2006). Rat PC12 cells, derived from adrenal gland, are used for neurobiological and neurochemical studies (Guan, et al. 2006). Interestingly, PCA from Acai showed cytoprotective activity in H_2O_2-stressed MCF-7 cells, a human estrogen dependent breast cancer cell line (Chin et al. 2008). This result suggests that PCA might reduce the effectiveness of therapeutic agents in vivo that function by producing oxidative stress.

Table 11.4 Anti-carcinogenic effects of protocatechuic acid and extract containing protocatechuic acid in vitro

Anti-cancer effect	Protocatechuic acid source	Concentration	Cells	Reference
Anti-oxidation				
↓ Liposome oxidation	Degradation product from tart cherry	50 μM	Human colon cancer cells	Seeram et al. (2001)
↑ Catalase and glutathione S-transferase activity	Grape seed extract	2.5–5 μg/ml	Human lymphocyte	Stanković et al. (2008)
↑ Catalase and glutathione	kernels of *Alpinia oxyphylla*	0.6–1.2 mM	Rat adrenal gland cells retaining dopaminergic characteristics and having been used for neurobiological and neurochemical studies	Guan et al. (2006)
Anti-cell proliferation				
↓ Proliferation	Rhus verniciflua stoke extract	10–100 μg/ml	Human B lymphoma cells	Lee et al. (2004)
↓ Proliferation	Rhus verniciflua stoke extract	10–100 μg/ml	Human osteosarcoma cells	Janng et al. (2005)
Induction of apoptosis				
↓ RB phosphorylation ↓ Bcl-2	*Hibiscus sabdariffa* L. extract	2 mM	Human leukemia cells	Tseng et al. (2000)
↑ DNA fragmentation	Rhus verniciflua stoke extract	100 μg/ml	Human B lymphoma cells	Lee et al. (2004)
↑ DNA fragmentation ↑ PARP cleavage, Caspase 8, Bax, release cytochrome c ↓ Bcl-2	Rhus verniciflua stoke extract	10–50 μg/ml	Human osteosarcoma cells	Janng et al. (2005)

Table 11.4 (continued)

Anti-cancer effect	Protocatechuic acid source	Concentration	Cells	Reference
↑ c-Jun N-terminal kinase (JNK) and p38	Synthetic	100 μmol/L	Human hepatocellular carcinoma cells	Yip et al. (2006)
↑ c-Jun N-terminal kinase (JNK) and p38 ↑ Fas signaling	Synthetic	6–8 mM	Human gastric carcinoma cells	Lin et al. (2007)
Anti-invasiveness				
↓ MMP2 ↓ NFκB ↓ RhoB/protein kinase Ce (PKCe) pathway ↓ Ras/Akt pathway	Synthetic	0.5–2 mM	Human gastric carcinoma cells	Lin et al. (2007)
↓ Cell adhesion ↓ ICAM-1, VEGF, IL-6, IL-8	Synthetic	2–8 μmol/L	Human breast, lung, liver, cervix, and prostate cancer cells	Yin et al. (2009)

PCA inhibits cell proliferation and induces apoptosis. *Rhus verniciflua* Stokes (RVS) is used as a food additive and a traditional herbal medicine. RVS extract containing PCA was shown to inhibit growth and induce apoptosis in Human B lymphoma (BJAB) (Lee et al. 2004) and human osteosarcoma (HOS) cells (Jang et al. 2005). In human leukemia HL-60 cells, PCA isolated from *Hibiscus sabdariffa L.*, a traditional Chinese rose tea, induced apoptosis via reduction of retinoblastoma (RB) phosphorylation and Bcl-2 expression (Tseng et al. 2000). Synthetic PCA suppressed cell viability through the induction of c-Jun N-terminal kinase (JNK) and p38 in human hepatocellular carcinoma (HepG2) cells (Yip et al. 2006). Similar findings were observed in human gastric carcinoma (AGS) cells (Lin et al. 2007). However, PCA did not induce apoptosis in human colon cancer colo 320 cells and had no significant effects on the BrdU labeling index (Zheng et al. 2002).

The ability of PCA to suppress cell motility and invasiveness has also been reported. PCA decreased motility and invasion of human gastric carcinoma AGS cells through inhibition of MMP-2 activity and inactivation of NF-κB, as well as inhibited RhoB/protein kinase Ce (PKCe) and Ras/Akt cascade pathways (Lin et al. 2007). PCA suppressed invasiveness of human MCF7 breast cancer cells, A549 lung cancer cells, HepG2 hepatoma cells, HeLa cervical cells, and LNCaP prostate cancer cells through decreasing cell adhesion and the expression levels of intercellular adhesion molecule-1 (ICAM-1, a cell adhesion molecule that participates in intercellular and cell–extracellular matrix interactions), VEGF, IL-6, and IL-8 (Yin et al. 2009).

11.5.2.2 Animal Studies

PCA has been evaluated extensively for its chemopreventive effects on aerodigestive tract cancers in rodents (Table 11.5). For example, PCA significantly inhibited colon tumor incidence and multiplicity in azoxymethane-treated F344 rats (Tanaka et al. 1993a). This was associated with decreases in cell proliferation as measured by bromodeoxyuridine (BrdU) labeling, counts of silver-stained nuclear organizer regions (AgNORs), and ornithine decarboxylase (ODC) activity. No toxicities were observed in this study. Using the same model, dietary PCA significantly decreased aberrant crypt foci in the colon (Kawamori et al. 1994). PCA also exhibits chemopreventive activity in the oral cavity as shown by its ability to reduce 7,12-dimethylbenz[a]anthracene (DMBA)-induced cheek pouch tumors in male Syrian golden hamsters (Ohnishi et al. 1997), and 4-nitroquinoline 1-oxide (4-NQO)- induced tongue tumors and preneoplastic lesions in F-344 rats (Tanaka et al. 1994). Further, PCA significantly reduced the numbers of diethylnitrosamine (DEN)-induced liver cell foci, adenomas and carcinomas in F344 rats (Tanaka et al. 1994). Hepatic ornithine decarboxylase activity was reduced in DEN-treated animals fed PCA diets compared to those given DEN alone (Tanaka et al. 1993b). Although PCA (500–1000 ppm in diet) did not alter the incidence and multiplicities of N-nitrosobis(2-oxopropyl)amine (BOP)-initiated pancreatic tumors in female hamsters, 1000 ppm PCA significantly reduced the incidence of advanced pancreatic tumors and reduced invasion of pancreatic tumor cells to adjacent tissues such as the diaphragm, spleen and stomach (Nakamura et al. 2000).

Table 11.5 Anti-carcinogenic effects of protocatechuic acid in vivo

Cancer types	Protocatechuic acid source	Concentration (in diet)	Mechanisms	Reference
Colon – tumor	Synthetic	500–1000 ppm	↓ Cell proliferation	Tanaka et al. (1993a)
Colon – aberrant crypt foci	Synthetic	1000–2000 ppm	ND	Kawamori et al. (1994)
Oral – cheek pouch	Synthetic	200 ppm	↓ Cell proliferation	Ohnishi et al. (1997)
Oral – tongue	Synthetic	500–2000 ppm	↓ Cell proliferation	Tanaka et al. (1994)
Liver	Synthetic	500–1000 ppm	↓ Ornithine decarboxylase activity	Tanaka et al. (1993b)
Pancreas	Synthetic	1000 ppm	ND	Nakamura et al. (2000)
Bladder	Synthetic	1000–2000 ppm	↓ Cell proliferation	Hirose et al. (1995)
Liver metastasis	Synthetic	20–40 mg/100 g body weight	↓ MMP2 ↓ RhoB/protein kinase Ce (PKCe) pathway ↓ Ras/Akt pathway	Lin et al. (2011)

ND not determined

Other than aerodigestive tract cancers, PCA has been shown to reduce N-butyl-N-(4-hydroxybutyl)nitrosamine (BBN)-induced bladder carcinogenesis in male F344 rats (Hirose et al. 1995). This was associated with a reduction in cell proliferation and in AgNORs. Finally, PCA inhibited metastasis of B16/F10 melanoma cells to the liver in mice (Lin et al. 2011). This was associated with inhibition of MMP-2 activity, and of RhoB/protein kinase Ce (PKCe) and Ras/Akt cascade pathways. PCA was not effective, however, in preventing 4-(methylnitrosamino)-1-(3-pyridyl)-1-butanone (NNK)-induced lung carcinogenesis in female A/J mice (Mori et al. 1999), 2-amino-1-methyl-6-phenylimidazo[4,5-b]pyridine (PhIP)-induced mammary carcinogenesis in female Sprague–Dawley rats (Mori et al. 1999), or N-methyl-N′-nitro-N-nitrosoguanidine (MNNG)-induced forestomach carcinogenesis in male F344 rats (Hirose, et al. 1992). Two studies showed different effects of PCA on skin tumorigenesis. In one study, topical application of PCA enhanced TPA-induced skin tumor promotion in female ICR mice (Nakamura et al. 2000). In another study, topical application of PCA isolated from *Hibiscus sabdariffa L.* significantly suppressed TPA-induced hyperplasia and tumor incidence in female CD-1 mouse skin (Tseng et al. 1998). The reasons for these different responses in skin have not been determined.

11.5.2.3 Human Studies

To date, no studies have evaluated naturally- occurring or synthesized PCA for chemopreventive effects in humans. However, bioavailability studies of PCA from different food sources have been conducted. Although PCA was the major compound measured in most of these studies, the reader should be aware that when humans consume fruit/berries containing different anthocyanins, the anthocyanins degrade to their corresponding phenolic acids derived from the B-ring (Fig. 11.1) of the anthocyanidin skeleton. For example, cyanidin degrades to PCA, malvidin to syringic acid, peonidin to vanillic acid, pelargonidin to 4-hydroxybenzoic acid, etc. Therefore, PCA is not the only phenolic acid produced from the anthocyanins.

The initial study reporting PCA as the major human metabolite of cyandin-glucoside (CyG) was published in 2007 (Vitaglione et al. 2007). Six healthy volunteers, 3 male and 3 female, 20–24 years old, took 1L of blood orange juice containing 71 mg CyG in ~15 min. Maximum serum CyG (1.9 ± 0.6 nmol/L) and PCA glucuronidated/methylated metabolites, but not PCA, were detected in urine. Both CyG and PCA were detected in fecal samples. The combined amount of PCA recovered in serum and in feces represented 72.5% of the consumed CyG indicating that PCA is the major metabolite of CyG. However, as stated above, PCA is found naturally in fruit, therefore, if the juice already contained PCA, the percentage conversion (72.5%) of CyG to PCA may have been overestimated. Recently, a randomized, placebo-controlled 8-week dietary intervention trial evaluating the bioavailability of berry polyphenols in 72 middle-aged subjects was reported (Koli et al. 2010). The average intake of berries (bilberries, lingonberries, black currants and chokeberries) in the berry group was 160 g/day of which total anthocyanin content was 515 mg and total PCA content was 10.4 mg. The control group consumed products that matched the energy intake in the berry group. Baseline PCA levels in plasma in both groups were ~110 nmol/L. After the 8-week intervention, the plasma PCA level increased significantly in the berry group (~125 nmol/L) and that in control group decreased to ~100 nmol/L. There was no difference in the urinary excretion of PCA in berry and control groups at baseline or after 8 weeks of intervention. A recent study investigated the effects of human oral mucosal tissue, saliva and oral microflora on intraoral metabolism and bioactivation of BRB anthocyanins (Mallery et al. 2011). Saliva samples from different time courses were collected following BRB rinses to assess local pharmacokinetics using LC-MS/MS. BRB anthocyanins were deglycosylated by microflora in saliva. PCA was detected in saliva for up to 4 h after rinsing and post-rinse saliva samples contained glucuronidated anthocyanin conjugates. This data demonstrated that comparable to the small intestine, the requisite hydrolytic, Phase II and efflux transporting enzymes necessary for local enteric recycling are present and functional in human oral mucosa.

11.6 Conclusion

Anthocyanins and protocatechuic acid, the major metabolite of cyanidin and also present naturally in plants and fruits, have been shown to exhibit anti-carcinogenic activity against multiple cancer cell types in vitro and tumor types in vivo. In vivo studies have shown that dietary anthocyanins inhibit cancers of the gastrointestinal tract and topically applied anthocyanins inhibit skin cancer, likely due to localized absorption of the compounds. Likewise, local absorption of protocatechuic acid is also important for its anti-cancer activities because it is especially effective in preventing aerodigestive tract cancers in rodents. Pharmacokinetic data indicate that the absorption of anthocyanins into the bloodstream of rodents (and humans) is minimal, however, dietary administration of these compounds appears to inhibit breast cancer in rats, and tumors produced in nude mice by xenotransplantation of lung and prostate cancer cells. Thus, in these model systems, the systemic administration of absorbed anthocyanins appears to be sufficient to confer protection. Measuring tissue-bound anthocyanins seems necessary for predicting their chemopreventive effects in different organs. In fact it was shown that the bioavailability of polyphenols can be much higher than we originally thought. A recent study comparing the uptake of quercetin and resveratrol in plasma and whole blood reported that up to 76% of the analyte, being associated with the cellular fraction in whole blood, was unaccounted for when only plasma was examined (Biasutto et al. 2010). This indicates the importance of analysing whole blood rather than plasma to avoid underestimating polyphenol absorption in bioavailability studies.

Although experimental studies have clearly demonstrated the anti-cancer activity of anthocyanins, epidemiological studies have not revealed protective effects in humans. This may be due to complexities associated with accurately determining anthocyanin uptake in human populations, and in separating anthocyanins' effects from those of other dietary factors. Further, to date, there is no study using metabolites, e.g., protocatechuic acid, for the prevention of cancer in humans. Future studies aimed at developing assays to extract anthocyanins binding to proteins are necessary to reflect the real bioavailability of these compounds which in turn determine their optimal doses in the chemoprevention of human cancer.

References

Afaq F, Malik A, Syed D et al (2005a) Pomegranate fruit extract modulates UV-B-mediated phosphorylation of mitogen-activated protein kinases and activation of nuclear factor kappa B in normal human epidermal keratinocytes. Photochem Photobiol 81:38–45

Afaq F, Saleem M, Kueger CG et al (2005b) Anthocyanin- and hydrolyzable tannin-rich pomegranate fruit extract modulates MAPK and NF-kappaB pathways and inhibits skin tumorigenesis in CD-1 mice. Int J Cancer 113:423–433

Aiyer HS, Gupta RC (2010) Berries and ellagic acid prevent estrogen-induced mammary tumorigenesis by modulating enzymes of estrogen metabolism. Cancer Prev Res 3:727–737

Andersen ØM, Jordheim M (2005) The anthocyanins. In: Andersen ØM, Markham KR (eds) Flavanoids: chemistry, biochemistry and applications, 1 st edn. CRC press, Boca Raton, FL

Bagchi D, Sen CK, Bagchi M et al (2004) Anti-angiogenic, antioxidant, and anti-carcinogenic properties of a novel anthocyanin rich berry extract formula. Biochemistry (Mosc) 69:75–80

Bajaj KL, Kansal BD, Chadha ML et al (1990) Chemical composition of some important varities of eggplant (*Solanum melongena* L). Tropical Sci 30:255–261

Bakker L, Timberlake CF (1985) The distribution and content of anthocyanins in young port wines as determined by high performance liquid chromatography. J Sci Food Agric 36:1325–1333

Biasutto L, Marotta E, Garbisa S et al (2010) Determination of quercetin and resveratrol in whole blood – implications for bioavailability studies. Molecules 15:6570–6579

Bode U, Hasan C, Hülsmann B.(1999) Recancostat compositum therapy does not prevent tumor progression in young cancer patients. Klin Padiatr 211:353–355

Bosetti C, Bravi F, Talamini R et al (2006) Flavonoids and prostate cancer risk: a study in Italy. Nutr Cancer 56:123–127

Boulton DW, Walle UK, Walle T (1999) Fate of the flavonoid quercetin in human cell lines: chemical instability and metabolism. J Pharm Pharmacol 51:353–359

Boyles MJ, Wrolstad RE (1993) Anthocyanins composition of red raspberry juice: influence of cultivar, processing and environmental factors. J Food Sci 58:1136–1141

Bridle P, Timberlake CF (1997) Anthocyanins as natural food colours-selected aspects. Food Chem 58:103–109

Cao G, Muccitelli H, Sanchez-Moreno C, Prior R (2001) Anthocyanins are absorbed in glycated forms in elderly women: a pharmacokinetic study. Am J Clin Nutr 73:920–926

Casado-Redin I, Fernández M, Vega FA (1992) Polyphenols in *Prunus spinosa* L fruits during ripening process. In: XVIe Journées Internationales Groupe Polyphénols and the Royal Soiciety of Chemistry, Lisbon. DTA, Lisbon, Portugal

Chen PN, Chu SC, Chiou HL et al (2005) Cyanidin 3-glucoside and peonidin 3-glucoside inhibit tumor cell growth and induce apoptosis in vitro and suppress tumor cell growth in vivo. Nutr Cancer 53:232–243

Chen PN, Chu SC, Chiou HL et al (2006a) Mulberry anthocyanins, cyanidin 3-rutinoside and cyanidin 3-glucoside, exhibited an inhibitory effect on the migration and invasion of a human lung cancer cell line. Cancer Lett 235:248–259

Chen PN, Kwo WH, Chiang CL et al (2006b) Black rice anthocyanins inhibit cancer cells invasion via repression of MMPs and u-PA expression. Chem Biol Interact 163:218–229

Chin Y-W, Chai H-B, Keller WJ et al (2008) Lignans and other constituents of the fruits of Euterpe oleracea (açai) with antioxidant and cytoprotective activities. J Agric Food Chem 56: 7759–7764

Clifford M (2000) Anthocyanins – nature, occurrence and dietary burden. J Sci Food Agric 80:1063–1072

Ding M, Feng, R, Wang, SY et al (2006) Cyanidin-3-glucoside, a natural product derived from blackberry, exhibits chemopreventive and chemotherapeutic activity. J Biol Chem 281: 17359–17368

Dreiseitel A, Oosterhius B, Vukman KV et al (2009) Berry anthocyanins and anthocyanidins exhibit distinct affinities for the efflux transporters BCRP and MDR1. Br J Pharmacol 158:1942–1950

Duthie SJ, Jenkinson AM, Crozier A et al (2006) The effects of cranberry juice consumption on antioxidant status and biomarkers relating to heart disease and cancer in healthy human volunteers. Eur J Nutr. 45:113–122

Favot L, Martin S, Keravis T et al (2003) Involvement of cyvlin-dependent pathway in the inhibitory effect of delphinidin on angiogenesis. Cardiovasc Res 59:479–487

Felgines C, Texier O, Besson C, Fraisse D, Lamaison JL, Rémésy C (2002) Blackberry anthocyanins are slightly bioavailable in rats. J Nutr 132:1249–1253

Felgines C, Talavera S, Gonthier MP et al (2003) Strawberry anthocyanins are recovered in urine as glucuro- and sulfoconjugates in humans. J Nutr 133:1296–1301

Felgines C, Talavera S, Texier O et al (2005) Blackberry anthocyanins are mainly recovered from urine as methylated and glucuronidated conjugates in humans. J Agric Food Chem 53: 7721–7727

Felgines C, Texier O, Garcin P et al (2009) Tissue distribution of anthocyanins in rats fed a blackberry anthocyanin-enriched diet. Mol Nutr Food Res 53:1098–1103

Field T, Lee D, Holbtook N (2001) Why leaves turn red in autumn. The role of anthocyanins in senescing leaves of Red-Osier Dogwood. Plant Physiol 127:566–574

Fimognari C, Berti F, Nüsse M et al (2004) Induction of apoptosis in two human leukemia cell lines as wall as differentiation in human promyelocytic cells by cyanidin-3-O-[beta]-glucopyranoside. Biochem Pharmacol 67:2047–2056

Francis FJ (1989) Food colorants: anthocyanins. Crit Rev Food Sci Nutr 28:273–314

Frankel EN, Waterhouse AL, Teissedre P-L (1995) Principal phenolic phytochemicals in selected California wines and their antioxidant activity in inhibiting oxidation of human low-density lipoproteins. J Agric Food Chem 43:890–894

Galvano F, La Fauci L, Lazzarino G et al (2004) Cyanidins: metabolism and biological properties. J Nutr Biochem 15:2–11

Gao L, Mazza G (1995) Characterization, quantitation and distribution of anthocyanins and colourless phenolics in sweet cherries. J Agric Food Chem 43:343–346

Gould K (2004) Nature's swiss army knife: the diverse protection roles of anthocyanins in leaves. J Biomed Biotechnol 5:314–320

Gould K, Lee D (2002) Anthocyanins in leaves. (Adv Bot Res 37). Academic, New York

Gould K, McKelvie J, Markham K (2002) Do anthocyanins function as antioxidants in leaves? Imaging of H_2O_2 in red and green leaves after mechanical injury. Plant Cell Environ 25: 1261–1269

Guan S, Bao YM, Jiang B et al (2006) Protective effect of protocatechuic acid from Alpinia oxyphylla on hydrogen peroxide-induced oxidative PC12 cell death. Eur J Pharmacol 538:73–79

Giusti MM, Jing P (2007) Natural pigments of berry fruits: functionality and application. In: Zhao Y (ed) Berry fruit: value-added products for health promotion, 1 st edn. Taylor & Francis, Boca Raton, FL

Giusti MM, Wrolsted RE (2003) Acylated anthocyanins from edible sources and their applications in food systems. Biochem Eng J 14:217–225

Hafeez BB, Siddiqi IA, Asim M et al. (2008) A dietary anthocyanidin delphinidin induces apoptosis of human prostate cancer PC3 cells in vitro and in vivo: involvement of nuclear factor-κB signaling. Cancer Res 68:8564–8572

Hakimuddin F, Paliyath G, Meekling K (2004) Selective cytotoxicity of a red grape wine flavonoid fraction against MCF-7 cells. Breast Cancer Res Treat 85:65–79

Harborne JB (1979) Correlations between flavanoid chemistry, anatomy and geography in the restionaceae from Australasia and South Africa. Phytochemistry 18:1323–1327

Herrmann K, (1992) Über die Gehalte der hauptsächtligen Pflanzenphenole im im Obst. Flüssiges Obst 59:66–70

Hirose M, Kawabe M, Shibata M et al (1992) Influence of caffeic acid and other o-dihydroxybenzene derivatives on N-methyl-N′-nitro-N-nitrosoguanidine-initiated rat forestomach carcinogenesis. Carcinogenesis 13:1825–1828

Hirose Y, Tanaka T, Kawamori T et al (1995) Chemoprevention of urinary bladder carcinogenesis by the natural phenolic compound protocatechuic acid in rats. Carcinogenesis 16:2337–2342

Hoch W, Singsaas E, McCown B (2003) Resorption protection. Anthocyanins facilitate nutrient recovery in autumn by shielding leaves from potentially damaging light levels. Plant Physiol 133:1296–1305

Jang H-S, Kook S-H, Son Y-O et al (2005) Flavonoids purified from Rhus verniciflua Stokes actively inhibit cell growth and induce apoptosis in human osteosarcoma cells. Biochim Biophys Acta 1726:309–316

Jing P, Giusti MM (2011) Contribution of berry anthocyanins to their chemopreventative properties. In: Stoner G, Seeram N (eds) Berries and cancer prevention. Springer, New York

Kawamori T, Tanaka T, Kojima T et al (1994) Suppression of azoxymethane-induced rat colon aberrant crypt foci by dietary protocatechuic acid. Jpn J Cancer Res 85:686–691

Kay CD, Mazza G, Holub BJ et al (2004) Anthocyanin metabolites in human urine and serum. Br J Nutr 91:933–942

Keppler, K, Humpf H (2005) Metabolism of anthocyanins and their phenolic degradation products by the intestinal microflora. Bioorg Med Chem 13:5195–5205

Keskitalo J, Bergquist G, Gardeström S (2005) A cellular timetable of autumn senescence. Plant Physiol 139:1635–1648

Koli R, Erlund I, Jula A et al (2010) Bioavailability of various polyphenols from a diet containing moderate amounts of berries. J Agric Food Chem 58:3927–3932

Kong J-M, Chia L-S, Goh N-K et al (2003) Analysis and biological activities of anthocyanins. Phytochemistry 64:923–933

Kovinich N, Saleem A, Arnason J, Miki B (2010) Functional characterization of a UDP-glucose: flavonoid 3-O-glucosyltransferase from the seed coat of black soybean (Glycine max (L.) Merr.). Phytochemistry 71:1253–1263

Kresty LA, Frankel WL, Hammond CD et al (2006) Transitioning from preclinical to clinical chemopreventive assessments of lyophilized black raspberries: interim results show berries modulate markers of oxidative stress in Barrett's esophagus patients. Nutr Cancer 54:148–156

Krikorian R, Shidler MD, Nash TA et al (2010) Blueberry supplementation improves memory in older adults. J Agric Food Chem 58:3996–4000

Lala G, Malik M, Zhao C et al (2006) Anthocyanin-rich extracts inhibit multiple biomarkers of colon cancer in rats. Nutr Cancer 54:84–93

Lee JC, Lee KY, Kim J et al (2004) Extract from Rhus verniciflua Stokes is capable of inhibiting the growth of human lymphoma cells. Food Chem Toxicol 42:1383–1388

Lin H-H, Chen J-H, Huang C-C et al (2007) Apoptotic effect of 3,4-dihydroxybenzoic acid on human gastric carcinoma cells involving JNK/p38 MAPK signaling activation. Int J Cancer 120:2306–2316

Lin H-H, Chen J-H, Chou F-P et al (2011) Protocatechuic acid inhibits cancer cell metastasis involving the down-regulation of Ras/Akt/NF-κB pathway and MMP-2 production by targeting RhoB activation. Br J Pharmacol 162:237–254

Mallery SR, Budendorf DE, Larsen MP et al (2011) Effects of human oral mucosal tissue, saliva and oral microflora on intraoral metabolism and bioactivation of black raspberry anthocyanins. Cancer Prev Res (Phila) 2011 May 10. [Epub ahead of print]

Mann J (1987) Secondary metabolism, 2nd edn. Clarendon Press, Oxford

Mazza G, Miniati E (1993) Anthocyanins in fruits, vegetables, and grains. CRC Press, Boca Raton, FL

McGhie TK, Hall HK, Ainge GD et al (2003) Anthocyanin glycosides from berry fruit are absorbed and excreted unmetabolized by both humans and rats. J Agric Food Chem 51:4539–4548

Miyazawa T, Nakagawa K, Kudo M, Muraishi (1999) Direct intestinal absorption of red fruit anthocyanins, cyanidin-3-glucoside and cyanidin-3,5-diglucoside into rats and humans. J Agric Food Chem 47:1083–1091

Mori H, Matsunaga K, Tanakamaru Y et al (1999) Effects of protocatechuic acid, S-methylmethanethiosulfonate or 5-hydroxy-4-(2-phenyl-(E)ethenyl)-2(5H)-furanone(KYN-54) on 4-(methylnitrosamino)-1-(3-pyridyl)-1-butanone-induced pulmonary carcinogenesis in mice. Cancer Lett 135:123–127

Mukhtar H, Adhami VM, Afaq F et al (2008) Delphinidin induces apoptosis and growth inhibition of prostate cancer PC-3 cells via inhibition of Notch-1 and NF-κB/PI3K pathways. Am Assoc Cancer Res Proc 48:375

Nakajima J, Tanaka Y, Yamazaki M, Saito K (2001) Reaction mechanism from leucoanthocyanidin to anthocyanidin 3-glucoside, a key reaction for coloring in anthocyanin biosynthesis. J Biol Chem 276 (28):25797–25803

Nakamura Y, Torikai K, Ohto Y et al (2000) A simple phenolic antioxidant protocatechuic acid enhances tumor promotion and oxidative stress in female ICR mouse skin: dose- and timing-dependent enhancement and involvement of bioactivation by tyrosinase. Carcinogenesis 21:1899–1907

Nemeth K, Plumb GW, Berrin JG et al (2003) Deglycosylation by small intestinal epithelial cell beta-glucosidases is a critical step in the absorption and metabolism of dietary flavonoid glycosidases in humans. Eur J Nutr 42:29–42

Ohnishi M, Yoshimi N, Kawamori T et al (1997) Inhibitory effects of dietary protocatechuic acid and costunolide on 7,12-dimethylbenz[a]anthracene-induced hamster cheek pouch carcinogenesis. Jpn J Cancer Res 88:111–119

Passamonti S, Vrhovsek U, Vanzo A, Mattivi F (2003) The stomach as a site for anthocyanins absorption from food. FEBS Lett 544:210–213

Ravoori S, Vadhanam MV, Kausar H et al (2008) Effect of select berries on estrogen-induced mammary tissue proliferation. Am Asso Cancer Res Proc 48:3821

Reddy MK, Alexander-Lindo RL, Nair MG (2005) Relative inhibition of lipid peroxidation, cyclooxygenase enzymes, and human tumor cell proliferation by natural food colors. J Agric Food Chem 53:9268–9273

Rodrigo KA, Rawal y, Renner RJ et al (2006) Suppression of the tumorigemic phenotype in human oral squamous cell carcinoma cells by an ethanol extract derived from freeze-dried black raspberries. Nutr Cancer 54:58–68

Rossi M, Garavello W, Talamini R et al (2007) Flavonoids and the risk of oral and pharyngeal cancer: a case-control study from Italy. Cancer Epidemiol Biomarkers Prev 16:1621–1625

Scalbert A, Williamson G (2000) Dietary intake and bioavailability of polyphenols. J Nutr 130:2073S–2085S

Seeram, NP (2008) Berry fruits: compositional elements, biochemical activities and the impact of their intake on human health, performance, and disease. J Agric Food Chem 56:627–629

Seeram NP, Bourquin LD, Nair MG (2001) Degradation products of cyanidin glycosides from tart cherries and their bioactivities. J Agric Food Chem 49:4924–4929

Singh J, Yao M, Jardine G, Dong Q (2008) Retardation of prostate cancer growth in vitro and in vivo by a dietary phytochemical cocktail. Am Asso Cancer Res Proc 48:5463

Singletary KW, Jung KJ, Giusti MM (2007) Anthocyanin-rich grape extract blocks breast cell DNA damage. J Med Food 10:244–251

Siriwoharn T, Wrolstad R, Finn C, Pereira C (2004) Influence of cultivar, maturity, and sampling on blackberry (Rubus L. Hybrids) anthocyanins, polyphenolics, and antioxidant properties. J Agric Food Chem 52:8021–8030

Skrede G, Wrolstad RE, Lea P et al (1992) Color stability of strawberry and blackcurrant syrups. J Food Sci 57:172–177

Stanković M, Tešević V, Vajs V et al (2008) Antioxidant properties of grape seed extract on human lymphocyte oxidative defence. Planta Med 74:730–735

Steyn W, Wand S, Holcroft D, Jacobs G (2002) Anthocyanins in vegetative tissues: a proposed unified function in photoprotection. New Phytol 155:349–361

Stoner GD, Sardo C, Aspeloff G et al (2005) Pharmacokinetics of anthocyanins and ellagic acid in healthy volunteers fed freeze-dried black raspberries daily for 7 days. J Clin Pharmacol 45:1153–1164

Stoner GD, Wang LS, Seguin C et al (2010) Multiple berry types prevent N-nitrosomethylbenzylamine-induced esophageal cancer in rats. Pharm Res 27:1138–1145

Sullivan J (1998) Anthocyanin.Carnivorous Plant Newsletter. September 1998. http://www.carnivorousplants.org/cpn/samples/Science273anthocyanin.htm. Accessed 19 June 2011

Talavéra S, Felgines C, Texier O, Besson C, Manach C, Lamaison JL, Rémésy C (2003) Anthocyanins are efficiently absorbed from the stomach of anesthetized.rats. J Nutr 133: 4178–4182

Talavéra S, Felgines C, Texier O, Besson C, Manach C, Lamaison JL, Rémésy C (2004) Anthocyanins are efficiently absorbed from the small intestine in rats. J Nutr 134:2275–2279

Tanaka T, Kojima T, Suzui M et al (1993a) Chemoprevention of colon carcinogenesis by the natural product of a simple phenolic compound protocatechuic acid: suppressing effects on tumor development and biomarkers expression of colon tumorigenesis. Cancer Res 53:3908–3913

Tanaka T, Kojima T, Kawamori T, Yoshimi N, Mori H (1993b) Chemoprevention of diethylnitrosamine-induced hepatocarcinogenesis by a simple phenolic acid protocatechuic acid in rats. Cancer Res 53:2775–2779

Tanaka T, Kawamori T, Ohnishi M et al (1994) Chemoprevention of 4-nitroquinoline 1-oxide-induced oral carcinogenesis by dietary protocatechuic acid during initiation and postinitiation phases. Cancer Res 54:2359–2365

Timberlake CF (1988) The biological properties of anthocyanins. Nat Assoc Colourers Quart Inf Bull 1:4–15

Torre LC, Barritt BH (1977) Quantative evaluation of *Rubus* fruit anthocyanin pigments. J Food Sci 42:488–490

Tseng T-H, Hsu J-D, Lo M-H et al (1998) Inhibitory effect of Hibiscus protocatechuic acid on tumor promotion in mouse skin. Cancer Lett 126:199–207

Tseng T-H, Kao T-W, Chu C-Y et al (2000) Induction of apoptosis by Hibiscus protocatechuic acid in human leukemia cells via reduction of retinoblastoma (RB) phosphorylation and Bcl-2 expression. Biochem Pharmacol 60:307–315

Tsuda T, Horio F, Osawa T (1999) Absorption and metabolism cyanidin 3-O-β-D-glucoside in rats. FEBS Lett 449:179–182

Vitaglione P, Donnarumma G, Napolitano A et al (2007) Protocatechuic acid is the major human metabolite of cyanidin-glucosides. J Nutr 137:2043–2048

Wang LS, Stoner GD (2008) Anthocyanins and their role in cancer prevention. Cancer Lett 269:281–190

Wang LS, Stoner GD (2009) Anthocyanidins. In: Knasmuller S, DeMarini DM, Johnson IT, Gerhauser C (eds) Chemoprevention of Cancer and DNA damage by dietary factors. Wiley-VCH, Weinheim, Germany

Wang LS, Hecht SS, Carmella SG et al (2009) Anthocyanins in black raspberries prevent esophageal tumors in rats. Cancer Prev Res 2:84–93

Wang LS, Dombkowski AA, Seguin C et al (2011a) Mechanistic basis for the chemopreventive effects of black raspberries at a late stage of rat esophageal carcinogenesis. Mol Carcinog 50:291–300

Wang LS, Arnold M, Huang YW et al (2011b) Modulation of genetic and epigenetic biomarkers of colorectal cancer in humans by black raspberries: a phase I pilot study. Clin Cancer Res 17:598–610

Weisel T, Baum M, Eisenbrand G et al (2006) An anthocyanin/polyphenolic-rich fruit juice reduces oxidative DNA damage and increases glutathione level in healthy probands. Biotechnol J 1:388–397

Wheldale M (1916) The anthocyanin pigments of plants. Cambridge University Press, Cambridge

Wilska-Jeszka J, Bos J, Pawlik M (1992) Wild plant fruits as a source of catechins and proanthocyanidins. In XVIe Journées Internationales Groupe Polyphénols and The Royal Society of Chemistry, Lisbon. DTA, Lisbon, Portugal

Wu X, Pittman H, Hager T, Hager A et al (2009) Phenolic acids in black raspberry and in the gastrointestinal tract of pigs following ingestion of black raspberry. Mol Nutr Food Res 53: S76–S84

Yin M-C, Lin C-C, Wu H-C et al (2009) Apoptotic effects of protocatechuic acid in human breast, lung, liver, cervix, and prostate cancer cells: potential mechanisms of action. J Agric Food Chem 57:6468–6473

Yip E, Chan A, Pang H et al (2006) Protocatechuic acid induces cell death in HepG2 hepatocellular carcinoma cells through a c-Jun N-terminal kinase-dependent mechanism. Cell Biol Toxicol 22:293–302

Zhang Y, Vareed SK, Nair MG (2005) Human tumor cell growth inhibition by nontoxic anthocyanidins, the pigments in fruits and vegetable. Life Sci 76:1465–1472

Zheng Q, Hirose Y, Yoshimi N et al (2002) Further investigation of the modifying effect of various chemopreventive agents on apoptosis and cell proliferation in human colon cancer cells. J Cancer Res Clin Oncol 128:539–546

Zikri NN, Riedl KM, Wang LS et al (2009) Black raspberry components inhibit proliferation, induce apoptosis, and modulate gene expression in rat esophageal epithelial cells. Nutr Cancer 61:816–826

Chapter 12
Slow but Steady Progress in Cancer Chemoprevention with Phenethyl Isothiocyanate: Fulfilled Promises and Translational Challenges

Anna A. Powolny, Ajay Bommareddy, and Shivendra V. Singh

Abstract Population-based observational studies continue to support the premise that intake of certain fruits and vegetables may lower the risk of cancer, and this association is quite persuasive for the cruciferous vegetables. Inverse association between cruciferous vegetable intake and the risk of cancer has been noted for different types of malignancies, including stomach, prostate, lung, breast, colon, and bladder cancers. Epidemiological observations in "FOLKS" have undoubtedly sparked interest among cancer biologists to conduct "FLASK"-based bench investigations to identify bioactive anticancer compounds from cruciferous vegetables as well as to determine their efficacy through "FUR"-based preclinical research in rodents. Cancer protective effect of cruciferous vegetables is partly attributed to organic isothiocyanates (ITC) with an $-N=C=S$ functional group. Elucidation of the mechanism by which ITCs impart protection against cancer has been the topic of intense research in the past few decades. This article reviews bench-cage-bedside evidence supporting cancer chemopreventive potential of one such ITC compound, phenethyl isothiocyanate (PEITC). Future directions and challenges in clinical translation for PEITC are also highlighted.

Abbreviations

4E-BP1	eIF4E binding protein
AR	androgen receptor
AUC	area under the curve
BP	benzo[*a*]pyrene
Cdk	cyclin-dependent kinase
C_{max}	maximal achievable concentration
CYP	cytochrome P450

S.V. Singh (✉)
Department of Pharmacology and Chemical Biology, University of Pittsburgh School of Medicine, University of Pittsburgh Cancer Institute, Pittsburgh, PA, USA
e-mail: singhs@upmc.edu

F.H. Sarkar (ed.), *Nutraceuticals and Cancer*, DOI 10.1007/978-94-007-2630-7_12,

eIF4E	eukaryotic translation initiation factor 4E
ER	estrogen receptor
ERK	extracellular signal-regulated kinase
GST	glutathione *S*-transferase
ITCs	isothiocyanates
JNK	c-Jun N-terminal kinase
MAPK	mitogen-activated protein kinase
MMP	matrix metalloproteinase
NAC	*N*-acetylcysteine
NF-κB	nuclear factor-κB
NNK	4-(methylnitrosamino)-1-(3-pyridyl)-1-butanone
Nrf2	NF-E2 related factor-2
PEITC	phenethyl isothiocyanate
QR	NAD(P)H:quinone oxidoreductase
ROS	reactive oxygen species
T_{max}	time to reach C_{max}
TRAMP	*tr*ansgenic *a*denocarcinoma of *m*ouse *p*rostate

12.1 Introduction

Cancer chemoprevention is a relatively new but rapidly emerging sub-discipline in oncology and signifies the use of natural (i.e., dietary constituents) or synthetic agents to prevent or delay the process of carcinogenesis (Sporn 1980, 2011). Evidence continues to mount to suggest that a diet rich in fruits and vegetables may be protective against cancer, and this association is quite credible for cruciferous vegetables (Verhoeven et al. 1996; Kolonel et al. 2000; Greenwald et al. 2001). Cruciferous vegetables commonly consumed by humans include broccoli, watercress, kale, cabbage, bok choy, collard greens, and horseradish. Increased consumption of cruciferous vegetables is inversely associated with the risk of different types of malignancies, including cancer of the stomach (Chyou et al. 1990), ovary (Pan et al. 2004), lung (Kvale et al. 1983; Steinmetz et al. 1993), prostate (Kolonel et al. 2000; Kirsh et al. 2007; Giovannucci et al. 2003), bladder (Michaud et al. 1999), non-Hodgkin's lymphoma (Zhang et al. 2000; Kelemen et al. 2008), and colon (Hara et al. 2003; Moy et al. 2008). Cancer protective effect of cruciferous vegetables is partly credited to isothiocyanates (ITCs), which occur naturally as thioglucoside conjugates (Hecht 2000; Cheung and Kong 2009). While many naturally-occurring ITCs have now been identified in plants (Fahey et al. 2001), evidence supporting chemopreventive effect is convincing only for a handful of compounds, including phenethyl isothiocyanate (PEITC) (Hecht 2000; Cheung and Kong 2009). This article highlights progress towards cancer chemoprevention by PEITC.

In cruciferous vegetables, PEITC is stored as a thioglucoside conjugate commonly known as gluconasturtiin (Fahey et al. 2001) (Fig. 12.1). Watercress is a rich

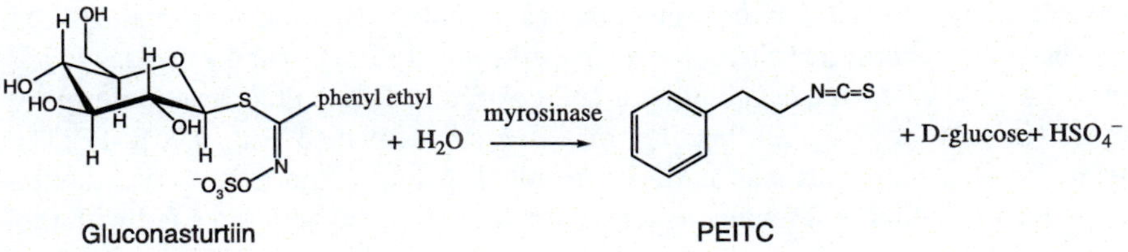

Fig. 12.1 Structure of phenethyl isothiocyanate (PEITC)

source of gluconasturtiin. Notably, glucosinolate content in the cruciferous plants varies depending on the species, climate, and soil upon which they grow (Kushad et al. 1999; Ciska et al. 2000). Tissue damage resulting from cutting or chewing of the cruciferous vegetables releases an enzyme (myrosinases), which is responsible for conversion of gluconasturtiin to PEITC (Hecht 2000; Fahey et al. 2001). Gluconasturtiin can also be converted to PEITC in the gut by intestinal microflora (Fahey et al. 2001).

12.2 In Vivo Evidence for Cancer Chemopreventive Effect of PEITC

12.2.1 Inhibition of Chemically-Induced Cancer in Rodents

PEITC has been shown to inhibit cancer in experimental rodents induced by a variety of chemicals (extensively reviewed in Hecht 2000). Cancer chemopreventive potential of PEITC was initially recognized by Wattenberg (Wattenberg 1977), who showed that PEITC administration 4 h before challenge with 7,12-dimethylbenz[a]anthracene inhibited mammary cancer development in female Sprague-Dawley rats. Addition of PEITC to a diet containing 7,12-dimethylbenz[a]anthracene inhibited neoplasm of the forestomach and pulmonary adenoma in female ICR/Ha mice (Wattenberg 1977). F344 rats fed diets containing 3 and 6 μmol PEITC/g diet, before as well as during treatment with the carcinogen *N*-nitrosobenzylmethylamine, developed 99–100% fewer esophageal tumors compared with rats on control diet (Stoner et al. 1991). Inhibitory effect of PEITC was observed on both preneoplastic (acanthosis and hyperkeratosis, leukoplakia, and leukokeratosis) and neoplastic lesions (papilloma and carcinoma) (Stoner et al. 1991). Lung tumorigenesis induced by the tobacco-derived carcinogen 4-(methylnitrosamino)-1-(3-pyridyl)-1-butanone (NNK) in male F344 rats was inhibited significantly by dietary administration of PEITC [8 mmol PEITC/kg diet (1304 ppm) and 4 mmol PEITC/kg diet (652 ppm)] for 22 weeks (1 week before to 1 week after the NNK treatment) (Chung et al. 1996). NNK-induced lung tumorigenesis in A/J mice was inhibited by *N*-acetylcysteine (NAC) conjugate of PEITC, which is the primary metabolic byproduct of PEITC excreted in urine (Jiao et al. 1997). Gavage of PEITC, three times/week for 8 weeks, inhibited azoxymethane-induced colonic aberrant crypt foci in F344 rats providing important laboratory evidence for a potential role of PEITC in the protection against colon cancer (Chung et al. 2000). Another study determined chemopreventive efficacy of PEITC using a mouse model involving azoxymethane as an initiator and dextran sodium sulfate as a tumor promoter (Cheung et al. 2010). Feeding of a diet supplemented with 0.05% PEITC before or after azoxymethane initiation resulted in lower tumor incidence, lower colon tumor multiplicities and smaller polyps, as compared with mice fed with the basal diet (Cheung et al. 2010). Adenoma growth inhibition by PEITC was associated with an increase in apoptosis (cleavage of caspase-3 and-7) and cell cycle arrest (induction of p21) (Cheung et al. 2010). To the contrary, Plate and Gallaher (Plate and Gallaher 2006) failed to observe PEITC-mediated prevention of aberrant crypt foci in F344 rats. Reasons for the discrepancy in results between these studies are unclear (Chung et al. 2000; Plate and Gallaher, 2006; Cheung et al. 2010). Yang and colleagues (Yang et al. 2002) showed inhibition of benzo(a)pyrene (BP)-induced lung tumorigenesis in A/J mice by dietary NAC conjugate of PEITC administered during the post-initiation phase that was associated with induction of mitogen-activated protein kinases (MAPK) and p53, and apoptosis. Malignant progression of lung adenoma in mice induced by a combination of BP and NNK was inhibited by PEITC and its NAC conjugate (Conaway et al. 2005). PEITC administration was shown to suppress *N*-nitrosomethylbenzylamine-induced cancer in hamster buccal pouch (Solt et al. 2003). Induction of preneoplastic lung lesions (alveolar hyperplasia and alveolar atypical dysplasia) in Wistar rats by a single intratracheal instillation of NNK was inhibited by PEITC in association with a decrease in NNK-induced cyclooxygenase-2 expression and suppression of proliferating cell nuclear antigen expression (Ye et al. 2007). In conclusion, these studies indicate that PEITC has protective effect against cancer in rodents induced by structurally diverse chemicals.

At the same time, a few studies suggest that PEITC may promote carcinogenesis. For example, PEITC administration in the diet (7 days prior to carcinogen treatment and then continuously throughout the duration of the bioassay) was shown to increase multiplicity of dimethylbenzanthracene-induced mammary cancer in rats (Lubet et al. 1997). PEITC has also been shown to promote bladder cancer in rodents (Ogawa et al. 1998, 2001; Hirose et al. 1998; Sugiura et al. 2003; Akagi et al. 2003; Takagi et al. 2005). Ogawa et al. (1998) reported that even though PEITC inhibited carcinogenesis at the initiation stage it promoted cancer when administered during the post-initiation phase. Further studies from this group showed that PEITC induced papillary or nodular hyperplasia, dysplasia, and transitional cell carcinomas in a dose dependent manner (Ogawa et al. 2001), but only after initiation with diethylnitrosamine and N-butyl-N-(4-hydroxybutyl) nitrosamine. However, whether PEITC alone acts as a carcinogen in the urinary bladder is unclear and controversial. Some studies suggested that PEITC promoted proliferation in normal looking epithelium and resulted in increased frequency of mutations in p53 in the treated animals, which ultimately led to irreversible dysplasia (Sugiura et al. 2003). Other studies indicated that PEITC treatment had only limited potential to initiate abnormal growth and did not effectively induce irreversible lesions in urinary bladder (Takagi et al. 2005). Clearly, further investigation is needed to resolve this issue.

12.2.2 Suppression of Spontaneous Cancer Development in Transgenic Mice

More recent studies have utilized transgenic mouse models to confirm chemopreventive efficacy of PEITC. For example, the $Apc^{Min/+}$ mice fed a diet supplemented with 0.05% PEITC for 3 weeks developed significantly less (31.7% reduction) and smaller polyps than those fed basal diet (Khor et al. 2008). PEITC-mediated polyp prevention in $Apc^{Min/+}$ mice was associated with an increase in apoptotic markers and p21 expression (Khor et al. 2008). Dietary feeding of 8 mmol PEITC/kg diet to polyoma middle-T antigen transgenic mice resulted in smaller mammary cancer lesions, although there was no effect on lung metastasis or survival (McCune et al. 2010). Feeding of a diet supplemented with 0.05% PEITC alone or 0.025% PEITC in combination with 1% curcumin, a constituent of turmeric, significantly decreased incidence of prostate tumor formation in Transgenic Adenocarcinoma of Mouse Prostate (TRAMP) mice (Barve et al. 2008). Immunohistochemistry revealed that significant inhibition of high-grade prostatic intraepithelial neoplasia by PEITC administration was associated with decreased proliferation and increased apoptotic index (Barve et al. 2008). Administration of 3 μmol PEITC/g diet decreased incidence as well as burden (affected area) of poorly differentiated tumors in the dorsolateral prostate of TRAMP mice, which was associated with induction of autophagy and overexpression of E-cadherin (Powolny et al. 2011). Most exciting discovery from this study was identification of plasma biomarkers potentially useful in future clinical trials to assess PEITC response. Two-dimensional gel electrophoresis followed by mass spectrometry revealed distinct changes in expression of several proteins in the plasma of representative PEITC-treated TRAMP mice compared with that of control mice (Powolny et al. 2011). Non-abundant proteins up-regulated in the plasma by dietary feeding of PEITC included alpha-fetoprotein, transferrin, actin filament associated protein 1-like 2, and apolipoprotein A-I (isoform CRA_b) (Powolny et al. 2011). Downregulated proteins in the plasma of PEITC-fed TRAMP mice in comparison with control included chain A, crystal structure of mouse transthyretin, plasminogen, isoform CRA_e, and clusterin (Powolny et al. 2011). One of these protein expression changes (clusterin) was verified using larger number of plasma specimens (Powolny et al. 2011). Clusterin (also known as apolipoprotein J and testosterone-repressed prostate message-2) is a highly conserved protein expressed in a variety of tissues, secreted in blood, and involved in regulation of apoptosis, cell adhesion, cell cycle regulation, and DNA repair (Shannan et al. 2006; Miyake et al. 2006). Increased levels of clusterin have been reported in several malignancies including breast, colon, lung, and prostate cancer (Shannan et al. 2006). Moreover, expression of clusterin was shown to correlates with Gleason score but not with prognosis in prostate cancer patients undergoing radical prostatectomy without neoadjuvant hormonal therapy (Miyake et al. 2006). These findings also underscore value of proteomics tool for discovery of biomarkers to assess response to potential chemopreventive agents. Discovery of biomarkers of response is highly desirable especially for cancer chemopreventive agents because cancer incidence is too rigorous of an end point for epithelial cancers with long latency.

12.2.3 Inhibition of Cancer Xenograft Growth

Efficacy of PEITC against in vivo cancer growth has also been determined using xenograft models. For example, growth of a cell line derived from spontaneously developing prostate tumor of a TRAMP mouse (TRAMP-C1 cells) subcutaneously implanted in male athymic mice was inhibited significantly by oral feeding of 9 and 12 μmol PEITC five times/week (Xiao et al. 2005b). Fifty days after starting therapy, the average tumor volume in control mice (567 ± 184 mm^3) was ~3-3.5-fold higher compared with mice receiving PEITC, reflecting a 67–71% reduction in tumor volume (Xiao et al. 2005b). Tumors from PEITC-treated mice, harvested at the termination of the experiment, exhibited significantly higher count of apoptotic bodies compared with tumors from control mice (Xiao et al. 2005b). A similar treatment regimen involving 12 μmol PEITC effectively inhibited growth of subcutaneously implanted PC-3 human prostate cancer cells in male athymic mice (Xiao et al. 2006). Body weights of the control and PEITC-treated mice did not differ significantly in both TRAMP-C1 and PC-3 xenograft studies (Xiao et al. 2005b, 2006). Dietary administration of NAC conjugate of PEITC (8 μmol PEITC-NAC/g diet) showed a significant reduction in subcutaneously implanted PC-3 tumor size in 100% of the mice during the 9-week treatment period in association with decreased mitosis and proliferation (Chiao et al. 2004). Growth inhibitory effect of dietary PEITC-NAC against PC-3 xenografts was accompanied by (a) increased apoptotic rate, (b) cleavage of poly-(ADP-ribose) polymerase, (c) upregulation of cyclin-dependent kinase inhibitors $p21^{WAF\text{-}1/Cip\text{-}1}$ and $p27^{Kip1}$, and (d) reduced expression of cyclin D and E, and phosphorylated retinoblastoma tumor suppressor (Chiao et al. 2004). Survival of nude mice inoculated intraperitoneally with T72Ras (*H-Ras*^{V12}-transformed) ovarian epithelial cells was increased by about 90% by intraperitoneal PEITC treatment (50 mg PEITC/kg, five times per week) (Trachootham et al. 2006). Together, these studies indicate that, in addition to prevention of chemically-induced or spontaneous carcinogenesis, PEITC effectively inhibits growth of xenografted cancer cells.

12.2.4 Inhibition of Angiogenesis and Metastasis

First clue for anti-angiogenic activity of PEITC came from a study showing inhibition of nuclear factor κB (NF-κB)-regulated expression of vascular endothelial growth factor, a well known pro-angiogenic factor, in prostate cancer cells (Xu et al. 2005). Since then several other groups have investigated the effect of PEITC treatment on angiogenesis. PEITC treatment was shown to reduce expression of vascular endothelial growth factor and inhibit capillary-like tube structures (a measure of neoangiogenesis) and migration in human umbilical vain endothelial cells (Xiao and Singh 2007). Furthermore, PEITC treatment inhibited angiogenesis ex vivo, as revealed by chicken egg chorioallantoic membrane assay (Xiao and Singh 2007). PEITC is an effective inhibitor of hypoxia inducible factor, which is a transcription factor that plays an important role in expression of pro-angiogenic factors (Wang et al. 2009). PEITC-mediated inhibition of cancer cell migration and invasion, and metastasis has also been documented (Hwang and Lee 2006; Wu et al. 2010; Yang et al. 2010; Lai et al. 2010). In gastric cancer AGS cells, PEITC-mediated inhibition of cell migration and invasion was accompanied by downregulation of urokinase-type plasminogen activator, matrix metalloproteinase (MMP)-2 and MMP-9 (Yang et al. 2010). Suppression of MMP-2 and MMP-9 along with inhibition of multiple signal transduction pathways, including MAPK, Akt, and protein kinase C was also observed in HT-29 human colon cancer cells that were susceptible to inhibition of cell migration and invasion by PEITC (Lai et al. 2010). PEITC-mediated prevention of prostate carcinogenesis in TRAMP mice was associated with a slight decrease in angiogenesis as judged by CD31 immunohistochemistry but the difference between control and PEITC groups was not significant (Powolny et al. 2011). Anti-angiogenic effects of dietary isothiocyanates, including PEITC, have been reviewed by Cavell et al. (2011).

Because angiogenesis plays an important role in metastasis, a previous study from our group determined the effect of PEITC administration on incidence and multiplicity of pulmonary metastasis in TRAMP model (Powolny et al. 2011). Overall incidence of pulmonary metastasis did not differ between the control and PEITC-treated TRAMP mice (Powolny et al. 2011). However, the number of lung metastasis per mouse in the mice fed the 3 μmol PEITC/g diet was 38.37% lower than that in mice fed the control diet. In addition, the area occupied by the pulmonary metastasis was generally smaller in PEITC-fed TRAMP mice compared with control, reflected by an approximate 60% reduction in mean pulmonary metastasis area (Powolny et al. 2011). Further work in other animal models is necessary for a full appreciation of anti-angiogenic and anti-metastatic efficacy of PEITC.

12.3 Bioavailability and Pharmacokinetics

Morris and co-workers have thoroughly studied pharmacokinetic parameters and bioavailability of PEITC using male Sprague-Dawley rats after intravenous dosing with PEITC (2, 10, 100, or 400 μmol/kg) or oral PEITC administration (10 or 100 μmol/kg) (Ji et al. 2005). With intravenous 2 μmol PEITC/kg, area under the curve (AUC) and $t_{1/2}$ values respectively were 2.96 ± 0.78 μM·h, and 3.52 ± 0.35 h (Ji et al. 2005). The AUC increased in a greater than proportional manner to 17.3 ± 9.3, 322 ± 149, and 807 ± 66.9 μM·h with intravenous 10, 100, and 400 μmol/kg PEITC respectively (Ji et al. 2005). Peak plasma concentration (C_{max}) was found to be 9.2 ± 0.6 and 42.1 ± 11.4 μM after oral doses of 10 and 100 μmol PEITC/kg, respectively. The AUC values obtained after intravenous and oral administration of 10- and 100-μmol PEITC/kg were not significantly different, which suggested that the oral bioavailability was close to 1 (Ji et al. 2005). Interestingly, modulation of pharmacokinetic behavior of PEITC upon repeated oral administration has been shown in rats (Konsue et al. 2010). Plasma levels of PEITC were determined in rats following oral treatment with 0.5, 1, and 5 mg PEITC/kg (Konsue et al. 2010).

Absolute bioavailability of PEITC was estimated to be about 77% (Konsue et al. 2010). Dose-associated decrease in bioavailability but modest increase in clearance was also observed. The C_{max} value did not rise proportionately to the PEITC dose (Konsue et al. 2010). At 1 and 5 mg PEITC/kg, repeated administration resulted in higher plasma C_{max} for PEITC (Konsue et al. 2010). In a human study involving three volunteers, the C_{max} value ranged between 0.64–1.40 μM after a single dose of 40 mg pure PEITC (Liebes et al. 2001). Time to reach C_{max} (T_{max}) for the three subjects was 3.1-, 5.5- and 5.2 h, whereas AUC (μM·h) was 7.76, 10.5, and 13.3 (Liebes et al. 2001). Data on tissue uptake of PEITC is limited, but we have shown recently that PEITC is detectable in the plasma (1.45 μM) as well as prostate (1138 nmol/kg tissue weight) of TRAMP mice fed 3 μmol PEITC/g diet (Powolny et al. 2011). Further work is necessary to determine uptake of PEITC in other tissues after oral or dietary administration.

12.4 Cancer Chemotherapy Sensitization

Evidence also exists to suggest that PEITC can sensitize cancer cells to chemotherapy drugs. Sub-lethal doses of PEITC sensitized Fas-resistant T24 bladder carcinoma cell line and Bcl-2 overexpressing Jurkat T cells to Fas-mediated apoptosis (Pullar et al. 2004). PEITC inhibited P-glycoprotein and multidrug-resistance protein 1-mediated efflux of daunomycin, which is a major mechanism of resistance for some anticancer agents (Tseng et al. 2002; Hu and Morris 2004). PEITC and/or its glutathione conjugates were suggested to be substrates for multidrug-resistance protein 1, but not P-glycoprotein (Hu and Morris 2004). Downregulation of protein kinase C and inhibition of telomerase activity were implicated in PEITC-mediated sensitization of PC-3 prostate cancer cells and HeLa cervical cancer cells to adriamycin and etoposide-induced apoptosis (Mukherjee et al. 2009a, b). PEITC sensitized non-small cell lung cancer cell line NCI-H596 to cisplatin independent of cellular platinum accumulation or DNA platination (Di Pasqua et al. 2010). Pharmacologic concentrations of PEITC augmented Docetaxel-induced apoptosis in PC-3 and DU145 cells in association with suppression of Bcl-2 and XIAP protein levels and induction of multidomain proapoptotic Bcl-2 family members Bax and Bak (Xiao and Singh 2010a). PEITC-Docetaxel combination was markedly more efficacious against PC-3 xenograft in vivo compared with PEITC or Docetaxel alone (Xiao and Singh 2010a). Furthermore, significantly higher count of apoptotic bodies was also observed in tumor sections from mice treated with the PEITC-Docetaxel combination in comparison with PEITC or Docetaxel alone (Xiao and Singh 2010a). PEITC-mediated reversal of resistance to histone deacetylase inhibitor vorinostat in leukemia cell lines and primary leukemia cells has been reported (Hu et al. 2010).

12.5 Human Studies with Watercress as a Source of PEITC

Human trials to determine biological effects of pure PEITC are still lacking. However, a few studies have attempted to determine the effect of watercress consumption as a source of PEITC on certain biological parameters. Consumption of 2 ounce (56.8 g) of watercress at each meal for 3 days inhibited oxidative metabolism of NNK in smokers ($n = 11$) (Hecht et al. 1995). In another study, effect of 85 g watercress consumption/day for 8 weeks ($n = 60$) on gene expression and enzymatic activity of glutathione peroxidase 1 and superoxide dismutase 2 was determined (Hofmann et al. 2009). Watercress intervention had no significant effect on gene expression or enzymatic activity of either glutathione peroxidase 1 or superoxide dismutase 2 due to high inter-individual variability (Hofmann et al. 2009).

We have shown previously that PEITC treatment inhibits phosphorylation of translation regulator 4E binding protein 4E-BP1 (Hu et al. 2007). Recently, in vivo significance of these observations was tested using peripheral blood mononuclear cells from subjects after ingestion of 80 g watercress (Syed Alwi et al. 2010). Phosphorylation of 4E-BP1 was significantly reduced 6 and 8 h after watercress ingestion in peripheral blood cells from four participants (Syed Alwi et al. 2010).

Stable reaction products with albumin and hemoglobin as biomarkers to monitor ITC exposure in humans have also been identified (Kumar and Sabbioni 2010; Kumar et al. 2010). Blood samples collected from one subject 1 day after ingestion of garden cress (60 g), watercress (100 g), and broccoli (300 g) revealed presence of PEITC-lysine adducts in both albumin and hemoglobin (Kumar and Sabbioni 2010). However, PEITC-lysine adducts were approximately 50 times lower in the hemoglobin than in albumin (Kumar and Sabbioni 2010). These results suggest that albumin-lysine adducts may be a sensitive biomarker to monitor ITC exposure (Kumar and Sabbioni 2010).

12.6 Molecular Insights into Cancer Chemopreventive Effects of PEITC

12.6.1 Alteration of Carcinogen Metabolism

Majority of carcinogens require cytochrome P450-dependent (Phase I) activation to exert their neoplastic effects (Guengerich 2000). At the same time, Phase II enzymes, including glutathione *S*-transferase (GST) and NAD(P)H:quinone oxidoreductase (QR), play an important role in detoxification of activated carcinogenic intermediates (Hayes and Pulford 1995). A large body of literature clearly demonstrates that ITCs can inhibit carcinogen activation due to inhibition of cytochrome P450 (CYP) as well as induction of Phase II enzymes. Alteration of carcinogen metabolism as a mechanism for chemopreventive response to PEITC has been reviewed extensively (Hecht 2000; Smith 2001; Keum et al. 2004). PEITC is capable of inhibiting the activation of carcinogenic nitrosamines including NNK

(Morse et al. 1991; Guo et al. 1992), *N*-nitrosodimethylamine (Ishizaki et al. 1990), and *N*-nitrosomethylbenzylamine (Stoner et al. 1991). Using a human CYP1A2 reconstituted system, PEITC was shown to decrease activity of methoxyresorufin *O*-dealkylase (a marker of CYP1A2 activity) with an IC_{50} of 340 nM (Smith et al. 1996). Activity of ethoxyresorufin *O*-deethylase was decreased in liver microsome of rodents treated with PEITC (Guo et al. 1992). Using microsome from baculovirus infected cells expressing human CYP isoforms, PEITC was shown to competitively inhibited CYP1A2, 2A6 and other isoforms (Nakajima et al. 2001). Natural and synthetic ITCs and their conjugates were examined for their effect on rat and human microsomal *N*-dimethylnitrosamine demethylase activity (Jiao et al. 1996). PEITC exhibited significant inhibition towards rat liver activity with an IC_{50} of 8.3 μM (Jiao et al. 1996). Glutathione and L-cysteine conjugates of PEITC were more potent inhibitors of *N*-dimethylnitrosamine demethylase activity in rat as well as human liver than NAC conjugate (Jiao et al. 1996). A recent study also showed that PEITC can antagonize the carcinogenicity of chemicals such as heterocyclic amines and polycyclic aromatic hydrocarbons which rely on the CYP1 family for their bioactivation (Konsue and Ioannides 2008). On the other hand, some reports provide contradicting results; for example, in one study using human primary hepatocytes, it was shown that PEITC dose-dependently up-regulated the expression levels of carcinogen activating enzymes CYP1A1 and CYP1A2 (Gross-Steinmeyer et al. 2004).

Induction of Phase II enzymes by PEITC has been well-documented both in vitro and in vivo. The effects of PEITC on Phase II enzymes are dose-dependent and tissue-specific with liver being most sensitive organ and lung generally resistant (Konsue and Ioannides 2008). An idea has also been floated that increased detoxification of carcinogens rather than cytochrome P450 inhibition may be the primary mechanism for chemopreventive activity of PEITC (Konsue and Ioannides 2008; Konsue and Ioannides 2010). PEITC was shown to activate antioxidant response element-mediated induction of Phase II enzymes *via* NF-E2 related factor-2 (Nrf2) and c-Jun N-terminal kinase1 (JNK1) pathways, and JNK acted as an upstream regulator of Nrf2 (Keum et al. 2003). In mouse skin papilloma PE cells, significant elevations of glutathione content, QR and GST activity induced by PEITC treatment were reported (Ye and Zhang 2001). Employing an oligonucleotide microarray approach, Hu et al. (2006) showed that PEITC treatment resulted in the induction of various GST isozymes. Collectively, these results suggest that ITCs function to prevent chemically-induced cancers not only by blocking carcinogen activation but also by increasing detoxification of activated carcinogenic intermediates.

Cellular uptake of ITCs, including PEITC, was demonstrated to occur predominantly, if not entirely, through conjugation to glutathione, and cellular GST promoted ITC uptake by augmenting the conjugation reaction (Zhang 2001). Role of glutathione in cytotoxicity of PEITC was studied further using human leukemia cells (Xu and Thornalley 2001a). Cysteinyl thiol group of glutathione was found to be an important site of thiocarbamoylation by PEITC (Xu and Thornalley 2001a).

More recently, the effect of PEITC administration on global gene expression has been investigated using microarray technology. *N*-nitrosomethylbenzylamine-induced changes in gene expression in rat esophagus were positively modulated to normal levels of expression by PEITC administration (Stoner et al. 2008). Effect of oral administration of PEITC for 7 days on the hepatic expression of genes important in drug metabolism and toxicity was studied using Sprague Dawley rats (Telang and Morris 2010). PEITC administration was found to significantly up-regulate UDP-glucuronosyltransferase 1A6 and strongly down-regulate nicotinamide N-methyltransferase (Telang and Morris 2010). Other significantly up-regulated genes included CYP2b15, the anti-apoptotic gene Bcl2l2, and the stress regulators Gadd45b, Dnajb9, Dnajb5 and Hspb1 (Telang and Morris 2010). Effect of dietary PEITC on environmental cigarette smoke-induced (neonatal mice were exposed to environmental cigarette smoke immediately after birth and for 2 weeks after weaning) alteration in expression of 576 miRNAs were evaluated by miRNA microarray in liver and lung (Izzotti et al. 2010b). Environmental cigarette smoke downregulated the expression of a number of miRNAs in lung, but mixed alterations were seen in the liver (Izzotti et al. 2010b). PEITC was shown to protect the lung from the environmental cigarette smoke-induced alterations of miRNA expression but exhibited some adverse effects in the liver (Izzotti et al. 2010b). However, physiological significance of these observations is unclear. In a follow-up study, it was shown that the main functions altered by environmental cigarette smoke and modulated by PEITC treatment included cell proliferation, apoptosis, differentiation, Ras activation, p53 functions, NF-κB pathway, transforming growth factor-related stress response, and angiogenesis (Izzotti et al. 2010a). Some miRNA known to be polymorphic in humans and downregulated by the environmental cigarette smoke were protected by PEITC (Izzotti et al. 2010a). Overall implication of these studies is that miRNA profiling may be a valuable tool for predicting safety and efficacy of cancer chemopreventive agents such as PEITC.

12.6.2 Inhibition of Cell Cycle Progression

Cell cycle progression is governed by cyclin-dependent kinases (Cdk) and their inhibitors, cip/kip family and INK4a/ARF (Nigg 1995). Hasegawa et al. (1993) were the first to report G2/M phase cell cycle arrest in HeLa cells upon treatment with 2.5–10 μM PEITC. With an exception of a few reports, most studies have shown G2/M phase cell cycle arrest in cancer cells upon treatment with PEITC (Xiao et al. 2004; Visanji et al. 2004; Jakubíková et al. 2005; Yin et al. 2009; Mi et al. 2010a; Hwang and Lee 2010; Wu et al. 2011). Molecular alterations associated with PEITC-mediated cell cycle arrest in cancer cells are summarized in Table 12.1. In HepG2 cells, PEITC-mediated G2/M phase cell cycle arrest was associated with a decrease in level of Cdk1 protein (also known as $p34^{cdc2}$) but induction of cyclin B1 protein expression (Rose et al. 2003). PEITC-mediated G2/M phase cell cycle arrest in PC-3 human prostate cancer cells correlated with reduction in Cdk1 and Cdc25C protein levels, leading to accumulation of Tyr^{15} phosphorylated (inactive) Cdk1

Table 12.1 Phenethyl isothiocyanate (PEITC)-mediated cell cycle arrest and associated molecular changes in cancer cells

Tumor type	Cell line	Arrest	Molecular changes	Reference
Liver	HepG2	G2/M	↑cyclin B1, ↓Cdk1	Rose et al. (2003)
Prostate	PC-3	G2/M	↓Cdk1, ↓Cdc25C, ↑pCdk1	Xiao et al. (2004)
Bladder	UM-UC-3, T24	S or G2/M	↓cyclin B1, ↓Cdk1, ↓cyclin A	Tang and Zhang (2004)
Colon	Caco-2	G2/M	↑pChk2, ↑p21	Visanji et al. (2004)
Colon	Caco-2	S, G1 or G2/M	Cell cycle arrest varied based on PEITC dose and treatment time, ↑pERK1/2	Jakubíková et al. (2005)
Prostate	LNCaP	G1	↑p21, ↑p27, ↓HDACs, ↓c-Myc	Wang et al. (2008)
Colon	HT-29	G1 arrest	↓cyclin A, ↓cyclin D, ↓cyclin E, ↓pRb ↑pp38 MAPK-attenuation of cell cycle arrest by p38 MAPK inhibitor	Cheung et al. (2008)
Lung	A549	G2/M	Disruption of microtubule polymerization covalent modification of cysteines in tubulin	Mi et al. (2008)
Prostate	DU145, LNCaP, PC-3, C4-2B	G2/M	↓α- and β-tubulin	Yin et al. (2009)
Prostate	LNCaP	G2/M	↓Cdk1, ↓cyclin B1	Hwang and Lee (2010)
Multiple myeloma	U266, RPMI-8226	G2/M	Inhibition of proteasome (20S and 26S)	Mi et al. (2010a)
Osteosarcoma	U-2OS	S or G2/M	↓cyclin A, ↓cyclin B1, ↑p53, ↑Chk1	Wu et al. (2011)

Cdk1 cyclin-dependent kinase 1, *Cdc25C* cell division cycle 25C, *pCdk1* phospho-Cdk1, *pChk2* phospho-checkpoint kinase 2, *pERK* phospho-extracellular signal-regulated kinase 1/2, *HDACs* histone deacetylases, *pRB* phospho-retinoblastoma, *MAPK* mitogen-activated protein kinase, *Chk1* checkpoint kinase 1

(Xiao et al. 2004). PEITC-mediated cell cycle arrest and downregulation of Cdk1 and Cdc25C were significantly attenuated in the presence of lactacystin suggesting that these proteins were degraded by the proteasome (Xiao et al. 2004). Reduction of α- and β-tubulin protein levels and G2/M phase cell cycle arrest was shown in a panel of human prostate cancer cells, including LNCaP (an androgen responsive cell line with wild-type p53) and PC-3 cells (an androgen-independent cell line lacking functional p53) (Yin et al. 2009). These results indicated that PEITC-mediated G2/M phase cell cycle arrest was not influenced by the androgen-responsiveness or the p53 status. In human bladder cancer cells, PEITC treatment resulted in cell cycle arrest at the G2/M and S phases coupled with downregulation of Cdk1 and cyclin A (Tang and Zhang 2004). PEITC-mediated G2/M phase arrest in Caco-2 cells was associated with increased phosphorylation of checkpoint kinase 2 and induction of Cdk1 inhibitor p21 (Visanji et al. 2004). Interestingly, PEITC treatment induced G1 phase cell cycle arrest in HT-29 human colon cancer cells, which was accompanied by downregulation of cyclin A, D, and E and reduced phosphorylation of retinoblastoma tumor suppressor (Cheung et al. 2008). PEITC-mediated cell cycle arrest and downregulation of cyclin A and D were attenuated by pharmacological inhibition of p38 MAPK (Cheung et al. 2008). Similarly, treatment of LNCaP cells with PEITC resulted in a concentration-dependent enrichment of G1 phase cells in association with induction of Cdk1 inhibitors p21 and p27 (Wang et al. 2008). Collectively, these results indicate that while G2/M phase cell cycle arrest is a more frequent cellular response to PEITC treatment in cancer cells, some cells are arrested in G1 phase. Biochemical basis for these discrepancies remains elusive.

12.6.3 Induction of Apoptosis

Two major cell destruction processes, apoptosis and autophagy, are extensively investigated for their potential benefits in cancer treatment. Notably, PEITC treatment induces both these cell death processes. Research over the past decade reveals that the molecular circuitry of PEITC-induced apoptosis is complex and utilizes a wide range of molecular mechanisms in order to promote apoptosis, including alterations in Bcl-2 family proteins, activation of MAPK, suppression of oncogenic signaling pathways, and activation of caspases (Table 12.2). Kong and colleagues (Yu et al. 1998) were the first to show apoptosis induction by PEITC in HeLa cells. During the same time period, Huang and colleagues (Huang et al. 1998) used mouse embryonic fibroblasts to demonstrate a critical role of p53 tumor suppressor in regulation of PEITC-induced apoptosis. This association was found to be unique to the mouse embryonic fibroblasts because PEITC treatment resulted in apoptosis induction in p53-deficient cancer cells (Xiao and Singh 2002). It is intriguing to note that PEITC treatment selectively depletes mutant p53, but not the wild-type p53, *via* a transcription-independent mechanism (Wang et al. 2011). Direct p53 binding followed by conformational change is implicated in PEITC-mediated depletion of mutant p53 (Wang et al. 2011). However, further studies

Table 12.2 Molecular changes in phenethyl isothiocyanate (PEITC)-induced apoptosis in cancer cells

Tumor type/cell line	PEITC conc.	Molecular changes	Functional studies1	Reference
Leukemia				
Jurkat	5–25 μM	↑pJNK	Attenuation of apoptosis by overexpression of dominant negative JNK1 and Bcl-2 or Bcl-xL	Chen et al. (1998)
HL60	10 μM	↑Bid cleavage, ↑pJNK	Attenuation of JNK activation by exogenous glutathione	Xu and Thornalley (2001b)
Jurkat	up to 60 μM	↓Bcl-xL	Bcl-2 and Bcl-xL overexpression did not protect against PEITC-induced apoptosis	Cuddihy et al. (2008)
Liver				
HepG2	5–20 μM	↑superoxide	No effect of antioxidants on apoptosis	Rose et al. (2003)
PLC/PRF/5	5 μM	↑p53, ↓XIAP, ↑Apaf-1 ↑Bid/t-Bid, ↑Bax, ↓Bcl-2, ↓Bcl-xL, ↓Mcl-1	Protection of apoptosis by antioxidants NAC and vitamin E	Wu et al. (2005)
HepG2	20 μM	↓complex III and IV, ↓O_2 consumption ↑Bax activation	No effect of mitochondrial permeability transition inhibitors on apoptosis	Rose et al. (2005)
Colon				
HT-29	5–100 μM	↑pJNK, ↑pERK, ↑pp38 MAPK	Attenuation of cytochrome c release and caspase-3 activation by JNK inhibitor	Hu et al. (2003)
Prostate				
LNCaP, PC-3 DU145, Tsu-Pr1	20 μM	↑pJNK		Chen et al. (2002)
PC-3	5–10 μM	↑pERK, ↑pp38	Attenuation of apoptosis by MEK1 inhibitor	Xiao and Singh (2002)
PC-3	2.5–10 μM	↓Bcl-2, ↓Bcl-xL	Bcl-2 overexpression had no effect on apoptosis	Xiao et al. (2004)
PC-3	5–7.5 μM	↓NF-κB, ↓Bcl-xL, ↓cyclin D1, ↓p65, ↓pp65		Xu et al. (2005)
LNCaP, DU145	5–10 μM	↑pERK, ↑pJNK	Attenuation of apoptosis by pharmacological and genetic inhibition of JNK only in DU145	Xiao et al. (2005a)
PC-3	5–10 μM	↓pPDK1, ↓pAkt, ↓pEGFR		Kim et al. (2006)
PC-3	5–10 μM	↑AP-1, ↑pERK, ↑pJNK, ↑pc-Jun	Attenuation of apoptosis by overexpression of dominant negative ERK2 and JNK1	Xu et al. (2006)

Table 12.2 (continued)

Tumor type/cell line	PEITC conc.	Molecular changes	Functional studies1	Reference
PC-3	1–7.5 μM	↑4E-BP1, ↓p4E-BP1 ↓cap-bound eIF4E ↓cap-dependent translation	Attenuation of apoptosis by overexpression of eIF4E (in HCT-116 colon cancer cell line)	Hu et al. (2007)
DU145, LNCaP	5–20 μM	↓pSTAT3, ↓pJAK2	PEITC-mediated inhibition of STAT3 activation was reversed by NAC	Gong et al. (2009)
PC-3, LNCaP	2.5–5 μM	↑ROS, ↓complex III, ↓OXPHOS, ↓ECAR, ↓ATP, ↑Bax activation	Attenuation of apoptosis by overexpression of Mn-SOD and Cu,Zn-SOD and Bax/Bak siRNA	Xiao et al. (2010)
Bladder				
UM-UC-3	7.5–30 μM	↑Mito.Bak		Tang and Zhang (2005)
Ovarian				
OVCAR-3	2.5–20 μM	↓Bcl-2, ↑Bax, ↑pJNK1/2, ↑pp38, ↓pERK1/2, ↓pAkt, ↓c-Myc	Reversal of PEITC cytotoxicity by inhibitors of JNK1/2 and p38	Satyan et al. (2006)
Lung				
A549	20–25 μM	↑protein binding		Mi et al. (2007)
Breast				
MCF-7	3–30 μM	↑Bax activation, ↑Mito.-Bad ↓Bcl-2, ↓XIAP		Lee and Cho (2008)
Osteosarcoma				
U-2OS	5–10 μM	↑ROS, ↑NO, ↑iNOS ↑AIF	Attenuation of cell growth inhibition and ROS by NAC	Wu et al. (2011)

JNK1 c-Jun NH_2-terminal kinase 1, *pJNK* phospho-JNK, *XIAP* X-linked inhibitor of apoptosis, *Apaf-1* apoptosis Protease activating factor 1, *NAC N*-acetylcysteine, *pERK* phospho-extracellular signal-regulated kinase, *MAPK* mitogen-activated protein kinase, *NF-κB* nuclear factor-κB, *MEK1* mitogen activated protein kinase 1, *pPDK1* phospho – phosphoinositide-dependent protein kinase 1, *pEGFR* phospho-epidermal growth factor receptor, *AP-1* activator protein-1, *4E-BP1* eukaryotic translation initiation factor 4E binding protein, *p4E-BP1* phospho-4E-BP1, *eIF4E* eukaryotic translation initiation factor 4E, *pSTAT3* phospho-signal transducer and activator of transcription 3, *pJAK2* phospho-Janus-activated kinase 2, *ROS* reactive oxygen species, *OXPHOS* oxidative phosphorylation, *ECAR* extracellular acidification rate (lactate production), *Mn-SOD* Mn-superoxide dismutase, *Cu,Zn-SOD* Cu,Zn-superoxide dismutase, *siRNA* small interfering RNA, *Mito.Bad* Bad in mitochondrial fraction, *NO* nitric oxide, *iNOS* inducible nitric oxide synthase, *AIF* apoptosis-inducing factor, *Mito.Bak* Bak in mitochondrial fraction

are needed to substantiate this speculation. It is interesting to note that the NAC conjugate of PEITC caused apoptosis more robustly in A549 cells stimulated with 12-*O*-tetradecanoyl phorbol-13-acetate than in un-stimulated cells (Yang et al. 2005).

Activation of MAPK by PEITC has been observed in different cancer cell types. Kong and colleagues (Chen et al. 1998) were the first to study the role of MAPK in PEITC-induced apoptosis. PEITC treatment resulted in sustained activation of JNK in Jurkat cells, and apoptosis induction by PEITC was suppressed by overexpression of dominant-negative mutant of JNK1, Bcl-2 and/or Bcl-xL (Chen et al. 1998). Subsequent work from the same group of investigators revealed that the JNK activation by PEITC was mediated by proteasomal degradation of a JNK-specific phosphatase (Chen et al. 2002). In HT-29 human colon cancer cells, PEITC treatment resulted in activation of JNK, extracellular signal-regulated kinase (ERK) and p38 MAPK (Hu et al. 2003). Importantly, JNK inhibitor SP600125, but not the ERK or p38 MAPK inhibitor, suppressed apoptosis induction by PEITC in HT-29 cells by attenuating both cytochrome *c* release and caspase-3 activation (Hu et al. 2003). To the contrary, ERK has been implicated in proapoptotic response to PEITC in PC-3 human prostate cancer cells (Xiao and Singh 2002; Xu et al. 2006). Thorough review of the literature suggests that involvement of MAPK in proapoptotic response to PEITC may be a cell line-specific response (Chen et al. 1998; Xiao and Singh 2002; Hu et al. 2003; Xiao et al. 2005a). For instance, exposure of DU145 and LNCaP human prostate cancer cells to growth suppressive concentrations of PEITC resulted in activation of ERK and JNK, but not p38 MAPK (Xiao et al. 2005a). In DU145 cells, the apoptosis induction by PEITC was significantly attenuated by pharmacological inhibition of JNK as well as overexpression of JNK binding domain of JNK-interacting protein-1 (Xiao et al. 2005a). On the other hand, inhibition of ERK activation with PD98059 failed to confer protection against PEITC-induced apoptosis in DU145 cells. In LNCaP cells, PEITC-induced cell death was not affected by pretreatment with either PD98059 or SP600125 or overexpression of JNK binding domain of JNK-interacting protein-1 (Xiao et al. 2005a). Besides MAPK activation, PEITC treatment has been shown to suppress different oncogenic signaling pathways including NF-κB (Xu et al. 2005), c-Myc (Wang et al. 2008), epidermal growth factor receptor (Kim et al. 2006), signal transducer and activator of transcription 3 (Gong et al. 2009), and Akt (Kim et al. 2006; Wu et al. 2010). PEITC treatment also downregulated X-linked inhibitor of apoptosis protein in MCF-7 human breast cancer cells (Lee and Cho 2008).

Several studies suggest that production of reactive oxygen species (ROS) is an important event in proapoptotic signal transduction by PEITC in cancer cells (Rose et al. 2005; Xiao et al. 2006, 2010; Trachootham et al. 2006, 2008; Zhang et al. 2008; Gong et al. 2009; Xiao and Singh 2010b; Powolny and Singh 2010; Wu et al. 2010). However, the mechanism of PEITC-induced ROS production as well as signal transduction downstream of ROS production in execution of PEITC-induced apoptosis is well-studied only in prostate cancer cells (Xiao et al. 2010; Xiao and Singh 2010b; Powolny and Singh 2010). PEITC-induced ROS production in PC-3 and LNCaP cells was associated with inhibition of oxidative phosphorylation and complex III activity leading to ATP depletion (Xiao et al. 2010). Notably, these effects were not observed in a representative normal human prostate epithelial cell line (PrEC) (Xiao et al. 2010). Furthermore, PEITC treatment differentially altered expression of oxidative stress and antioxidant defense genes in PC-3 *versus* PrEC cells (Powolny and Singh 2010), which may also partly explain differential sensitivity of these cells to ROS production by PEITC. A role for adapter protein p66^{Shc} has also been established in ROS production and apoptosis induction by PEITC (Xiao and Singh 2010b). Mechanism downstream of ROS activation in PEITC-induced apoptosis in prostate cancer cells involves activation of Bax, which is evident in wild-type LNCaP and PC-3 cells, but not in their respective Rho-0 variants lacking normal oxidative phosphorylation (Xiao et al. 2010). PEITC-mediated inhibition of complex III and oxygen consumption coupled with activation of Bax have also been observed in hepatoma HepG2 cells (Rose et al. 2005). In HepG2 cells, however, PEITC-mediated apoptosis was not prevented by either pre- or co-treatment with various free radical scavengers, including Trolox, ascorbate, mannitol, uric acid and a superoxide dismutase mimetic (Rose et al. 2003). The reasons for discrepancies in results between HepG2 cells and prostate cancer cells concerning ROS-dependence of PEITC-induced apoptosis are unclear (Rose et al. 2003; Xiao et al. 2010). However, the concentration of PEITC used in this study was rather high at 20 μM (Rose et al. 2003) raising a possibility that ROS-independent mechanism(s) may predominate at high PEITC concentrations.

Many studies have relied on pharmacological approaches using NAC to show attenuation of PEITC-induced ROS production and apoptosis (Wu et al. 2005; Zhang et al. 2008; Trachootham et al. 2006, 2008). However, caution must be exercised in interpretation of results using NAC because PEITC being electrophilic in nature is capable of reacting with nucleophiles, and the protection observed with NAC against apoptosis may simply be a consequence of unavailability of free PEITC (Mi et al. 2010b).

Bcl-2 family proteins has emerged as critical regulator of cell death process either by acting as promoters (e.g., Bax, Bak, Bid, Bim) or inhibitors of apoptosis (e.g., Bcl-2, Bcl-xL, Mcl-1) (Chao and Korsmeyer 1998; Adams and Cory 2007; Akiyama et al. 2009). PEITC-mediated apoptosis in different cellular systems is associated with down regulation of anti-apoptotic Bcl-2, Bcl-xL, and/or Mcl-1 (Xiao et al. 2004, 2005b; Xu et al. 2005; Wu et al. 2005; Satyan et al. 2006; Lee and Cho 2008; Trachootham et al. 2008), increased levels of phosphorylated Bcl-2 (Tang and Zhang 2005), activation and/or induction of multidomain proapoptotic proteins Bax and/or Bak (Rose et al. 2005; Tang and Zhang 2005; Wu et al. 2005; Xiao et al. 2005b; Satyan et al. 2006; Lee and Cho 2008), suppression of X-linked inhibitor of apoptosis protein (Wu et al. 2005; Lee and Cho 2008), cleavage of Bid (Xu and Thornalley 2001b; Wu et al. 2005), and activation of caspases (Xiao et al. 2004; Tang and Zhang 2005; Wu et al. 2005; Satyan et al. 2006; Lee and Cho 2008). In PC-3 prostate cancer cells, however, Bcl-2 overexpression failed to confer protection against PEITC-induced apoptosis (Xiao et al. 2004). Consistent with these results, PEITC triggered apoptosis in Jurkat cells made resistant to other drugs by overexpression of Bcl-2 and Bcl-xL (Thomson et al. 2006; Cuddihy et al. 2008). Genetic knockdown of Bax and/or Bak has been shown to confer significant protection against PEITC-induced cell death (Xiao et al. 2005b).

Inhibition of cap-dependent translation in proapoptotic response to PEITC has also been described (Hu et al. 2007). Treatment of HCT-116 human colorectal cancer cells and PC-3 cells, but not a normal prostate epithelial cell line (PrEC), with PEITC resulted in an increase in expression of the eukaryotic translation initiation factor 4E (eIF4E) binding protein (4E-BP1) and inhibition of 4E-BP1 phosphorylation. Pull-down assays using 7-methyl-GTP Sepharose 4B beads indicated that PEITC treatment reduced cap-bound eIF4E, confirming that increased 4E-BP1 expression and inhibition of 4E-BP1 phosphorylation indeed reduced the availability of eIF4E for translation initiation (Hu et al. 2007). Results from in vivo translation using luciferase reporter assay indicated PEITC-mediated inhibition of cap-dependent translation, in particular translation of mRNA with secondary stem-loop structure (Hu et al. 2007). Furthermore, ectopic expression of eIF4E prevented PEITC-induced translation inhibition and conferred significant protection against PEITC-induced apoptosis (Hu et al. 2007). This study suggested that inhibition of cap-dependent translation might be an important mechanism in PEITC-induced apoptosis.

12.6.4 Induction of Autophagy

Autophagy is an evolutionarily conserved process for bulk degradation and recycling of cellular proteins and organelles. The role of autophagy in cancer development is complex and may, depending on circumstances, have opposite consequences for tumor development (Apel et al. 2009). The connection between apoptotic and autophagic cell death in the context of cancer therapy is still unresolved but in some models autophagy is a protective mechanism against therapy-induced apoptosis. For example, inhibition of autophagy by chloroquine was demonstrated to increase activity of an alkylating agent cyclophosphamide in a Myc-driven model of lymphoma (Amaravadi et al. 2007). Furthermore, autophagy inhibitors 3-methyladenine (3-MA) and chloroquine synergistically augmented the pro-apoptotic response to a histone deacetylase inhibitor (Carew et al. 2007). At the same time, autophagy has been shown to promote apoptosis by some agents (Kanzawa et al. 2003). Recent studies from our laboratory have revealed that autophagy induction by PEITC in prostate cancer cells is not a protective mechanism against apoptotic cell death (Bommareddy et al. 2009). PEITC-induced autophagy in prostate cancer cells is partially dependent on ROS production (Xiao et al. 2010) and Atg5-12, but not mammalian target of rapamycin and Akt (Bommareddy et al. 2009). It is unclear if the autophagic cell death caused by PEITC is unique to the prostate cancer cells. Interestingly, formation of aggresome-like structures by PEITC treatment has been documented (Mi et al. 2009). Functional connection, if any, between PEITC-induced autophagy and aggresome-like structure formation remains to be determined.

12.6.5 Histone Modification

PEITC was reported to inhibit histone deacetylase activity in LNCaP and its androgen-independent variant (Wang et al. 2007, 2008). PEITC treatment resulted in a concentration-dependent increase in selective histone acetylation, chromatin re-organization, and activation of p21 expression in the prostate cancer cells (Wang et al. 2008). PEITC-treated LNCaP cells exhibited a concentration-dependent enhancement of acetylation of histone H3 similar to those mediated by sodium butyrate, a known histone deacetylase inhibitor (Wang et al. 2008). PEITC treatment selectively increased the levels of mono/di/trimethylation at lysine 4 of histone H3, but decreased the level of trimethylated lysine 9 of H3. Methylated histone H3 lysine 4 is a marker of activated chromatin, whereas methylation of histone H3 lysine 9 signifies heterochromatin (Kondo et al. 2004). Additionally, PEITC was able to restore epigenetically silenced expression of GSTP1 gene by causing promoter demethylation (Wang et al. 2007). These findings indicate that PEITC may impact the process of carcinogenesis through alteration of histone acetylation and promoter methylation leading to altered expression of genes involved in cell cycle progression and/or carcinogen metabolism. Further studies are needed to test in vivo relevance of these observations.

12.6.6 Protein Binding

More recent studies have documented direct covalent modification of various proteins by PEITC (Mi et al. 2007, 2008; Cross et al. 2007, 2009; Brown et al. 2009). Idea of protein binding as a mechanism to explain cellular chemopreventive response to PEITC was first put forward by Chung and colleagues (Mi et al. 2007). A novel affinity reagent for detection of protein modification by PEITC was used in competition assays to monitor direct modification of MEKK1 by ITC (Cross et al. 2007). PEITC inhibited the MEKK1 protein kinase in a manner dependent on a specific cysteine residue in the ATP binding pocket, which was due to direct, covalent and irreversible modification of the MEKK1 protein itself (Cross et al. 2007). Tubulin is another major binding target for PEITC (Mi et al. 2008). PEITC treatment disrupted microtubule polymerization in vitro and in vivo leading to mitotic arrest (Mi et al. 2008). Mass spectrometry showed that specific cysteine in tubulin were covalently modified by PEITC (Mi et al. 2008). Two research groups independently reported direct and covalent modification of macrophage migration inhibitory factor by PEITC (Brown et al. 2009; Cross et al. 2009). PEITC was shown to covalently modify N-terminal proline residue of macrophage migration inhibitory factor, which resulted in complete loss of catalytic tautomerase activity. Monoclonal antibody binding to plasma macrophage migration inhibitory factor was disrupted in humans consuming watercress (Brown et al. 2009). These observations are significant considering emerging role of macrophage migration inhibitory factor in control of malignant cell growth.

12.7 Suppression of Hormone Receptors

Role of androgen-receptor (AR) in prostate cancer and that of estrogen receptor (ER) α in human breast cancer is well-accepted. Studies have shown that PEITC can repress levels of these receptors in cancer cells (Wang et al. 2006; Kang et al. 2009; Kang and Wang 2010). For example, PEITC repressed mRNA and protein levels of AR in androgen-dependent and androgen-independent prostate cancer cells (Wang et al. 2006) through dual effects at the transcriptional and post-translational levels involving inhibition of the transcription factor Sp1 and protein degradation (Wang et al. 2006). In a rat model of testosterone (hormone)-induced prostatic cell growth, PEITC nullified this effect through downregulation of AR (Beklemisheva et al. 2007). PEITC treatment resulted in suppression of ERα and its novel variant ERα36 in human breast cancer cells in MCF-7 and T47D cells in a dose- and time-dependent manner (Kang et al. 2009; Kang and Wang 2010). In addition, PEITC also abrogated the transcriptional activity of ERα and hence inhibited estrogen-stimulated expression of the estrogen responsive gene, pS2 (Kang et al. 2009). Thus suppression of hormone receptors may be an important mechanism in anticancer effects of PEITC against hormonally-regulated cancers. It is tempting to speculate that PEITC may inhibit emergence of androgen-independent (castration-resistant) prostate cancer because of involvement of AR in this process (Feldman and Feldman 2001).

12.8 Concluding Remarks and Future Directions

Research over the past few decades has provided valuable insights into how cruciferous vegetables and their constituents (e.g., PEITC) inhibit cancer development. It is commendable that emerging technologies and research tools (e.g., omics, imaging etc) are now frequently employed in cancer chemoprevention research. Willingness of clinicians to entertain the idea of cancer prevention with diet derived agents is equally laudable. Clinical development of PEITC as a chemopreventive agent against cancer seems more plausible today, mainly because of knowledge acquired in past few decades. At the same time, a few obvious hurdles in clinical development of PEITC as a chemopreventive agent can't be ignored. First, a formulation of pure PEITC suitable for clinical investigations is not yet easily available. Second, PEITC is cleared rapidly and clinical trial designs must consider pharmacokinetic attributes of this agent, requiring multiple daily dosing regimens. Third, human chemoprevention trials with cancer incidence as the primary end point are too expensive requiring substantial resources and thousands of subjects. Instead, a few trials with biomarker-based outcomes are urgently needed to pace translation for this agent. Finally, the question of whether PEITC is a promoter of bladder cancer requires further investigation, both population-based studies and laboratory-based investigations, because this may turn out to be a major impediment in long-term usage of PEITC necessary for cancer prevention in high-risk subjects.

Acknowledgements Work cited from our laboratory was supported by the US PHS grant CA101753, awarded by the National Cancer Institute. Contributions of the present (Eun-Ryeong Hahm, Su-Hyeong Kim, Anuradha Sehrawat, Julie A Arlotti) and past members (Dong Xiao, Yan Zeng, Sunga Choi) of the Singh laboratory for preclinical studies on PEITC cited in this article are greatly appreciated.

References

Adams JM, Cory S (2007) The Bcl-2 apoptotic switch in cancer development and therapy. Oncogene 26:1324–1337

Akagi K, Sano M, Ogawa K et al (2003) Involvement of toxicity as an early event in urinary bladder carcinogenesis induced by phenethyl isothiocyanate, benzyl isothiocyanate, and analogues in F344 rats. Toxicol Pathol 31:388–396

Akiyama T, Dass CR, Choong PF (2009) Bim-targeted cancer therapy: a link between drug action and underlying molecular changes. Mol Cancer Ther 8:3173–3180

Amaravadi RK, Yu D, Lum JJ, Bui T et al (2007) Autophagy inhibition enhances therapy-induced apoptosis in a Myc-induced model of lymphoma. J Clin Invest 117:326–336

Apel A, Zentgraf H, Buchler MW et al (2009) Autophagy-A double-edged sword in oncology. Int J Cancer 125:991–995

Barve A, Khor TO, Hao X et al (2008) Murine prostate cancer inhibition by dietary phytochemicals-curcumin and phenyethylisothiocyanate. Pharm Res 25:2181–2189

Beklemisheva AA, Feng J, Yeh YA et al (2007) Modulating testosterone stimulated prostate growth by phenethyl isothiocyanate via Sp1 and androgen receptor down-regulation. Prostate 67: 863–870

Bommareddy A, Hahm ER, Xiao D et al (2009) Atg5 regulates phenethyl isothiocyanate-induced autophagic and apoptotic cell death in human prostate cancer cells. Cancer Res 69:3704–3712

Brown KK, Blaikie FH, Smith RA et al (2009) Direct modification of the proinflammatory cytokine macrophage migration inhibitory factor by dietary isothiocyanates. J Biol Chem 284: 32425–32433

Carew JS, Nawrocki ST, Kahue CN et al (2007) Targeting autophagy augments the anticancer activity of the histone deacetylase inhibitor SAHA to overcome Bcr-Abl-mediated drug resistance. Blood 110:313–322

Cavell BE, Alwi SSS, Donlevy A et al (2011) Anti-angiogenic effects of dietary isothiocyanates: mechanisms of action and implications for human health. Biochem Pharmacol 81:327–336

Chao DT, Korsmeyer SJ (1998) Bcl-2 family: regulators of cell death. Annu Rev Immunol 16: 395–419

Chen YR, Wang W, Kong AN et al (1998) Molecular mechanisms of c-Jun N-terminal kinase-mediated apoptosis induced by anticarcinogenic isothiocyanates. J Biol Chem 273:1769–1775

Chen YR, Han J, Kori R et al (2002) Phenylethyl isothiocyanate induces apoptotic signaling via suppressing phosphatase activity against c-Jun N-terminal kinase. J Biol Chem 277:39334–39342

Cheung KL, Kong AN (2009) Molecular targets of dietary phenethyl isothiocyanate and sulforaphane for cancer chemoprevention. AAPS J 12:87–97

Cheung KL, Khor TO, Yu S et al (2008) PEITC induces G1 cell cycle arrest on HT-29 cells through the activation of p38 MAPK signaling pathway. AAPS J 10:277–281

Cheung KL, Khor TO, Huang MT et al (2010) Differential in vivo mechanism of chemoprevention of tumor formation in azoxymethane/dextran sodium sulfate mice by PEITC and DBM. Carcinog 31:880–885

Chiao JW, Wu H, Ramaswamy G et al (2004) Ingestion of an isothiocyanate metabolite from cruciferous vegetables inhibits growth of human prostate cancer cell xenografts by apoptosis and cell cycle arrest. Carcinog 25:1403–1408

Chung FL, Kelloff G, Steele V et al (1996) Chemopreventive efficacy of arylalkyl isothiocyanates and N-acetylcysteine for lung tumorigenesis in Fischer rats. Cancer Res 15(56):772–778
Chung FL, Conaway CC, Rao CV et al (2000) Chemoprevention of colonic aberrant crypt foci in Fischer rats by sulforaphane and phenethyl isothiocyanate. Carcinog 21:2287–2291
Chyou PH, Nomura AM, Hankin JH et al (1990) A case-cohort study of diet and stomach cancer. Cancer Res 50:7501–7504
Ciska E, Martyniak-Przybyszewska B, Kozlowska H (2000) Content of glucosinolates in cruciferous vegetables grown at the same site for two years under different climatic conditions. J Agric Food Chem 48:2862–2867
Conaway CC, Wang CX, Pittman B et al (2005) Phenethyl isothiocyanate and sulforaphane and their N-acetylcysteine conjugates inhibit malignant progression of lung adenomas induced by tobacco carcinogens in A/J mice. Cancer Res 65:8548–8557
Cross JV, Foss FW, Rady JM et al (2007) The isothiocyanate class of bioactive nutrients covalently inhibit the MEKK1 protein kinase. BMC Cancer 7:183
Cross JV, Rady JM, Foss FW et al (2009) Nutrient isothiocyanates covalently modify and inhibit the inflammatory cytokine macrophage migration inhibitory factor (MIF). Biochem J 423: 315–321
Cuddihy SL, Brown KK, Thomson SJ et al (2008) Induction of apoptosis by phenethyl isothiocyanate in cells overexpressing Bcl-X_L. Cancer Lett 271:215–221
Di Pasqua AJ, Hong C, Wu MY et al (2010) Sensitization of non-small cell lung cancer cells to cisplatin by naturally occurring isothiocyanates. Chem Res Toxicol 23:1307–1309
Fahey JW, Zalcmann AT, Talalay P (2001) The chemical diversity and distribution of glucosinolates and isothiocyanates among plants. Phytochem 56:5–51
Feldman BJ, Feldman D (2001) The development of androgen-independent prostate cancer. Nat Rev Cancer 1:34–45
Giovannucci E, Rimm EB, Liu Y et al (2003) A prospective study of cruciferous vegetables and prostate cancer. Cancer Epidemiol Biomarkers Prev 12:1403–1409
Gong A, He M, Vanaja DK et al (2009) Phenethyl isothiocyanate inhibits STAT3 activation in prostate cancer cells. Mol Nutr Food Res 53:878–886
Greenwald P, Clifford CK, Milner JA (2001) Diet and cancer prevention. Eur J Cancer 37:948–965
Gross-Steinmeyer K, Stapleton PL, Liu F et al (2004) Phytochemical-induced changes in gene expression of carcinogen-metabolizing enzymes in cultured human primary hepatocytes. Xenobiotica 34:619–632
Guengerich FP (2000) Metabolism of chemical carcinogens. Carcinog 21:345–351
Guo Z, Smith TJ, Wang E et al (1992) Effects of phenethyl isothiocyanate, a carcinogenesis inhibitor, on xenobiotic-metabolizing enzymes and nitrosamine metabolism in rats. Carcinog 13:2205–2210
Hara M, Hanaoka T, Kobayashi M et al (2003) Cruciferous vegetables, mushrooms, and gastrointestinal cancer risks in a multicenter, hospital-based case-control study in Japan. Nutr Cancer 46:138–147
Hasegawa T, Nishino H, Iwashima A (1993) Isothiocyanates inhibit cell cycle progression of HeLa cells at G2/M phase. Anti-cancer drugs 4:273–279
Hayes JD, Pulford DJ (1995) The glutathione *S*-transferase supergene family: regulation of GST*and the contribution of the isoenzymes to cancer chemoprotection and drug resistance. Crit Rev Biochem Mol Biol 30:445–600
Hecht SS (2000) Inhibition of carcinogenesis by isothiocyanates. Drug Metab Rev 32:395–411
Hecht SS, Chung FL, Richie JP Jr et al (1995) Effects of watercress consumption on metabolism of a tobacco-specific lung carcinogen in smokers. Cancer Epidemiol Biomarkers Prev 4:877–884
Hirose M, Yamaguchi T, Kimoto N et al (1998) Strong promoting activity of phenylethyl isothiocyanate and benzyl isothiocyanate on urinary bladder carcinogenesis in F344 male rats. Int J Cancer 77:773–777

Hofmann T, Kuhnert A, Schubert A et al (2009) Modulation of detoxification enzymes by watercress: in vitro and in vivo investigations in human peripheral blood cells. Eur J Nutr 48:483–491

Hu K, Morris ME (2004) Effects of benzyl-, phenethyl-, and alpha-naphthyl isothiocyanates on P-glycoprotein- and MRP1-mediated transport. J Pharm Sci 93:1901–1911

Hu R, Kim BR, Chen C et al (2003) The roles of JNK and apoptotic signaling pathways in PEITC-mediated responses in human HT-29 colon adenocarcinoma cells. Carcinog 24:1361–1367

Hu R, Xu C, Shen G, Jain MR et al (2006) Identification of Nrf2-regulated genes induced by chemopreventive isothiocyanate PEITC by oligonucleotide microarray. Life Sci 79:1944–1955

Hu J, Straub J, Xiao D et al (2007) Phenethyl isothiocyanate, a cancer chemopreventive constituent of cruciferous vegetables, inhibits cap-dependent translation by regulating the level and phosphorylation of 4E-BP1. Cancer Res 67:3569–3573

Hu Y, Lu W, Chen G et al (2010) Overcoming resistance to histone deacetylase inhibitors in human leukemia with the redox modulating compound β-phenylethyl isothiocyanate. Blood 116: 2732–2741

Huang C, Ma WY, Li J et al (1998) Essential role of p53 in phenethyl isothiocyanate-induced apoptosis. Cancer Res 58:4102–4106

Hwang ES, Lee HJ (2006) Phenylethyl isothiocyanate and its N-acetylcysteine conjugate suppress the metastasis of SK-Hep1 human hepatoma cells. J Nutr Biochem 17:837–846

Hwang ES, Lee HJ (2010) Effects of phenethyl isothiocyanate and its metabolite on cell-cycle arrest and apoptosis in LNCaP human prostate cancer cells. Int J Food Sci Nutr 61:324–336

Ishizaki H, Brady JF, Ning SM et al (1990) Effect of phenethyl isothiocyanate on microsomal N-nitrosodimethylamine metabolism and other monooxygenase activities. Xenobiotica 20: 255–264

Izzotti A, Calin GA, Steele VE et al (2010a) Chemoprevention of cigarette smoke-induced alterations of MicroRNA expression in rat lungs. Cancer Prev Res 3:62–72

Izzotti A, Larghero P, Cartiglia C et al (2010b) Modulation of microRNA expression by budesonide, phenethyl isothiocyanate and cigarette smoke in mouse liver and lung. Carcinog 31:894–901

Jakubíková J, Sedlák J, Bacon J et al (2005) Effects of MEK1 and PI3K inhibitors on allyl-, benzyl- and phenylethyl-isothiocyanate-induced G2/M arrest and cell death in Caco-2 cells. Int J Oncol 27:1449–1458

Ji Y, Kuo Y, Morris ME (2005) Pharmacokinetics of dietary phenethyl isothiocyanate in rats. Pharm Res 22:1658–1666

Jiao D, Conaway CC, Wang MH et al (1996) Inhibition of *N*-nitrosodimethylamine demethylase in rat and human liver microsomes by isothiocyanates and their glutathione, L-cysteine, and *N*-acetyl-L-cysteine conjugates. Chem Res Toxicol 9:932–938

Jiao D, Smith TJ, Yang CS et al (1997) Chemopreventive activity of thiol conjugates of isothiocyanates for lung tumorigenesis. Carcinog 18:2143–2147

Kanzawa T, Kondo Y, Ito H et al (2003) Induction of autophagic cell death in malignant glioma cells by arsenic trioxide. Cancer Res 63:2103–2108

Kang L, Wang ZY (2010) Breast cancer cell growth inhibition by phenethyl isothiocyanate is associated with down-regulation of oestrogen receptor-α36. J Cell Mol Med 14:1485–1493

Kang L, Ding L, Wang ZY (2009) Isothiocyanates repress estrogen receptor alpha expression in breast cancer cells. Oncol Rep 21:185–192

Kelemen LE, Wang SS, Lim U et al (2008) Vegetables- and antioxidant-related nutrients, genetic susceptibility, and non-Hodgkin lymphoma risk. Cancer Causes Control 19:491–503

Keum YS, Owuor ED, Kim BR et al (2003) Involvement of Nrf2 and JNK1 in the activation of antioxidant responsive element (ARE) by chemopreventive agent phenethyl isothiocyanate (PEITC). Pharm Res 20:1351–1356

Keum YS, Jeong WS, Kong AN (2004) Chemoprevention by isothiocyanates and their underlying molecular signaling mechanisms. Mutat Res 555:191–202

Khor TO, Cheung WK, Prawan A et al (2008) Chemoprevention of familial adenomatous polyposis in *Apc*$^{Min/+}$ mice by phenethyl isothiocyanate (PEITC). Molecular carcinogenesis 47:321–325
Kim JH, Xu C, Keum YS et al (2006) Inhibition of EGFR signaling in human prostate cancer PC-3 cells by combination treatment with beta-phenylethyl isothiocyanate and curcumin. Carcinog 27:475–482
Kirsh VA, Peters U, Mayne ST et al (2007) Prospective study of fruit and vegetable intake and risk of prostate cancer. J Natl Cancer Inst 99:1200–1209
Kolonel LN, Hankin JH, Whittemore AS et al (2000) Vegetables, fruits, legumes and prostate cancer: a multiethnic case-control study. Cancer Epidemiol Biomarkers Prev 9:795–804
Kondo Y, Shen L, Yan PS et al (2004) Chromatin immunoprecipitation microarrays for identification of genes silenced by histone H3 lysine 9 methylation. Proc Natl Acad Sci USA 101:7398–7403
Konsue N, Ioannides C (2008) Tissue differences in the modulation of rat cytochromes P450 and phase II conjugation systems by dietary doses of phenethyl isothiocyanate. Food Chem Toxicol 46:3677–3683
Konsue N, Ioannides C (2010) Modulation of carcinogen-metabolising cytochromes P450 in human liver by the chemopreventive phytochemical phenethyl isothiocyanate, a constituent of cruciferous vegetables. Toxicol 268:184–190
Konsue N, Kirkpatrick J, Kuhnert N et al (2010) Repeated oral administration modulates the pharmacokinetic behavior of the chemopreventive agent phenethyl isothiocyanate in rats. Mol Nutr Food Res 54:426–432
Kumar A, Sabbioni G (2010) New biomarkers for monitoring the levels of isothiocyanates in humans. Chem Res Toxicol 23:756–765
Kumar A, Vineis P, Sacerdote C et al (2010) Determination of new biomarkers to monitor the dietary consumption of isothiocyanates. Biomarkers 15:739–745
Kushad MM, Brown AF, Kurilich AC et al (1999) Variation of glucosinolates in vegetable crops of Brassica oleracea. J Agric Food Chem 47:1541–1548
Kvale G, Bjelke E, Gart JJ (1983) Dietary habits and lung cancer risk. Int J Cancer 31:397–405
Lai KC, Hsu SC, Kuo CL et al (2010) Phenethyl isothiocyanate inhibited tumor migration and invasion via suppressing multiple signal transduction pathways in human colon Cancer HT29 cells. J Agric Food Chem 58:11148–11155
Lee JW, Cho MK (2008) Phenethyl isothiocyanate induced apoptosis via down regulation of Bcl-2/XIAP and triggering of the mitochondrial pathway in MCF-7 cells. Arch Pharm Res 31: 1604–1612
Liebes L, Conaway CC, Hochster H et al (2001) High-performance liquid chromatography-based determination of total isothiocyanate levels in human plasma: application to studies with 2-phenethyl isothiocyanate. Anal Biochem 291:279–289
Lubet RA, Steele VE, Eto I et al (1997) Chemopreventive efficacy of anethole trithione, N-acetyl-L-cysteine, miconazole and phenethylisothiocyanate in the DMBA-induced rat mammary cancer model. Int J Cancer 72:95–101
McCune K, Mehta R, Thorat MA et al (2010) Loss of ERα and FOXA1 expression in a progression model of luminal type breast cancer: insights from PyMT transgenic mouse model. Oncol Rep 24:1233–1239
Mi L, Wang X, Govind S et al (2007) The role of protein binding in induction of apoptosis by phenethyl isothiocyanate and sulforaphane in human non-small lung cancer cells. Cancer Res 67:6409–6416
Mi L, Xiao Z, Hood BL et al (2008) Covalent binding to tubulin by isothiocyanates. A mechanism of cell growth arrest and apoptosis. J Biol Chem 283:22136–22146
Mi L, Gan N, Chung FL (2009) Aggresome-like structure induced by isothiocyanates is novel proteasome-dependent degradation machinery. Biochem Biophys Res Commun 388:456–462
Mi L, Gan N, Chung FL (2010a) Isothiocyanates inhibit proteasome activity and proliferation of multiple myeloma cells. Carcinog 32:216–223

Mi L, Sirajiddin P, Gan N et al (2010b) A cautionary note on using N-acetylcysteine as an antagonist to assess isothiocyanate-induced reactive oxygen species-mediated apoptosis. Anal Biochem 405:269–271

Michaud DS, Spiegelman D, Clinton SK et al (1999) Fruit and vegetable intake and incidence of bladder cancer in a male prospective cohort. J Natl Cancer Inst 91:605–613

Miyake H, Muramaki M, Kurahashi T et al (2006) Expression of clusterin in prostate cancer correlates with Gleason score but not with prognosis in patients undergoing radical prostatectomy without neoadjuvant hormonal therapy. Urology 68:609–614

Morse MA, Eklind KI, Hech SS et al (1991) Structure-activity relationships for inhibition of 4-(methylnitrosamino)-1-(3-pyridyl)-1-butanone lung tumorigenesis by arylalkyl isothiocyanates in A/J mice. Cancer Res 51:1846–1850

Moy KA, Yuan JM, Chung FL et al (2008) Urinary total isothiocyanates and colorectal cancer: a prospective study of men in Shanghai, China. Cancer Epidemiol Biomarkers Prev 17: 1354–1359

Mukherjee S, Bhattacharya RK, Roy M (2009a) Targeting protein kinase C (PKC) and telomerase by phenethyl isothiocyanate (PEITC) sensitizes PC-3 cells towards chemotherapeutic drug-induced apoptosis. J Environ Pathol Toxicol Oncol 28:269–282

Mukherjee S, Dey S, Bhattacharya RK et al (2009b) Isothiocyanates sensitize the effect of chemotherapeutic drugs via modulation of protein kinase C and telomerase in cervical cancer cells. Mol Cell Biochem 330:9–22

Nakajima M, Yoshida R, Shimada N et al (2001) Inhibition and inactivation of human cytochrome P450 isoforms by phenethyl isothiocyanate. Drug Metab Disp 29:1110–1113

Nigg EA (1995) Cyclin-dependent protein kinases: key regulators of the eukaryotic cell cycle. Bioessays 17:471–480

Ogawa K, Futakuchi M, Hirose M et al (1998) Stage and organ dependent effects of 1-O-hexyl-2,3,5-trimethylhydroquinone, ascorbic acid derivatives, n-heptadecane-8-10-dione and phenylethyl isothiocyanate in a rat multiorgan carcinogenesis model. Int J Cancer 76:851–856

Ogawa K, Hirose M, Sugiura S et al (2001) Dose-dependent promotion by phenylethyl isothiocyanate, a known chemopreventer, of two-stage rat urinary bladder and liver carcinogenesis. Nutr Cancer 40:134–139

Pan SY, Ugnat AM, Mao Y et al (2004) A case-control study of diet and the risk of ovarian cancer. Cancer Epidemiol Biomarkers Prev 13:1521–1527

Plate AYA, Gallaher DD (2006) Effects of indole-3-carbinol and phenethyl isothiocyanate on colon carcinogenesis induced by azoxymethane in rats. Carcinog 27:287–292

Powolny AA, Singh SV (2010) Differential response of normal (PrEC) and cancerous human prostate cells (PC-3) to phenethyl isothiocyanate-mediated changes in expression of antioxidant defense genes. Pharm Res 27:2766–2775

Powolny AA, Bommareddy A, Hahm ER et al (2011) Chemopreventative potential of the cruciferous vegetable constituent phenethyl isothiocyanate in a mouse model of prostate cancer. J Natl Cancer Inst 103:571–584

Pullar JM, Thomson SJ, King MJ et al (2004) The chemopreventive agent phenethyl isothiocyanate sensitizes cells to Fas-mediated apoptosis. Carcinogenesis 25:765–772

Rose P, Whiteman M, Huang SH et al (2003) β-Phenylethyl isothiocyanate-mediated apoptosis in hepatoma HepG2 cells. Cell Mol Life Sci 60:1489–1503

Rose P, Armstrong JS, Chua YL et al (2005) β-phenylethyl isothiocyanate mediated apoptosis; contribution of Bax and the mitochondrial death pathway. Int J Biochem Cell Biol 37:100–119

Satyan KS, Swamy N, Dizon DS et al (2006) Phenethyl isothiocyanate (PEITC) inhibits growth of ovarian cancer cells by inducing apoptosis: role of caspase and MAPK activation. Gynecol Oncol 103:261–270

Shannan B, Seifert M, Leskov K et al (2006) Challenge and promise: roles for clusterin in pathogenesis, progression and therapy of cancer. Cell Death Differ 13:12–19

Smith TJ (2001) Mechanisms of carcinogenesis inhibition by isothiocayantes. Expert Opin Investig Drugs 10:2167–2174

Smith TJ, Guo Z, Guengerich FP et al (1996) Metabolism of 4-(methylnitrosamino)-1-(3-pyridyl)-1-butanone (NNK) by human cytochrome P450 1A2 and its inhibition by phenethyl isothiocyanate. Carcinog 17:809–813

Solt DB, Chang K, Helenowski I et al (2003) Phenethyl isothiocyanate inhibits nitrosamine carcinogenesis in a model for study of oral cancer chemoprevention. Cancer Lett 202:147–152

Sporn MB (1980) Combination chemoprevention of cancer. Nature 287:107–108

Sporn MB (2011) Perspective: the big C- for chemoprevention. Nature 471:S10–S11

Steinmetz KA, Potter JD, Folsom AR (1993) Vegetables, fruit, and lung cancer in the Iowa Women's Health Study. Cancer Res 53:536–543

Stoner GD, Morrissey DT, Heur YH et al (1991) Inhibitory effects of phenethyl isothiocyanate on *N*-nitrosobenzylmethylamine carcinogenesis in the rat esophagus. Cancer Res 51:2063–2068

Stoner GD, Dombkowski AA, Reen RK et al (2008) Carcinogen-altered genes in rat esophagus positively modulated to normal levels of expression by both black raspberries and phenylethyl isothiocyanate. Cancer Res 68:6460–6467

Sugiura S, Ogawa K, Hirose M et al (2003) Reversibility of proliferative lesions and induction of non-papillary tumors in rat urinary bladder treated with phenylethyl isothiocyanate. Carcinog 24:547–553

Syed Alwi SS, Cavell BE, Telang U et al (2010) *In vivo* modulation of 4E binding protein 1 (4E-BP1) phosphorylation by watercress: a pilot study. Br J Nutr 104:1288–1296

Takagi H, Shibutani M, Uneyama C et al (2005) Limited tumor-initiating activity of phenylethyl isothiocyanate by promotion with sodium L-ascorbate in a rat two-stage urinary bladder carcinogenesis model. Cancer Lett 219:147–153

Tang L, Zhang Y (2004) Dietary isothiocyanates inhibit the growth of human bladder carcinoma cells. J Nutr 134:2004–2010

Tang L, Zhang Y (2005) Mitochondria are the primary target in isothiocyanate-induced apoptosis in human bladder cancer cells. Mol Cancer Ther 4:1250–1259

Telang U, Morris ME (2010) Effect of orally administered phenethyl isothiocyanate on hepatic gene expression in rats. Mol Nutr Food Res 54:1802–1806

Thomson SJ, Brown KK, Pullar JM et al (2006) Phenethyl isothiocyanate triggers apoptosis in Jurkat cells made resistant by the overexpression of Bcl-2. Cancer Res 66:6772–6777

Trachootham D, Zhou Y, Zhang H et al (2006). Selective killing of oncogenically transformed cells through a ROS-mediated mechanism by β-phenylethyl isothiocyanate. Cancer Cell 10:241–252

Trachootham D, Zhang H, Zhang W et al (2008) Effective elimination of fludarabine-resistant CLL cells by PEITC through a redox-mediated mechanism. Blood 112:1912–1922

Tseng E, Kamath A, Morris ME (2002) Effect of organic isothiocyanates on the P-glycoprotein- and MRP1-mediated transport of daunomycin and vinblastine. Pham Res 19:1509–1515

Verhoeven DT, Goldbohm RA, van Poppel G et al (1996) Epidemiological studies on brassica vegetables and cancer risk. Cancer Epidemiol Biomarkers Prev 5:733–748

Visanji JM, Duthie SJ, Pirie L et al (2004) Dietary isothiocyanates inhibit Caco-2 cell proliferation and induce G2/M phase cell cycle arrest, DNA damage, and G2/M checkpoint activation. J Nutr 134:3121–3126

Wang LG, Liu XM, Chiao JW (2006) Repression of androgen receptor in prostate cancer cells by phenethyl isothiocyanate. Carcinogenesis 27:2124–2132

Wang LG, Beklemisheva A, Liu XM et al (2007) Dual action on promoter demethylation and chromatin by an isothiocyanate restored GSTP1 silenced in prostate cancer. Mol Carcinog 46:24–31

Wang LG, Liu XM, Fang Y et al (2008) De-repression of the p21 promoter in prostate cancer cells by an isothiocyanate via inhibition of HDACs and c-Myc. Int J Oncol 33:375–380

Wang XH, Cavell BE, Syed Alwi SS et al (2009) Inhibition of hypoxia inducible factor by phenethyl isothiocyanate. Biochem Pharmacol 78:261–272

Wang X, Di Pasqua AJ, Govind S et al (2011) Selective depletion of mutant p53 by cancer chemopreventive isothiocyanates and their structure-activity relationships. J Med Chem 54:809–816

Wattenberg LW (1977) Inhibition of carcinogenic effects of polycyclic hydrocarbons by benzyl isothiocyanate and related compounds. J Natl Cancer Inst 58:395–398

Wu SJ, Ng LT, Lin CC (2005) Effects of antioxidants and caspase-3 inhibitor on the phenylethyl isothiocyanate-induced apoptotic signaling pathways in human PLC/PRF/5 cells. Eur J Pharmacol 518:96–106

Wu X, Zhu Y, Yan H et al (2010) Isothiocyanates induce oxidative stress and suppress the metastasis potential of human non-small cell lung cancer cells. BMC Cancer 10:269

Wu CL, Huang AC, Yang JS et al (2011) Benzyl isothiocyanate (BITC) and phenethyl isothiocyanate (PEITC)-mediated generation of reactive oxygen species causes cell cycle arrest and induces apoptosis via activation of caspase-3, mitochondria dysfunction and Nitric Oxide (NO) in human osteogenic sarcoma U-2 OS cells. J Orthp Res 29:1199–1209

Xiao D, Singh SV (2002) Phenethyl isothiocyanate-induced apoptosis in p53-deficient PC-3 human prostate cancer cell line is mediated by extracellular signal-regulated kinases. Cancer Res 62:3615–3619

Xiao D, Singh SV (2007) Phenethyl isothiocyanate inhibits angiogenesis *in vitro* and *ex vivo*. Cancer Res 7:2239–2246

Xiao D, Singh SV (2010a) Phenethyl isothiocyanate sensitizes androgen-independent human prostate cancer cells to docetaxel-induced apoptosis *in vitro* and *in vivo*. Pharm Res 27:722–731

Xiao D, Singh SV (2010b) p66Shc is indispensable for phenethyl isothiocyanate-induced apoptosis in human prostate cancer cells. Cancer Res 70:3150–3158

Xiao D, Johnson CS, Trump DL et al (2004) Proteasome-mediated degradation of cell division cycle 25C and cyclin-dependent kinase 1 in phenethyl isothiocyanate-induced G2-M-phase cell cycle arrest in PC-3 human prostate cancer cells. Mol Cancer Ther 3:567–575

Xiao D, Choi S, Lee YJ et al (2005a) Role of mitogen-activated protein kinases in phenethyl isothiocyanate-induced apoptosis in human prostate cancer cells. Mol Carcinog 43:130–140

Xiao D, Zeng Y, Choi S et al (2005b) Caspase-dependent apoptosis induction by phenethyl isothiocyanate, a cruciferous vegetable-derived cancer chemopreventive agent, is mediated by Bak and Bax. Clin Cancer Res 11:2670–2679

Xiao D, Lew KL, Zeng Y et al (2006) Phenethyl isothiocyanate-induced apoptosis in PC-3 human prostate cancer cells is mediated by reactive oxygen species-dependent disruption of the mitochondrial membrane potential. Carcinog 27:2223–2234

Xiao D, Powolny AA, Moura MB et al (2010) Phenethyl isothiocyanate inhibits oxidative phosphorylation to trigger reactive oxygen species-mediated death of human prostate cancer cells. J Biol Chem 285:26558–26569

Xu K, Thornalley PJ (2001a) Involvement of glutathione metabolism in the cytotoxicity of the phenethyl isothiocyanate and its cysteine conjugate to human leukaemia cells in vitro. Biochem Pharmacol 61:165–177

Xu K, Thornalley PJ (2001b) Signal transduction activated by the cancer chemopreventive isothiocyanates: cleavage of BID protein, tyrosine phosphorylation and activation of JNK. Br J Cancer 84:670–673

Xu C, Shen G, Chen C et al (2005) Suppression of NF-κB and NF-κB-regulated gene expression by sulforaphane and PEITC through IκBα, IKK pathway in human prostate cancer PC-3 cells. Oncogene 24:4486–4495

Xu C, Shen G, Yuan X et al (2006) ERK and JNK signaling pathways are involved in the regulation of activator protein 1 and cell death elicited by three isothiocyanates in human prostate cancer PC-3 cells. Carcinog 27:437–445

Yang YM, Conaway CC, Chiao JW et al (2002) Inhibition of benzo(a)pyrene-induced lung tumorigenesis in A/J mice by dietary N-acetylcysteine conjugates of benzyl and phenethyl isothiocyanates during the postinitiation phase is associated with activation of mitogen-activated protein kinases and p53 activity and induction of apoptosis. Cancer Res 62:2–7

Yang YM, Jhanwar-Uniyal M, Schwartz J et al (2005) N-acetylcysteine conjugate of phenethyl isothiocyanate enhances apoptosis in growth-stimulated human lung cells. Cancer Res 65:8538–8547

Yang MD, Lai KC, Lai TY et al (2010) Phenethyl isothiocyanate inhibits migration and invasion of human gastric cancer AGS cells through suppressing MAPK and NF-kappaB signal pathways. Anticancer Res 30:2135–2143

Ye L, Zhang Y (2001) Total intracellular accumulation levels of dietary isothiocyanates determine their activity in elevation of cellular glutathione and induction of Phase 2 detoxification enzymes. Carcinogenesis 22:1987–1992

Ye B, Zhang YX, Yang F et al (2007) Induction of lung lesions in Wistar rats by 4-(methylnitrosamino)-1-(3-pyridyl)-1-butanone and its inhibition by aspirin and phenethyl isothiocyanate. BMC Cancer 7:90

Yin P, Kawamura T, He M et al (2009) Phenethyl isothiocyanate induces cell cycle arrest and reduction of α- and β- tubulin isotypes in human prostate cancer cells. Cell Biol Int 33:57–64

Yu R, Mandlekar S, Harvey KJ et al (1998) Chemopreventive isothiocyanates induce apoptosis and caspase-3-like protease activity. Cancer Res 58:402–408

Zhang Y (2001) Molecular mechanism of rapid cellular accumulation of anticarcinogenic isothiocyanates. Carcinogenesis 22:425–431

Zhang SM, Hunter DJ, Rosner BA et al (2000) Intakes of fruits, vegetables, and related nutrients and the risk of non-Hodgkin's lymphoma among women. Cancer Epidemiol Biomarkers Prev 9:477–485

Zhang H, Trachootham D, Lu W et al (2008) Effective killing of Gleevec-resistant CML cells with T315I mutation by a natural compound PEITC through redox-mediated mechanism. Leukemia 22:1191–1199

Chapter 13
Skin Cancer Chemoprevention: Current Status and Future Potential

Imtiaz A. Siddiqui, Vaqar M. Adhami, and Hasan Mukhtar

Abstract Skin is an organ of vital importance; however, it is under intense and relentless physical and chemical stress that ultimately lead to many skin related disorders including cancer. With continuous increase in the incidence of skin cancer, currently advocated methods such as the use of sunscreens and wearing protective clothing have not proven useful in reversing this trend. Chemoprevention is one promising strategy where the process of carcinogenesis can be slowed or entirely stopped by the utilization of natural or synthetic agents. Chemoprevention is particularly suited for skin cancers because the skin is continuously exposed to ultraviolet radiations (UVR) from the sun that cause DNA damage and genetic mutations that subsequently lead to skin cancer. In this article, we provide a brief overview on the skin cancer chemopreventive potential and mechanism of action of tested natural and synthetic agents. Many of these agents are present in daily diet and are supplemented or topically applied against prevention of various stages of skin cancer. Use of already advocated strategies in combination with chemoprevention could be an effective strategy to reduce the incidence of skin cancer.

13.1 Introduction

Skin is an extremely important organ because of the fact that in an adult human it covers an enormous surface area of 1.5–2.0 m^2 and it is the most accessible organ to environmental contaminants and thus is constantly exposed to a variety of physical and chemical insults (Leiter and Garbe 2008; Green et al. 1999a). It is universally accepted that the process of skin carcinogenesis is multi-step and is comprised of initiation, promotion and progression where ultraviolet (UV) radiations from the sun and environmental toxins are considered to play major roles (Agarwal and Mukhtar 1996; Yuspa et al. 1996; Leiter and Garbe 2008). For human skin cancer the major etiologic factor is chronic exposure UV radiation. UV radiations is subdivided into ultraviolet-A(UVA) (315–400 nm), ultraviolet-B (UVB) (280–315 nm) and ultraviolet-C (UVC) (100–280 nm) with 90–98% of solar UV

H. Mukhtar (✉)
Department of Dermatology, University of Wisconsin-Madison, Madison, WI 53706, USA
e-mail: hmukhtar@wisc.edu

F.H. Sarkar (ed.), *Nutraceuticals and Cancer*, DOI 10.1007/978-94-007-2630-7_13,

reaching the earth being UVA. Since UVC does not reach the earth the causative UV radiations responsible for human skin cancers are UVA and UVB. One study indicated that 65–90% of melanomas are attributable to UV radiations (Glanz et al. 2007) with several studies indicating a positive correlation of UV radiation and skin cancer. UV exposure, particularly the UVB can cause a marked sunburn reaction that leads to severe edema and blistering of the skin (Kornhauser et al. 2009; Suh et al. 2007) while the chronic exposure results in premature skin aging, wrinkling, alterations in immune response and cancer (Situm et al. 2008; Gonzaga 2009; Adhami et al. 2008; Katiyar 2007). The damaging effects of UV on the skin are thought to be caused by direct cellular damage and alterations in immunologic function. UV produces DNA damage in the form of cyclobutane pyrimidine dimers, gene mutations, immunosuppression, oxidative stress and inflammation, all of which are thought to have important roles in photoaging of skin and skin cancer (Meeran et al. 2008). The American Academy of Dermatology advocates use of sunscreens and protective clothing to protect against UV associated damage however it has not resulted in significant protection against the growing incidence of skin cancers. It is also thought that certain xenobiotics such as industrial chemicals, arsenic, pesticides, cigarette smoke or pollutants also contribute to increasing episodes of skin related occupational health problems and skin cancer (Rockley et al. 1994a, b).

According to WHO, the incidence of both non-melanoma and melanoma skin cancers has been increasing over the past decades. Currently, between 2 and 3 million non-melanoma skin cancers and 132,000 melanoma skin cancers occur globally each year (Katiyar 2011) and http://www.who.int/uv/faq/skincancer/en/index1.html. One in every three cancers diagnosed is a skin cancer and, according to Skin Cancer Foundation Statistics, one in every five Americans will develop skin cancer in their lifetime. In the United States skin cancer is the most common malignancy with >1 million new cases of non-melanoma skin cancer (NMSC), predominantly basal cell carcinoma (BCC) and squamous cell carcinoma (SCC) identified each year (Bailey et al. 2010; Jemal et al. 2010). NMSC poses a significant public health concern despite the fact that it is associated with low mortality as compared to other malignancies. The most important risk factor for NMSC is chronic exposure to solar UV radiations (Bailey et al. 2010; Jemal et al. 2010). BCC and SCC are usually found in sun exposed areas like head and neck regions and are positively related to amount of UV received and inversely proportional to the degree of skin pigmentation (Suarez et al. 2007; Narayanan et al. 2010).

Current preventive methods against UV radiation are to wear protective clothing to limit UV exposure, use of sunscreens with good sun protection factor (SPF) and avoiding sun and tanning beds. Although these factors are absolutely important but none of these have been able to reverse the trend mostly due to the fact that their practical compliance is always a problem. Novel strategies are thus urgently required to prevent UV radiation associated skin cancer because of the increasing incidence of patients suffering from this disease throughout the world.

13.2 Concept of Chemoprevention

The skin is known to possess an elaborate antioxidant defense system to protect itself from the deleterious effects of oxidative stress (McCullough and Kelly 2006; Pugliese 1998; Kohen 1999). An excessive exposure to reactive oxygen species could shift the prooxidant–antioxidant balance of skin toward a more oxidative state. Under these circumstances, exogenous supplementation of the antioxidants through natural or synthetic source may provide protection against skin cancer (Katiyar 2007; Adhami et al. 2008; Kornhauser et al. 2009; Agarwal and Mukhtar 1996; Ren and Lien 1997; Pezzuto 1997; Baliga and Katiyar 2006). This exogenous supplementation is often achieved by '*chemoprevention*'. Chemoprevention by definition *is the use of one or more synthetic or dietary entities to prevent the initiation of premalignant lesions or their progression to cancer* (Surh 2003; Russo 2007; Siddiqui et al. 2007; Adhami et al. 2003b). However, we define chemoprevention as slowing the process of carcinogenesis. This approach is promising because the therapy and surgery have not been fully effective against the high incidence or low survival rate of most of the cancer types (Surh 2003; Russo 2007; Siddiqui et al. 2007; Adhami et al. 2003b). Chemoprevention via the use of synthetic and naturally occurring non-toxic agents has emerged as a conceivable approach of cancer management (Surh 2003; Siddiqui et al. 2008). Among many diversified chemopreventive agents known for human cancer risk reduction, bioactive food components are most practical and hold extreme potential mostly due to their low toxicity and relative safety (Pezzuto 1997; Cragg and Suffness 1988; Wang 1998; Dragsted et al. 1993; Ames 1983; Surh 2003; Russo 2007; Khan and Mukhtar 2007; Adhami et al. 2003b). Furthermore, this approach appears to have practical implications in reducing cancer risk because unlike the carcinogenic factors that are difficult to control, individuals can easily modify their choice for the food and beverage they consume or utilize the synthetic agents for a better life.

At present several agents with proven cancer chemopreventive effects are known, many of which may have practical implications in reducing cancer incidence in individuals at high risk (Khan et al. 2006; Ren and Lien 1997; Pezzuto 1997; Cragg and Suffness 1988; Wang 1998; Dragsted et al. 1993; Ames 1983; Surh 2003; Russo 2007; Khan and Mukhtar 2007; Adhami et al. 2003b). Most of the experimental studies conducted in the last four decades have suggested that plant derived products are the most acceptable and promising agents that could inhibit or delay various types of cancers (Bode and Dong 2009). This information is also supported by the fact that epidemiological studies also suggest that consumption of fresh fruits and yellow-green vegetables reduce the cancer incidence and mortality (Amin et al. 2009; Bode and Dong 2009; Greenwald 2004). Some of the well-identified chemopreventive agents, in addition to possessing preventive effects, are also showing therapeutic potential and often they enhance the therapeutic efficacy of established chemotherapeutic agents. One misconception about chemoprevention is the concept of complete prevention of cancer, an unachievable goal. Since the process of cancer development is 'carcinogenesis' we believe that our aim should be to prevent carcinogenesis and not cancer. We, therefore, define chemoprevention as 'slowing the process of carcinogenesis', a goal that can be met.

13.2.1 Synthetic Agents for Skin Cancer Chemoprevention

13.2.1.1 Sunscreens

Sunscreens are chemicals that absorb UV radiation and attenuate the amount and nature of UV radiation reaching viable cells in the skin. They were originally developed to minimize erythema (Dennis et al. 2003). Chemical sunscreens act by filtering UV transmission to the epidermis and dermis of skin (Wolf 2003). The effectiveness of a topical sunscreen is assessed by its effectiveness in preventing acute erythema (sunburn), which is caused by solar radiation. This effectiveness is measured in the SPF of a sunscreen which is an experimentally derived number. SPF is not an amount of protection per se. Rather, it indicates how long it will take for UVB rays to redden skin when using a sunscreen, compared to how long skin would take to redden without the product. Overall the effectiveness of sunscreens is based on two different mechanisms of action, either the absorption of photons, or scattering of photons through physical reflection (Fourtanier et al. 2008; Moyal and Fourtanier 2008; Heenen 1999). The most widely used photon absorbing agents are para-aminobenzoic acid (PABA), PABA esters, benzophenones, dibenzomethanes, salicylates and cinnamates (Elmets and Anderson 1996). The other types of sunscreen are based on photon blocking agents such as zinc oxide, titanium dioxide and calamine. There have been numerous studies on prevention of skin cancers through sunscreen use (Bouknight et al. 2010; Diffey 2009; Fallon and Murphy 2009; Bens 2008). In a study it was concluded that regular use of sunscreens prevents the development of solar keratoses and, by implication, possibly reduces the risk of skin cancer in the long term (Thompson et al. 1993). In another study, using a mathematical model based on epidemiologic data, Stern et al. quantified the potential benefits of using a sunscreen with a sun protective factor of 15 and concluded that regular use of such a sunscreen during the first 18 years of life reduces the lifetime incidence of these tumors by 78%. The study further concluded that sunscreen use during childhood reduced the risk of sunburn, retarded the pace of skin aging, and possibly reduced melanoma risk (Stern et al. 1986). In a study, the authors observed that regular application of sunscreen has prolonged preventive effects on SCC but with no clear benefit in reducing BCC (van der Pols et al. 2006). A randomized controlled trial was performed with daily sunscreen application and beta carotene supplementation and this study concluded that there was no harmful effect of daily use of sunscreen. Cutaneous SCC, but not BCC seems to be amenable to prevention through the routine use of sunscreen by adults for 4.5 years. There was no beneficial or harmful effect on the rates of either type of skin cancer, as a result of beta carotene supplementation (Green et al. 1999b).

Despite these positive correlations of sunscreens, conflicting reports include claims that sunscreen increases risk for melanoma. The current major issue surrounding sunscreens involves their ability to prevent other potential deleterious effects of UV radiation on the skin (Vainio and Bianchini 2000). An international workshop of leading cancer scientists on the use of sunscreens and sun protection was held at the International Agency for Research on Cancer (IARC) in Lyon to evaluate the effectiveness of sunscreens in preventing skin cancer, and produced public health advice (Vainio et al. 2000). The workshop concluded that sunscreens prevent sunburns and do have the capacity to reduce squamous-cell carcinoma, however no conclusions were drawn regarding melanoma and basal-cell carcinoma. The picture seems different in cases of intentional exposure to sun, when the use of sunscreen does not seem to affect the occurrence of sunburn (Autier et al. 1999; Epstein 2006). Several epidemiologic studies have also reported moderately increased risks of cutaneous melanoma and basal-cell carcinoma in association with the use of sunscreens (Vainio et al. 2000), a result suggesting that sunscreen use could be a risk factor, rather than a protective factor. Nonetheless the use of sunscreens to provide protection from adverse effects of solar, in particular UV radiation is considered an effective strategy for prevention against skin cancer (Ulrich et al. 2008; Wolf 2003; Rigel 2002; Wolf et al. 2001). Although sunscreen use does not fit within strict definition of chemoprevention, but to our thinking it is chemoprevention because sunscreen is nothing but topically applied chemicals.

13.2.1.2 Antioxidant Vitamins

Antioxidants could be considered to act as potential anticarcinogens at multiple stages of skin carcinogenesis because of the fact that reactive oxygen species have been implicated in variety of disorders that mostly lead to skin diseases. These antioxidant agents are mostly vitamins that are present in the daily diet in the green and yellow vegetables and fruits (Singh and Lippman 1998a, b; Keller and Fenske 1998). These comprise of α- and β-carotene, lutein, lycopene, zeaxanthium, β-cryptoxanthin, etc. These agents are also available as synthetic analogs and have been tested in several models of mouse skin cancer. Number of laboratory studies has suggested that β-carotene may protect against UVB- and chemically-induced carcinogenesis in murine models of skin cancer (Savoure et al. 1995, 1996; Katsumura et al. 1996; Jones et al. 1994). However, studies conducted in humans are debatable in exhibiting protective or potentially harmful role in human skin (Biesalski and Obermueller-Jevic 2001).

Another potent antioxidant is vitamin C that has generated interest as a potential cancer preventive compound (D'Agostini et al. 2005; Berton et al. 1996; Pauling 1991; Pauling et al. 1982). Topical application of ascorbic acid and ascorbyl palmitate leads to inhibition of TPA-induced ODC activity, DNA synthesis and tumor promotion in mouse skin (Smart and Crawford 1991). In a recent study, a stable topical formulation of 15% L-ascorbic acid, 1% alpha-tocopherol, and 0.5% ferulic acid (CEFer) provided substantial UV photoprotection for skin. It was found to be particularly effective for reducing thymine dimer mutations known to be associated with skin cancer (Murray et al. 2008). These studies are consistent with epidemiological data where a correlation between low dietary levels of vitamin C and skin cancer has been observed (Dreher and Maibach 2001). A study from this laboratory has demonstrated that addition of vitamin C to biomelanin antioxidants result in significant inhibition in the generation of in vitro lipid peroxides (Kalka et al. 2000). Numbers of studies have also shown that topical application of vitamin E protects against acute and chronic photodamage and tumor formation in UVB-induced and chemical skin carcinogenesis models (Burke et al. 2000, 2003; Perchellet et al. 1987). Studies have also suggested that vitamin E may act as effective sunscreen in vivo that inhibits cyclobutane pyrimidine dimmer (CPD) formation in p53 gene as a consequence of UV irradiation (Chen et al. 1997).

13.2.1.3 Vitamin D

An organic compound, Vitamin D is fat-soluble (meaning some dietary fat is necessary for its absorption). Humans obtain Vitamin D through the diet and by synthesis in the skin upon exposure to ultraviolet B. Vitamin D are then converted by the liver to 25-hydroxyvitamin D, its major circulating form. Under the influence of parathyroid hormone, the kidney then converts 25-hydroxyvitamin D to 1,25-dihydroxyvitamin D, the biologically active, hormonal form of the nutrient which is expressed in bones and various cells in the skin (Shahriari et al. 2010). In addition, many cell types convert circulating 25-hydroxyvitamin D to 1,25-dihydroxyvitamin D for local use. This metabolite has been shown to exert potent effects on cellular differentiation, cellular proliferation, and immune regulation. It is theorized that by these mechanisms vitamin D and its analogues are effective treatment options for psoriasis and other skin diseases (Shahriari et al. 2010). Insufficient vitamin D nutritional status has been associated with a host of other diseases, most notably cancer. There is evidence that supplementation with vitamin D reduces the overall incidence of cancer, although current evidence is insufficient to prove a causative effect. Sunscreen use blocks the ability of the skin to photosynthesize vitamin D, although the effect this has on the vitamin D status of the general population is unclear (Shahriari et al. 2010). Vitamin D3 is effective in the treatment of nontumor hyper-proliferation skin disease, psoriasis (van De Kerkhof 2001). Topical application of vitamin D analogs for treating skin cancer has been controversial and is hampered due to its toxicity (Reichrath 2001). However, the combined application of vitamin D analog with retinoids and other biological active compounds such as cytokines and growth factors appears to be more beneficial (Carlberg and Saurat 1996).

13.2.1.4 Retinoids

Vitamin A, its physiologic metabolites, and synthetic derivatives (retinoids) have been shown to have protective effects against the development of certain types of cancer (Niles 2000). In addition, pharmacologic amounts of retinoids have been used with some success in the treatment of a few human tumors. The chemoprevention effect of retinoids is most likely exerted at the tumor-promotion phase of carcinogenesis. Retinoids have been assessed to block tumor promotion by inhibiting proliferation, inducing apoptosis, inducing differentiation, or a combination of these actions (Niles 2000). Retinoids suppress transformation of cells in vitro and inhibit carcinogenesis in various organs in animal models including in mouse skin carcinogenesis model (Lotan 1996; Niles 2000). Retinoids are known to block skin tumor promotion by inhibiting proliferation, causing apoptosis and inducing differentiation (Hansen et al. 2000; Niles 2000). Supplementation of retinoids in the diet reduces COX-2 expression and PGE(2) biosynthesis and inhibits papilloma and carcinoma formation in DMBA–TPA-promoted murine skin carcinogenesis model (Kanekura et al. 2000). Recent microarray analyses of the chemopreventive effect of all-trans retinoic acid (ATRA), one of the primary naturally occurring biologically active retinoids, in the two-stage mouse skin chemical carcinogenesis model have provided novel insight into their action. Comparison of the gene expression profiles of control skin and skin subjected to the two-stage protocol for 3 wk, with or without ATRA, has shown that approximately half of the genes regulated by 12-o-tetradecanoylphorbol-13-acetate (TPA) are oppositely regulated when ATRA is co-administered with TPA. It was further shown the Raf/Mek/Erk branch of mitogen-activated protein (MAP) kinase pathway contains a disproportionate number of oppositely regulated genes, thereby implicating it as one of the key pathways involved in tumor promotion by TPA, which is blocked by ATRA (Cheepala et al. 2007). In another study Mrass et al. observed that retinoic acid increased the expression of p53 and proapoptotic caspases and sensitized keratinocytes to apoptosis (Mrass et al. 2004). Two chemoprevention randomized clinical trials were begun in 1984 to evaluate retinoids in the prevention of skin cancers. Moderate risk subjects with a history of at least 10 actinic keratoses and at most two prior skin cancers were enrolled in the SKICAP-AK trial and randomized to 25,000 IU retinol or placebo daily for 5 years. High risk subjects with a history of at least four prior skin cancers were enrolled in the SKICAP-S/B trial and randomized to receive 25,000 IU retinol, 5–10 mg isotretinoin or placebo daily for 3 years. Data from the SKICAP-AK trial indicate that retinol reduces incidence of first new squamous cell skin cancers but had no effect on the incidence of first new basal cell skin cancer. The effect of retinoids had no significant benefit on squamous or basal cell skin cancers in the high risk subjects on the SKICAP-S/B trial, although intervention duration was less than planned. Daily retinol was effective in preventing squamous cell cancers in moderate risk subjects.

13.2.1.5 Other Agents

Oral or topical application of α-difluoromethylornithine (DFMO), an irreversible inhibitor of ODC has been demonstrated to suppress UVB-induced and chemical skin carcinogenesis in murine models (Lan et al. 2000; Einspahr et al. 2003; Fischer et al. 2001, 2003). Studies have also demonstrated that inhibition of ODC by DFMO in turn reduces tumor vascularization and epidermal carcinogenesis in transgenic mouse models of skin cancer (Arbeit et al. 1999; Lan et al. 2000). Our laboratory has demonstrated that oral consumption of DFMO to ODC transgenic mice results in complete prevention of UVB-mediated tumorigenesis and substantial decrease in the formation of pigmented cysts (Ahmad et al. 2001b). Based on our data we suggested supplementing of human skin care products with inhibitors of ODC preferably DFMO. Our observations are supported by various human clinical trials conducted with DFMO which have shown encouraging results for skin cancer prevention (Einspahr et al. 2003; Bailey et al. 2010; Einspahr et al. 2002; Alberts et al. 2000). Both COX-2 specific (celecoxib) and non-specific (indomethacin and iboprufen) inhibitors have been shown to possess protective effects against UVB mediated cutaneous inflammation and reduction in tumor yield in murine models (Fischer et al. 1999; Pentland et al. 1999; Wilgus et al. 2000). Specific inhibitors of COX-2 have been shown to reduce UVB-mediated inflammation including edema, dermal neutrophil infilteration, prostaglandin E2 levels and formation of sunburn cells (Kochevar et al. 1993; Muller-Decker et al. 1998). Almost similar results were observed with lipoxygenase inhibitor TMK688, which significantly inhibited different inflammatory mediators in both UVB-induced and murine models of chemical skin carcinogenesis (Jiang et al. 1994, 1996; Kochevar et al. 1993). A recent study evaluated the efficacy and safety of celecoxib, a COX-2 inhibitor, as a chemopreventive agent for actinic keratoses, the premalignant precursor of nonmelanoma skin cancers. In this double-blind placebo-controlled randomized trial involving 240, patients were randomly assigned to receive 200 mg of celecoxib or placebo administered orally twice daily for 9 months. There was no difference in the incidence of actinic keratoses between the two groups at 9 months after randomization. However, at 11 months after randomization, there were fewer nonmelanoma skin cancers in the celecoxib arm than in the placebo arm. After adjusting for age, sex, Fitzpatrick skin type, history of actinic keratosis at randomization, nonmelanoma skin cancer history, and patient time on study, the number of nonmelanoma skin cancers was lower in the celecoxib arm than in the placebo arm. The study concluded that Celecoxib may be effective for prevention of SCCs and BCCs in individuals who have extensive actinic damage and are at high risk for development of nonmelanoma skin cancers (Elmets et al. 2010).

Selenium, a dietary trace mineral has been a surge of interest because of its demonstrated anti-carcinogenic and anti-inflammatory properties (Brown and Arthur 2001). Dietary selenium is known to protect skin against UV-induced damage and cancer and its topical application improves skin surface parameters in humans, while selenium deficiency compromises protective antioxidant enzymes in skin. Furthermore, skin and hair abnormalities in humans and rodents may be caused by selenium deficiency, which are overcome by dietary selenium supplementation (Sengupta et al. 2010). A recent study concluded that 5-chloroacetyl-2-piperidino-1,3-selenazole (CS1), a novel selenium-containing compound, could be a useful candidate for the treatment of skin hyperpigmentation (Lee et al. 2010). Selenium was also found to inhibit the metastasis of murine melanoma cells through the induction of cell cycle arrest and cell death (Song et al. 2009). A study concluded that PBISe, a novel selenium-containing drug is a potent chemotherapeutic agent with novel properties enabling the targeting of iNOS, Akt3, and MAPK signaling, thereby promoting melanoma cell apoptosis and inhibition of proliferation (Madhunapantula et al. 2008). Studies have also suggested that dietary supplementation and topical application of selenium dramatically reduces the induction and growth of UVB- and chemically-induced skin tumors in mice (Bansal and Gupta 1988; Overvad et al. 1985).

13.2.2 Natural Agents for Skin Cancer Chemoprevention

Studies from ours and other laboratories worldwide have shown that bioactive food components afford protection against the development of skin cancer, both under in vitro as well as in vivo situations (Sharma and Katiyar 2010; Mehta et al. 2010; Robbins et al. 2010; Afaq and Mukhtar 2006; Khan et al. 2008; Sarfaraz et al. 2008). Utilization of bioactive food components in reducing skin-cancer risk appears to have practical implications because unlike the carcinogenic environmental factors that are difficult to control, individuals can modify their lifestyle by modifying dietary habits and use of skin care products.

13.2.2.1 Green Tea Polyphenols

Tea, made from the leaves of *Camellia sinensis*, an evergreen shrub of the Theaceae family, is a beverage of choice in many countries around the world (Siddiqui et al. 2007). Tea contains several polyphenolic components, which are antioxidant in nature, and many studies have shown that tea polyphenols possess the ability to prevent oxidant-induced cellular damage (Yamamoto et al. 2003; Chung et al. 2003a). In recent years, studies from ours and many laboratories around the world, conducted in various organ specific animal bioassay systems, have shown that tea and its polyphenolic constituents are capable of affording protection against a variety of cancer types (Siddiqui et al. 2006; Surh 2003; Chung et al. 2003a; Yamamoto et al. 2003). Although majority of the studies conducted have used green tea, a limited number of studies have also shown the anti-cancer efficacy of black tea. The polyphenolic catechins, which are the major antioxidants present in green tea are thought to be responsible for its chemopreventive potential (Siddiqui et al. 2004, 2009). Studies have shown that the antioxidant activity of green tea polyphenol EGCG is much higher than the well-known antioxidants viz. vitamin E and vitamin C (Rice-Evans et al. 1995; Ahmad and Mukhtar 2001). Since the first study suggesting that green tea might have preventive effects against UV-induced skin cancers, tea has come a long way to demonstrate its efficacy (Wang et al. 1991). We, in one of the first studies demonstrated that there is a significant protection by green tea polyphenols against skin tumorigenicity in a complete two-stage skin tumorigenesis protocol (Wang et al. 1989). Later EGCG was shown to inhibit the binding of ^{3}H-labelled polycyclic aromatic hydrocarbons to epidermal DNA. In sencar mice, the application of EGCG before DMBA also resulted in significant reduction both in the percentage of mice with tumors and the number of tumors per mouse (Katiyar et al. 1992).

Exposure to UV radiation is the most important risk factor for the development of skin cancer (LeBlanc et al. 2008). Researchers from laboratories worldwide have demonstrated the usefulness of green tea against UV-induced carcinogenesis. Numerous studies indicate that green tea has multiple biological effects that ameliorate the damaging effects of ultraviolet radiation. It is effective through topical application on the skin as well as through oral administration in drinking water. In a study that used brewed green tea as the sole source of drinking fluid during UVB- or DMBA-initiated and UVB-or TPA-promoted carcinogenesis, brewed green tea at concentrations similar to human consumption, significantly inhibited UVB- or TPA-induced tumorigenesis (Wang et al. 1992b). Another study demonstrated that oral administration of green tea to mice not only inhibited skin tumorigenesis but also reduced fatty tissues in the dermis (Conney et al. 2002). Oral administration or intraperitoneal injection of GTP inhibited the growth of UV-induced skin papillomas (Wang et al. 1992c) or TPA-induced cyclooxygenase 2 in rodent models (Kundu et al. 2003). Conney et al. (1999) have reported that oral administration of green tea, black tea, or EGCG inhibited the growth of well-established skin tumors and, in some cases also resulted in a tumor regression. When black tea was administered to papilloma-bearing mice, a complete regression was observed and the growth of nonmalignant tumors, squamous cell carcinomas and tumor volume decreased significantly. Oral administration of GTP reduced UVB-induced skin tumor incidence, tumor multiplicity, and tumor growth in SKH-1 mice. There was also reduced expression of the matrix metalloproteinases (MMP)-2 and MMP-9, CD31, vascular endothelial growth factor (VEGF), and proliferating cell nuclear antigen (PCNA) in the GTP-treated group. Additionally, there were more cytotoxic CD8(+)T cells and greater activation of caspase-3 in the tumors of the GTP group, indicating the apoptotic death of the tumor cells (Mantena et al. 2005). This laboratory has also demonstrated that topical application of green tea polyphenols resulted in a significant decrease in UVB-induced skin thickness, skin edema, infiltration of leukocytes, and inhibition of MAPK and NFκB pathways in SKH-1 hairless mice (Afaq et al. 2003b). EGCG treatment was also observed to induce a dose-dependent decrease in the viability and growth of A-375 amelanotic malignant melanoma and Hs-294T metastatic melanoma cell lines (Nihal et al. 2005).

Green tea and its individual constituents have been demonstrated to protect against many of the other damaging effects of UV radiation. Both systemic and topical administration of GTP and EGCG were demonstrated to protect against the UV-induced sunburn response (Katiyar et al. 1999a), immunosuppression, (Katiyar et al. 1995a, 1999a) and photoaging of the skin (Wang et al. 1992a). Direct examination of UV-irradiated skin that had been pretreated in vivo with topical EGCG reduced the number of apoptotic keratinocytes as detected by TUNEL staining (Chung et al. 2003b; Elmets et al. 2001). The in vivo observations are supported by in vitro studies in which cultured normal human keratinocytes were exposed to UVB radiation (Xia et al. 2005). In contrast to its effect on normal keratinocytes, EGCG is known to stimulate apoptosis in UV-induced pre-malignant papillomas and invasive squamous cell carcinomas (Chen et al. 1998; Chung et al. 2003b). GTP is also shown to inhibit UVB-induced markers of oxidative stress in vivo, when applied topically or given orally, pretreatment with EGCG or GTP before UVB radiation protects against depletion of glutathione and catalase, decreases UV-induced lipid peroxidation and inhibits UVB-induced protein oxidation (Vayalil et al. 2004). EGCG is also shown to protect against UV-induced oxidative stress in humans. When it was applied to the skin just before exposure to a 4x minimal erythema dose (MED) of UVB radiation, EGCG significantly decreased the production of hydrogen peroxide and nitric oxide production as well as lipid peroxidation in the dermis and epidermis (Katiyar et al. 2001b). In an in vitro study using cultured human cells (lung fibroblasts, skin fibroblasts, and epidermal keratinocytes), EGCG resulted in a dose-dependent reduction in UV-induced DNA damage (Morley et al. 2005). Green tea polyphenols also significantly inhibited the UVB-induced DNA damage when applied topically to the mouse epidermis, using a ^{32}P post-labeling technique (Chatterjee et al. 1996). Studies have also demonstrated that oral administration of green tea to SKH-1 hairless mice enhanced UV-induced increases in the number of p53- and p21/WAF1-positive cells in the epidermis following UV exposure (Lu et al. 2000) suggesting that the photo protective effect of green tea on UV-induced carcinogenesis may be mediated through stimulation of UV-induced increases in the levels of p53 and p21/WAF1. EGCG was also shown to selectively decrease both proliferation and survival of primary cultures of ODC overexpressing transgenic keratinocytes but not keratinocytes from normal littermates or ras-infected keratinocytes (Paul et al. 2005).

Studies conducted in our laboratory and in many other laboratories around the world have shown the chemopreventive potential of antioxidant polyphenols present in green tea against skin cancer development in various types of protocols employed in mouse skin (Nihal et al. 2005; Lu et al. 2002; Wang et al. 1994; Khan et al. 1988). It is important to mention that the cancer chemopreventive properties of green tea was first demonstrated from our laboratory in a protocol where initiation accomplished by topical application of (+/—)-7 beta, 8 alpha-dihydroxy-9 alpha, 10 alpha-epoxy-7,8,9,10-tetrahydrobenzo[a]pyrene (BPDE-2) and promotion accomplished by 12-O-tetradecanoyl phorbol-13-acetate (TPA) in SENCAR mouse model of chemical carcinogenesis (Khan et al. 1988). Subsequent studies from our laboratory and elsewhere have shown the anti-tumor potential of green tea in several other models of skin cancer. Further studies have suggested that topical application of GTP significantly protects against TPA-induced hyperplasia in the ear skin, neutrophil infiltration as well as malignant conversion of chemically-induced benign skin papillomas to squamous cell carcinoma in SENCAR mice (Conney et al. 1992; Agarwal et al. 1992; Katiyar et al. 1993). In many mouse skin tumor models, the topical application or oral consumption of GTP was shown to afford protection against UVB-induced skin carcinogenesis and inflammatory responses (Kim et al. 2001; Katiyar et al. 2001a; Record and Dreosti 1998; Katiyar and Mukhtar 2001). Topical application of GTP on mouse skin prior to UV exposure also resulted in a decreased UV-induced (i) hyperplastic response, (ii) myeloperoxidase activity, (iii) infiltration of inflammatory leukocytes and (iv) inhibition of the contact hypersensitivity response (Katiyar et al. 1995a; Katiyar and Mukhtar 2001). Studies have shown that oral feeding of GTP to SKH-1 hairless mice as a sole source of drinking fluid resulted in significant inhibition of UV-related skin tumors (Agarwal et al. 1993; Conney et al. 1992). Studies have suggested that UVB radiation mediated modulation of cytokines may play key role in UVB-responses including photocarcinogenesis (Halliday et al. 1998; Katiyar et al. 1995b, 1999a). Studies from our laboratory have demonstrated the relevance of the extensive in vitro and in vivo laboratory data showing the preventive effects of GTP against UV radiation-mediated damages to humans (Katiyar et al. 1999b, 2000, 2001b). In another study from this laboratory, we evaluated the effect of topical application of GTP against UV light-induced DNA damage in the form of CPDs in the human skin (Katiyar et al. 2000). DNA damage in the form of CPDs is a critical event in tumor initiating activity of UV radiation. GTP treatment was found to inhibit UVB-induced erythema response as well as CPD formation in skin (Katiyar et al. 2000). The inhibition of UVB-induced CPDs by GTP treatment may be, at least in part, responsible for the inhibition of photocarcinogenesis.

A recent study evaluated the GTP mediated induction of IL-12 and DNA repair in human cells. In this study KB cells and normal human keratinocytes were exposed to GTP 5 h before and after UVB treatment. UVB-induced apoptosis was reduced in UVB-exposed cells treated with GTP and GTP was also found to induce the secretion of IL-12 in keratinocytes. The reduction in UV-induced cell death by GTP was almost completely reversed upon addition of an anti-IL-12-antibody, indicating that the reduction of UV-induced cell death by GTP is mediated via IL-12 (Schwarz et al. 2008). A recent study by Kundu et al. suggested that EGCG inhibits TPA-induced DNA binding of NF-kappaB and CREB by blocking activation of p38 MAPK, which may provide a molecular basis of COX-2 inhibition by EGCG in mouse skin in vivo (Kundu and Surh 2007). We also demonstrated that EGCG protects against the adverse effects of UV radiation via modulations in NF-kappaB pathway, and provided a molecular basis for the photochemopreventive effect of EGCG (Afaq et al. 2003a). UV radiation induced infiltrating leukocytes, depletion of antigen-presenting cells, and oxidative stress in the skin play an important role in the induction of immune suppression and photocarcinogenesis. We demonstrated that EGCG treatment to mouse skin prevents UVB-induced infiltration of leukocytes, depletion of antigen-presenting cells, and oxidative stress (Katiyar and Mukhtar 2001). We also demonstrated that EGCG has the potential to inhibit UVB-induced oxidative stress-mediated phosphorylation of MAPK signaling pathways, suggesting that EGCG could be useful in attenuation of oxidative stress-mediated and MAPK-caused skin disorders in humans (Katiyar et al. 2001a).

13.2.2.2 Resveratrol

Resveratrol (trans-3, 5,4-trihydroxystilbene), a naturally occurring polyphenolic compound with strong antioxidant properties, is abundantly found in grapes, berries, nuts and red wine (Jang et al. 1997; Aziz et al. 2005). The cancer chemopreventive property of resveratrol was first reported in 1997, by Jang et al. (Jang et al. 1997), when the authors demonstrated that resveratrol possesses antimutagenic and anticarcinogenic effects and can effectively block all the three stages of carcinogenesis. This study demonstrated that resveratrol acts as an antioxidant and anti-mutagen and induces phase II drug-metabolizing enzymes (anti-initiation activity). In addition, resveratrol was found to mediate anti-inflammatory effects and inhibited cyclooxygenase and hydroperoxidase functions (anti-promotion activity), and it also induced the differentiation of human promyelocytic leukemia cell (anti-progression activity). Following this important study by Jang et al., other studies evaluated and established the cancer chemopreventive and/or therapeutic potential of resveratrol (Baur and Sinclair 2006; Shankar et al. 2007; Delmas et al. 2006; Aziz et al. 2005). Another study suggested that resveratrol inhibits tumorigenesis in mouse skin through interference with pathways of reactive oxidants and possibly by modulating the expression of c-fos and TGF-beta1. In this study, the application of TPA to mouse skin resulted in significant generation of H_2O_2, enhanced levels of myeloperoxidase and oxidized glutathione reductase activities, and decrease in glutathione levels and superoxide dismutase activity. A pre-treatment of skin with resveratrol resulted in reversal of these effects (Jang and Pezzuto 1998). A published study from this laboratory (Ahmad et al. 2001a) has shown that resveratrol treatment of human epidermoid carcinoma A431 cells resulted in inhibition of cell growth, G(1)-phase arrest of the cell cycle and induction of apoptosis. Later, we demonstrated the involvement of the pRb-E2F/DP pathway as an important contributor of resveratrol-mediated cell cycle arrest and apoptosis (Adhami et al. 2001). Consistently She et al. demonstrated that resveratrol induced activation of p53 and apoptosis is mediated by extracellular-signal-regulated protein kinases and p38 kinase in a mouse JB6 epidermal cell line (She et al. 2001).

Adhami et al. demonstrated that in the normal human epidermal keratinocytes, resveratrol blocks UVB-mediated activation of NF-kappaB in a dose-dependent as well as time-dependent fashion (Adhami et al. 2003a). This study further showed that resveratrol treatment of keratinocytes inhibits UVB-mediated phosphorylation and degradation of IkappaBalpha, and activation of IKKalpha. In another study, topical application of resveratrol was observed to result in significant decrease in UVB-induced bi-fold skin thickness, hyperplasia, and infiltration of leukocytes. The study further showed that multiple exposures to UVB radiations cause significant upregulation in: (i) proliferating cell nuclear antigen (PCNA), a marker of cellular proliferation, and (ii) cyclin-dependent kinase (cdk)-2, -4 and -6, cyclin-D1, and cyclin-D2. Resveratrol treatment resulted in significant downregulation in UV-mediated increases in these critical cell cycle regulatory proteins (Reagan-Shaw et al. 2004). An interesting observation of this study was that resveratrol treatment resulted in a further stimulation of UVB-mediated increases in cyclin kinase inhibitor WAF1/p21 and tumor suppressor p53. The result from a study (Seve et al. 2005) indicated that resveratrol potentiates the production of significant amounts of 8-oxo-7,8-dihydro-2′-deoxyguanosine in UVA-irradiated genomic DNA. Moreover, the combination of resveratrol with UVA significantly enhances the induction of DNA strand breaks and cell death in HaCaT keratinocytes. Roy et al. (2009) recently demonstrated that chemopreventive efficacy of resveratrol is reflected by delay in onset of tumorigenesis, reduced cumulative number of tumors, and reduction in tumor volume. This study also demonstrated that resveratrol treatment increased the DMBA suppressed p53 and Bax while decreased the expression of Bcl-2 and Survivin. Further, resveratrol supplementation resulted in release of cytochrome C, caspases activation, and increase in apoptotic protease-activating factor-1 (Apaf-1) as mechanism of apoptosis induction (Roy et al. 2009). In another study Yusuf et al. observed that resveratrol enhances cell-mediated immune response to DMBA through toll-like receptor4 and prevents DMBA induced cutaneous carcinogenesis (Yusuf et al. 2009).

13.2.2.3 Curcumin

Curcumin (diferuloylmethane), the naturally occurring yellow pigment in turmeric and curry, is isolated from the rhizomes of the plant *Curcuma longa Linn.* It has been extensively investigated for its cancer chemopreventive potential in many tumor model systems (Goel et al. 2008; Aggarwal et al. 2003; Huang et al. 1992; Azuine and Bhide 1992; Conney et al. 1991). Topical application of curcumin to mouse skin has been demonstrated to enhance glutathione content and glutathione-S-transferase activity and inhibits lipid peroxidation and arachidonic acid metabolism in mouse skin (Iersel et al. 1996). Further, topical application of curcumin has been shown to decrease the induction of ODC in mouse skin (Lu et al. 1993). Studies have also shown that curcumin exhibits anti-mutagenic activity in the Ames Salmonella test and possesses anti-carcinogenic activity as it inhibits chemically-induced neoplastic lesions in many organs including skin, probably via an antioxidant mechanism (Lu et al. 1993; Huang et al. 1991). The results from a recent study demonstrated the crucial role of PKC in TPA-mediated cellular responses in skin and this study further showed that curcumin modulates transmembrane signal transduction via PKC to affect TPA-induced biochemical and molecular alterations in mouse skin (Garg et al. 2008). In a recent study Iersel et al. demonstrated that curcumin was the most potent inhibitor of glutathione S-transferase, the major pi-class GST subunit P1 activity, towards 1-chloro-2,4-dinitrobenzene in intact human IGR-39 melanoma cells (Iersel et al. 1996). Curcumin has also been shown to decrease superoxide radical formation in normal human keratinocytes leading to lower levels of cytotoxic hydrogen peroxide, which could be proposed as an explanation for this protective effect against UV radiation (Kuttan et al. 1987). A previous study by Ishizaki et al. has demonstrated that UVA irradiation significantly enhanced ODC induction after topical application of TPA in the epidermis of CD-1 mice, and aggravated TPA-mediated dermatitis (Ishizaki et al. 1996). A pre-treatment of skin with curcumin was found to significantly inhibit these UVA-enhancing effects (Ishizaki et al. 1996). In another recent study by Jee et al. has shown that curcumin induces apoptosis in human BCC cells in a dose- and time- dependent manner where p53-associated signaling pathway is critically involved in curcumin-mediated apoptotic cell death (Jee et al. 1998). These studies suggest that curcumin may impart beneficial effect against the responses of UV radiation in skin and in vitro models of skin cancer. Curcumin supplemented cosmetics are sold in many parts of the world especially in India. More studies are needed to examine the effect of curcumin on photocarcinogenesis.

13.2.2.4 Diallyl Sulfide

Diallyl sulfide (DAS) is a naturally occurring compound present in garlic and onion, which is known to possess strong antioxidant potential (Adhami et al. 2008; Agarwal and Mukhtar 1996; Baliga and Katiyar 2006; Dragsted et al. 1993; Khan et al. 2008; Pezzuto 1997; Surh 2003; Wang 1998). Studies have indicated that DAS, diallyl disulfide and diallyl trisulfide has potential chemopreventive effects against variety of cancers including cancer of the skin. Initial studies by Perchellet et al. have shown inhibition of DMBA-induced mouse skin tumorigenesis by garlic oil and inhibition of two tumor-promotion stages by garlic and onion oils (Perchellet et al. 1986). A single 2-mg dose of garlic oil applied 30 min before a single carcinogenic dose of 7,12-dimethylbenz[a]-anthracene (DMBA) inhibited papilloma production in Sencar mice. This study further showed that onion and garlic oils inhibited the TPA-stimulated DNA synthesis when given as single doses of 5 mg 1 h before TPA. The stimulatory effects of these oils on epidermal GSH peroxidase activity were found to be concentration-dependent and long lasting. These oils completely abolished the prolonged inhibitory effect of TPA on this enzyme (Perchellet et al. 1986). Further, garlic oil significantly inhibited TPA-induced ODC activity in the same epidermal cell system and enhanced GSH peroxidase activity in the presence of various non-phorbol ester tumor promoters. Based on this study, it was suggested that some of the inhibitory effects of garlic and onion oils on skin tumor promotion may result from their enhancement of the natural GSH dependent antioxidant protective system of the epidermal cells. Studies have implicated DAS as a chemopreventive agent against a variety of cancer types including skin cancer. In a similar study by Sadhana et al., the authors observed that when garlic oil was topically applied during the initiation phase of benzo[a]pyrene (B(a)P)-induced skin carcinogenesis in random bred adult female Swiss albino mice of two different substrains, there was a decline in the number of tumor-bearing mice as well as in the mean number of tumors per effective mouse (Sadhana et al. 1988). In another study, Perchellet et al. showed that garlic oil and onion oils inhibited skin tumor-promotion in SENCAR mice (Perchellet et al. 1990). This study further revealed that garlic oil inhibited DMBA-induced mouse skin tumorigenesis. In a study from this laboratory we demonstrated that topical application of DAS resulted in an inhibition of benzoyl peroxide-mediated tumor promotion in 7,12-dimethylbenz(a)anthracene initiated skin of SENCAR mice (Athar et al. 1990). Dwivedi et al. in a study found that topical applications of DAS and diallyl disulfide to the skin of SENCAR mouse resulted in significant inhibition of DMBA-induced and TPA-promoted skin tumor formation (Dwivedi et al. 1992). Further, Singh & Shukla demonstrated that diallyl sulfide inhibits BaP- and DMBA-induced carcinogenesis (Singh and Shukla 1998a, b). Further studies from this group suggested that

DAS is a potential chemopreventive agent capable of modulating and regulating the tumor suppressor p53 along with its downstream effective molecule, p21/waf1 in 7,12-dimethylbenz[a]anthracene-induced skin tumors by diallyl sulfide in Swiss albino mice (Arora et al. 2004). In a recent study Nigam et al. demonstrated that DAS application results in a significant protection in DMBA-induced DNA strand breaks. Pre-treatment of DAS (10 mg/kg body-weight) showed 68.35% protection and post-treatment showed 59.49% protection, at an intermittent period of 48 h, against DMBA-induced DNA strand breakage (Nigam and Shukla 2007).

13.2.2.5 Silymarin

Silymarin a flavonoid extracted from the seeds of *Silybum marianum*, is a mixture of three structural isomers: silybinin, silydianin and silychristin. Amongst the three, silybinin is the most active component (Agarwal et al. 1994). We demonstrated silymarin as an antioxidant compound with skin cancer chemopreventive properties (Agarwal et al. 1994). In a study from this laboratory, Chatterjee et al., demonstrated that topical application of silymarin or green tea polyphenols as well as sunscreen containing ethylhexyl-pmethoxycinnamate resulted in a protection against UVB exposure-mediated formation of pyrimidine dimers in mouse skin (Chatterjee et al. 1996). In another study from our laboratory we evaluated the protective effects of silymarin against UVB radiation induced NMSC in mice in long-term and short-term studies (Katiyar et al. 1997). In this study, we utilized a three way approach and the female SKH-1 hairless mice were subjected to (i) UVB-induced tumor initiation followed by TPA-mediated tumor promotion, (ii) DMBA-induced tumor initiation followed by UVB-mediated tumor promotion, and (iii) UVB induced complete carcinogenesis. Silymarin was topically applied prior to UVB exposure, and its effects on tumor incidence, tumor multiplicity, and average tumor volume per mouse were recorded. This study demonstrated that in all the protocols employed, silymarin treatment was found to result in significant protection against skin tumorigenesis in the mice. Later, in short-term experiments, silymarin application was found to result in significant inhibition in UVB-induced (i) formation of sunburn and apoptotic cell, (ii) skin edema, (iii) depletion of catalase activity, and (iv) induction of COX and ODC activities and ODC mRNA expression (Zhao et al. 1999, 2000). These studies suggested that silymarin may provide protection against different stages of UVB-induced carcinogenesis, possibly via its antioxidant properties. As a mechanism of UV-induced photooxidative damage silymarin has shown ability to modulate the activation of the transcription factors nuclear factor kappa B (NF-kappaB) and activator protein-1 (AP-1) in HaCaT keratinocytes (Saliou et al. 1999). Silymarin was found to inhibit NF-kappaB activation induced by UV radiation in a dose-dependent manner in human keratinocytes (Saliou et al. 1999). These results indicated that silymarin can efficiently modulate the cellular response to UV through their selective action on NF-kappaB activation. In a study Gu et al. demonstrated that dietary feeding of silibinin affords strong protection against UVB-induced damages in skin epidermis possibly via silibinin-caused up-regulation of p53 and p21/cip1 as major UVB-damage control sensors (Gu et al. 2005). Studies from this group later suggested that silibinin prevents skin tumor promotion by inhibiting UVB- and EGF-induced mitogenic and cell survival signal involving both AP-1 and NF-kappaB (Singh et al. 2006). Recently in a study flavonolignans from *Silybum marianum* were observed to moderate UVA-induced oxidative damage to HaCaT keratinocytes (Svobodova et al. 2007). In this study, application of the flavonolignans (1–50 micromol/l) led to an increase in cell viability of irradiated (20 J/cm^2) HaCaT keratinocytes. The agents also suppressed intracellular ATP and GSH depletion, ROS production and peroxidation of membrane lipids. UVA-induced caspases-3 activity/activation was suppressed by treatment with the agents. Lower concentrations of the agents (10 micromol/l) were seen to significantly reduce cellular DNA single strand break formation. In a recent study performed in mouse skin, CD11b$^+$ cell population from UV-irradiated skin resulted in significantly higher production of ROS in both epidermis and dermis than CD11b$^-$ cell population, and silymarin was found to inhibit UV-induced oxidative stress through targeting infiltrating the CD11b$^+$ cell type in the skin.

13.2.2.6 Genistein

A soy-derived isoflavone (4-,5,7-Trihydroxyisoflavone) has attracted much attention and has been shown to possess antioxidant and anticarcinogenic effects for skin (Wei et al. 1993, 1995, 1998). Genistein treatment has been shown to suppress H_2O_2 production by TPA stimulated human polymorphonuclear leukocytes (PMNs) and HL-60 cells in a dose-dependent manner (Wei et al. 1993). In in vivo CD-1 mouse skin model, genistein strongly inhibited TPA-induced oxidant formation, edema, and PMN infiltration in mouse skin. It was suggested that inhibition of TPA-mediated H_2O_2 in vivo may result from decreased cell-derived H_2O_2 formation, scavenging of H_2O_2 produced, and/or suppression of PMN infiltration into the dermis (Miller et al. 1994; Wei et al. 1998). This study established the antioxidant property of genistein that may be responsible for its anti-carcinogenic effects. In a two-stage skin carcinogenesis study, low levels of genistein significantly prolong tumor latency and decrease tumor multiplicity by approximately 50%. Further, dietary feeding of genistein significantly increases the activities of catalase, superoxide dismutase, glutathione peroxidase and glutathione reductase in skin (Cai and Wei 1996). In another study dietary administration of genistein significantly enhanced the activities of antioxidant enzymes in the skin of SENCAR mice. Further this study demonstrated that genistein significantly inhibits TPA-induced proto-oncogene expression (c-fos) in mouse skin in a dose-dependent manner. In another study it was shown that topical application of genistein before UVB radiation reduced c-fos and c-jun expression in the SENCAR mouse skin in dose-dependent manner (Wang et al. 1998). In this study genistein exhibited more inhibition of c-fos than that of c-jun. Further, genistein application after UVB exposure down-regulated the expressions of c-fos and c-jun, but to a lesser extent compared with pre-application. These authors later suggested that UVB irradiation elicit a series of oxidative events, which can be substantially inhibited by isoflavonoid genistein through either direct quenching of reactive oxygen species or indirect antiinflammatory effects (Wei et al. 2002).

In another study genistein has been shown to significantly inhibit 7,12-dimethylbenz[a]anthracene initiated and TPA-promoted skin tumorigenesis in a two-stage carcinogenesis model on SENCAR mouse skin (Wei et al. 1998). Topical application of genistein was shown to reduce tumor incidence and multiplicity. Further, genistein treatment inhibited DMBA-induced bulky DNA adduct formation and substantially suppressed TPA-stimulated H_2O_2 and inflammatory responses in mouse skin (Wei et al. 1998). These results suggest that genistein exerts its anti-initiation and anti-promotion effects on skin carcinogenesis probably through blockage of DNA adduct formation and inhibition of oxidative and inflammatory events in vivo. Studies on the possible mechanisms of genistein against UV-mediated stress have shown that genistein down-regulated the UVB-mediated phosphorylation of TPK-dependent EGF-R in a dose-dependent manner in human epidermoid carcinoma A431 cells (Miller et al. 1994). Suppression of UVB-induced protooncogene expression in SENCAR mouse skin suggests that genistein may serve as a potential preventive agent against photo damage and photocarcinogenesis (Wang et al. 1998). In a study the authors examined the effects of Bifidobacterium-fermented soy milk extract (BE) containing genistein and daidzein on the hyaluronic acid (HA) content and rheological and physiological properties of hairless mouse and/or human skin. Topical application of BE for 6 weeks significantly restored changes in the elasticity and viscoelasticity of mouse skin, increased the HA content, and hydrated and thickened mouse skin. Also, topical application of a gel formula containing 10% BE to the human forearm for 3 months significantly lessened the decrease in skin elasticity (Miyazaki et al. 2004). Photoprotective effect of isoflavone genistein on ultraviolet B-induced pyrimidine dimer formation and PCNA expression in human reconstituted skin and its implications in dermatology and prevention of cutaneous carcinogenesis was studied recently (Moore et al. 2006). In this study skin samples were pre-treated with three concentrations of genistein (10, 20 and 50 microM) 1 h prior to UVB radiation at 20 and 60 mJ/cm2. Proliferating cell nuclear antigen (PCNA) and pyrimidine dimer (PD) expression profiles were localized using immunohistochemical analysis. Genistein was observed to dose dependently preserve proliferating cell populations with increasing genistein concentrations and noticeable paucity in PCNA immunoreactivity in the absence of genistein. Genistein was also found to inhibit UV-induced DNA damage. In a different study nutritional concentration of genistein were found to protect human dermal fibroblasts from oxidative stress-induced collagen biosynthesis inhibition through IGF-I receptor-mediated signaling (Sienkiewicz et al. 2008). In a recent study genistein was observed to protect UVB-induced senescence-like characteristics in human dermal fibroblasts via maintenance of antioxidant enzyme activities and modulation of mitochondrial oxidative stress through down-regulation of a p66Shc-dependent signaling pathway (Wang et al. 2010).

13.2.2.7 Ginger Compounds

Ginger rhizome (*Zingiber officinale*), known commonly as ginger, is consumed worldwide in cookeries as a spice and a flavoring agent. The skin cancer chemopreventive properties of ginger have been demonstrated previously (Lamson and Brignall 2001; Safe et al. 1999). A study from our laboratory for the first time evaluated the anti-tumor-promoting effects of ethanol extract of ginger in a mouse skin tumorigenesis model. We demonstrated that a pre-application of ethanol extract of ginger on the skin of SENCAR mice resulted in significant inhibition of TPA-caused induction of epidermal ornithine decarboxylase, cyclooxygenase and lipoxygenase activities and ODC mRNA expression (Katiyar et al. 1996). In this study, preapplication of ginger extract to mouse skin also afforded significant inhibition of TPA-caused epidermal edema (56%) and hyperplasia (44%). In long-term tumor studies, topical application of extract 30 min prior to that of each TPA application to 7,12-dimethylbenz(a)anthracene-initiated SENCAR mice resulted in a highly significant protection against skin tumor incidence and its subsequent multiplicity. Subsequent studies by Park et al. evaluated the anti-tumor promotional activity of 6-gingerol, the major pungent constituent of ginger, in a two-stage mouse skin carcinogenesis model (Park et al. 1998). The topical application of 6-gingerol on the dorsal shaven skin of female ICR mice significantly inhibited DMBA-initiated TPA-promoted skin papilloma formation, as well as TPA-induced epidermal ornithine decarboxylase activity and inflammation in mouse skin. Based on many studies, it is believed that gingerol is a good scavenger of peroxyl radicals generated by pulse radiolysis. In another recent study Bode et al. demonstrated the effect of two structurally related compounds of the ginger family, [6]-gingerol and [6]-paradol, on EGF-induced cell transformation and AP-1 activation in mouse epidermal JB6 cell lines (Bode et al. 2001). The results indicate that [6]-gingerol and [6]-paradol block EGF-induced cell transformation and although closely related structurally, act through different mechanisms. [6]-Gingerol inhibited EGF-induced AP-1 transactivation by blocking EGF-induced AP-1 DNA binding activity in a concentration-dependent manner, and in contrast, [6]-paradol had no effect on AP-1 activation.

Topical application of [6]-gingerol was found to inhibit PMA-induced COX-2 expression and suppress NF-kappaB DNA binding activity in mouse skin. In addition, [6]-gingerol inhibited the phoshorylation of p38 mitogen-activated protein kinase which may account for its inactivation of NF-kappaB and suppression of COX-2 expression (Kim et al. 2004). Later these authors demonstrated that topical application of [6]-gingerol inhibits COX-2 expression in mouse skin stimulated with TPA. The study further demonstrated that pretreatment with [6]-gingerol resulted in a decrease in both TPA-induced DNA binding and transcriptional activities of NF-kappaB through suppression of IkappaBalpha degradation and p65 nuclear translocation. Phosphorylation of both IkappaBalpha and p65 was also substantially blocked by [6]-gingerol. In addition, [6]-gingerol inhibited TPA-stimulated interaction of phospho-p65-(Ser-536) with cAMP response element binding protein-binding protein, a transcriptional coactivator of NF-kappaB (Kim et al. 2005). Recently [6]-gingerol was assessed for its anti-apoptotic effects in human epidermoid carcinoma A431 cells. [6]-Gingerol treatment exhibited considerable cytotoxicity as indicated by growth inhibition of A431 cells mediated via generation of ROS. Increase in ROS led to decrease in mitochondrial membrane potential and subsequent induction of apoptosis. Results revealed that perturbations in mitochondrial membrane are associated with deregulation of Bax/Bcl-2 ratio at gene transcriptional level as well as protein level, where treatment with [6]-gingerol leads to up-regulation of Cytochrome-c and Apaf-1 subsequently culminating in triggering of Caspase cascade (Nigam et al. 2009). In a very recent study the anti-inflammatory effect of water extract of Zingiber officinale, gingerol, and shogaol was investigated on UVB-induced skin damage in the human keratinocyte cell line HaCaT and C57BL/6 mice. The water extract of Z. officinale, gingerol, and shogaol was found to inhibit the production of cytokines in UVB-irradiated HaCaT cells. Further, treatment with Z. officinale attenuated UVB-induced hyperplasia, infiltration of leukocytes, and dilation of blood vessels in the dermis of the mice (Guahk et al. 2010).

13.2.2.8 Apigenin

Apigenin is flavonoid (5,7,4-trihydroxyflavone) in nature and widely present in herbs (endives, cloves), fruits (apples, cherries, grapes), vegetables (beans, broccoli, celery, leeks, onions, barley, parsley, tomatoes) and beverages (tea, wine) (Lepley et al. 1996; Janssen et al. 1998). Apigenin has been shown to possess anti-inflammatory, anti-carcinogenic effects for skin (Birt et al. 1986, 1997). In one of these studies, the authors (Birt et al. 1997) reported that topical application of apigenin prior to UV irradiation prevents UV-induced tumorigenesis in mice. In this study they also observed that apigenin treatment to mouse skin resulted in inhibition of UV-induced increase of ornithine decarboxylase activity, which is considered as a biomarker of tumor promotion, and reduced tumor incidence as well as increased tumor-free survival in mice. Apigenin is also considered a potent inhibitor of epidermal ornithine decarboxylase induction by TPA and significantly inhibited the incidence and numbers of carcinoma in SENCAR mice (Wei et al. 1990). Apigenin has also been shown to suppress PKC activity and nuclear oncogene expression in TPA-induced tumor promotion that might contribute to the molecular mechanisms of skin cancer inhibition (Lin et al. 1997). As a mechanism of apigenin action in human diploid fibroblasts produced a (i) G1 cell-cycle arrest by inhibiting cdk2 kinase activity, (ii) phosphorylation of retinoblastoma protein, (iii) induction the cdk inhibitor p21/WAF1, and (iv) stabilization of tumor suppressor gene p53 (McVean et al. 2000; Lepley and Pelling 1997; Lepley et al. 1996). In another in vivo study apigenin treatment was found to be effective in the prevention of UVB light induced skin carcinogenesis in SKH-1 mice (Birt et al. 1997). In another study apigenin was found to prevent UVB-induced cyclooxygenase 2 expression, coupled mRNA stabilization and translational inhibition (Tong et al. 2007). In a different study apigenin suppressed the UVB-induced increase in COX-2 protein and mRNA in mouse and human keratinocyte cell lines. UVB radiation of keratinocytes transfected with a mouse COX-2 promoter/luciferase reporter plasmid resulted in a threefold increase in transcription from the promoter, and apigenin inhibited the UV-induced promoter activity at doses of 5–50 microM. Overall this study suggested that one pathway by which apigenin inhibited COX-2 expression was through modulation of USF transcriptional activity (Van Dross et al. 2007). Further, a study utilized three models of human keratinocytes to study the effect of apigenin treatment on UVB-induced apoptosis: HaCaT human keratinocyte cells, primary keratinocyte cultures isolated from human neonatal foreskin, and human organotypic keratinocyte cultures (Abu-Yousif et al. 2008). Each keratinocyte model was exposed to a moderate dose of UVB (300–1,000 J/m^2), then treated with apigenin (0–50 micromol/L). Apigenin treatment was observed to enhance UVB-induced apoptosis >2-fold in each of the models tested. In this study when keratinocytes were exposed to UVB, apigenin treatment stimulated changes in Bax localization and increased the release of cytochrome c from the mitochondria compared with UVB exposure alone. Overexpression of the antiapoptotic protein Bcl-2 and expression of a dominant-negative form of Fas-associated death domain led to a reduction in the ability of apigenin to enhance UVB-induced apoptosis. Overall the data from this study suggested that enhancement of UVB-induced apoptosis by apigenin treatment involves both the intrinsic and extrinsic apoptotic pathways (Abu-Yousif et al. 2008).

13.3 Future Prospects of Skin Cancer Chemoprevention

Non melanoma skin cancer for which the chemoprevention seems applicable is associated with significant morbidity and some mortality in human population. The incidence of skin cancer is on the rise escalating each year especially in Caucasian populations (Shore 2001; Leiter and Garbe 2008; English et al. 1997). Skin cancer is estimated to attack one out of every five Americans each year, making it the most prevalent form of cancer (Jemal et al. 2010). More than a million new cases of non-melanoma skin cancers are diagnosed annually in the USA and in individuals with a history of skin cancer there appears to be an increased risk for other lethal cancer types. Thus there is an urgent necessity of developing mechanism-based approaches for prevention of these cancers. Recently, the concept of chemoprevention is being increasingly accepted by research investigators and is gaining popularity by the public (Fig. 13.1). This is well evident from the fact that a variety of cosmetic products supplemented with synthetic or botanical antioxidant are available at the drug stores, supermarkets and departmental stores and are increasingly consumed by the human population. Products supplemented with botanicals such as green tea and other agents include but are not limited to depilatory creams, cleansing lotions, shampoos, moisturizing creams, toothpastes, scented sprays, body lotions etc. Most of the synthetic agents and most of the naturally occurring antioxidant compounds discussed in this review have not been adequately tested for their effectiveness and safety for humans in the clinical trials. Safety of naturally occuring agents is less of a concern because only small concentrations are used in skin care products. The

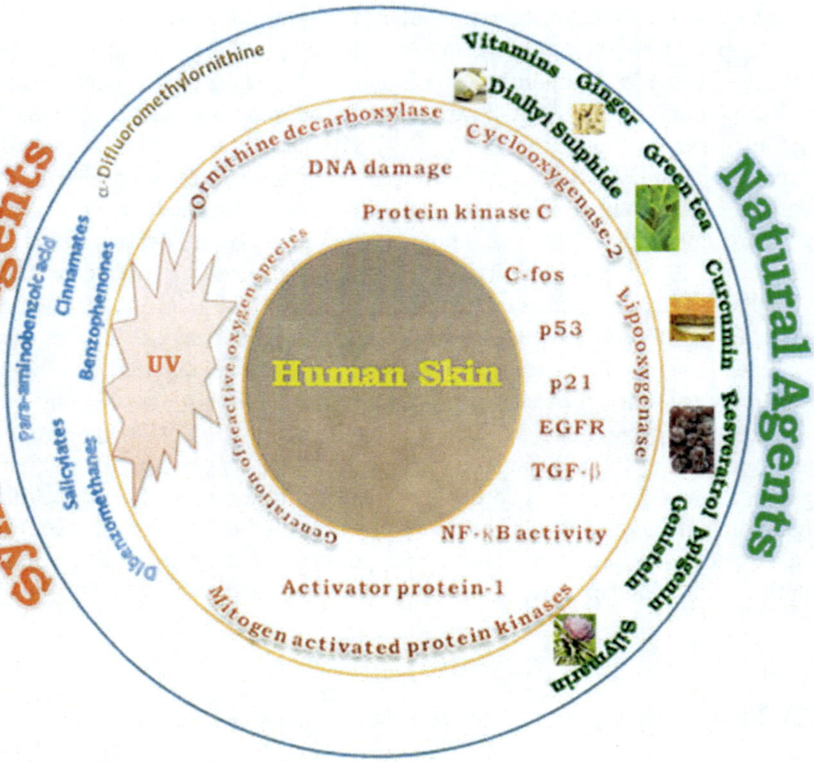

Fig. 13.1 Chemoprevention of skin cancer: human skin (represented by the *inner circle*), is continuously exposed to environmental hazards including ultraviolet light that contribute substantially to the production of reactive oxygen species, DNA damage and modulation of signal transduction pathways (represented by the *middle circle*) leading to escalation of the skin related disorders including skin cancer. Natural and synthetic agents (represented by the *outer circle*) have been used to counter the effects of environmental hazards that the skin is exposed to. Synthetic agents commonly work by blocking the ultraviolet light with the exception of α-difluoromethylornithine which is an irreversible inhibitor of ornithine decarboxylase and suppresses UVB- and chemical -induced skin carcinogenesis. In contrast natural agents work in many ways by modulating and repairing damaged signaling pathways

scope of future skin cancer chemoprevention could be broadened considerably by combining chemoprevention approaches using combination of agents working on distinct pathways responsible for cancer outcome. Such a combination could then be supplemented in skin care products of natural and/or synthetic agents. A greater emphasis should be given to the use of natural agents as they target multi-facet actions and possess minimal toxicity. Such strategies may reduce skin cancer incidence and mortality through early intervention for individuals who are at high risk of developing skin cancer. Further, there is a need to initiate clinical trials for selected antioxidants for skin cancer chemoprevention.

13.4 Conclusions

The in depth understanding of the biology of skin cancer encourages the investigation of compounds that could be used to intervene in the process of carcinogenesis; after the initial ultraviolet damage has taken place but before the tumor develops. Evidence indicates that many cancers are preventable, especially because diet and environment are essential factors in the modulation of cancer risk. Green tea polyphenols are known to target many enzymes directly associated with cancer (the proteasome, telemorase, several growth factors, etc) (Wright et al. 2006; Hsu 2005).

Despite the remarkable beneficial properties of bioactive food components, standard delivery systems for topical application have not been established. Most of these natural agents are easily oxidized in the environment and gradually lose their activities if not used immediately after preparation. Thus, maintaining the stability of these antioxidants is the primary goal for topical formulations. Another potential challenge is penetration of these agents through the epidermis. With the exception of traumatic open wounds, infections (pathogenic lesions) or other such abnormal conditions, the human skin is a waterproof barrier protected by multilayers of cornified keratinocytes. This is especially true for green tea polyphenols, tests using in vitro delivery models have shown that after a 24-h period, solutions saturated with green tea extract failed to deliver the polyphenols in a solution higher than the maximum serum concentration (Batchelder et al. 2004). Also, a higher concentration of EGCG (such as 10%) has not been tested for long term toxicity. Additionally, higher concentrations of any agent in a formulation would increase the cost considerably. We believe that research should continue on synthesizing and evaluating analogs of the natural agents that have potent efficacy and could be made readily available to the skin. Apart from the single agent approach, studies are also required with natural and synthetic products as a complex mixture, a cocktail approach, which together may have synergistic anti-cancer benefits. This approach should continue to be explored in vitro and in vivo as well as in clinical and epidemiological studies in the future. Integrating new molecular findings into clinical practice is a major challenge of cancer prevention. A fundamental understanding in this area is important for the rational design of future human intervention trials and cohort studies to elucidate the relationship studies between bioactive food components and skin cancer.

Acknowledgement Imtiaz Siddiqui was supported by T32 AR 055893.

References

Abu-Yousif AO, Smith KA, Getsios S, Green KJ, Van Dross RT, Pelling JC (2008) Enhancement of UVB-induced apoptosis by apigenin in human keratinocytes and organotypic keratinocyte cultures. Cancer Res 68(8):3057–3065

Adhami VM, Afaq F, Ahmad N (2001) Involvement of the retinoblastoma (pRb)-E2F/DP pathway during antiproliferative effects of resveratrol in human epidermoid carcinoma (A431) cells. Biochem Biophys Res Commun 288(3):579–585

Adhami VM, Afaq F, Ahmad N (2003a) Suppression of ultraviolet B exposure-mediated activation of NF-kappaB in normal human keratinocytes by resveratrol. Neoplasia 5(1):74–82
Adhami VM, Ahmad N, Mukhtar H (2003b) Molecular targets for green tea in prostate cancer prevention. J Nutr 133(7 Suppl):2417S-2424S
Adhami VM, Syed DN, Khan N, Afaq F (2008) Phytochemicals for prevention of solar ultraviolet radiation-induced damages. Photochem Photobiol 84(2):489–500
Afaq F, Adhami VM, Ahmad N, Mukhtar H (2003a) Inhibition of ultraviolet B-mediated activation of nuclear factor kappaB in normal human epidermal keratinocytes by green tea Constituent (-)-epigallocatechin-3-gallate. Oncogene 22(7):1035–1044
Afaq F, Ahmad N, Mukhtar H (2003b) Suppression of UVB-induced phosphorylation of mitogen-activated protein kinases and nuclear factor kappa B by green tea polyphenol in SKH-1 hairless mice. Oncogene 22(58):9254–9264
Afaq F, Mukhtar H (2006) Botanical antioxidants in the prevention of photocarcinogenesis and photoaging. Exp Dermatol 15(9):678–684
Agarwal R, Mukhtar H (1996) Chemoprevention of photocarcinogenesis. Photochem Photobiol 63(4):440–444
Agarwal R, Katiyar SK, Zaidi SI, Mukhtar H (1992) Inhibition of skin tumor promoter-caused induction of epidermal ornithine decarboxylase in SENCAR mice by polyphenolic fraction isolated from green tea and its individual epicatechin derivatives. Cancer Res 52(13): 3582–3588
Agarwal R, Katiyar SK, Khan SG, Mukhtar H (1993) Protection against ultraviolet B radiation-induced effects in the skin of SKH-1 hairless mice by a polyphenolic fraction isolated from green tea. Photochem Photobiol 58(5):695–700
Agarwal R, Katiyar SK, Lundgren DW, Mukhtar H (1994) Inhibitory effect of silymarin, an anti-hepatotoxic flavonoid, on 12-O-tetradecanoylphorbol-13-acetate-induced epidermal ornithine decarboxylase activity and mRNA in SENCAR mice. Carcinogenesis 15(6):1099–1103
Aggarwal BB, Kumar A, Bharti AC (2003) Anticancer potential of curcumin: preclinical and clinical studies. Anticancer Res 23(1A):363–398
Ahmad N, Mukhtar H (2001) Cutaneous photochemoprotection by green tea: a brief review. Skin Pharmacol Appl Skin Physiol 14(2):69–76
Ahmad N, Adhami VM, Afaq F, Feyes DK, Mukhtar H (2001a) Resveratrol causes WAF-1/p21-mediated G(1)-phase arrest of cell cycle and induction of apoptosis in human epidermoid carcinoma A431 cells. Clin Cancer Res 7(5):1466–1473
Ahmad N, Gilliam AC, Katiyar SK, O'Brien TG, Mukhtar H (2001b) A definitive role of ornithine decarboxylase in photocarcinogenesis. Am J Pathol 159(3):885–892
Alberts DS, Dorr RT, Einspahr JG, Aickin M, Saboda K, Xu MJ, Peng YM, Goldman R, Foote JA, Warneke JA, Salasche S, Roe DJ, Bowden GT (2000) Chemoprevention of human actinic keratoses by topical 2-(difluoromethyl)-dl-ornithine. Cancer Epidemiol Biomarkers Prev 9(12):1281–1286
Ames BN (1983) Dietary carcinogens and anticarcinogens. Oxygen radicals and degenerative diseases. Science 221(4617):1256–1264
Amin AR, Kucuk O, Khuri FR, Shin DM (2009) Perspectives for cancer prevention with natural compounds. J Clin Oncol 27(16):2712–2725
Arbeit JM, Riley RR, Huey B, Porter C, Kelloff G, Lubet R, Ward JM, Pinkel D (1999) Difluoromethylornithine chemoprevention of epidermal carcinogenesis in K14-HPV16 transgenic mice. Cancer Res 59(15):3610–3620
Arora A, Siddiqui IA, Shukla Y (2004) Modulation of p53 in 7,12-dimethylbenz[a]anthracene-induced skin tumors by diallyl sulfide in Swiss albino mice. Mol Cancer Ther 3(11):1459–1466
Athar M, Raza H, Bickers DR, Mukhtar H (1990) Inhibition of benzoyl peroxide-mediated tumor promotion in 7,12-dimethylbenz(a)anthracene-initiated skin of Sencar mice by antioxidants nordihydroguaiaretic acid and diallyl sulfide. J Invest Dermatol 94(2):162–165

Autier P, Dore JF, Negrier S, Lienard D, Panizzon R, Lejeune FJ, Guggisberg D, Eggermont AM (1999) Sunscreen use and duration of sun exposure: a double-blind, randomized trial. J Natl Cancer Inst 91(15):1304–1309

Aziz MH, Reagan-Shaw S, Wu J, Longley BJ, Ahmad N (2005) Chemoprevention of skin cancer by grape constituent resveratrol: relevance to human disease? FASEB J 19(9):1193–1195

Azuine MA, Bhide SV (1992) Chemopreventive effect of turmeric against stomach and skin tumors induced by chemical carcinogens in Swiss mice. Nutr Cancer 17(1):77–83

Bailey HH, Kim K, Verma AK, Sielaff K, Larson PO, Snow S, Lenaghan T, Viner JL, Douglas J, Dreckschmidt NE, Hamielec M, Pomplun M, Sharata HH, Puchalsky D, Berg ER, Havighurst TC, Carbone PP (2010) A randomized, double-blind, placebo-controlled phase 3 skin cancer prevention study of {alpha}-difluoromethylornithine in subjects with previous history of skin cancer. Cancer Prev Res (Phila) 3(1):35–47

Baliga MS, Katiyar SK (2006) Chemoprevention of photocarcinogenesis by selected dietary botanicals. Photochem Photobiol Sci 5(2):243–253

Bansal MP, Gupta G (1988) Influence of selenium on 3-methylcholanthrene induced skin carcinogenesis in mice. J Environ Pathol Toxicol Oncol 8(7 Spec No):49–53

Batchelder RJ, Calder RJ, Thomas CP, Heard CM (2004) In vitro transdermal delivery of the major catechins and caffeine from extract of Camellia sinensis. Int J Pharm 283(1–2):45–51

Baur JA, Sinclair DA (2006) Therapeutic potential of resveratrol: the in vivo evidence. Nat Rev Drug Discov 5(6):493–506

Bens G (2008) Sunscreens. Adv Exp Med Biol 624:137–161

Berton TR, Fischer SM, Conti CJ, Locniskar MF (1996) Comparison of ultraviolet light-induced skin carcinogenesis and ornithine decarboxylase activity in sencar and hairless SKH-1 mice fed a constant level of dietary lipid varying in corn and coconut oil. Nutr Cancer 26(3):353–363

Biesalski HK, Obermueller-Jevic UC (2001) UV light, beta-carotene and human skin–beneficial and potentially harmful effects. Arch Biochem Biophys 389(1):1–6

Birt DF, Walker B, Tibbels MG, Bresnick E (1986) Anti-mutagenesis and anti-promotion by apigenin, robinetin and indole-3-carbinol. Carcinogenesis 7(6):959–963

Birt DF, Mitchell D, Gold B, Pour P, Pinch HC (1997) Inhibition of ultraviolet light induced skin carcinogenesis in SKH-1 mice by apigenin, a plant flavonoid. Anticancer Res 17(1A):85–91

Bode AM, Dong Z (2009) Cancer prevention research – then and now. Nat Rev Cancer 9(7): 508–516

Bode AM, Ma WY, Surh YJ, Dong Z (2001) Inhibition of epidermal growth factor-induced cell transformation and activator protein 1 activation by [6]-gingerol. Cancer Res 61(3):850–853

Bouknight P, Bowling A, Kovach FE (2010) Sunscreen use for skin cancer prevention. Am Fam Physician 82(8):989–990

Brown KM, Arthur JR (2001) Selenium, selenoproteins and human health: a review. Public Health Nutr 4(2B):593–599

Burke KE, Clive J, Combs GF Jr, Commisso J, Keen CL, Nakamura RM (2000) Effects of topical and oral vitamin E on pigmentation and skin cancer induced by ultraviolet irradiation in Skh:2 hairless mice. Nutr Cancer 38(1):87–97

Burke KE, Clive J, Combs GF, Jr., Nakamura RM (2003) Effects of topical L-selenomethionine with topical and oral vitamin E on pigmentation and skin cancer induced by ultraviolet irradiation in Skh:2 hairless mice. J Am Acad Dermatol 49(3):458–472

Cai Q, Wei H (1996) Effect of dietary genistein on antioxidant enzyme activities in SENCAR mice. Nutr Cancer 25(1):1–7

Carlberg C, Saurat JH (1996) Vitamin D-retinoid association: molecular basis and clinical applications. J Investig Dermatol Symp Proc 1(1):82–86

Chatterjee ML, Agarwal R, Mukhtar H (1996) Ultraviolet B radiation-induced DNA lesions in mouse epidermis: an assessment using a novel 32P-postlabelling technique. Biochem Biophys Res Commun 229(2):590–595

Cheepala SB, Syed Z, Trutschl M, Cvek U, Clifford JL (2007) Retinoids and skin: microarrays shed new light on chemopreventive action of all-trans retinoic acid. Mol Carcinog 46(8):634–639

Chen W, Barthelman M, Martinez J, Alberts D, Gensler HL (1997) Inhibition of cyclobutane pyrimidine dimer formation in epidermal p53 gene of UV-irradiated mice by alpha-tocopherol. Nutr Cancer 29(3):205–211

Chen ZP, Schell JB, Ho CT, Chen KY (1998) Green tea epigallocatechin gallate shows a pronounced growth inhibitory effect on cancerous cells but not on their normal counterparts. Cancer Lett 129(2):173–179

Chung FL, Schwartz J, Herzog CR, Yang YM (2003a) Tea and cancer prevention: studies in animals and humans. J Nutr 133(10):3268S–3274S

Chung JH, Han JH, Hwang EJ, Seo JY, Cho KH, Kim KH, Youn JI, Eun HC (2003b) Dual mechanisms of green tea extract (EGCG)-induced cell survival in human epidermal keratinocytes. FASEB J 17(13):1913–1915

Conney AH, Lysz T, Ferraro T, Abidi TF, Manchand PS, Laskin JD, Huang MT (1991) Inhibitory effect of curcumin and some related dietary compounds on tumor promotion and arachidonic acid metabolism in mouse skin. Adv Enzyme Regul 31:385–396

Conney AH, Wang ZY, Huang MT, Ho CT, Yang CS (1992) Inhibitory effect of green tea on tumorigenesis by chemicals and ultraviolet light. Prev Med 21(3):361–369

Conney AH, Lu Y, Lou Y, Xie J, Huang M (1999) Inhibitory effect of green and black tea on tumor growth. Proc Soc Exp Biol Med 220(4):229–233

Conney AH, Lu YP, Lou YR, Huang MT (2002) Inhibitory effects of tea and caffeine on UV-induced carcinogenesis: relationship to enhanced apoptosis and decreased tissue fat. Eur J Cancer Prev 11 Suppl 2:S28–36

Cragg G, Suffness M (1988) Metabolism of plant-derived anticancer agents. Pharmacol Ther 37(3):425–461

D'Agostini F, Balansky RM, Camoirano A, De Flora S (2005) Modulation of light-induced skin tumors by N-acetylcysteine and/or ascorbic acid in hairless mice. Carcinogenesis 26(3): 657–664

Delmas D, Lancon A, Colin D, Jannin B, Latruffe N (2006) Resveratrol as a chemopreventive agent: a promising molecule for fighting cancer. Curr Drug Targets 7(4):423–442

Dennis LK, Beane Freeman LE, VanBeek MJ (2003) Sunscreen use and the risk for melanoma: a quantitative review. Ann Intern Med 139(12):966–978

Diffey B (2009) Sunscreens: expectation and realization. Photodermatol Photoimmunol Photomed 25(5):233–236

Dragsted LO, Strube M, Larsen JC (1993) Cancer-protective factors in fruits and vegetables: biochemical and biological background. Pharmacol Toxicol 72 Suppl 1:116–135

Dreher F, Maibach H (2001) Protective effects of topical antioxidants in humans. Curr Probl Dermatol 29:157–164

Dwivedi C, Rohlfs S, Jarvis D, Engineer FN (1992) Chemoprevention of chemically induced skin tumor development by diallyl sulfide and diallyl disulfide. Pharm Res 9(12):1668–1670

Einspahr JG, Nelson MA, Saboda K, Warneke J, Bowden GT, Alberts DS (2002) Modulation of biologic endpoints by topical difluoromethylornithine (DFMO), in subjects at high-risk for nonmelanoma skin cancer. Clin Cancer Res 8(1):149–155

Einspahr JG, Bowden GT, Alberts DS (2003) Skin cancer chemoprevention: strategies to save our skin. Recent Results Cancer Res 163:151–164; discussion 264–156

Elmets CA, Anderson CY (1996) Sunscreens and photocarcinogenesis: an objective assessment. Photochem Photobiol 63(4):435–440

Elmets CA, Singh D, Tubesing K, Matsui M, Katiyar S, Mukhtar H (2001) Cutaneous photoprotection from ultraviolet injury by green tea polyphenols. J Am Acad Dermatol 44(3):425–432

Elmets CA, Viner JL, Pentland AP, Cantrell W, Lin HY, Bailey H, Kang S, Linden KG, Heffernan M, Duvic M, Richmond E, Elewski BE, Umar A, Bell W, Gordon GB (2010) Chemoprevention of nonmelanoma skin cancer with celecoxib: a randomized, double-blind, placebo-controlled trial. J Natl Cancer Inst

English DR, Armstrong BK, Kricker A, Fleming C (1997) Sunlight and cancer. Cancer Causes Control 8(3):271–283

Epstein H (2006) Sunscreen savvy: why do sunscreens fail to protect? Clin Dermatol 24(5): 463–464

Fallon J, Murphy GM (2009) Sunscreens and sun protection. Cancer Treat Res 146:425–432

Fischer SM, Lo HH, Gordon GB, Seibert K, Kelloff G, Lubet RA, Conti CJ (1999) Chemopreventive activity of celecoxib, a specific cyclooxygenase-2 inhibitor, and indomethacin against ultraviolet light-induced skin carcinogenesis. Mol Carcinog 25(4):231–240

Fischer SM, Lee M, Lubet RA (2001) Difluoromethylornithine is effective as both a preventive and therapeutic agent against the development of UV carcinogenesis in SKH hairless mice. Carcinogenesis 22(1):83–88

Fischer SM, Conti CJ, Viner J, Aldaz CM, Lubet RA (2003) Celecoxib and difluoromethylornithine in combination have strong therapeutic activity against UV-induced skin tumors in mice. Carcinogenesis 24(5):945–952

Fourtanier A, Moyal D, Seite S (2008) Sunscreens containing the broad-spectrum UVA absorber, Mexoryl SX, prevent the cutaneous detrimental effects of UV exposure: a review of clinical study results. Photodermatol Photoimmunol Photomed 24(4):164–174

Garg R, Ramchandani AG, Maru GB (2008) Curcumin decreases 12-O-tetradecanoylphorbol-13-acetate-induced protein kinase C translocation to modulate downstream targets in mouse skin. Carcinogenesis 29(6):1249–1257

Glanz K, Buller DB, Saraiya M (2007) Reducing ultraviolet radiation exposure among outdoor workers: state of the evidence and recommendations. Environ Health 6:22

Goel A, Kunnumakkara AB, Aggarwal BB (2008) Curcumin as "Curecumin": from kitchen to clinic. Biochem Pharmacol 75(4):787–809

Gonzaga ER (2009) Role of UV light in photodamage, skin aging, and skin cancer: importance of photoprotection. Am J Clin Dermatol 10 Suppl 1:19–24

Green A, Whiteman D, Frost C, Battistutta D (1999a) Sun exposure, skin cancers and related skin conditions. J Epidemiol 9(6 Suppl):S7–13

Green A, Williams G, Neale R, Hart V, Leslie D, Parsons P, Marks GC, Gaffney P, Battistutta D, Frost C, Lang C, Russell A (1999b) Daily sunscreen application and betacarotene supplementation in prevention of basal-cell and squamous-cell carcinomas of the skin: a randomised controlled trial. Lancet 354(9180):723–729

Greenwald P (2004) Clinical trials in cancer prevention: current results and perspectives for the future. J Nutr 134(12 Suppl):3507S–3512S

Gu M, Dhanalakshmi S, Singh RP, Agarwal R (2005) Dietary feeding of silibinin prevents early biomarkers of UVB radiation-induced carcinogenesis in SKH-1 hairless mouse epidermis. Cancer Epidemiol Biomarkers Prev 14(5):1344–1349

Guahk GH, Ha SK, Jung HS, Kang C, Kim CH, Kim YB, Kim SY (2010) Zingiber officinale protects HaCaT cells and C57BL/6 mice from ultraviolet B-induced inflammation. J Med Food 13(3):673–680

Halliday GM, Bestak R, Yuen KS, Cavanagh LL, Barnetson RS (1998) UVA-induced immunosuppression. Mutat Res 422(1):139–145

Hansen LA, Sigman CC, Andreola F, Ross SA, Kelloff GJ, De Luca LM (2000) Retinoids in chemoprevention and differentiation therapy. Carcinogenesis 21(7):1271–1279

Heenen M (1999) [Photoprotection, cancer protection and solar protection factor]. Rev Med Brux 20(3):143–146

Hsu S (2005) Green tea and the skin. J Am Acad Dermatol 52(6):1049–1059

Huang MT, Lysz T, Ferraro T, Abidi TF, Laskin JD, Conney AH (1991) Inhibitory effects of curcumin on in vitro lipoxygenase and cyclooxygenase activities in mouse epidermis. Cancer Res 51(3):813–819

Huang MT, Wang ZY, Georgiadis CA, Laskin JD, Conney AH (1992) Inhibitory effects of curcumin on tumor initiation by benzo[a]pyrene and 7,12-dimethylbenz[a]anthracene. Carcinogenesis 13(11):2183–2186

Iersel ML, Ploemen JP, Struik I, van Amersfoort C, Keyzer AE, Schefferlie JG, van Bladeren PJ (1996) Inhibition of glutathione S-transferase activity in human melanoma cells by alpha,beta-unsaturated carbonyl derivatives. Effects of acrolein, cinnamaldehyde, citral, crotonaldehyde, curcumin, ethacrynic acid, and trans-2-hexenal. Chem Biol Interact 102(2):117–132

Ishizaki C, Oguro T, Yoshida T, Wen CQ, Sueki H, Iijima M (1996) Enhancing effect of ultraviolet A on ornithine decarboxylase induction and dermatitis evoked by 12-o-tetradecanoylphorbol-13-acetate and its inhibition by curcumin in mouse skin. Dermatology 193(4):311–317

Jang M, Pezzuto JM (1998) Effects of resveratrol on 12-O-tetradecanoylphorbol-13-acetate-induced oxidative events and gene expression in mouse skin. Cancer Lett 134(1):81–89

Jang M, Cai L, Udeani GO, Slowing KV, Thomas CF, Beecher CW, Fong HH, Farnsworth NR, Kinghorn AD, Mehta RG, Moon RC, Pezzuto JM (1997) Cancer chemopreventive activity of resveratrol, a natural product derived from grapes. Science 275(5297):218–220

Janssen K, Mensink RP, Cox FJ, Harryvan JL, Hovenier R, Hollman PC, Katan MB (1998) Effects of the flavonoids quercetin and apigenin on hemostasis in healthy volunteers: results from an in vitro and a dietary supplement study. Am J Clin Nutr 67(2):255–262

Jee SH, Shen SC, Tseng CR, Chiu HC, Kuo ML (1998) Curcumin induces a p53-dependent apoptosis in human basal cell carcinoma cells. J Invest Dermatol 111(4):656–661

Jemal A, Siegel R, Xu J, Ward E (2010) Cancer statistics, 2010. CA Cancer J Clin 60(5):277–300

Jiang H, Yamamoto S, Kato R (1994) Inhibition of two-stage skin carcinogenesis as well as complete skin carcinogenesis by oral administration of TMK688, a potent lipoxygenase inhibitor. Carcinogenesis 15(5):807–812

Jiang H, Yamamoto S, Ozawa S, Shimada M, Yamazoe Y, Kato R (1996) Inhibitory effect of TMK688 on skin tumor initiation caused by 7,12-dimethylbenz[a]anthracene in relation to inhibition of aryl hydrocarbon hydroxylase activity and Cyp1a1 mRNA induction. Pharmacology 53(2):123–132

Jones CS, Sly L, Chen LC, Ben T, Brugh-Collins M, Lichti U, De Luca LM (1994) Retinol and beta-carotene concentrations in skin, papillomas and carcinomas, liver, and serum of mice fed retinoic acid or beta-carotene to suppress skin tumor formation. Nutr Cancer 21(1):83–93

Kalka K, Mukhtar H, Turowski-Wanke A, Merk H (2000) Biomelanin antioxidants in cosmetics: assessment based on inhibition of lipid peroxidation. Skin Pharmacol Appl Skin Physiol 13(3–4):143–149

Kanekura T, Higashi Y, Kanzaki T (2000) Inhibitory effects of 9-cis-retinoic acid and pyrrolidinedithiocarbamate on cyclooxygenase (COX)-2 expression and cell growth in human skin squamous carcinoma cells. Cancer Lett 161(2):177–183

Katiyar SK (2007) UV-induced immune suppression and photocarcinogenesis: chemoprevention by dietary botanical agents. Cancer Lett 255(1):1–11

Katiyar SK (2011) Green tea prevents non-melanoma skin cancer by enhancing DNA repair. Arch Biochem Biophys 508(2):152–158

Katiyar SK, Mukhtar H (2001) Green tea polyphenol (-)-epigallocatechin-3-gallate treatment to mouse skin prevents UVB-induced infiltration of leukocytes, depletion of antigen-presenting cells, and oxidative stress. J Leukoc Biol 69(5):719–726

Katiyar SK, Agarwal R, Wang ZY, Bhatia AK, Mukhtar H (1992) (-)-Epigallocatechin-3-gallate in Camellia sinensis leaves from Himalayan region of Sikkim: inhibitory effects against biochemical events and tumor initiation in Sencar mouse skin. Nutr Cancer 18(1):73–83

Katiyar SK, Agarwal R, Mukhtar H (1993) Protection against malignant conversion of chemically induced benign skin papillomas to squamous cell carcinomas in SENCAR mice by a polyphenolic fraction isolated from green tea. Cancer Res 53(22):5409–5412

Katiyar SK, Elmets CA, Agarwal R, Mukhtar H (1995a) Protection against ultraviolet-B radiation-induced local and systemic suppression of contact hypersensitivity and edema responses in C3H/HeN mice by green tea polyphenols. Photochem Photobiol 62(5):855–861

Katiyar SK, Rupp CO, Korman NJ, Agarwal R, Mukhtar H (1995b) Inhibition of 12-O-tetradecanoylphorbol-13-acetate and other skin tumor-promoter-caused induction of epidermal interleukin-1 alpha mRNA and protein expression in SENCAR mice by green tea polyphenols. J Invest Dermatol 105(3):394–398

Katiyar SK, Agarwal R, Mukhtar H (1996) Inhibition of tumor promotion in SENCAR mouse skin by ethanol extract of Zingiber officinale rhizome. Cancer Res 56(5):1023–1030

Katiyar SK, Korman NJ, Mukhtar H, Agarwal R (1997) Protective effects of silymarin against photocarcinogenesis in a mouse skin model. J Natl Cancer Inst 89(8):556–566

Katiyar SK, Challa A, McCormick TS, Cooper KD, Mukhtar H (1999a) Prevention of UVB-induced immunosuppression in mice by the green tea polyphenol (-)-epigallocatechin-3-gallate may be associated with alterations in IL-10 and IL-12 production. Carcinogenesis 20(11): 2117–2124

Katiyar SK, Matsui MS, Elmets CA, Mukhtar H (1999b) Polyphenolic antioxidant (-)-epigallocatechin-3-gallate from green tea reduces UVB-induced inflammatory responses and infiltration of leukocytes in human skin. Photochem Photobiol 69(2):148–153

Katiyar SK, Perez A, Mukhtar H (2000) Green tea polyphenol treatment to human skin prevents formation of ultraviolet light B-induced pyrimidine dimers in DNA. Clin Cancer Res 6(10):3864–3869

Katiyar SK, Afaq F, Azizuddin K, Mukhtar H (2001a) Inhibition of UVB-induced oxidative stress-mediated phosphorylation of mitogen-activated protein kinase signaling pathways in cultured human epidermal keratinocytes by green tea polyphenol (-)-epigallocatechin-3-gallate. Toxicol Appl Pharmacol 176(2):110–117

Katiyar SK, Afaq F, Perez A, Mukhtar H (2001b) Green tea polyphenol (-)-epigallocatechin-3-gallate treatment of human skin inhibits ultraviolet radiation-induced oxidative stress. Carcinogenesis 22(2):287–294

Katsumura N, Okuno M, Onogi N, Moriwaki H, Muto Y, Kojima S (1996) Suppression of mouse skin papilloma by canthaxanthin and beta-carotene in vivo: possibility of the regression of tumorigenesis by carotenoids without conversion to retinoic acid. Nutr Cancer 26(2):203–208

Keller KL, Fenske NA (1998) Uses of vitamins A, C, and E and related compounds in dermatology: a review. Journal of the American Academy of Dermatology 39(4 Pt 1):611–625

Khan N, Mukhtar H (2007) Tea polyphenols for health promotion. Life Sci 81(7):519–533

Khan WA, Wang ZY, Athar M, Bickers DR, Mukhtar H (1988) Inhibition of the skin tumorigenicity of (+/-)-7 beta,8 alpha-dihydroxy-9 alpha,10 alpha-epoxy-7,8,9,10-tetrahydrobenzo[a]pyrene by tannic acid, green tea polyphenols and quercetin in Sencar mice. Cancer Lett 42(1–2):7–12

Khan N, Afaq F, Saleem M, Ahmad N, Mukhtar H (2006) Targeting multiple signaling pathways by green tea polyphenol (-)-epigallocatechin-3-gallate. Cancer Res 66(5):2500–2505

Khan N, Afaq F, Mukhtar H (2008) Cancer chemoprevention through dietary antioxidants: progress and promise. Antioxid Redox Signal 10(3):475–510

Kim J, Hwang JS, Cho YK, Han Y, Jeon YJ, Yang KH (2001) Protective effects of (-)-epigallocatechin-3-gallate on UVA- and UVB-induced skin damage. Skin Pharmacol Appl Skin Physiol 14(1):11–19

Kim SO, Chun KS, Kundu JK, Surh YJ (2004) Inhibitory effects of [6]-gingerol on PMA-induced COX-2 expression and activation of NF-kappaB and p38 MAPK in mouse skin. Biofactors 21(1–4):27–31

Kim SO, Kundu JK, Shin YK, Park JH, Cho MH, Kim TY, Surh YJ (2005) [6]-Gingerol inhibits COX-2 expression by blocking the activation of p38 MAP kinase and NF-kappaB in phorbol ester-stimulated mouse skin. Oncogene 24(15):2558–2567

Kochevar IE, Moran M, Lyon N, Flotte T, Siebert E, Gange RW (1993) Effects of systemic indomethacin, meclizine, and BW755C on chronic ultraviolet B-induced effects in hairless mouse skin. J Invest Dermatol 100(2):186–193

Kohen R (1999) Skin antioxidants: their role in aging and in oxidative stress–new approaches for their evaluation. Biomed Pharmacother 53(4):181–192

Kornhauser A, Wei RR, Yamaguchi Y, Coelho SG, Kaidbey K, Barton C, Takahashi K, Beer JZ, Miller SA, Hearing VJ (2009) The effects of topically applied glycolic acid and salicylic acid

on ultraviolet radiation-induced erythema, DNA damage and sunburn cell formation in human skin. J Dermatol Sci 55(1):10–17
Kundu JK, Surh YJ (2007) Epigallocatechin gallate inhibits phorbol ester-induced activation of NF-kappa B and CREB in mouse skin: role of p38 MAPK. Ann N Y Acad Sci 1095:504–512
Kundu JK, Na HK, Chun KS, Kim YK, Lee SJ, Lee SS, Lee OS, Sim YC, Surh YJ (2003) Inhibition of phorbol ester-induced COX-2 expression by epigallocatechin gallate in mouse skin and cultured human mammary epithelial cells. J Nutr 133(11 Suppl 1):3805S–3810S
Kuttan R, Sudheeran PC, Josph CD (1987) Turmeric and curcumin as topical agents in cancer therapy. Tumori 73(1):29–31
Lamson DW, Brignall MS (2001) Natural agents in the prevention of cancer, part two: preclinical data and chemoprevention for common cancers. Altern Med Rev 6(2):167–187
Lan L, Trempus C, Gilmour SK (2000) Inhibition of ornithine decarboxylase (ODC) decreases tumor vascularization and reverses spontaneous tumors in ODC/Ras transgenic mice. Cancer Res 60(20):5696–5703
LeBlanc WG, Vidal L, Kirsner RS, Lee DJ, Caban-Martinez AJ, McCollister KE, Arheart KL, Chung-Bridges K, Christ S, Clark J 3rd, Lewis JE, Davila EP, Rouhani P, Fleming LE (2008) Reported skin cancer screening of US adult workers. J Am Acad Dermatol 59(1):55–63
Lee EH, Lim YJ, Ha SK, Kang TH, Koketsu M, Kang C, Kim SY, Park JH (2010) Inhibitory effects of 5-chloroacetyl-2-piperidino-1,3-selenazole, a novel selenium-containing compound, on skin melanin biosynthesis. J Pharm Pharmacol 62(3):352–359
Leiter U, Garbe C (2008) Epidemiology of melanoma and nonmelanoma skin cancer–the role of sunlight. Adv Exp Med Biol 624:89–103
Lepley DM, Pelling JC (1997) Induction of p21/WAF1 and G1 cell-cycle arrest by the chemopreventive agent apigenin. Mol Carcinog 19(2):74–82
Lepley DM, Li B, Birt DF, Pelling JC (1996) The chemopreventive flavonoid apigenin induces G2/M arrest in keratinocytes. Carcinogenesis 17(11):2367–2375
Lin JK, Chen YC, Huang YT, Lin-Shiau SY (1997) Suppression of protein kinase C and nuclear oncogene expression as possible molecular mechanisms of cancer chemoprevention by apigenin and curcumin. J Cell Biochem Suppl 28–29:39–48
Lotan R (1996) Retinoids in cancer chemoprevention. FASEB J 10(9):1031–1039
Lu YP, Chang RL, Huang MT, Conney AH (1993) Inhibitory effect of curcumin on 12-O-tetradecanoylphorbol-13-acetate-induced increase in ornithine decarboxylase mRNA in mouse epidermis. Carcinogenesis 14(2):293–297
Lu YP, Lou YR, Li XH, Xie JG, Brash D, Huang MT, Conney AH (2000) Stimulatory effect of oral administration of green tea or caffeine on ultraviolet light-induced increases in epidermal wild-type p53, p21(WAF1/CIP1), and apoptotic sunburn cells in SKH-1 mice. Cancer Res 60(17):4785–4791
Lu YP, Lou YR, Xie JG, Peng QY, Liao J, Yang CS, Huang MT, Conney AH (2002) Topical applications of caffeine or (-)-epigallocatechin gallate (EGCG) inhibit carcinogenesis and selectively increase apoptosis in UVB-induced skin tumors in mice. Proc Natl Acad Sci USA 99(19):12455–12460
Madhunapantula SV, Desai D, Sharma A, Huh SJ, Amin S, Robertson GP (2008) PBISe, a novel selenium-containing drug for the treatment of malignant melanoma. Mol Cancer Ther 7(5):1297–1308
Mantena SK, Meeran SM, Elmets CA, Katiyar SK (2005) Orally administered green tea polyphenols prevent ultraviolet radiation-induced skin cancer in mice through activation of cytotoxic T cells and inhibition of angiogenesis in tumors. J Nutr 135(12):2871–2877
McCullough JL, Kelly KM (2006) Prevention and treatment of skin aging. Ann N Y Acad Sci 1067:323–331
McVean M, Xiao H, Isobe K, Pelling JC (2000) Increase in wild-type p53 stability and transactivational activity by the chemopreventive agent apigenin in keratinocytes. Carcinogenesis 21(4):633–639

Meeran SM, Punathil T, Katiyar SK (2008) IL-12 deficiency exacerbates inflammatory responses in UV-irradiated skin and skin tumors. J Invest Dermatol 128(11):2716–2727

Mehta RG, Murillo G, Naithani R, Peng X (2010) Cancer chemoprevention by natural products: how far have we come? Pharm Res 27(6):950–961

Miller CC, Hale P, Pentland AP (1994) Ultraviolet B injury increases prostaglandin synthesis through a tyrosine kinase-dependent pathway. Evidence for UVB-induced epidermal growth factor receptor activation. J Biol Chem 269(5):3529–3533

Miyazaki K, Hanamizu T, Sone T, Chiba K, Kinoshita T, Yoshikawa S (2004) Topical application of Bifidobacterium-fermented soy milk extract containing genistein and daidzein improves rheological and physiological properties of skin. J Cosmet Sci 55(5):473–479

Moore JO, Wang Y, Stebbins WG, Gao D, Zhou X, Phelps R, Lebwohl M, Wei H (2006) Photoprotective effect of isoflavone genistein on ultraviolet B-induced pyrimidine dimer formation and PCNA expression in human reconstituted skin and its implications in dermatology and prevention of cutaneous carcinogenesis. Carcinogenesis 27(8):1627–1635

Morley N, Clifford T, Salter L, Campbell S, Gould D, Curnow A (2005) The green tea polyphenol (-)-epigallocatechin gallate and green tea can protect human cellular DNA from ultraviolet and visible radiation-induced damage. Photodermatol Photoimmunol Photomed 21(1):1522

Moyal DD, Fourtanier AM (2008) Broad-spectrum sunscreens provide better protection from solar ultraviolet-simulated radiation and natural sunlight-induced immunosuppression in human beings. J Am Acad Dermatol 58(5 Suppl 2):S149–S154

Mrass P, Rendl M, Mildner M, Gruber F, Lengauer B, Ballaun C, Eckhart L, Tschachler E (2004) Retinoic acid increases the expression of p53 and proapoptotic caspases and sensitizes keratinocytes to apoptosis: a possible explanation for tumor preventive action of retinoids. Cancer Res 64(18):6542–6548

Muller-Decker K, Kopp-Schneider A, Marks F, Seibert K, Furstenberger G (1998) Localization of prostaglandin H synthase isoenzymes in murine epidermal tumors: suppression of skin tumor promotion by inhibition of prostaglandin H synthase-2. Mol Carcinog 23(1):36–44

Murray JC, Burch JA, Streilein RD, Iannacchione MA, Hall RP, Pinnell SR (2008) A topical antioxidant solution containing vitamins C and E stabilized by ferulic acid provides protection for human skin against damage caused by ultraviolet irradiation. J Am Acad Dermatol 59(3):418–425

Narayanan DL, Saladi RN, Fox JL (2010) Ultraviolet radiation and skin cancer. Int J Dermatol 49(9):978–986

Nigam N, Shukla Y (2007) Preventive effects of diallyl sulfide on 7,12-dimethylbenz[a]anthracene induced DNA alkylation damage in mouse skin. Mol Nutr Food Res 51(11):1324–1328

Nigam N, Bhui K, Prasad S, George J, Shukla Y (2009) [6]-Gingerol induces reactive oxygen species regulated mitochondrial cell death pathway in human epidermoid carcinoma A431 cells. Chem Biol Interact 181(1):77–84

Nihal M, Ahmad N, Mukhtar H, Wood GS (2005) Anti-proliferative and proapoptotic effects of (-)-epigallocatechin-3-gallate on human melanoma: possible implications for the chemoprevention of melanoma. Int J Cancer 114(4):513–521

Niles RM (2000) Recent advances in the use of vitamin A (retinoids) in the prevention and treatment of cancer. Nutrition 16(11–12):1084–1089

Overvad K, Thorling EB, Bjerring P, Ebbesen P (1985) Selenium inhibits UV-light-induced skin carcinogenesis in hairless mice. Cancer Lett 27(2):163–170

Park KK, Chun KS, Lee JM, Lee SS, Surh YJ (1998) Inhibitory effects of [6]-gingerol, a major pungent principle of ginger, on phorbol ester-induced inflammation, epidermal ornithine decarboxylase activity and skin tumor promotion in ICR mice. Cancer Lett 129(2):139–144

Paul B, Hayes CS, Kim A, Athar M, Gilmour SK (2005) Elevated polyamines lead to selective induction of apoptosis and inhibition of tumorigenesis by (-)-epigallocatechin-3-gallate (EGCG) in ODC/Ras transgenic mice. Carcinogenesis 26(1):119–124

Pauling L (1991) Effect of ascorbic acid on incidence of spontaneous mammary tumors and UV-light-induced skin tumors in mice. Am J Clin Nutr 54(6 Suppl):1252S–1255S

Pauling L, Willoughby R, Reynolds R, Blaisdell BE, Lawson S (1982) Incidence of squamous cell carcinoma in hairless mice irradiated with ultraviolet light in relation to intake of ascorbic acid (vitamin C) and of D, L-alpha-tocopheryl acetate (vitamin E). Int J Vitam Nutr Res Suppl 23:53–82

Pentland AP, Schoggins JW, Scott GA, Khan KN, Han R (1999) Reduction of UV-induced skin tumors in hairless mice by selective COX-2 inhibition. Carcinogenesis 20(10):1939–1944

Perchellet JP, Perchellet EM, Abney NL, Zirnstein JA, Belman S (1986) Effects of garlic and onion oils on glutathione peroxidase activity, the ratio of reduced/oxidized glutathione and ornithine decarboxylase induction in isolated mouse epidermal cells treated with tumor promoters. Cancer Biochem Biophys 8(4):299–312

Perchellet JP, Abney NL, Thomas RM, Guislain YL, Perchellet EM (1987) Effects of combined treatments with selenium, glutathione, and vitamin E on glutathione peroxidase activity, ornithine decarboxylase induction, and complete and multistage carcinogenesis in mouse skin. Cancer Res 47(2):477–485

Perchellet JP, Perchellet EM, Belman S (1990) Inhibition of DMBA-induced mouse skin tumorigenesis by garlic oil and inhibition of two tumor-promotion stages by garlic and onion oils. Nutr Cancer 14(3–4):183–193

Pezzuto JM (1997) Plant-derived anticancer agents. Biochem Pharmacol 53(2):121–133

Pugliese PT (1998) The skin's antioxidant systems. Dermatol Nurs 10(6):401–416; quiz 417–408

Reagan-Shaw S, Afaq F, Aziz MH, Ahmad N (2004) Modulations of critical cell cycle regulatory events during chemoprevention of ultraviolet B-mediated responses by resveratrol in SKH-1 hairless mouse skin. Oncogene 23(30):5151–5160

Record IR, Dreosti IE (1998) Protection by black tea and green tea against UVB and UVA + B induced skin cancer in hairless mice. Mutat Res 422(1):191–199

Reichrath J (2001) Will analogs of 1,25-dihydroxyvitamin D(3) (calcitriol) open a new era in cancer therapy? Onkologie 24(2):128–133

Ren S, Lien EJ (1997) Natural products and their derivatives as cancer chemopreventive agents. Prog Drug Res 48:147–171

Rice-Evans CA, Miller NJ, Bolwell PG, Bramley PM, Pridham JB (1995) The relative antioxidant activities of plant-derived polyphenolic flavonoids. Free Radic Res 22(4):375–383

Rigel DS (2002) The effect of sunscreen on melanoma risk. Dermatol Clin 20(4):601–606

Robbins D, Gu X, Shi R, Liu J, Wang F, Ponville J, McCord JM, Zhao Y (2010) The chemopreventive effects of Protandim: modulation of p53 mitochondrial translocation and apoptosis during skin carcinogenesis. PLoS One 5(7):e11902

Rockley PF, Trieff N, Wagner RF, Jr., Tyring SK (1994a) Nonsunlight risk factors for malignant melanoma. Part I: chemical agents, physical conditions, and occupation. Int J Dermatol 33(6):398–406

Rockley PF, Trieff N, Wagner RF Jr, Tyring SK (1994b) Nonsunlight risk factors for malignant melanoma. Part II: immunity, genetics, and workplace prevention. Int J Dermatol 33(7): 462–467

Roy P, Kalra N, Prasad S, George J, Shukla Y (2009) Chemopreventive potential of resveratrol in mouse skin tumors through regulation of mitochondrial and PI3K/AKT signaling pathways. Pharm Res 26(1):211–217

Russo GL (2007) Ins and outs of dietary phytochemicals in cancer chemoprevention. Biochem Pharmacol 74(4):533–544

Sadhana AS, Rao AR, Kucheria K, Bijani V (1988) Inhibitory action of garlic oil on the initiation of benzo[a]pyrene-induced skin carcinogenesis in mice. Cancer Lett 40(2):193–197

Safe S, Wargovich MJ, Lamartiniere CA, Mukhtar H (1999) Symposium on mechanisms of action of naturally occurring anticarcinogens. Toxicol Sci 52(1):1–8

Saliou C, Kitazawa M, McLaughlin L, Yang JP, Lodge JK, Tetsuka T, Iwasaki K, Cillard J, Okamoto T, Packer L (1999) Antioxidants modulate acute solar ultraviolet radiation-induced NF-kappa-B activation in a human keratinocyte cell line. Free Radic Biol Med 26(1–2):174–183

Sarfaraz S, Siddiqui IA, Syed DN, Afaq F, Mukhtar H (2008) Guggulsterone modulates MAPK and NF-kappaB pathways and inhibits skin tumorigenesis in SENCAR mice. Carcinogenesis 29(10):2011–2018

Savoure N, Briand G, Amory-Touz MC, Combre A, Maudet M, Nicol M (1995) Vitamin A status and metabolism of cutaneous polyamines in the hairless mouse after UV irradiation: action of beta-carotene and astaxanthin. Int J Vitam Nutr Res 65(2):79–86

Savoure N, Maudet M, Nicol M, Pelissier MA, Albrecht R, Briand G, Combre A (1996) Modulation of ultraviolet light-induced oxidative stress in mice skin related to dietary vitamin A and selenium intake. Int J Vitam Nutr Res 66(4):306–315

Schwarz A, Maeda A, Gan D, Mammone T, Matsui MS, Schwarz T (2008) Green tea phenol extracts reduce UVB-induced DNA damage in human cells via interleukin-12. Photochem Photobiol 84(2):350–355

Sengupta A, Lichti UF, Carlson BA, Ryscavage AO, Gladyshev VN, Yuspa SH, Hatfield DL (2010) Selenoproteins are essential for proper keratinocyte function and skin development. PLoS One 5(8):e12249

Seve M, Chimienti F, Devergnas S, Aouffen M, Douki T, Chantegrel J, Cadet J, Favier A (2005) Resveratrol enhances UVA-induced DNA damage in HaCaT human keratinocytes. Med Chem 1(6):629–633

Shahriari M, Kerr PE, Slade K, Grant-Kels JE (2010) Vitamin D and the skin. Clin Dermatol 28(6):663–668

Shankar S, Singh G, Srivastava RK (2007) Chemoprevention by resveratrol: molecular mechanisms and therapeutic potential. Front Biosci 12:4839–4854

Sharma SD, Katiyar SK (2010) Dietary grape seed proanthocyanidins inhibit UVB-induced cyclooxygenase-2 expression and other inflammatory mediators in UVB-exposed skin and skin tumors of SKH-1 hairless mice. Pharm Res 27(6):1092–1102

She QB, Bode AM, Ma WY, Chen NY, Dong Z (2001) Resveratrol-induced activation of p53 and apoptosis is mediated by extracellular-signal-regulated protein kinases and p38 kinase. Cancer Res 61(4):1604–1610

Shore RE (2001) Radiation-induced skin cancer in humans. Med Pediatr Oncol 36(5):549–554

Siddiqui IA, Afaq F, Adhami VM, Ahmad N, Mukhtar H (2004) Antioxidants of the beverage tea in promotion of human health. Antioxid Redox Signal 6(3):571–582

Siddiqui IA, Adhami VM, Saleem M, Mukhtar H (2006) Beneficial effects of tea and its polyphenols against prostate cancer. Mol Nutr Food Res 50(2):130–143

Siddiqui IA, Saleem M, Adhami VM, Asim M, Mukhtar H (2007) Tea beverage in chemoprevention and chemotherapy of prostate cancer. Acta Pharmacol Sin 28(9):1392–1408

Siddiqui IA, Afaq F, Adhami VM, Mukhtar H (2008) Prevention of prostate cancer through custom tailoring of chemopreventive regimen. Chem Biol Interact 171(2):122–132

Siddiqui IA, Tarapore RS, Mukhtar H (2009) Prevention of skin cancer by green tea: past, present and future. Cancer Biol Ther 8(13):1288–1291

Sienkiewicz P, Surazynski A, Palka J, Miltyk W (2008) Nutritional concentration of genistein protects human dermal fibroblasts from oxidative stress-induced collagen biosynthesis inhibition through IGF-I receptor-mediated signaling. Acta Pol Pharm 65(2):203–211

Singh DK, Lippman SM (1998a) Cancer chemoprevention. Part 1: retinoids and carotenoids and other classic antioxidants. Oncology (Williston Park) 12(11):1643–1653, 1657–1648; discussion 1659–1660

Singh DK, Lippman SM (1998b) Cancer chemoprevention. Part 2: hormones, nonclassic antioxidant natural agents, NSAIDs, and other agents. Oncology (Williston Park) 12(12):1787–1800; discussion 1802, 1805

Singh A, Shukla Y (1998a) Antitumor activity of diallyl sulfide in two-stage mouse skin model of carcinogenesis. Biomed Environ Sci 11(3):258–263

Singh A, Shukla Y (1998b) Antitumour activity of diallyl sulfide on polycyclic aromatic hydrocarbon-induced mouse skin carcinogenesis. Cancer Lett 131(2):209–214

Singh RP, Dhanalakshmi S, Mohan S, Agarwal C, Agarwal R (2006) Silibinin inhibits UVB- and epidermal growth factor-induced mitogenic and cell survival signaling involving activator protein-1 and nuclear factor-kappaB in mouse epidermal JB6 cells. Mol Cancer Ther 5(5):1145–1153

Situm M, Buljan M, Bulat V, Lugovic Mihic L, Bolanca Z, Simic D (2008) The role of UV radiation in the development of basal cell carcinoma. Coll Antropol 32(Suppl 2):167–170

Smart RC, Crawford CL (1991) Effect of ascorbic acid and its synthetic lipophilic derivative ascorbyl palmitate on phorbol ester-induced skin-tumor promotion in mice. Am J Clin Nutr 54(6 Suppl):1266S–1273S

Song H, Hur I, Park HJ, Nam J, Park GB, Kong KH, Hwang YM, Kim YS, Cho DH, Lee WJ, Hur DY (2009) Selenium inhibits metastasis of murine melanoma cells through the induction of cell cycle arrest and cell death. Immune Netw 9(6):236–242

Stern RS, Weinstein MC, Baker SG (1986) Risk reduction for nonmelanoma skin cancer with childhood sunscreen use. Arch Dermatol 122(5):537–545

Suarez B, Lopez-Abente G, Martinez C, Navarro C, Tormo MJ, Rosso S, Schraub S, Gafa L, Sancho-Garnier H, Wechsler J, Zanetti R (2007) Occupation and skin cancer: the results of the HELIOS-I multicenter case-control study. BMC Public Health 7:180

Suh KS, Roh HJ, Choi SY, Jeon YS, Doh KS, Bae JH, Kim ST (2007) Long-term evaluation of erythema and pigmentation induced by ultraviolet radiations of different wavelengths. Skin Res Technol 13(2):154–161

Surh YJ (2003) Cancer chemoprevention with dietary phytochemicals. Nat Rev Cancer 3(10): 768–780

Svobodova A, Zdarilova A, Walterova D, Vostalova J (2007) Flavonolignans from Silybum marianum moderate UVA-induced oxidative damage to HaCaT keratinocytes. J Dermatol Sci 48(3):213–224

Thompson SC, Jolley D, Marks R (1993) Reduction of solar keratoses by regular sunscreen use. N Engl J Med 329(16):1147–1151

Tong X, Van Dross RT, Abu-Yousif A, Morrison AR, Pelling JC (2007) Apigenin prevents UVB-induced cyclooxygenase 2 expression: coupled mRNA stabilization and translational inhibition. Mol Cell Biol 27(1):283–296

Ulrich C, Degen A, Patel MJ, Stockfleth E (2008) Sunscreens in organ transplant patients. Nephrol Dial Transplant 23(6):1805–1808

Vainio H, Bianchini F (2000) Cancer-preventive effects of sunscreens are uncertain. Scand J Work Environ Health 26(6):529–531

Vainio H, Miller AB, Bianchini F (2000) An international evaluation of the cancer-preventive potential of sunscreens. Int J Cancer 88(5):838–842

van De Kerkhof PC (2001) New developments in the treatment of psoriasis. Skin Pharmacol Appl Skin Physiol 14(3):129–135

van der Pols JC, Williams GM, Pandeya N, Logan V, Green AC (2006) Prolonged prevention of squamous cell carcinoma of the skin by regular sunscreen use. Cancer Epidemiol Biomarkers Prev 15(12):2546–2548

Van Dross RT, Hong X, Essengue S, Fischer SM, Pelling JC (2007) Modulation of UVB-induced and basal cyclooxygenase-2 (COX-2) expression by apigenin in mouse keratinocytes: role of USF transcription factors. Mol Carcinog 46(4):303–314

Vayalil PK, Mittal A, Hara Y, Elmets CA, Katiyar SK (2004) Green tea polyphenols prevent ultraviolet light-induced oxidative damage and matrix metalloproteinases expression in mouse skin. J Invest Dermatol 122(6):1480–1487

Wang HK (1998) Plant-derived anticancer agents currently in clinical use or in clinical trials. IDrugs 1(1):92–102

Wang ZY, Khan WA, Bickers DR, Mukhtar H (1989) Protection against polycyclic aromatic hydrocarbon-induced skin tumor initiation in mice by green tea polyphenols. Carcinogenesis 10(2):411–415

Wang ZY, Agarwal R, Bickers DR, Mukhtar H (1991) Protection against ultraviolet B radiation-induced photocarcinogenesis in hairless mice by green tea polyphenols. Carcinogenesis 12(8):1527–1530

Wang ZY, Hong JY, Huang MT, Reuhl KR, Conney AH, Yang CS (1992a) Inhibition of N-nitrosodiethylamine- and 4-(methylnitrosamino)-1-(3-pyridyl)-1-butanone-induced tumorigenesis in A/J mice by green tea and black tea. Cancer Res 52(7):1943–1947

Wang ZY, Huang MT, Ferraro T, Wong CQ, Lou YR, Reuhl K, Iatropoulos M, Yang CS, Conney AH (1992b) Inhibitory effect of green tea in the drinking water on tumorigenesis by ultraviolet light and 12-O-tetradecanoylphorbol-13-acetate in the skin of SKH-1 mice. Cancer Res 52(5):1162–1170

Wang ZY, Huang MT, Ho CT, Chang R, Ma W, Ferraro T, Reuhl KR, Yang CS, Conney AH (1992c) Inhibitory effect of green tea on the growth of established skin papillomas in mice. Cancer Res 52(23):6657–6665

Wang ZY, Huang MT, Lou YR, Xie JG, Reuhl KR, Newmark HL, Ho CT, Yang CS, Conney AH (1994) Inhibitory effects of black tea, green tea, decaffeinated black tea, and decaffeinated green tea on ultraviolet B light-induced skin carcinogenesis in 7,12-dimethylbenz[a]anthracene-initiated SKH-1 mice. Cancer Res 54(13):3428–3435

Wang Y, Zhang X, Lebwohl M, DeLeo V, Wei H (1998) Inhibition of ultraviolet B (UVB)-induced c-fos and c-jun expression in vivo by a tyrosine kinase inhibitor genistein. Carcinogenesis 19(4):649–654

Wang YN, Wu W, Chen HC, Fang H (2010) Genistein protects against UVB-induced senescence-like characteristics in human dermal fibroblast by p66Shc down-regulation. J Dermatol Sci 58(1):19–27

Wei H, Tye L, Bresnick E, Birt DF (1990) Inhibitory effect of apigenin, a plant flavonoid, on epidermal ornithine decarboxylase and skin tumor promotion in mice. Cancer Res 50(3): 499–502

Wei H, Wei L, Frenkel K, Bowen R, Barnes S (1993) Inhibition of tumor promoter-induced hydrogen peroxide formation in vitro and in vivo by genistein. Nutr Cancer 20(1):1–12

Wei H, Bowen R, Cai Q, Barnes S, Wang Y (1995) Antioxidant and antipromotional effects of the soybean isoflavone genistein. Proc Soc Exp Biol Med 208(1):124–130

Wei H, Bowen R, Zhang X, Lebwohl M (1998) Isoflavone genistein inhibits the initiation and promotion of two-stage skin carcinogenesis in mice. Carcinogenesis 19(8):1509–1514

Wei H, Zhang X, Wang Y, Lebwohl M (2002) Inhibition of ultraviolet light-induced oxidative events in the skin and internal organs of hairless mice by isoflavone genistein. Cancer Lett 185(1):21–29

Wilgus TA, Ross MS, Parrett ML, Oberyszyn TM (2000) Topical application of a selective cyclooxygenase inhibitor suppresses UVB mediated cutaneous inflammation. Prostaglandins Other Lipid Mediat 62(4):367–384

Wolf P (2003) [Sunscreens. Protection against skin cancers and photoaging]. Hautarzt 54(9): 839–844

Wolf R, Wolf D, Morganti P, Ruocco V (2001) Sunscreens. Clin Dermatol 19(4):452–459

Wright TI, Spencer JM, Flowers FP (2006) Chemoprevention of nonmelanoma skin cancer. J Am Acad Dermatol 54(6):933–946; quiz 947–950

Xia J, Song X, Bi Z, Chu W, Wan Y (2005) UV-induced NF-kappaB activation and expression of IL-6 is attenuated by (-)-epigallocatechin-3-gallate in cultured human keratinocytes in vitro. Int J Mol Med 16(5):943–950

Yamamoto T, Hsu S, Lewis J, Wataha J, Dickinson D, Singh B, Bollag WB, Lockwood P, Ueta E, Osaki T, Schuster G (2003) Green tea polyphenol causes differential oxidative environments in tumor versus normal epithelial cells. J Pharmacol Exp Ther 307(1):230–236

Yuspa SH, Dlugosz AA, Denning MF, Glick AB (1996) Multistage carcinogenesis in the skin. J Investig Dermatol Symp Proc 1(2):147–150

Yusuf N, Nasti TH, Meleth S, Elmets CA (2009) Resveratrol enhances cell-mediated immune response to DMBA through TLR4 and prevents DMBA induced cutaneous carcinogenesis. Mol Carcinog 48(8):713–723

Zhao J, Sharma Y, Agarwal R (1999) Significant inhibition by the flavonoid antioxidant silymarin against 12-O-tetradecanoylphorbol 13-acetate-caused modulation of antioxidant and inflammatory enzymes, and cyclooxygenase 2 and interleukin-1alpha expression in SENCAR mouse epidermis: implications in the prevention of stage I tumor promotion. Mol Carcinog 26(4):321–333

Zhao J, Lahiri-Chatterjee M, Sharma Y, Agarwal R (2000) Inhibitory effect of a flavonoid antioxidant silymarin on benzoyl peroxide-induced tumor promotion, oxidative stress and inflammatory responses in SENCAR mouse skin. Carcinogenesis 21(4):811–816

Chapter 14
Dietary Phytochemicals and Chemoprevention of Solar Ultraviolet Radiation-Induced Skin Cancer

Farrukh Afaq and Santosh K. Katiyar

Abstract Preclinical, clinical and epidemiological studies suggest that exposure of skin to solar ultraviolet (UV) radiation induces harmful effects and leads to various skin diseases including melanoma and non-melanoma skin cancers. Solar UV radiation-induced skin cancers are caused by depletion in antioxidant defense system, inflammation, DNA damage, oxidation of lipids and proteins, disturbances in apoptotic machinery, deregulation of signaling pathways, mutation in critical target genes and immunosuppression. Therefore, for reducing the incidence of skin cancer the use of phytochemicals that possess the abilities to inhibit these events is gaining considerable attention as photoprotective agents. These phytochemicals are widely distributed in plant kingdom which includes fruits, vegetables, seeds, flowers and bark; and belong to several classes that include polyphenols, flavonoids, isoflavonoids, proanthocyanidins, phytoalexins, anthocyanidins and carotenoids. This chapter presents and discusses key findings from studies on the photoprotective effects of some selected phytochemicals, such as, green tea polyphenols, pomegranate fruit extract, grape seed proanthocyanidins, silymarin, resveratrol, genistein, honokiol, quercetin, delphinidin, curcumin, sulforaphone, lycopene and lutein/zeaxanthin on UV-induced skin inflammation, oxidative stress, immunosuppression, DNA damage and dysregulation of important cellular signaling pathways for the management of skin cancer.

Abbreviations

BCC	basal cell carcinomas
CHS	contact hypersensitivity
COX-2	cyclooxygenase-2
CPD	cyclobutane pyrimidine dimers
ECG	(-)-epicatechin gallate

S.K. Katiyar (✉)
Department of Dermatology, Comprehensive Cancer Center, Nutrition Obesity Research Center, University of Alabama at Birmingham, Birmingham, AL 35294, USA

Birmingham VA Medical Center, Birmingham, AL, USA
e-mail: skatiyar@uab.edu

F.H. Sarkar (ed.), *Nutraceuticals and Cancer*, DOI 10.1007/978-94-007-2630-7_14,

EGC	(-)-epigallocatechin
EGCG	(-)-epigallocatechin-3-gallate
GPx	glutathione peroxidase
GSH	reduced glutathione
GSPs	grape seed proanthocyanidins
GTPs	green tea polyphenols
H_2O_2	hydrogen peroxide
IL	interleukin
MAPK	mitogen-activated protein kinase
NER	nucleotide excision repair
NFκB	nuclear factor-kappaB
PCNA	proliferating cell nuclear antigen
PFE	pomegranate fruit extract
PG	prostaglandin
PGE_2	prostaglandin E2
ROS	reactive oxygen species
SCC	squamous cell carcinomas
TNFα	tumor necrosis factor alpha
UV	ultraviolet
XPA	xeroderma pigmentosum complementation group A

14.1 Introduction

Epidemiologic, clinical and laboratory studies have revealed that bioactive phytochemicals present in fruit and vegetables consumed by the human population afford photoprotection against melanoma and non-melanoma skin cancers (Nichols and Katiyar 2010; Adhami et al. 2008; Surh 2003). Thus, a concept of what to consume and what to avoid is of paramount interest for maintaining healthy skin and protecting it from potentially harmful biological and environmental insults, including the harmful effects of solar ultraviolet (UV) radiation. The use of dietary phytochemicals that possesses antioxidant, anti-inflammatory, immunomodulatory, DNA repair capability, and that can correct undesired cellular functions has gained considerable attention as photoprotective and/or photochemopreventive agents (Katiyar 2007; Afaq 2011; Nichols and Katiyar 2010; Surh 2003). Because of these properties dietary phytochemicals are gaining popularity as more and more skin care products containing botanical ingredients are introduced in the market for the protection of human skin from the damaging effects of solar UV radiation. Phytochemicals which are medicinally bioactive are widely distributed in fruits, vegetables, seeds, flowers and bark; and belong to several classes that include polyphenols, flavonoids, isoflavonoids, proanthocyanidins, phytoalexins, phenols, anthocyanidins and carotenoids. Some of these phytochemicals are: polyphenols from green tea (GTPs), anthocyanidins from fruit extract of pomegranate (PFE), grape seed proanthocyanidins (GSPs), silymarin, resveratrol, genistein, delphinidin, curcumin, honokiol, sulforaphane, quercetin, lycopene and lutein/zeaxanthin (Table 14.1). Studies have suggested that many of these phytochemicals play multiple roles in ameliorating the process of photocarcinogenesis (Katiyar 2007; Afaq 2011; Nichols and Katiyar 2010; Surh 2003). Thus, the photochemopreventive approach appears to be a practical strategy in reducing the risk

Table 14.1 Structures and common sources of phytochemicals discussed in this book chapter

Phytochemicals	Structure	Source
EGCG	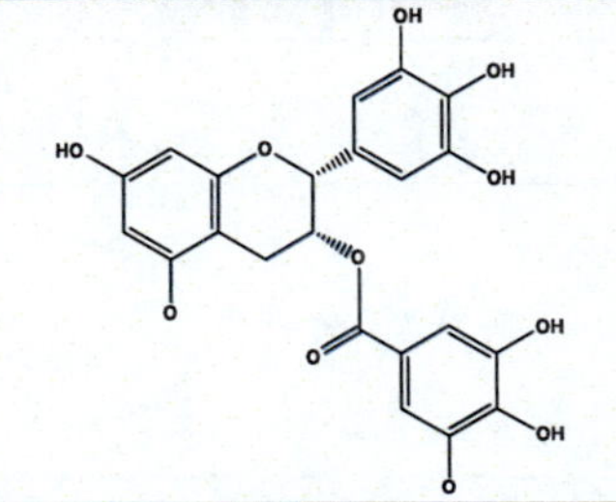	Tea leaves *(Camellia sinensis)*
Proanthocyanidins	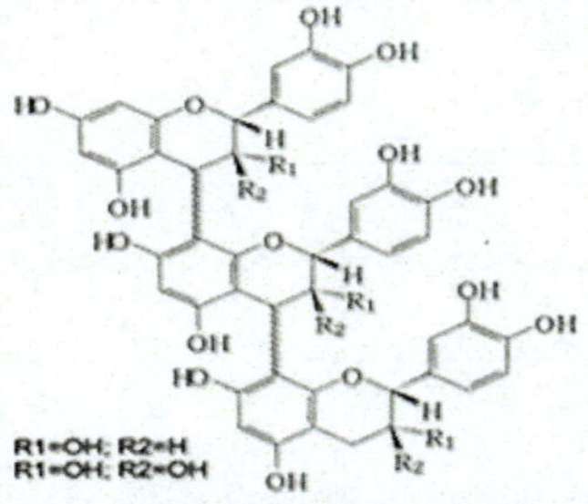	Grape seeds
Silymarin/silibinin	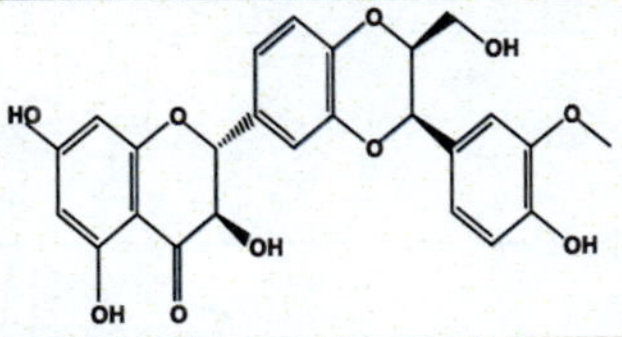	Milk thistle *(Silybum marianum)*
Resveratrol	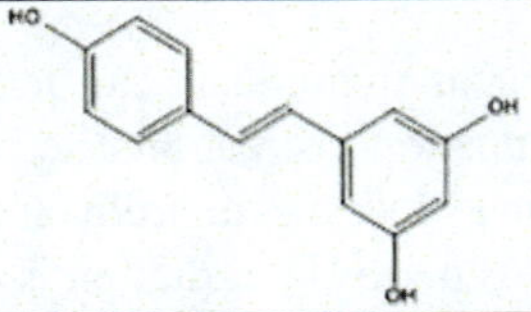	Grape skins, Red wine and Peanuts
Genistein	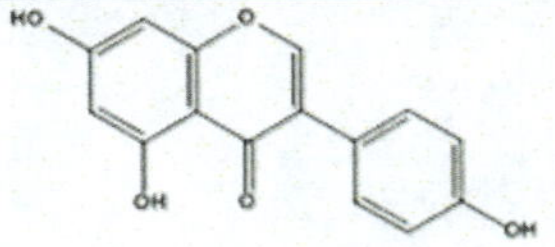	Soybeans

Table 14.1 (continued)

Delphinidin	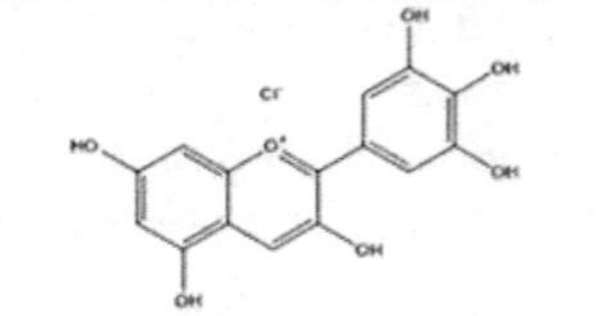	Berries and pomegrantes
Curcumin	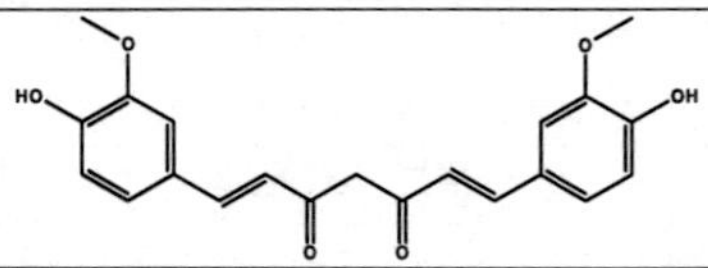	Turmeric
Sulforaphane	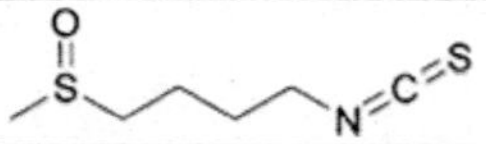	Broccoli sprouts, cabbages and kales
Quercetin	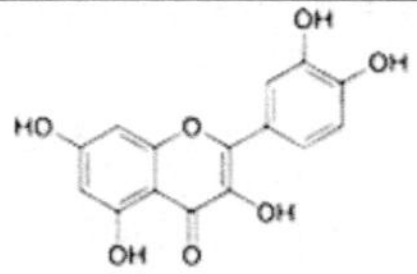	Fruits, vegetables and grains
Honokiol	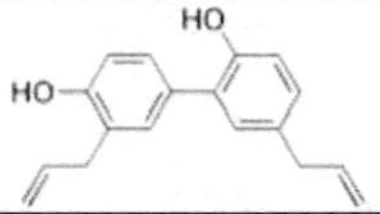	*Magnolia* species
Lycopene	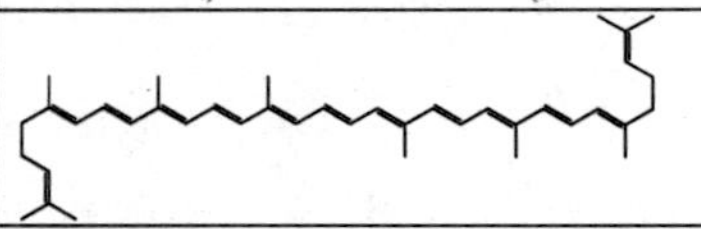	Tomatoes
Lutein	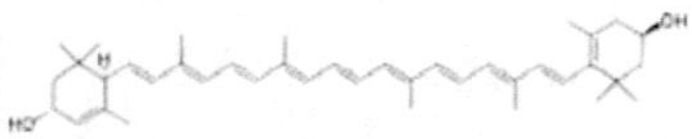	Spinach and Kales
Zeaxanthin	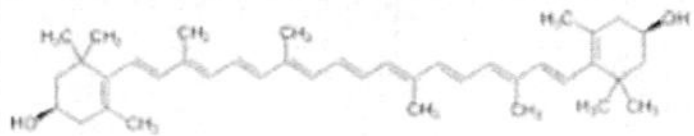	Zea mays

of non-melanoma skin cancer as individuals can modify their dietary habits and lifestyle (such as outdoor occupation, recreational activity and use of tanning parlor) in combination with careful use of skin care products supplemented with non-toxic phytochemicals, because exposure to UV radiation is difficult to control.

14.2 Solar UV Spectrum

Solar UV radiation is the most prominent and ubiquitous carcinogen in our environment that leads to various skin diseases including the risk of melanoma and non-melanoma skin cancers comprising of basal cell carcinomas (BCCs) and squamous cell carcinomas (SCCs) (Jemal et al. 2010; Bowden 2004; Katiyar 2007). The cause of these effects is contingent upon the UV dose, time of exposure and the wavelength of UV radiation. Solar UV spectrum is primarily divided into three regions depending on the wavelength: UVC (200–280 nm), UVB (280–320 nm), and UVA (320–400 nm). UVC is the short wavelength of the UV spectrum and is the most biologically damaging region of UV radiation. It has enormous energy and can penetrate the skin to a depth of approximately 60–80 micrometer. However, it is prevented from reaching the Earth's surface as it is almost completely absorbed by the stratospheric ozone layer. Therefore, the role of UVC in human skin pathogenesis is insignificant. UVB radiation of the UV spectrum constitutes about 5% of total UV radiation and can penetrates the skin to a depth of approximately 160–180 micrometer. UVB radiation has both direct and indirect effects on the skin that includes DNA damage, protein oxidation, depletion of cutaneous antioxidants enzymes, DNA damage, inflammation, immunosuppression and premature aging of the skin (Rundhaug et al. 2007; Halliday 2005; Melnikova and Ananthaswamy 2005; Clydesdale et al. 2001; Afaq 2011; Adhami et al. 2008; Nichols and Katiyar 2010). UVB also can act as a tumor initiator (Kligman et al. 1980), tumor promoter (Katiyar et al. 1997a), and co-carcinogen (Donawho and Kripke 1991; Ziegler et al. 1994). In addition, UVB radiation is responsible for a variety of skin diseases including non-melanoma and melanoma skin cancers (Jemal et al. 2010). Studies have suggested that in UV skin tumorigenesis approximately 90% of the carcinogenic dose of solar light is derived from UVB. UVA is the long wavelength part of the UV spectrum and constitutes about 90–95% of the total solar UV radiation reaching the Earth's surface. Because of its longer wavelength, UVA can penetrate the skin to a depth of approximately 1000 micrometer. UVA accounts for at least 10% of the carcinogenic dose of the solar light. UVA irradiation leads to generation of reactive oxygen species (ROS) such as hydrogen peroxide (H_2O_2), and hydroxyl radical, singlet oxygen etc. that can cause damage to cellular proteins, lipids and DNA (Nichols and Katiyar 2010; Adhami et al. 2008). The formation of ROS results in oxidative stress and imbalance the antioxidant defense capacity of skin cells leading to inflammation, immunosuppression, photoaging, and skin cancer (Bachelor and Bowden 2004; Nichols and Katiyar 2010; Ullrich 1995).

14.3 Solar UV Radiation and Adverse Effects on the Skin

Skin is the largest organ of the body, covers an enormous surface area (1.5–2.0 m^2) and situated at the interface between the body and its environment, directly suffers from the deleterious effects of solar UV radiation (Afaq and Mukhtar 2006; Katiyar 2007). Solar UV radiation jeopardizes the integrity of the skin that is critical for cellular homeostasis by the formation of ROS that react with proteins, lipids and DNA (Afaq et al. 2005; Nichols and Katiyar 2010). Exposure of the skin to solar UV radiation has been implicated in the initiation of several skin disorders, such as fine and coarse wrinkling, rough skin texture, dryness, mottled pigment abnormalities, skin aging and skin cancer (Mukhtar and Elmets 1996; Quan et al. 2009; Gonzaga 2009). The incidence of UV-induced skin cancers has increased dramatically worldwide accounting for more than 40% of all human cancers in the United States, with about 1.3 million new cases being diagnosed annually. A considerable body of evidence suggests that exposure to UVB plays a major role in the development of non-melanoma skin cancers comprising of BCCs and SCCs, the most frequently diagnosed cutaneous malignancies. Approximately 80% of non-melanoma skin cancers are BCCs, and 20% are SCCs. On the other hand, malignant melanoma, the deadliest form of skin cancer accounts approximately 4% of all skin cancers (Jemal et al. 2010). Studies have shown that the average erythemal UV doses of Americans are about 25,000 J/m^2/year, or about 33,000 J/m^2/year, including a conservative continental US vacation (about 8,000 J/m^2/year) (Godar et al. 2001).

14.4 Dietary Phytochemicals and Prevention of Photocarcinogenesis

Accumulating evidences suggest that it is possible to prevent cutaneous malignancies and other skin disorders caused by over exposure of UV radiation which share common pathogenetic mechanisms, such as DNA damage, oxidative stress, and chronic inflammation (Katiyar 2007; Afaq 2011; Nichols and Katiyar 2010). A palpable approach is avoidance of exposure to solar UV radiation. As complementary strategies, it is possible to render the skin cells more resistant to solar UV radiation and/or to inhibit progression of the disease by administering naturally occurring chemopreventive agents known as phytochemicals. Intake of fruits, vegetables, spices and whole grains may reduce the incidence of skin cancer and this has been attributed to these foods being rich sources of numerous bioactive phytochemicals (Surh 2003; Afaq 2011; Nichols and Katiyar 2010). Dietary phytochemicals are generally regarded as being safe and some of them may even have efficacy for preventing or reversing premalignant lesions and/or reducing tumor incidence. Because of these reasons phytochemicals present in the human diet and in beverages have gained considerable attention for the prevention of UV-induced skin photodamage and can be exploited as ideal chemopreventive agents. These phytochemicals may work in different ways by: (i) reducing oxidative DNA damage, (ii) enhancing DNA repair, (iii) reducing inflammation, (iv) stimulating the immune response, (v) inducing oncogene suppression, (vi) inducing expression of tumor suppressor genes, and (vii) modulating cellular signaling pathways. Many of these phytochemicals play multiple roles in ameliorating the process of photocarcinogenesis. In this chapter, we have discussed the biological effects and postulated mechanism(s) of some of the selected phytochemicals (such as GTPs, PFE, GSPs, silymarin, resveratrol, genistein, delphinidin, curcumin, honokiol, sulforaphone, quercetin, lycopene and lutein/zeaxanthin) in relation to their protective and chemopreventive potentials against UV radiation-mediated skin damages (Table 14.2). Various animal models have been used to study the anti-photocarcinogenic effects of phytochemicals.

Table 14.2 A summary of biological effects and molecular mechanism(s) of selected dietary phytochemicals in prevention of UV-induced skin cancer

Phytochemicals	Biological effects/molecular mechanism(s)	References
Green tea polyphenols/EGCG	Reduction in tumor incidence and tumor multiplicity in mice.	Wang et al. (1991), Mantena et al. (2005), Mantena and Katiyar (2006), Meeran et al. (2009)
	Regression of established experimentally-induced non-malignant skin papilloma in mice.	Wang et al. (1992b)
	Inhibition of UVB radiation-induced cutaneous edema in mice.	Afaq et al. (2003b)
	Inhibition of UVB radiation-induced inflammatory biomarkers (COX-2, PGE_2, PCNA, cyclin D1) and proinflammatory cytokines (TNF-α, IL-6, IL-1β) in mice.	Meeran et al. (2009)
	Reduction in UVB-mediated induction of myeloperoxidase activity as well as the production of H_2O_2 and nitric oxide in both epidermis and dermis of mouse skin.	Katiyar and Mukhtar (2001)
	Inhibition of UVB-induced phosphorylation of MAPKs in NHEK.	Katiyar et al. (2001a)
	Protection from UVB-induced depletion of antioxidant enzymes, induction of lipid peroxidation and oxidation of proteins in mouse skin.	Agarwal et al. (1993), Vayalil et al. (2003)
	Reduction in UVB-induced infiltration of $CD11b^+$ cells and IL-10 production. Induction of IL-12 production in UVB-exposed skin.	Katiyar et al. (1999a)
	Reduction in UVB-induced DNA damage through IL-12 dependent functional NER mechanism in mouse skin.	Meeran et al. (2009)
	Inhibition of UVB-mediated formation of CPD^+ cells in mouse skin.	Katiyar et al. (2010)
	Inhibition of UVB-mediated DNA damage through IL-12 dependent induction of DNA repairs in human reconstitituted skin.	Schwarz et al. (2008)
	Reduction in UVB-mediated formation of CPDs in both epidermis and dermis of human skin.	Katiyar et al. (2000)

Table 14.2 (continued)

Phytochemicals	Biological effects/molecular mechanism(s)	References
	Inhibition of UVB-induced production of prostaglandin metabolites, particularly PGE_2, in human skin.	Katiyar et al. (1999b)
	Inhibition of UV-induced production of H_2O_2 and nitric oxide as well as lipid peroxidation in both epidermis and dermis. Protection against UVB-induced depletion of antioxidant enzymes.	Katiyar et al. (2001b)
Grape seed proanthocyanidins	Reduction in tumor incidence, tumor multiplicity and tumor size. Prevention/delay in malignant transformation of UVB-induced papillomas to carcinomas in mice.	Mittal et al. (2003)
	Inhibition of UVB-mediated infiltration and accumulation of activated macrophages and neutrophils, myeloperoxidase activity, COX-2, cyclin D1, PCNA, PGE_2, TNF-α, IL-6 and IL-1β in mouse skin.	Sharma and Katiyar (2010)
	Restoration of UVB-induced depletion of GPx, GSH, and catalase; and suppression of oxidative stress in terms of H_2O_2 and nitric oxide production, lipid peroxidation and protein oxidation in mouse skin.	Sharma et al. (2007)
	Inhibition of UVB-induced phosphorylation of MAPKs and activation of NF-κB signaling pathway in mouse skin.	Sharma et al. (2007)
	Protection against UVB-mediated enhanced production of IL-10 by the epidermal and dermal cells of the skin, and in the draining lymph nodes. Increase in the production of IL-12 in the draining lymph nodes.	Sharma and Katiyar (2006)
	Inhibition of UVB-induced immunosuppression by activating $CD8^+$ effector T cells and inhibiting $CD4^+$ regulatory T cells.	Vaid et al. (2010b)
	Repair of UV-induced CPDs is mediated through stimulation of IL-12.	Vaid et al. (2010b)
Siymarin/silibinin	Effective in protecting the skin from UV-induced tumor initiation, tumor promotion, and complete carcinogenesis in mice.	Katiyar et al. (1997a)
	Inhibition of UVB-induced infiltration of $CD11b^+$ cells and myeloperoxidase activity in mouse skin.	Katiyar et al. (2008)
	Inhibition of UVB-induced expression of COX-2 and prostaglandin metabolites in mouse skin.	Katiyar et al. (1997a)

Table 14.2 (continued)

Phytochemicals	Biological effects/molecular mechanism(s)	References
	Reduction in UVB-mediated COX-2 protein expression by targeting transcription factors such as STAT3 and NF-κB in mouse skin.	Gu et al. (2007)
	Reduction in the number of UVB-induced H_2O_2 producing cells, inducible nitric oxide synthase expressing cells concomitant with decrease in H_2O_2 and nitric oxide production. Inhibition of UVB-induced myeloperoxidase activity, IL-10 producing cells and the levels of IL-10 in mouse skin.	Katiyar (2002)
	Reduction in UVB-induced CPDs positive cells in mouse epidermis and this may be mediated via an activation of p53-p21/Cip1 cascade.	Dhanalakshmi et al. (2004), Gu et al. (2005)
Pomegranate fruit extract	Result in reduced tumor incidence, delay in the latency period of tumor appearance, and lower tumor body burden in mice.	Afaq et al. (2008)
	Inhibition of UVB-induced skin edema, hyperplasia, infiltration of leukocytes, lipid peroxidation, COX-2 expression, hydrogen peroxide generation and protein oxidation in mouse skin.	Afaq et al. (2007b, 2010)
	Reduction in UVB-mediated formation of CPDs, and 8-oxodG in mouse skin.	Afaq et al. (2010)
	Protection of HaCaT cells from UVB-mediated depletion of endogenous GSH. Inhibition of UVB-induced lipid peroxidation.	Zaid et al. (2007)
	Reduction in UVB -induced formation of CPDs and 8-oxodG in reconstituted human skin.	Afaq et al. (2009)
Resveratrol	Inhibition of UVB-radiation induced tumor incidence and delay in the onset of skin tumorigenesis in mice.	Aziz et al. (2005)
	Reduction in the average number of skin tumors, average tumor volume and in the number of SCCs in mice.	Kim et al. (2011)
	Reduction in UVB-mediated infiltration of leukocytes, skin edema, H_2O_2 production and PG metabolites, especially PGE_2 and PGD_2.	Afaq et al. (2003a)
	Inhibition of UVB-mediated activation of NF-κB pathway in NHEK.	Adhami et al. (2003)

Table 14.2 (continued)

Phytochemicals	Biological effects/molecular mechanism(s)	References
Genistein	Reduction in UVB-induced formation of sunburn cells in mouse skin.	Brand and Jendrzejewski, (2008)
	Inhibition of UVB-stimulated PGE_2 synthesis and phosphorylation of EGFR at tyrosine residues in cell culture.	Miller et al. (1994)
	Modulation of UVB-induced mitochondrial oxidative stress through down-regulation of p66Shc-dependent signaling pathway in human dermal fibroblasts.	Wang et al. (2010)
	Inhibition of UVB-induced H_2O_2 generation and malondialdehyde production in mouse skin.	Wei et al. (2002)
	Inhibition of UVB-induced CPDs formation in human reconstituted skin	Moore et al. (2006)
Delphinidin	Suppression of UVB-induced COX-2 expression and PGE_2 production in JB6 P^+ mouse epidermal cells.	Kwon wt al. (2009)
	Reduction in UVB-mediated DNA damage in the form of CPDs and 8-oxodG in mouse skin. Inhibition of UVB-mediated increase in lipid peroxidation.	Afaq et al. (2007a)
Curcumin	Inhibition of UVB-induced expression of COX-2 mRNA and protein as well as activation of p38 and JNK in HaCaT cells.	Cho et al. (2005)
	Inhibition of the proliferation-associated MAPKs ERK1/2 and protein kinase B when applied in combination with UVA or visible light. Inhibition of EGFR, an upstream regulator of both kinases.	Dujic et al. (2007)
Sulforaphane	Inhibition of UV radiation-induced skin carcinogenesis in initiated high-risk mice.	Dinkova-Kostova et al. (2006)
	Reduction in UVB-induced AP-1 activation in HCL14 cells.	Zhu et al. (2004)
	Inhibition of UVB-mediated increase in IL-6, IL-1β, COX-2 and PGE_2 levels in HaCaT cells.	Shibata et al. (2010)
	Inhibition of UV-induced inflammation and edema in mice.	Talalay et al. (2007)

Table 14.2 (continued)

Phytochemicals	Biological effects/molecular mechanism(s)	References
	In healthy human subjects elevates cytoprotective NAD(P)H:quinone oxidoreductase 1.	Dinkova-Kostova et al. (2006)
	Reduction in susceptibility to erythema in humans.	Talalay et al. (2007)
Quercetin	Reduction in UVB-induced transactivation of AP-1, NF-κB and phosphorylation of MAPKs in JB6 cells.	Ding et al. (2010)
	Inhibition of UVB-mediated increase in myeloperoxidase activity, GSH depletion and proteinases secretion/activity in mouse skin.	Casagrande et al. (2006)
Honokiol	Result in a significant protection against photocarcinogenesis both in terms of tumor multiplicity and tumor volume per tumor-bearing mouse. Inhibit/delayed the conversion of papillomas to carcinoma in mice.	Vaid et al. (2010a)
	Inhibition of UVB-induced expression of COX-2, PGE_2 and proinflammatory cytokines in the skin and in skin tumors of mice.	Vaid et al. (2010a)
Lycopene	Inhibition of UVB-mediated induction of myeloperoxidase activity and skin swelling in mice.	Fazekas et al. (2003)
	Capable of decreasing UV-induced formation of thiobarbituric acid-reactive substances in skin fibroblasts.	Eichler et al. (2002)
	Protection against UV-light-induced erythema in human.	Aust et al. (2005), Stahl et al. (2001)
Lutein/zeaxanthin	Reduction in tumor multiplicity and total tumor volume in mice.	Astner et al. (2007)
	Prevention of the deleterious effects of UVR on CHS in the systemic model of UV-induced immunosuppression.	Lee et al. (2004)
	Provides the highest degree of antioxidant protection in clinical trial.	Palombo et al. (2007)

Here, we will summarize and discuss the recent advancement in the area of anti-photocarcinogenic potential of some selected phytochemicals employing various mouse models as test systems.

Following standard photocarcinogenesis protocols, it has been shown that topical application or oral administration of GTPs (which primarily contained a mixture of polyphenolic ingredients) in drinking water of mice reduced tumor burden in terms of tumor incidence and tumor multiplicity in these animals compared to non-GTPs-fed control group of mice (Wang et al. 1991; Agarwal et al. 1993; Katiyar et al. 1997b; Mantena et al. 2005; Meeran et al. 2009). Oral feeding of GTPs to mice was found to inhibit the growth and/or caused the regression of established experimentally-induced nonmalignant skin papilloma in mice (Wang et al. 1992b), and also showed marked inhibitory effect on the formation of UVB-induced keratoacanthomas and carcinomas (Wang et al. 1994). Oral consumption of brewed green tea by SKH-1 hairless mice at concentrations similar to human consumption (1.25% and 2.5%) significantly inhibited UVB -induced tumorigenesis (Wang et al. 1992a). Since IL-12 has been shown to have anti-tumor activity and DNA repair ability in mice, Meeran et al. (2006b) employed interleukin-12 knockout (IL-12 KO) mouse model to elucidate whether the induction of IL-12 by (-)-epigallocatchin-3-gallate (EGCG) is associated with its protective effect against photocarcinogenesis. It was found that topical application of EGCG to wild-type mice resulted in a significant inhibition of UVB-induced skin carcinogenesis both in terms of tumor incidence and tumor multiplicity compared with non-EGCG-treated wild-type mice. On the other hand, topical application of EGCG to IL-12KO mice did not protect the mice from photocarcinogenesis. These observations imply that the chemopreventive effect of EGCG against photocarcinogenesis requires IL-12 or mediated through IL-12-based mechanism.

Skin application of silymarin, a flavonoid from milk thistle (*Silybum marianum*), to SKH-1 hairless mice prior to UVB exposure was effective in protecting the skin against all the stages of photocarcinogenesis such as UV-induced tumor initiation, tumor promotion, and complete carcinogenesis protocol (initiation + promotion) (Katiyar et al. 1997a). Silibinin, a major component of silymarin, afforded protection against photocarcinogenesis in mice when applied topically or in the diet (Gu et al. 2007; Mallikarjuna et al. 2004). It has been shown that the topical application of mouse skin with resveratrol (both pre- and post- UV irradiation) resulted in inhibition of UVB radiation-induced tumor incidence and delay in the onset of skin tumorigenesis. The post- and pre-treatment of resveratrol was found to impart equal protection, suggesting that resveratrol-mediated responses may not be due to sunscreen effects (Aziz et al. 2005). Treatment of $p53^{+/-}$/SKH-1 hairless mice with resveratrol reduced the average number of skin tumors and the average tumor volume compared with non-resveratrol treated and UV-exposed control mice. The number of SCCs in resveratrol-treated mice was less than non-resveratrol treated control mice (Kim et al. 2011). Consumption of GSPs-supplemented AIN76 control diet of SKH-1 hairless mice significantly inhibited photocarcinogenesis in terms of tumor incidence, tumor multiplicity and tumor growth (Mittal et al. 2003). Dietary feeding of GSPs also resulted in prevention as well as delay of malignant transformation of UVB-induced papillomas to carcinomas as compared to the malignant progression observed in non-GSPs-treated UVB-exposed control mice (Mittal et al. 2003).

Topical treatment of mice with honokiol, a phytochemical from the *Magnolia* plant, in a hydrophilic cream-based topical formulation before or after UVB irradiation resulted in a significant protection against photocarcinogenesis both in terms of tumor multiplicity and tumor volume per tumor-bearing mouse. Honokiol treatment also delayed the latency period of tumor appearance by almost 3 weeks when compared to non-honokiol-treated UVB-irradiated mice. In addition, honkiol treatment also inhibited and delayed the conversion of papillomas to carcinoma (Vaid et al. 2010a). Oral feeding of PFE, a rich source of anthocyanins, ellagitannins and hydrolyzable tannins, to SKH-1 hairless mice resulted in reduced tumor incidence, delay in the latency period of tumor appearance, and lower tumor body burden compared to that of water-fed UVB-irradiated control animals (Afaq et al. 2008). Studies have shown that UV radiation-induced skin carcinogenesis in 'initiated high-risk mice' was substantially inhibited by topical application of broccoli sprout extracts containing sulforaphane (Dinkova-Kostova et al. 2006). Treatment of SKH-1 hairless mice with lutein/zeaxanthin, carotenoids found in green leafy vegetables, resulted in increased tumor-free survival time; reduced UVB-induced tumor multiplicity and tumor volume in comparison with control UVB-irradiated animals fed the standard diet (Astner et al. 2007). These studies suggest that phytochemicals have the potential to protect the skin from UVB-induced photocarcinogenesis.

14.5 Mechanistic Studies

14.5.1 Anti-inflammatory Effects

UV radiation-induced inflammatory responses play an important role in the development of skin cancer by enhancing erythema, edema and hyperplastic epithelial responses through proinflammatory cytokines, growth factors, and induction of the cyclooxygenase-2 (COX-2) enzyme resulting in increased prostaglandin (PG) levels (Nichols and Katiyar 2010; Mukhtar and Elmets 1996). COX-2, a rate-limiting enzyme, catalyzes the conversion of arachidonic acid to PG metabolites, and aberrant COX-2 expression has been linked to the pathophysiology of inflammation and skin cancer (Langenbach et al. 1999; Rundhaug and Fischer 2008). Studies have demonstrated the overexpression of COX-2 in hyperplastic skin, benign papillomas and in SCCs after chronic UV exposure (Buckman et al. 1998; An et al. 2002). Cellular signaling pathways (such as NF-κB, AP-1, STAT, MAPK and PI3K/AKT) act independently or coordinately to regulate expression of target genes involved in inflammation (Nichols and Katiyar 2010; Afaq 2011).

Studies have revealed that oral administration or topical application of GTPs to SKH-1 hairless mice resulted in significant inhibition of UVB radiation-induced biomarkers of inflammation such as cutaneous edema, erythema, and bi-fold skin thickness (Afaq et al. 2003b). Meeran et al. (2009) have shown that the levels of inflammation associated biomarkers (COX-2, PGE_2, PCNA, cyclin D1) and proinflammatory cytokines (TNF-α, IL-6, IL-1β) were higher in chronically UVB-exposed skin and skin tumors of IL-12 KO mouse skin compared to that of UVB-exposed skin of their wild-type counterparts. This study provide evidence that IL-12-deficiency may be a contributing factor in inducing inflammation and because of this early occurrence and rapid development of skin tumors was observed in IL-12 KO mice. Administration of GTPs in drinking water of mice significantly reduced the levels of biomarkers of inflammation and proinflammatory cytokines in UVB-exposed skin and skin tumors in the wild-type mice but had a non-significant effect in IL-12 KO mice. This study indicates that photoprotective effect of GTPs on UV-induced skin tumor development is mediated through IL-12 (Meeran et al. 2009). Topical treatment of EGCG to C3H/HeN mice before an acute exposure of UVB inhibited UVB-induced infiltration of leukocytes, myeloperoxidase activity, the number of H_2O_2-producing cells and inducible nitric oxide synthase-expressing cells as well as the production of H_2O_2 and nitric oxide in both epidermis and dermis of mouse skin (Katiyar and Mukhtar 2001). Topical application of silymarin to C3H/HeN mice inhibited UVB-induced infiltration of $CD11b^+$ cells. In addition, reduction in myeloperoxidase activity also indicated that silymarin significantly decreased UVB-induced infiltration of leukocytes (Katiyar et al. 2008). Topical application of silymarin also inhibited UVB-induced expression of COX-2 and its prostaglandin metabolites in mouse skin (Katiyar et al. 1997a). Silibinin treatment to SKH-1 hairless mouse skin reduced UVB-mediated COX-2 overexpression by targeting transcription factors such as STAT3 and NF-κB (Gu et al. 2007). Treatment of mice with honokiol in a hydrophilic cream-based topical formulation before or after UVB irradiation significantly inhibited UVB-induced expression of COX-2, PGE_2 and proinflammatory cytokines (TNFα, IL-1β and IL-6) in the skin and in skin tumors (Vaid et al. 2010a). Similar observation was found when mice were fed with dietary GSPs (Sharma and Katiyar 2010). These data collectively suggest that anti-photocarcinogenic activity of GTPs, honokiol, GSPs, silymarin is associated with the inhibition of UVB-induced inflammation and mediators of inflammatory responses.

Treatment of mice skin with resveratrol reduced UVB-induced infiltration of leukocytes, skin edema, H_2O_2 production and PG metabolites, especially PGE_2 and PGD_2 (Afaq et al. 2003a). Topical application of genistein, a soy-derived isoflavone, to mouse skin before UVB irradiation reduced UVB-induced sunburn cell formation (Brand and Jendrzejewski 2008). Pretreatment of irradiated cultures with genistein blocked UVB-stimulated PGE_2 synthesis and phosphorylation of EGFR at tyrosine residues (Miller et al. 1994). Topical application of genistein protects pig skin from solar-simulated UV-induced photodamage, as measured by sunburn cell formation and/or erythema (Lin et al. 2008). Treatment of HaCaT cells with curcumin, a natural compound extracted from the rhizome of *Curcuma longa*, inhibited UVB-induced expression of COX-2 mRNA and protein as well as activation of p38 and JNK. The DNA binding activity of transcription factor AP-1 was also markedly decreased with curcumin treatment in UVB-irradiated HaCaT cells. Collectively, these results suggest that curcumin inhibits COX-2 expression by suppressing p38 and JNK activities in UVB-irradiated HaCaT cells (Cho et al. 2005). Curcumin at low concentrations inhibited the proliferation-associated MAPKs ERK1/2 and protein kinase B when applied in combination with UVA or visible light. Combination of curcumin and UVA light induced apoptosis of human keratinocytes as shown by an increase in fragmented cell nuclei, release of cytochrome *c*, activation of caspases-9 and -8, and inhibition of NF-κB activity. In addition, EGFR, an upstream regulator of both kinases, was inhibited indicating that apoptosis is induced due to blockage of survival- and proliferation-associated signal cascades at the receptor level (Dujic et al. 2007).

The treatment of HCL14 cells with sulforaphane, an isothiocyanate found in cruciferous vegetables, such as broccoli and broccoli sprouts, dose-dependently reduced UVB-induced AP-1 activation, and this appears to be at least, in part, due to the direct inhibition of AP1-DNA binding activity (Zhu et al. 2004). Treatment of HaCaT cells with sulforaphane inhibited UVB-mediated increases in the levels of IL-6, IL-1β, COX-2 and PGE_2. In addition, sulforaphane inhibited UVB-mediated activation of p38, ERK and SAPK/JNK, demonstrating that the inhibition of MAPKs by sulforaphane would attenuate the expression of COX-2, thereby reducing inflammatory responses (Shibata et al. 2010). Topical application of sulforaphane-rich extracts of broccoli sprouts protected UV-induced inflammation and edema in mice. These studies provide evidence that broccoli sprout extracts containing sulforaphane may reduce UV-induced skin damage (Talalay et al. 2007). Topical application of lycopene reduced UVB-mediated induction of myeloperoxidase activity, and significantly reduced bifold skin thickness in a dose-dependent manner (Fazekas et al. 2003). Supplementation with tomato-based products increases lycopene levels in human serum and protects from solar UV-induced erythema (Aust et al. 2005). The skin bi-fold thickness and number of infiltrating mast cells following UVB irradiation were significantly reduced in lutein/zeaxanthin-treated mice when compared to UVB alone irradiated control mice (Astner et al. 2007).

Quercetin induced c-Fos mRNA and protein expression through activation of p38 and cAMP-responsive element binding protein, and also potentiated UVB-induced c-Fos expression in human keratinocyte cell line, HaCaT. Conversely, addition of ascorbic acid in cell culture media stablized quercetin and completely prevented both quercetin- and UVB-induced *c-fos* expression, a cellular event important for the promotion phase of tumor development (Olson et al. 2010). Treatment of JB6 cells with quercetin reduced UVB-induced transactivation of AP-1, NF-κB and phosphorylation of MAPKs. This study suggests that quercetin contributes to the inhibition of neoplastic transformation by blocking the cellular signaling pathway (Ding et al. 2010). Treatment of JB6 P^+ mouse epidermal cells with delphinidin suppressed UVB-induced COX-2 expression and PGE_2 production. These effects were mediated by blocking the MAPKK4 and PI3K pathways and subsequently suppressing activities of AP-1 and NF-κB (Kwon wt al. 2009). Anthocyanins inhibited UVB-induced COX-2 and PGE_2 production through suppression of nuclear

NF-κB-dependent pathway and regulation of the PI3K/Akt pathway in HaCaT cells. Moreover, topical application of anthocyanins to hairless mice inhibited UVB-mediated induction of COX-2 and PGE_2 (Tsoyi et al. 2008).

14.5.2 Anti-oxidant Effects

The skin cells possess a versatile endogenous antioxidant defense system to counterbalance UV-induced production of ROS. Endogenous antioxidant defense system includes ROS detoxifying enzymes (such as, superoxide dismutase, glutathione peroxidase, catalase and thioredoxin reductase), and low-molecular-mass antioxidant molecules (such as glutathione, tocopherol and ascorbic acid). However, excessive and chronic exposure to UV radiation jeopardizes the integrity of the skin by increased generation of ROS that overwhelms the antioxidant defense mechanisms of the cells leading to oxidative stress. UV-induced production of ROS can result in single- or double-stranded DNA breaks, purine, pyrimidine, or deoxyribose modifications, DNA cross-links, and oxidation of proteins and lipids. Furthermore, persistent damage to critical cellular molecules, such as, proteins, lipids and DNA can result in arrest or induction of transcription factors, induction of signal transduction pathways, genomic instability and replication errors that may result in immunosuppression, premature aging of the skin and development of melanoma and non-melanoma skin cancers (Afaq 2011; Nichols and Katiyar 2010).

Treatment of normal human epidermal keratinocytes (NHEK) with EGCG prior to UVB exposure inhibited UVB-induced H_2O_2 production and H_2O_2-mediated phosphorylation of MAPKs. These studies suggest that EGCG could be useful in attenuation of oxidative stress and MAPK-mediated skin disorders in humans (Katiyar et al. 2001a). In addition, topical application of GTPs or its most active constituent EGCG to mouse skin afforded significant protection from UVB-induced depletion of antioxidant enzymes such as glutathione peroxidase (GPx), catalase and glutathione (GSH) level (Agarwal et al. 1993; Vayalil et al. 2003). Furthermore, treatment of mouse skin with GTPs inhibited UVB-induced epidermal lipid peroxidation (Vayalil et al. 2003). Treatment of guinea pig skin with EGCG also inhibited UVB-induced lipid peroxidation (Kim et al. 2001). These studies suggest that both GTPs and EGCG can induce photoprotective effects by acting at different active sites within the cascade of events that generate ROS.

Treatment of immortalized HaCaT cells with PFE prior to UVB exposure protected cells from UVB-mediated depletion of endogenous GSH and decreased UVB-induced lipid peroxidation (Zaid et al. 2007). Treatment of HaCaT cells with delphinidin, one of the major anthocyanidins present in pomegranate, inhibited UVB-mediated increase in lipid peroxidation (Afaq et al. 2007a). Treatment of NHEK with GSPs inhibited UVB-induced H_2O_2 production, lipid peroxidation, and depletion of antioxidant defense components, such as GPx, catalase, superoxide dismutase, and GSH (Mantena and Katiyar 2006). Feeding of dietary GSPs to SKH-1 hairless mice exposed either acutely or chronically UVB irradiation resulted in restoration of UVB-induced depletion of endogenous antioxidant defense enzymes, such as GPx, GSH, and catalase; and suppression of oxidative stress in terms of H_2O_2 and nitric oxide production, and lipid peroxidation (Sharma et al. 2007). As UVB-induced oxidative stress mediates activation of MAPK and NF-κB signaling pathways, the effects of GSPs on these pathways were analyzed in the same mouse model. It was found that the treatment with GSPs inhibited UVB-induced phosphorylation of ERK1/2, JNK1/2 and p38 proteins of the MAPK family, which seemed to be mediated through reactivation of MAPK phosphatases. In addition, GSPs inhibited UVB-induced activation of NF-κB through inhibition of degradation of IκBα and activation of IKK (Sharma et al. 2007). Topical application of silymarin to C3H/HeN mice resulted in significant reduction of the number of UVB-induced H_2O_2 producing cells and inducible nitric oxide synthase expressing cells concomitant with decrease in H_2O_2 and nitric oxide production when compared with the non-silymarin-treated UVB exposed control mice. The inhibition of the UVB-induced oxidative stress was associated with significant inhibition of UV-induced infiltration of activated macrophages and neutrophils (Katiyar 2002).

The oxidation of amino acids, such as lysine, arginine and proline, leads to the formation of carbonyl derivatives that affect the function of the proteins (Stadtman 2001). Under conditions of oxidative stress, the presence of carbonyl groups in proteins has become a widely accepted measure of oxidative damage of proteins. Multiple exposures of the mouse skin to UVB radiation enhance the formation of protein carbonyls in comparison to non-UV exposed skin. Topical treatment with EGCG, GTPs, GSPs or PFE significantly inhibited acute or chronic UV irradiation-induced protein oxidation in mouse skin (Vayalil et al. 2003; Sharma et al. 2007, Afaq et al. 2007b).

Pretreatment of NHEK with resveratrol, a polyphenolic antioxidant from grape skin, inhibited UVB-mediated activation of the NF-κB pathway (Adhami et al. 2003). Single topical application of resveratrol to SKH-1 hairless mice prior to UVB irradiation inhibited UVB-induced generation of H_2O_2, infiltration of leukocytes and lipid peroxidation (Afaq et al. 2003a). Inhibition of these critical molecules or events by resveratrol may be associated with the prevention of UV radiation-induced skin damage in these mice. Genistein treatment protected human dermal fibroblast against UVB-induced senescence via maintenance of antioxidant enzyme activities and modulation of mitochondrial oxidative stress through down-regulation of a p66Shc-dependent signaling pathway (Wang et al. 2010). Genistein significantly inhibited UVB-induced H_2O_2 generation and malondialdehyde production in mouse skin. These results suggest that UVB irradiation elicit a series of oxidative events that can be substantially inhibited by genistein through direct quenching of ROS (Wei et al. 2002). Application of topical formulations containing quercetin onto the skin of hairless mice inhibited UVB-mediated myeloperoxidase activity, GSH depletion and proteinases secretion/activity (Casagrande et al. 2006). These data suggest the possible usefulness of topical formulations containing quercetin against UVB radiation induced skin damages. Eichler et al. (2002) using multilamellar liposomes as a vehicle to deliver lycopene to skin fibroblasts showed that lycopene was capable of decreasing UV-induced formation of thiobarbituric acid-reactive substances. Single exposure of a small area of one volar forearm to solar-simulated light resulted in reduction in skin lycopene concentration compared with an adjacent non-exposed area. This study suggests that lycopene plays an important role in mitigating oxidative damage in tissues (Ribaya-Mercado et al. 1995).

14.5.3 Prevention of Immunosuppression

Immunosuppression is important biological consequence of UVB exposure that has been implicated in skin cancer (Meunier et al. 1998; Yoshikawa et al. 1990). In addition, suppression of immune system by UVB exposure exacerbates infectious diseases and initiates skin cancer (Katiyar 2007; Chapman et al. 1995). This hypothesis is supported by the facts that chronically immunosuppressed patients living in regions of intense sun exposure experience a remarkably high rate of skin cancer (Kinlen et al. 1979). Exposure of skin to UVB radiation suppresses the development of allergic contact hypersensitivity; a prototypic T-cell-mediated immune response through both local and systemic effects (Kripke 1990). Topical application of EGCG to C3H/HeN mice before UVB exposure prevented UVB-induced inhibition of the contact hypersensitivity (CHS) response and tolerance induction to the contact sensitizer 2, 4-dinitrofluorobenzene. In addition, EGCG protected UVB-induced immunosuppression and tolerance induction by blocking UVB-induced infiltration of $CD11b^+$ cells, reducing IL-10 production, and markedly increasing IL-12 production (Katiyar et al. 1999a). Pre- and Post-application of GTPs to C3H/HeN mice afforded a significant protection against UVB-mediated local and systemic suppression of CHS response (Katiyar et al. 1995). Oral consumption of GTPs by mice in drinking water inhibited the immunosuppressive effects of UV radiation in local and systemic models of CHS. In addition, GTPs have the ability to prevent UVB-induced immune tolerance in mice and can protect for a longer period of time even after ceasing it consumption. These studies suggest that green tea, specifically polyphenols present therein, may be useful against immunosuppression caused by UVB radiation, at least in part, by protection of IL-12 and a reduction in IL-10 (Katiyar et al. 2010).

Inclusion of GSPs in the diet of mice inhibited UVB-induced suppression of CHS responses in a local model of immunosuppression but had only moderate inhibitory effect in a systemic model of immunosuppression. GSPs supplemented diet provided significant protection against UVB-induced enhanced production of IL-10 by the epidermal and dermal cells of the skin, and in the draining lymph nodes compared with mice that did not receive GSPs. Interestingly, dietary GSPs enhanced the production of immunostimulatory cytokine IL-12 in the draining lymph nodes. Intra-peritoneal injection of GSPs-fed mice with anti-IL-12 antibody reduced the protective effects of the GSPs against UVB-induced suppression of the CHS response (Sharma and Katiyar 2006). Vaid et al. (2010b) recently used an adoptive transfer approach to define the cell population liable for the GSPs-mediated inhibition of UVB-induced immunosuppression and to delineate the role of IL-12 in this process. The levels of Th1 cytokines (IFNγ, IL-2) were much higher in $CD8^+$ T cells from GSPs treated mice, whereas the Th2 cytokines (IL-4 and IL-10) in

$CD4^+$ T cells were barely detectable. These data indicate that GSPs inhibit UVB-induced immunosuppression by activating CD8+ effector T cells and inactivating $CD4^+$ regulatory T cells.

Topical application of silymarin to C3H/HeN mice reduced UVB-induced suppression of CHS and this was associated with the inhibition of infiltrating leukocytes, particularly $CD11b^+$ cell type, and myeloperoxidase activity. In addition, silymarin was found to reduce UVB-mediated increase in the immunosuppressive cytokine, IL-10 producing cells and the levels of IL-10 (Katiyar et al. 2002). This study was further extended to determine whether topical application of silymarin or silibinin (a major component of silymarin) has effect on UVB-induced suppression of CHS response in local and in systemic models of contact hypersensitivity. It was found that both silymarin and silibinin inhibited UVB-induced local and systemic immunosuppression. However, the magnitude of the immunoprotective effect of silymarin or silibinin in the systemic CHS model was lower than that in the local CHS model (Meeran et al. 2006a). Topical application of silymarin reduced UVB-mediated increases in the level of IL-10 in the skin and draining lymph nodes and enhanced the levels of IL-12. In addition, treatment of mice with anti-IL-12 antibody abrogated the ability of silymarin to protect UVB-induced suppression of the CHS response in a local model of CHS. Moreover, topical application of silymarin to mice did not protect against UVB-induced immunosupression of the CHS response in IL-12 knockout mice but prevented it in their wild-type counterparts (Meeran et al. 2006a). Mice exposed to UVB radiation and then sensitized to dinitrofluorobenzene at the site of irradiation showed a decreased CHS response upon challenge. This suppression by UVB radiation was significantly inhibited by feeding mice with lutein-supplemented diet. Conversely, dietary lutein did not prevent the deleterious effects of UVR on CHS in the systemic model of UV-induced immunosuppression (Lee et al. 2004).

14.5.4 Prevention or Repair of UV-Induced DNA Damage

UVB radiation is the most damaging component of the solar radiation and acts mainly on the epidermal cell layers of the skin and induces DNA damage by formation of cyclobutane pyrimidine dimers (CPDs) and primidyne-(6-4)-pyrimidone photoproducts (Melnikova and Ananthaswamy 2005; Afaq et al. 2007a). However, 8-oxo-7,8-dihydro-2'-deoxyguanosine (8-oxodG) is formed by ROS and plays an important role in carcinogenesis (Arad et al. 2008). CPDs are formed immediately in the skin after the interaction of photons with the DNA molecule and are thought be an important molecular trigger for the induction of immunosuppression and initiation of photocarcinogenesis (Kripke et al. 1992; Yarosh et al. 1992). Studies have shown that GTPs and EGCG protected skin fibroblasts and epidermal keratinocytes from UVB-induced DNA damage (Morley et al. 2005). Meeran et al. (2006b) investigated whether EGCG prevents UVB-induced photocarcinogenesis through an IL-12-dependent DNA repair mechanism by employing IL-12 KO and WT mice. UVB-induced DNA damage was resolved more rapidly in the skin of wild-type mice that were topically treated with EGCG than untreated control mice. However, the extent of UVB-induced DNA damage in mouse skin was almost similar in the EGCG-treated IL-12 KO mice and their respective untreated UVB-irradiated control mice. EGCG was found to induce repair of UVB-induced CPDs in xeroderma pigmentosum complementation group A (*XPA*)-proficient cells but does not reduce the numbers of UVB-induced CPDs in *XPA*-deficient cells. This study suggests that EGCG-induced DNA repair in the form of CPDs is mediated through IL-12 dependent functional NER mechanism (Meeran et al. 2006b). GTPs containing EGCG reduced UVB-induced DNA damage in human reconstituted skin and this effect appear to be mediated *via* IL-12, most likely through induction of DNA repair (Schwarz et al. 2008).

Studies have shown that dietary GSPs did not inhibit UVB-induced CPDs formation immediately after UVB irradiation. However, the numbers of CPD-positive cells were significantly reduced or repaired in the GSPs-treated mouse skin samples obtained at 24 h or 48 h after UVB exposure compared to the control group of mice which were not treated with GSPs. Dietary GSPs did not remove or repair UV-induced CPDs in the skin of IL-12 KO mice but repaired CPDs in the skin of their wild-type counterparts. These studies suggest that the rapid repair of UV-induced CPDs by GSPs was mediated through stimulation of IL-12 (Vaid et al. 2010b). Employing human reconstituted skin, Afaq et al. (2009) have shown that pomegranate derived products were effective in reducing UVB -induced formation of CPDs and 8-oxodG. In another study, it was shown that oral feeding of PFE in drinking water to SKH-1 hairless mice reduced the number of CPDs and 8-oxodG positive cells and these may be due to enhanced DNA repair. In addition PFE also enhanced UVB-mediated increase in p53 and p21 proteins in SKH-1 hairless mouse skin, therefore shutting off cell replication and DNA synthesis and allowing extended time for DNA repair (Afaq et al. 2010). Treatment of HaCaT cells with delphinidin or topical application of delphinidin (pre- and post-application) to SKH-1 hairless mouse skin reduced UVB-mediated DNA damage in the form of CPDs and 8-oxodG (Afaq et al. 2007a). Wei et al. (1998) have shown by computer modeling that genistein intercalate into DNA and interrupt the production of oxidizing species, and subsequently reduce the formation of UV-induced oxidative DNA damage. Treatment of human reconstituted skin with genistein prior to UVB irradiation inhibited UVB-mediated CPDs formation (Moore et al. 2006). The study suggests that genistein possesses photoprotective efficacy and minimized the harmful effect of UVB irradiation in reconstituted skin. Oral feeding or topical application of silibinin to SKH-1 hairless mice prior to, or immediately after, UVB irradiation significantly reduced UVB-induced CPDs positive cells in epidermis and this may be mediated via an activation of p53-p21/Cip1 cascade (Dhanalakshmi et al. 2004; Gu et al. 2005).

14.6 Bioavailability of Dietary Phytochemicals

A comparative pharmacokinetics studies using equimolar doses of pure EGC, ECG, and EGCG in 10 healthy volunteers revealed that the average peak plasma concentrations after intake of a single dose of 1.5 mmol were 5.0 μmol/L for EGC,

3.1 μmol/L for ECG, and 1.3 μmol/L for EGCG. The plasma concentration of EGC and EGCG returned to baseline after 24 h, but plasma ECG remained elevated even after 24 h (Higdon and Frei 2003). A phase-I study revealed that the serum concentration of curcumin peaked at 1 to 2 h after oral intake of crucumin and gradually declined within 12 h. A trend was seen with the average peak serum concentrations after taking 4,000 mg, 6,000 mg and 8,000 mg of curcumin were 0.51 ± 0.11 μM, 0.63 ± 0.06 μM and 1.77 ± 1.87 μM, respectively. In addition, there was no treatment-related toxicity up to 8,000 mg/day (Cheng et al. 2001). The pharmacokinetic study of genistein was determined in healthy women by giving a single-bolus dose of 50 mg of genistein and the data revealed that the mean t_{max} for peak plasma concentration was 9.33 ± 1.33 h, with a mean C_{max} for genistein of 341 ± 74 ng/mL (1.26 ± 0.27 μmol/L) (Setchell et al. 2001). A two-period, open-label, single-arm control study in eight healthy subjects who were given trans-resveratrol 2000 mg twice daily revealed that the mean area under the plasma concentration-time curve from 0 to 12 h AUC(12) and maximum plasma concentration Cmax of trans-resveratrol were 3558 (2195) ng/mL and 1274 (790) ng/mL, respectively (la Porte et al. 2010). Recent studies have shown that a daily supplement of 15 mg lycopene given for 4 wk as beadlet preparations containing synthetic lycopene (Lycovit 10%) or tomato oleoresin (Lyc- O-Mato) resulted in a marked increase in serum cis-, trans- and total lycopene. Both synthetic and tomato-lycopene resulted in an increase in serum total lycopene by 0.58 and 0.57 μmol/L, trans-lycopene by 0.34 and 0.41 μmol/L, and total-cis-lycopene by 0.24 and 0.16 μmol/L respectively. This study indicates that both sources had the same bioavailability (Hoppe et al. 2003). Healthy volunteers received 180 ml pomegranate juice concentrate and their blood samples were collected after 6 h. Ellagic acid was detected in plasma of all subjects with a maximum concentration of 0.06 ± 0.01 μmol/L, area under concentration time curve of 0.17 ± 0.02 (μmol × h) × L(-1), time of maximum concentration of 0.98 ± 0.06 h, and elimination half-life of 0.71 ± 0.08 h. EA metabolites, including dimethylellagic acid glucuronide and hydroxy-6H-benzopyran-6-one derivatives, were also detected in plasma in conjugated and free forms (Seeram et al. 2006). A study conducted in seven healthy volunteers who received 12 gm of an anthocyanin extract revealed that the anthocyanins were detected in their intact form in both plasma and urine samples (Garcia-Alonso et al. 2009). These observations suggest the bioavailability of phytochemicals.

14.7 Translation of Animal Studies to Human System

Studies revealed that EGCG protects UV-induced oxidative stress in humans as well. When it was applied topically to human skin before exposure to a 4x minimal erythema dose of UVB radiation, it significantly decreased UV-induced production of H_2O_2 and nitric oxide as well as lipid peroxidation in both epidermis and dermis in a time-dependent manner (Katiyar et al. 2001b). In addition, topical application of EGCG to human skin afforded significant protection against UVB-induced depletion of antioxidant enzymes such as GPx, catalase and GSH levels (Katiyar et al. 2001b). Topical application of EGCG to human skin also inhibited UVB-induced production of prostaglandin metabolites, particularly PGE_2, which play a critical role in inflammatory disorders and in proliferative skin diseases (Katiyar et al. 1999b), and thus may be able to inhibit UVB-induced production of ROS as these infiltrating leukocytes are the major source of nitric oxide and H_2O_2 production. Treatment of human skin with GTPs prior to UVB irradiation reduced the formation of CPDs in both epidermis and dermis (Katiyar et al. 2000). Topical application of sulforaphane-rich extracts of broccoli sprouts reduced susceptibility to erythema in humans (Talalay et al. 2007). Dietary intake of tomato paste rich in lycopene for 10 weeks protected against UV-induced erythema formation in humans (Stahl et al. 2001). Supplementation with tomato-based products increases lycopene levels in human serum and protects against UV-light-induced erythema (Aust et al. 2005). Topical application of broccoli sprout extracts containing sulforaphane to the skin of mice and healthy human subjects elevates cytoprotective NAD(P)H:quinone oxidoreductase 1 (Dinkova-Kostova et al. 2006). In a clinical trial, lutein and zeaxanthin were administered orally, topically, or in combination. It was found that the combined oral and topical administration of lutein and zeaxanthin provided the highest degree of antioxidant protection. Oral administration of lutein provided better protection than that afforded by topical application of this antioxidant when measured by changes in lipid peroxidation and photoprotective activity in the skin following UV light irradiation (Palombo et al. 2007). Together, these studies reveal that the phytochemicals are not only beneficial in animal model but also in human system.

Acknowledgments The work highlighted from author's laboratory was supported by funds from the National Institutes of Health [(R21 AT002429-02, F.A.) (CA104428, CA140832, AT002536, S.K.K.)] and Veterans Administration Merit Review Award (S.K.K.). The content of this article does not necessarily reflect the views or policies of the funding agencies.

References

Adhami VM et al (2003) Suppression of ultraviolet B exposure-mediated activation of NF-kappaB in normal human keratinocytes by resveratrol. Neoplasia 5:74–82

Adhami VM et al (2008) Phytochemicals for prevention of solar ultraviolet radiation-induced damages. Photochem Photobiol 84:489–500

Afaq F (2011) Natural agents: cellular and molecular mechanisms of photoprotection. Arch Biochem Biophys 508:144–151

Afaq F, Mukhtar H (2006) Botanical antioxidants in the prevention of photocarcinogenesis and photoaging. Exp Dermatol 15:678–684

Afaq F et al (2003a). Prevention of short-term ultraviolet B radiation-mediated damages by resveratrol in SKH-1 hairless mice. Toxicol Appl Pharmacol 186:28–37

Afaq F et al (2003b) Suppression of UVB-induced phosphorylation of mitogen-activated protein kinases and nuclear factor kappa B by green tea polyphenol in SKH-1 hairless mice. Oncogene 22:9254–9264

Afaq F et al (2005) Photochemoprevention of ultraviolet B signaling and photocarcinogenesis. Mutat Res 571:153–173

Afaq F et al (2007a) Delphinidin, an anthocyanidin in pigmented fruits and vegetables, protects human HaCaT keratinocytes and mouse skin against UVB-mediated oxidative stress and apoptosis. J Invest Dermatol 127:222–232

Afaq F et al (2007b) Pomegranate fruit extract inhibits UVB-induced activation of NFκB and MAPK leading to decreased expression of matrix metalloprotenaises in SKH-1 mouse skin. Proc Amer Assoc Cancer Res 48:2571

Afaq F et al (2008) Inhibitory effect of oral feeding of pomegranate fruit extract on UVB-induced skin carcinogenesis in SKH-1 hairless mice. Proc Am Assoc Cancer Res 49:1246

Afaq F et al (2009) Protective effect of pomegranate-derived products on UVB-mediated damage in human reconstituted skin. Exp Dermatol 18:553–561

Afaq F et al (2010) Oral feeding of pomegranate fruit extract inhibits early biomarkers of UVB radiation-induced carcinogenesis in SKH-1 hairless mouse epidermis. Photochem Photobiol 86:1318–1326

Agarwal R et al (1993) Protection against ultraviolet B radiation-induced effects in the skin of SKH-1 hairless mice by a polyphenolic fraction isolated from green tea. Photochem Photobiol 58:695–700

An KP et al (2002) Cyclooxygenase-2 expression in murine and human nonmelanoma skin cancers: Implications for therapeutic approaches. Photochem Photobiol 76:73–80

Arad S et al (2008) Topical thymidine dinucleotide treatment reduces development of ultraviolet-induced basal cell carcinoma in Ptch-1+/- mice. Am J Pathol 172:1248–1255

Astner S et al (2007) Dietary lutein/zeaxanthin partially reduces photoaging and photocarcinogenesis in chronically UVB-irradiated Skh-1 hairless mice. Skin Pharmacol Physiol 20:283–291

Aust O et al (2005) Supplementation with tomato-based products increases lycopene, phytofluene, and phytoene levels in human serum and protects against UV-light-induced erythema. Int J Vitam Nutr Res 75:54–60

Aziz MH et al (2005) Chemoprevention of skin cancer by grape constituent resveratrol: relevance to human disease? FASEB J 19:1193–1195

Bachelor MA, Bowden GT (2004) UVA-mediated activation of signaling pathways involved in skin tumor promotion and progression. Semin Cancer Biol 14:131–138

Bowden GT (2004) Prevention of non-melanoma skin cancer by targeting ultraviolet-B-light signalling. Nat Rev Cancer 4:23–35

Brand RM, Jendrzejewski JL (2008) Topical treatment with (-)-epigallocatechin-3-gallate and genistein after a single UV exposure can reduce skin damage. J Dermatol Sci 50:69–72

Buckman SY et al (1998) COX-2 expression is induced by UVB exposure in human skin: Implications for the development of skin cancer. Carcinogenesis 19:723–729

Casagrande R et al (2006) Protective effect of topical formulations containing quercetin against UVB-induced oxidative stress in hairless mice. J Photochem Photobiol B 84:21–27

Chapman RS et al (1995) Solar ultraviolet radiation and the risk of infectious disease. Photochem Photobiol 61:223–247

Cheng AL et al (2001) Phase I clinical trial of curcumin, a chemopreventive agent, in patients with high-risk or pre-malignant lesions. Anticancer Res 21:2895–2900

Cho JW et al (2005) Curcumin inhibits the expression of COX-2 in UVB-irradiated human keratinocytes (HaCaT) by inhibiting activation of AP-1: p38 MAP kinase and JNK as potential upstream targets. Exp Mol Med 37:186–192

Clydesdale GJ et al (2001) Ultraviolet light induced injury: immunological and inflammatory effects. Immunol Cell Biol 79:547–568

Dhanalakshmi S et al (2004) Silibinin prevents ultraviolet radiation-caused skin damages in SKH-1 hairless mice via a decrease in thymine dimer positive cells and an up-regulation of p53-p21/Cip1 in epidermis. Carcinogenesis 25:1459–1465

Ding M et al (2010) Inhibition of AP-1 and MAPK signaling and activation of Nrf2/ARE pathway by quercitrin. Int J Oncol 36:59–67

Dinkova-Kostova AT et al (2006) Protection against UV-light-induced skin carcinogenesis in SKH-1 high-risk mice by sulforaphane-containing broccoli sprout extracts. Cancer Lett 240:243–252

Dinkova-Kostova AT et al (2007) Induction of the phase 2 response in mouse and human skin by sulforaphane-containing broccoli sprout extracts. Cancer Epidemiol Biomarkers Prev 16: 847–851

Donawho CK, Kripke ML (1991) Evidence that the local effect of ultraviolet radiation on the growth of murine melanomas is immunologically mediated. Cancer Res 51:4176–4181

Dujic J et al (2007) Low concentrations of curcumin induce growth arrest and apoptosis in skin keratinocytes only in combination with UVA or visible light. J Invest Dermatol 127:1992–2000

Eichler O et al (2002) Divergent optimum levels of lycopene, beta-carotene and lutein protecting against UVB irradiation in human fibroblastst. Photochem Photobiol 75:503–506

Fazekas Z et al (2003) Protective effects of lycopene against ultraviolet B-induced photodamage. Nutr Cancer 47:181–187

Garcia-Alonso M et al (2009) Red wine anthocyanins are rapidly absorbed in humans and affect monocyte chemoattractant protein 1 levels and antioxidant capacity of plasma. J Nutr Biochem 20:521–529

Godar DE et al (2001) UV doses of Americans. Photochem Photobiol 73:621–629

Gonzaga ER (2009) Role of UV light in photodamage, skin aging, and skin cancer: importance of photoprotection. Am J Clin Dermatol Suppl 1:19–24

Gu M et al (2005) Dietary feeding of silibinin prevents early biomarkers of UVB radiation-induced carcinogenesis in SKH-1 hairless mouse epidermis. Cancer Epidemiol. Biomarkers Prev 14:1344–1349

Gu M et al (2007) Silibinin inhibits inflammatory and angiogenic attributes in photocarcinogenesis in SKH-1 hairless mice. Cancer Res 67:3483–3491

Halliday GM (2005) Inflammation, gene mutation and photoimmunosuppression in response to UVR-induced oxidative damage contributes to photocarcinogenesis. Mutat Res 571:107–120

Higdon JV, Frei B (2003) Tea catechins and polyphenols: health effects, metabolism, and antioxidant functions. Crit Rev Food Sci Nutr 43:89–143

Hoppe PP et al (2003) Synthetic and tomato-based lycopene have identical bioavailability in humans. Eur J Nutr 42:272–278

Jemal A et al (2010) Cancer statistics, 2010. CA Cancer J Clin 60:277–300

Katiyar SK (2002) Treatment of silymarin, a plant flavonoid, prevents ultraviolet light-induced immune suppression and oxidative stress in mouse skin. Int J Oncol 21:1213–1222

Katiyar SK (2007) UV-induced immune suppression and photocarcinogenesis: chemoprevention by dietary botanical agents. Cancer Lett 255:1–11

Katiyar SK, Mukhtar H (2001) Green tea polyphenol (-)-epigallocatechin-3-gallate treatment to mouse skin prevents UVB-induced infiltration of leukocytes, depletion of antigen-presenting cells, and oxidative stress. J Leukoc Biol 69:719–726

Katiyar SK et al (1995) Protection against ultraviolet-B radiation-induced local and systemic suppression of contact hypersensitivity and edema responses in C3H/HeN mice by green tea polyphenols. Photochem Photobiol 62:855–861

Katiyar SK et al (1997a) Protective effects of silymarin against photocarcinogenesis in a mouse skin model. J Natl Cancer Inst 89:556–566

Katiyar SK et al (1997b) Protection against induction of mouse skin papillomas with low and high risk of conversion to malignancy by green tea polyphenols. Carcinogenesis 18:497–502

Katiyar SK et al (1999a) Prevention of UVB-induced immunosuppression in mice by the green tea polyphenol (-)-epigallocatechin-3-gallate may be associated with alterations in IL-10 and IL-12 production. Carcinogenesis 20:2117–2124

Katiyar SK et al (1999b) Polyphenolic antioxidant (-)-epigallocatechin-3-gallate from green tea reduces UVB-induced inflammatory responses and infiltration of leukocytes in human skin. Photochem Photobiol 69:148–153

Katiyar SK et al (2000) Green tea polyphenol treatment to human skin prevents formation of ultraviolet light B-induced pyrimidine dimers in DNA. Clin Cancer Res 6:3864–3869
Katiyar SK et al (2001a) Inhibition of UVB-induced oxidative stress-mediated phosphorylation of mitogen-activated protein kinase signaling pathways in cultured human epidermal keratinocytes by green tea polyphenol (-)-epigallocatechin-3-gallate. Toxicol Appl Pharmacol 176:110–117
Katiyar SK et al (2001b) Green tea polyphenol (-)-epigallocatechin-3-gallate treatment of human skin inhibits ultraviolet radiation-induced oxidative stress. Carcinogenesis 22:287–294
Katiyar SK et al (2008) Silymarin, a flavonoid from milk thistle (Silybum marianum L.), inhibits UV-induced oxidative stress through targeting infiltrating $CD11b^+$ cells in mouse skin. Photochem Photobiol 84:266–271
Katiyar SK et al (2010) Green tea polyphenols prevent UV-induced immunosuppression by rapid repair of DNA damage and enhancement of nucleotide excision repair genes. Cancer Prev Res 3:179–189
Kim J et al (2001) Protective effects of (-)-epigallocatechin-3-gallate on UVA- and UVB-induced skin damage. Skin Pharmacol Appl Skin Physiol 14:11–19
Kim KH et al (2011) Resveratrol targets transforming growth factor-β2 signaling to block UV-induced tumor progression. J Invest Dermatol 131:195–202
Kinlen L et al (1979) Collaborative United Kingdom-Australia study of cancer in patients treated with immunosuppressive drugs. Br J Med II:1461–1466
Kligman LH et al (1980) Sunscreens prevent ultraviolet photocarcinogenesis. J Am Acad Dermatol 3:30–35
Kripke ML (1990) Photoimmunology. Photochem Photobiol 52:919–924
Kripke ML et al (1992) Pyrimidine dimers in DNA initiated systemic immunosuppression in UV-irradiated mice. Proc Natl Acad Sci USA 89:7516–7520
Kwon JY et al (2009) Delphinidin suppresses ultraviolet B-induced cyclooxygenases-2 expression through inhibition of MAPKK4 and PI-3 kinase. Carcinogenesis 30:1932–1940
Langenbach R et al (1999) Cyclooxygenase-deficient mice. A summary of their characteristics and susceptibilities to inflammation and carcinogenesis. Ann N Y Acad Sci 889:52–61
la Porte C et al (2010) Steady-State pharmacokinetics and tolerability of trans-resveratrol 2000 mg twice daily with food, quercetin and alcohol (ethanol) in healthy human subjects. Clin Pharmacokinet 49:449–454
Lee EH et al (2004) Dietary lutein reduces ultraviolet radiation-induced inflammation and immunosuppression. J Invest Dermatol 122:510–517
Lin JY et al (2008) Topical isoflavones provide effective photoprotection to skin. Photodermatol Photoimmunol Photomed 24:61–66
Mallikarjuna G et al (2004) Silibinin protects against photocarcinogenesis via modulation of cell cycle regulators, mitogen-activated protein kinases, and Akt signaling. Cancer Res 64: 6349–6356
Mantena SK, Katiyar SK (2006) Grape seed proanthocyanidins inhibit UV-radiation-induced oxidative stress and activation of MAPK and NF-kappaB signaling in human epidermal keratinocytes. Free Radic Biol Med 40:1603–1614
Mantena SK et al (2005) Orally administered green tea polyphenols prevent ultraviolet radiation-induced skin cancer in mice through activation of cytotoxic T cells and inhibition of angiogenesis in tumors. J Nutr 135:2871–2877
Meeran SM et al (2006a) Silymarin inhibits UV radiation-induced immunosuppression through augmentation of interleukin-12 in mice. Mol Cancer Ther 5:1660–1668
Meeran SM et al (2006b) (-)-Epigallocatechin-3-gallate prevents photocarcinogenesis in mice through interleukin-12-dependent DNA repair. Cancer Res 66:5512–5520
Meeran SM et al (2009) Inhibition of UVB-induced skin tumor development by drinking green tea polyphenols is mediated through DNA repair and subsequent inhibition of inflammation. J Invest Dermatol 129:1258–1270

Melnikova VO, Ananthaswamy HN (2005) Cellular and molecular events leading to the development of skin cancer. Mutat Res 571:91–106
Meunier L et al (1998) UV-induced immunosuppression and skin cancers. Rev Med Interne 19:247–254
Miller CC et al (1994) Ultraviolet B injury increases prostaglandin synthesis through a tyrosine kinase-dependent pathway. Evidence for UVB-induced epidermal growth factor receptor activation. J Biol Chem 269:3529–3533
Mittal A et al (2003) Dietary feeding of proanthocyanidins from grape seeds prevents photocarcinogenesis in SKH-1 hairless mice: relationship to decreased fat and lipid peroxidation. Carcinogenesis 24:1379–1388
Moore JO et al (2006) Photoprotective effect of isoflavone genistein on ultraviolet B-induced pyrimidine dimer formation and PCNA expression in human reconstituted skin and its implications in dermatology and prevention of cutaneous carcinogenesis. Carcinogenesis 27:1627–1635
Morley N et al (2005) The green tea polyphenol (-)-epigallocatechin gallate and green tea can protect human cellular DNA from ultraviolet and visible radiation-induced damage. Photodermatol Photoimmunol Photomed 21:15–22
Mukhtar H, Elmets CA (1996) Photocarcinogenesis: Mechanisms, models and human health implications. Photochem Photobiol 63:355–447
Nichols JA, Katiyar SK (2010) Skin photoprotection by natural polyphenols: anti-inflammatory, antioxidant and DNA repair mechanisms. Arch Dermatol Res 302:71–83
Olson ER et al(2010) Quercetin potentiates UVB-Induced c-Fos expression: implications for its use as a chemopreventive agent. Cancer Prev Res. (Phila) 3:876–884
Palombo P et al (2007) Beneficial long-term effects of combined oral/topical antioxidant treatment with the carotenoids lutein and zeaxanthin on human skin: a double-blind, placebo-controlled study. Skin Pharmacol Physiol 20:199–210
Quan T et al (2009) Matrix-degrading metalloproteinases in photoaging. J Investig Dermatol Symp Proc 14:20–24
Ribaya-Mercado JD et al (1995) Skin lycopene is destroyed preferentially over beta-carotene during ultraviolet irradiation in humans. J Nutr 125:1854–1859
Rundhaug JE, Fischer SM (2008) Cyclo-oxygenase-2 plays a critical role in UV-induced skin carcinogenesis. Photochem Photobiol 84:322–329
Rundhaug JE et al (2007) A role for cyclooxygenase-2 in ultraviolet light-induced skin carcinogenesis. Mol Carcinog 46:692–698
Schwarz A et al (2008) Green tea phenol extracts reduce UVB-induced DNA damage in human cells via interleukin-12. Photochem Photobiol 84:350–355
Seeram NP et al (2006) Pomegranate juice ellagitannin metabolites are present in human plasma and some persist in urine for up to 48 hours. J Nutr 136:2481–2485
Setchell KD et al (2001) Bioavailability of pure isoflavones in healthy humans and analysis of commercial soy isoflavone supplements. J Nutr 131:1362S-1375S
Sharma SD, Katiyar SK (2006) Dietary grape-seed proanthocyanidin inhibition of ultraviolet B-induced immune suppression is associated with induction of IL-12. Carcinogenesis 27:95–102
Sharma SD, Katiyar SK (2010) Dietary grape seed proanthocyanidins inhibit UVB-induced cyclooxygenase-2 expression and other inflammatory mediators in UVB-exposed skin and skin tumors of SKH-1 hairless mice. Pharm Res 27:1092–1102
Sharma SD et al (2007) Dietary grape seed proanthocyanidins inhibit UVB-induced oxidative stress and activation of mitogen-activated protein kinases and nuclear factor-kappaB signaling in in vivo SKH-1 hairless mice. Mol Cancer Ther 6:995–1005
Shibata A et al (2010) Sulforaphane suppresses ultraviolet B-induced inflammation in HaCaT keratinocytes and HR-1 hairless mice. J Nutr Biochem 21:702–709
Stadtman ER (2001) Protein oxidation in aging and age-related diseases. Ann N Y Acad Sci 928:22–38

Stahl W et al (2001) Dietary tomato paste protects against ultraviolet light-induced erythema in humans. J Nutr 131:1449–1451

Surh YJ (2003) Cancer chemoprevention with dietary phytochemicals. Nat Rev Cancer 3:768–780

Talalay P et al (2007) Sulforaphane mobilizes cellular defenses that protect skin against damage by UV radiation. Proc Natl Acad Sci USA 104:17500–17505

Tsoyi K et al (2008) Anthocyanins from black soybean seed coats inhibit UVB-induced inflammatory cylooxygenase-2 gene expression and PGE2 production through regulation of the nuclear factor-kappaB and phosphatidylinositol 3-kinase/Akt pathway. J Agric Food Chem 56:8969–8974

Ullrich SE (1995) Potential for immunotoxicity due to environmental exposure to ultraviolet radiation. Hum Exp Toxicol 14:89–91

Vaid M et al (2010a) Honokiol, a phytochemical from the Magnolia plant, inhibits photocarcinogenesis by targeting UVB-induced inflammatory mediators and cell cycle regulators: development of topical formulation. Carcinogenesis 31:2004–2011

Vaid M et al (2010b) Proanthocyanidins inhibit photocarcinogenesis through enhancement of DNA repair and xeroderma pigmentosum group A-dependent mechanism. Cancer Prev Res (Phila) 3:1621–1629

Vayalil PK et al (2003) Treatment of green tea polyphenols in hydrophilic cream prevents UVB-induced oxidation of lipids and proteins, depletion of antioxidant enzymes and phosphorylation of MAPK proteins in SKH-1 hairless mouse skin. Carcinogenesis 24:927–936

Wang ZY et al (1991) Protection against ultraviolet B radiation-induced photocarcinogenesis in hairless mice by green tea polyphenols. Carcinogenesis 12:1527–1530

Wang ZY et al (1992a) Inhibitory effect of green tea in the drinking water on tumorigenesis by ultraviolet light and 12-O-tetradecanoylphorbol-13-acetate in the skin of SKH-1 mice. Cancer Res 52:1162–1170

Wang ZY et al (1992b) Inhibitory effect of green tea on the growth of established skin papillomas in mice. Cancer Res 52:6657–6665

Wang ZY et al (1994) Inhibitory effects of black tea, green tea, decaffeinated black tea, and decaffeinated green tea on ultraviolet B light-induced skin carcinogenesis in 7, 12-dimethylbenz[a]anthracene-initiated SKH-1 mice. Cancer Res 54:3428–3435

Wang YN et al (2010) Genistein protects against UVB-induced senescence-like characteristics in human dermal fibroblast by p66Shc down-regulation. J Dermatol Sci 58:19–27

Wei H et al (1998) DNA structural integrity and base composition affect ultraviolet light-induced oxidative DNA damage. Biochemistry 37:6485–6490

Wei H Y et al (2002) Inhibition of ultraviolet light-induced oxidative events in the skin and internal organs of hairless mice by isoflavone genistein. Cancer Lett 185:21–29

Yarosh D et al (1992) Pyrimidine dimer removal enhanced by DNA repair liposomes reduces the incidence of UV skin cancer in mice. Cancer Res 52:4227–4231

Yoshikawa T et al (1990) Susceptibility to effects of UVB radiation on induction of contact hypersensitivity as a risk factor for skin cancer in humans. J Invest Dermatol 95:530–536

Zaid MA et al (2007) Inhibition of UVB-mediated oxidative stress and markers of photoaging in immortalized HaCaT keratinocytes by pomegranate polyphenol extract POMx. Photochem Photobiol 83:882–888

Zhu M et al (2004) Phase II enzyme inducer, sulforaphane, inhibits UVB-induced AP-1 activation in human keratinocytes by a novel mechanism. Mol Carcinog 41:179–186

Ziegler A et al (1994) Sunburn and p53 in the onset of skin cancer. Nature 372:773–776

Chapter 15
The Role of Vitamin E Forms in Cancer Prevention and Therapy – Studies in Human Intervention Trials and Animal Models

Silvia Y. Moya-Camarena and Qing Jiang

Abstract Vitamin E is a generic term of eight structurally related molecules including α-, β-, γ-, δ-tocopherol and α-, β-, γ-, δ-tocotrienol, all of which are potent lipophilic antioxidants. Despite eight forms in the vitamin E family, most studies have traditionally focused on α-tocopherol (αT) until the last couple of decades. The role of αT in modulation of carcinogenesis and especially its supplementation in chemoprevention has been extensively investigated in numerous animal and human studies including large clinical trials. These studies have yielded inconsistent and disappointing outcomes regarding the protective role of αT in cancer. On the other hand, other vitamin E forms, despite low in tissues, are rich in different diets and have recently been shown to have unique properties independent of antioxidant activities which likely play a role in cancer prevention. Here we review recent development in the field of different forms of vitamin E and cancer development with emphasis on the results from large clinical intervention trials and animal cancer models. In addition, potential mechanisms of the actions by different vitamin E forms are discussed.

15.1 Introduction

Vitamin E is a generic term of eight structurally related molecules including α-, β-, γ-, δ-tocopherol (αT, βT, γT and δT) and α-, β-, γ-, δ-tocotrienol (Fig. 15.1), all of which are potent lipophilic antioxidants. Despite eight forms in the vitamin E family, most studies have traditionally focused on α-tocopherol (αT) until the last couple of decades. This is because αT is the predominant form of vitamin E in tissues and its deficiency results in vitamin E deficiency associated ataxia, increased risk of atherosclerosis and possibly immune dysfunction (Brigelius-Flohe and Traber 1999; Jiang et al. 2001; Reiter et al. 2007). The role of αT in modulation of carcinogenesis and especially its supplementation in chemoprevention has also been extensively investigated in animal and numerous human studies including large clinical trials. These studies have yielded inconsistent and disappointing outcomes regarding the

Q. Jiang (✉)
Department of Nutrition Science, Purdue University, West Lafayette, IN 47907, USA
e-mail: qjiang@purdue.edu

F.H. Sarkar (ed.), *Nutraceuticals and Cancer*, DOI 10.1007/978-94-007-2630-7_15,

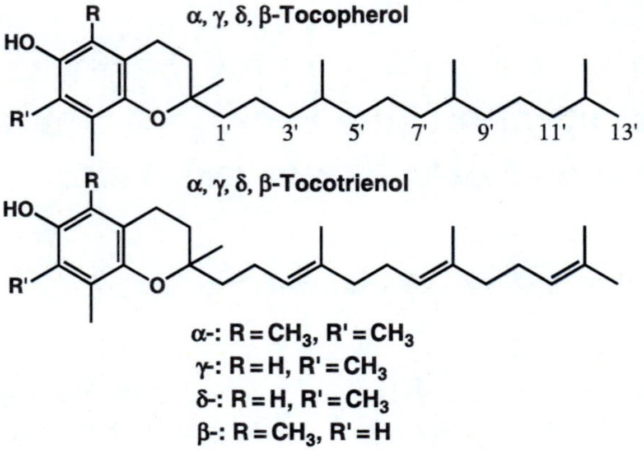

Fig. 15.1 Naturally occurring forms of vitamin E

protective role of αT in cancer. On the other hand, other vitamin E forms, despite low in tissues, are rich in different diets (Jiang et al. 2001) and have recently been shown to have unique properties independent of antioxidant activities which likely play a role in cancer prevention. In this chapter, we review recent development in the study of different forms of vitamin E and cancer development with emphasis on the results from large clinical intervention trials and animal cancer models. In addition, potential mechanisms of the actions by different vitamin E forms are briefly discussed.

15.2 Human Intervention Studies on the Role of Alpha-Tocopherol in Cancer Prevention and Therapy

15.2.1 Alpha-Tocopherol in Large Randomized Clinical Trials

All the clinical intervention studies related to vitamin E and cancer have exclusively focused on αT. Since 1994, eight large randomized clinical trials have been reported to investigate the role of αT or its combinations with other nutrition factors in cancer risk (summarized in Table 15.1). Four of these studies are primary prevention trials with apparently healthy subjects, i.e., SUVIMAX (Hercberg et al. 2004), WHS (Lee et al. 2005), SELECT (Lippman et al. 2009) and PHS II (Gaziano et al. 2009). The Linxian study (Blot et al. 1993) and the ATBC trial (The Alpha-Tocopherol BCCPSG, 1994) were conducted in high risk individuals for cancer including subjects with modest malnutrition or heavy smokers, respectively. In HOPE/HOPE-TOO (Lonn et al. 2005) and HPS (HPSCG, 2002) studies, participants with coronary diseases or diabetes were included. Since all these studies include relatively large population and provide valuable data in different populations (Table 15.1), it is important to reviewing them in great depth.

Linxian Study – The micronutrient intervention trial in Linxian, China (Blot et al. 1993) was designed to determine if supplementation with vitamins and minerals can lower cancer incidence, cancer mortality and mortality from other chronic diseases (primary outcomes). Linxian has a population with high rates of esophageal/gastric

Table 15.1 α-Tocopherol supplementation and the risk of cancer in large intervention trials

Study and locations	Characteristics of the subjects	Intervention	Major outcomes measured
Linxian study – Nutrition Intervention Trials. In Linxian, China. (Blot et al. 1993)	29,584 individuals aged from 40 to 69 years. Subclinical deficiencies of several micronutrients.	15 mg β-carotene, 30 mg α-tocopherol, and 50 μg selenium.	*Primary*: cancer incidence and mortality. *Secondary*: mortality from other diseases.
The α-Tocopherol, β-Carotene Cancer Prevention Study (ATBC). Southwestern, Finland. (The Alpha-Tocopherol 1994)	29,133 men aged from 50 to 69 years. Heavy smokers.	50 mg/day *dl*-α-tocopheryl acetate. 50 mg/day *dl*-α-tocopheryl acetate + 20 mg/day β-carotene.	*Primary*: lung cancer. *Secondary*: prostate, bladder, colon and rectum, stomach, other.
Heart Protection Study MRC/BHF (HPS) United Kingdom. (HPSCG 2002)	20,536 individuals of aged from 40 to 80 years. Coronary disease, occlusive arterial disease, or diabetes.	600 mg vitamin E, 250 mg vitamin C, 20 mg β-carotene daily	*Primary*: major coronary events and fatal or non-fatal vascular events. *Secondary*: cancer and other major morbidity.
Supple 'mentation en Vitamines et Miéraux Antioxydants (SUVIMAX) France. (Hercberg et al. 2004)	13,017 adults (women aged 35–60 years or men aged 45–60 years). Overall healthy	120 mg of ascorbic acid, 30 mg of vitamin E, 6 mg of β-carotene, 100 μg of selenium, and 20 mg of zinc, daily.	*Primary*: incidence of cancer and ischemic cardiovascular disease.
Women's Health Study (WHS). United States. (Lee et al. 2005)	39,876 apparently healthy US women $\geq$ 45 years. No previous history of coronary hearth disease, cerebro-vascular disease or cancer (except nonmelanoma skin cancer) or other major chronic illness.	600 IU natural source of α-tocopherol.	*Primary*: first major cardiovascular event. *Secondary*: individual cardiovascular events, stroke, and cardiovascular death and breast, lung and colon cancers.

Table 15.1 (continued)

Study and locations	Characteristics of the subjects	Intervention	Major outcomes
The Heart Outcomes Prevention Evaluation and The HOPE-The Ongoing Outcomes (HOPE and HOPE-TOO). Multi European countries and US. (Lonn et al. 2005)	7,030 patients ≥ 55 years with vascular disease or diabetes mellitus from the initial HOPE trial (1993–1999) and the HOPE-TOO extension (1999–2003).	400 IU/d RRR-α-tocopherol acetate.	*Primary*: cancer incidence, cancer deaths and major cardiovascular events.
Selenium and vitamin E Cancer Prevention Trial (SELECT). Canada, Puerto Rico, US. (Lippman et al. 2009)	35,533 men ≥50 y (African American) and ≥ 55 y (others). PSA ≤4 ng/ml and not suspicious for prostate cancer.	400 mg IU *all rac*-α-tocopheryl acetate. 200 μg/d L-selenomethionine + 400 mg IU *all rac*-α-tocopheryl acetate.	*Primary*: prostate cancer. *Secondary*: Lung, colorectal and overall primary cancer.
Physician's Health Study II (PHSII) United States. (Gaziano et al. 2009)	14,641 physicians ≥ 50 y including 1,307 men with history of prior cancer.	400 IU synthetic α-tocopherol every other day and vitamin C 500 mg daily.	*Primary*: prostate cancer for vitamin E and total cancer for vitamin C. *Secondary*: total cancer for vitamin E.

cardia cancer and persistently low intake of several micronutrients. As summarized in Table 15.1, one of the four treatments in the study included 15 mg β-carotene, 30 mg αT, and 50 μg selenium. This regimen led to a significant reduction in total mortality, mainly due to a lowered risk of cancer. Interestingly, this beneficial effect was still observed up to 10 years after the termination of supplementation (Qiao et al. 2009).

Despite the positive outcomes, the authors suggest caution in extrapolating the findings to other populations due to the special characteristics of Linxian with relatively low micronutrients. In addition, as mentioned before, αT was given in combination with β-carotene and selenium, and therefore the effects found can not be attributed to a specific micronutrient. In an extended analysis of the Linxian trial (follow-up 13 years after intervention), liver cancer mortality was examined (Qu et al. 2007). No effect was found on liver cancer mortality among the supplements studied, including the combination of β-carotene, αT, and selenium.

The ATBC study – The α-Tocopherol, β-Carotene Cancer Prevention Study (ATBC) (The Alpha-Tocopherol BCCPSG, 1994) was designed to determine the effect of daily supplementation of αT alone or in combination with β-carotene on the incidence of lung (primary outcome) and other cancers, in male heavy smokers (20 cigarettes/day). Randomly assigned participants received 50 mg/day *dl*-α-tocopheryl acetate ($n = 7{,}286$), 20 mg/day β-carotene ($n = 7{,}282$), both supplements ($n = 7{,}278$) and placebo ($n = 7{,}287$) capsules. Compared with placebo controls, no significant effect of αT on the incidence of lung cancer was found, whereas β-carotene unexpectedly increased the risk of lung cancer and total mortality (1994). Interestingly, significant reduction in prostate cancer incidence by 32% was seen in participants receiving αT supplementation ($n = 14{,}564$) compared with those not receiving it ($n = 14{,}569$) (Heinonen et al. 1998). Mortality from prostate cancer was found to be 41% lower among men receiving αT than those non-recipients. It is noteworthy that the reduction was evident in clinical prostate cancer (stage II-IV) but not in relatively early stages (stage 0–1) (Heinonen et al. 1998). α-Tocopherol had no effect on total mortality, while men allocated in the αT group seemed to have more death from hemorragic stroke when compared to no αT group.

An additional report from ATBC study indicated increased colorectal cancer risk in those participants receiving αT supplementation as compared with those that did not receive it. However, the authors suspected of bias in the diagnostic process because supplementation with αT also caused more rectal bleeding and intestinal pain leading to more colonoscopies, which may consequently led to increased detection of the incidence of polyps (Malila et al. 1999). In addition, αT supplementation had no effect on the incidence of gastric cancer (Malila et al. 2002; Varis et al. 1998), urinary tract cancer (Virtamo et al. 2000), colorectal cancer (Albanes et al. 2000), aero digestive tract cancer (Wright et al. 2007) and oral mucosal lesions (Liede et al. 1998).

Although the protective effects on prostate cancer were observed with αT during its supplementation, in the 6–8 year ATBC post-intervention follow-up study aiming to valuate the duration of the intervention, the beneficial effects of αT and the adverse effects of β-carotene disappeared (Virtamo et al. 2003). This suggests that the protective effect of αT may be transient and diminishing rapidly after termination of supplementation.

One of the caveats discussed in the literature for the ATBC study is that prostate cancer was not a pre-specified end point in the trial, and therefore the results could be due to confounding bias (Gann 2009). In addition, the ATBC study group suspected that the intervention period may be too short to inhibit the development of cancers resulting from life-long exposure to cigarette smoke and other carcinogens, and the dose of αT may be low (50 mg/day) (1994), especially if male smokers have inadequate vitamin E status previous to the supplementation.

Supplementary analysis from the ATBC trial, looking at baseline or serum levels of αT and other forms of vitamin E, have been reported. In a report during the trial intervention with only 317 cases, the relationship between baseline serum αT levels and prostate cancer risk was not significant (Hartman et al. 1998). But later, the ATBC group reported a significant inverse association between baseline serum αT and prostate cancer risk. A nested case-control analysis from ATBC trial reported that higher baseline serum levels of γ-tocopherol were also associated with lower prostate cancer risk in supplemented individuals (with αT or β-carotene) (Weinstein et al. 2005). In addition, a strong inverse relationships between baseline serum αT and prostate or pancreatic cancer risk were reported based on the data obtained from 19 years follow-up after ATBC intervention (Stolzenberg-Solomon et al. 2009; Weinstein et al. 2007).

The Heart Protection Study (HPSCG) (2002) was designed to investigate the effect of daily supplementation with a combination of antioxidant vitamins including αT on vascular events as the primary endpoints. Non-vascular events including cancer and other major morbidity were evaluated as secondary endpoints. The study included 20,536 British adults who had coronary diseases, other occlusive arterial disease or diabetes. These participants were randomly assigned to receive a combination of 600 mg vitamin E, 250 mg vitamin C, and 20 mg β-carotene daily ($n = 10{,}241$) or matching placebo ($n = 10{,}228$). After 5-year treatment, although this regime substantially increased blood concentrations of αT, ascorbate and β-carotene, no protective effect of the antioxidant vitamin combination was found on all-cause mortality, cancer incidence, cancer mortality, cancer in specific sites or other non-vascular outcomes. On the other hand, the authors concluded that the supplement appeared to be safe in the high-risk individuals studied. It is important to note that the primary endpoint of this study was vascular events (but not cancer incidence), which accordingly determined the time of intervention and follow-up time. As a result, the follow-up period may be too short for cancer events (incidence and mortality). Although the authors mentioned that the participants in this trial would be followed for several years, but to our knowledge no report has been published to date.

The Supple'mentation en Vitamines et Miéraux Antioxydants (SU.VI.MAX) (Hercberg et al. 2004) was designed to test the effect of what the authors called 'an adequate and well balanced intake of antioxidant nutrients' on the incidence of cancers and ischemic cardiovascular disease (CVD) in a middle-aged general population. The study included 13,017 apparently healthy adults (35–60 years old) in France. Participants were randomly assigned to take a single daily capsule of a low-dose antioxidant supplementation containing ascorbic acid (20 mg), αT (30 mg), β-carotene (6 mg), selenium (100 μg) and zinc (20 mg), or a placebo in the controls. After a medium 7.5-year intervention, this low-dose antioxidant supplementation lowered total cancer incidence and all cause mortality in men but not in women. Interestingly, like the Linxian study in China, nutritional intake and concentrations of baseline β-carotene was lower in men than in women, which may potentially explain the effects limited to men (Blot et al. 1993).

In a post intervention analysis of the SUVIMAX study, the beneficial effects found in men disappeared during 5-year follow-up after antioxidant supplementation ceased (Hercberg et al. 2010). In contrast, the risk of skin cancer appeared to increase in women during the period of supplementation in SUVIMAX (Hercberg et al. 2007), although after a 5-year post-intervention follow up no increased risk of skin cancer was observed for either gender (Ezzedine et al. 2010).

The Heart Outcomes Prevention Evaluation (HOPE) and HOPE–The Ongoing Outcomes (HOPE-TOO) (Lonn et al. 2005) – HOPE trial was conducted for 4–5 years to test potential protective effects of αT supplementation on cardiovascular events and revealed a neutral effect on cardiovascular outcomes (Yusuf et al. 2000). HOPE-TOO study was 4-year extension of the HOPE study to assess whether longer duration of αT supplementation trial would prevent cancer and cardiovascular disease. The original HOPE study was an international, multicenter, double-blind, randomized, 2×2 factorial design trial that evaluates ramipril (10 mg/day) and vitamin E (RRR-α-tocopheryl acetate, 400 UI/day) in patients with high risk for cardiovascular events. The use of increased dose of αT (compared with Linxian and ATBC studies) was because of the lack of relation between vitamin E and coronary heart disease in the Linxian and ATBC studies (Yusuf et al. 2000). After the initial 5-year study showing significant beneficial effects from ramipril, the HOPE-TOO was extended for 4 more years with recommendation of ramipril for all participants. The primary outcomes in the HOPE-TOO trial included cancer incidence, cancer deaths, and major cardiovascular events. In final HOPE-TOO analysis, all patients from HOPE were included (final $n = 9{,}541$). No significant effect of αT supplementation was found on the incidence of cancers, cancer deaths, or major cardiovascular events, in patients with cardiovascular disease or diabetes mellitus. However, higher rates of heart failure and hospitalizations for heart failure were found in the αT supplementation group.

The Women's Health Study (WHS) (Lee et al. 2005) – The study was designed to test whether vitamin E supplementation for 10 years decreases the risk of major cardiovascular diseases (nonfatal myocardial infarction, nonfatal stroke or cardiovascular death) and total invasive cancer (primary outcomes) in healthy women (39,876 women aged al least 45 y). In a 2×2 factorial design, apparently healthy US women were randomly assigned to receive 600 IU natural source of αT or placebo and 100 mg of aspirin or placebo every other day. The use of 600 IU was based on previous reports where individuals with high vitamin E intake have lower rates of cardiovascular disease and cancer than those with low vitamin E intake

(Rexrode et al. 2000). After 10-year supplementation, αT did not show significant effect on the incidences of major cardiovascular events (myocardial infarction, stroke, or ischemic or hemorrhagic stroke) or incidences of cancer or cancer deaths, including total invasive cancer or main site-specific cancers (lung, breast, colon cancers). Although there was a significant 24% reduction of cardiovascular death in αT supplemented group, the authors concluded that this observation was likely due to chance arising from multiple comparisons as no effects on the incidence of any major cardiovascular events were observed in the current study or other previous studies (Eidelman et al. 2004; Vivekananthan et al. 2003). It is interesting to note that unlike observations in ATBC, HOPE-TOO studies or meta-analysis (Miller et al. 2005), no significant adverse effects, e.g., increased hemorrhagic strokes or all-cause mortality, were observed related to αT supplementation in the WHS.

The Selenium and Vitamin E Cancer Prevention Trial (SELECT) – The SELECT trial (Lippman et al. 2009) was prompted by the reported beneficial effects of αT in the ATBC study (1994) and selenium in the Nutritional Prevention of Cancer (Clark et al. 1996), as well as the reduction of overall cancer mortality in the Linxian study by supplementation of selenium, αT and β-carotene (Blot et al. 1993). The main objective of SELECT was to assess whether selenium (200 μg/day from L-selenomethionine), vitamin E (400 UI/day of all *rac-α*-tocopheryl acetate) or their combination could prevent prostate cancer and other diseases in healthy men. The study included healthy, low-cancer-risk men who have prostate specific antigen (PSA) values $\leq$ 4 ng/ml, have no prior prostate cancer diagnosis and are not suspicious for cancer during a digital rectal examination. Prostate cancer incidences were reported by participants and were further confirmed by medical records, prostate biopsy and pathology laboratory. After 5.46-year supplementation, there were no differences in the rates of prostate cancer among the treatment groups and placebo; Specifically, 416 prostate cancer cases were diagnosed during the trial in the patients receiving placebo, 473 receiving αT alone, 432 in the selenium alone group, and 437 in the group that received the combination of αT and selenium. Among all groups, more than 95% diagnosed prostate cancer was in early stage, e.g., ~70 and 25% in stage T1 and T2, respectively. In sharp contrast to the ATBC study, there was a non-significant ($P = 0.06$) increase in stage-one prostate cancer in αT alone group.

In addition, no effect of treatments was found for any pre-specified secondary cancer endpoints including lung, colorectal and overall primary cancer. The numbers of deaths from any cause were similar in all treatment groups. No significant effects were found on the overall incidence of cardiovascular events.

The Physicians' Health Study II (PHS II) – Unlike the SELECT trial that is focused on low-risk subjects, the PHS II (Gaziano et al. 2009) was designed to test whether αT prevents prostate cancer in men, regardless current risk of prostate cancer or previous history of cancer. PHS II included 14,641 male physicians at 50 years or older from the American Medical Association, approximately 9% of whom have previous history of cancer, myocardial infarction or stroke. The main goal of the study was to evaluate whether long-term vitamin E (400 IU αT every other day) or vitamin C (500 mg ascorbic acid daily) decreases the risk of prostate cancer or total cancer among men. After the mean 8 years follow-up, neither αT nor vitamin C supplementation reduced the risk of prostate cancer, total cancer, and site-specific cancer incidence or total mortality. On the other hand, a greater number of hemorrhagic strokes were observed among those assigned to vitamin E (39 *vs.* 23 events; HR, 1.74; 95% CI, 1.04–2.91) compared with placebo. Similar adverse effects were also reported in the ATBC (1994) and the HOPE-TOO study (Lonn et al. 2005).

15.2.2 Summary of Large Intervention Studies

Three out of the eight large intervention studies have found that αT or its combination with other antioxidants reduced cancer risk, which include the Linxian study in China where supplementation of β-carotene, αT and selenium significantly reduced total cancer incidence and mortality of cancer, the ATBC study which showed reduction in the incidence of prostate cancer among heavy smokers, and the SUVIMAX where reduction of total cancer incidence and all mortality cause was seen in men but not women. It is important to note that these studies were conducted in different but yet very specific populations with distinct characteristics; Specifically, the Linxian study has population with subclinical deficiencies of micronutrients (Blot et al. 1993), and the subjects in the ATBC and SUVIMAX include heavy smokers who likely have increased oxidative stress, or men with low plasma levels of antioxidant levels, respectively. Interestingly, compared with other large trials, these three used low doses of αT (e.g., 30–50 mg of αT) alone or combined with other nutrients. The protective effects of low-dose supplementation on cancer in high cancer-risk populations can be explained by the notion that mild malnutrition or unbalanced antioxidant status due to heavy smoking may result in increased DNA damage and compromised DNA repair system, which may consequently lead to increased risk for cancer development compared with healthy populations (Ames et al. 2002). It is therefore conceivable that in these 'abnormal' populations, supplementation of even low-dose αT and/or its combinations with other nutrients would be sufficient to suppress the increased risk.

In contrast to the subjects with sub-adequate nutrient or unbalanced antioxidant characteristics, participants in the other large trials have sufficient nutrients with limited number of current smokers. The subjects in the SELECT trial, the WHS and PHS II include low-risk and apparently healthy individuals, although the PHS II also included less than 9% men with previous cancer or vascular diseases. Unlike the ATBC, which has 100% heavy smokers, the SELECT and PHS II included <8% current smokers. In these studies, long-term supplementation of high doses of αT (>400 IU) or its combination with other antioxidants failed to show any beneficial effects on cancer risk or cancer mortality. Similarly, in the HOPE-TOO and HPS study where subjects are patients with vascular diseases or diabetes mellitus, high doses of αT did not show any benefits to cancer or cardiovascular incidence. These results are consistent with animal studies (Sections below) showing that high-dose supplementations with αT do not seem to show consistent protective effects on cancer development compared with controls, which have adequate dietary intake of αT.

It is worth mentioning that four of the eight large trials indicate potential adverse effects from high-dose αT supplementation, including greater number of hemorrhagic strokes (PHS II), and ATBC, non-significant ($P = 0.06$) increase in stage-one prostate cancer in αT alone group (SELECT), or higher rates of heart failure and hospitalizations for heart failure in the αT supplementation group (HOPE-TOO). Interestingly, potential adverse effects associated with higher dose of αT, e.g., 400 IU or higher, were also pointed out by a meta analyses that take consideration of large and small clinical trials (Miller et al. 2005). Since high dose of αT has been shown to modulate the expression of cytochrome P450s and pregnane-X-receptor (Brigelius-Flohe 2005), which are among the key players for drug metabolism, it is reasonable to speculate that high dose of αT may potentially modulate drug metabolism. This may partially explain adverse effects in patients on multiple drugs due to high-dose αT supplementation. In addition, αT supplementation is known to suppress γ-tocopherol (Jiang et al. 2001), which has been shown to have unique health benefits based on mechanistic and animal studies (Jiang et al. 2001; Reiter et al. 2007).

The protective effects of low-dose αT supplementation in subjects with moderate malnutrition or heavy smokers underscores the importance of long-term maintenance of healthy nutrient status in prevention of cancer and possibly other chronic diseases. This aspect has been proven by other nutrition factors including folate whose deficiency has been shown to increase the risk of cancer (Ames et al. 2002; Kim 2008). In the meanwhile, the lack of significant protection from high-dose supplementation of αT strongly suggests that essential nutrient factors may have limited role in directly intervening carcinogenesis that is promoted by factors beyond nutrient deficiency. These notions are elaborated in an elegant study by Suarna et al. (2006) showing that low-dose supplementation of αT significantly attenuated αT-deficiency induced exaggeration of atherosclerosis development, whereas high-dose supplementation of αT did not offer further benefits.

15.3 Case-Control Studies of Different Vitamin E Forms

The evidence of beneficial effect of tocopherols on cancer in case-control studies is controversial. From 21 studies reviewed (number of cases ranging from 67 to 1,072), seven showed that higher αT levels were associated with reduced risk of various types of cancer, such as bladder (Liang et al. 2008), cervical neoplasia (Cho et al. 2009), esophagus and noncardia (Taylor et al. 2003), gastric (Jenab et al. 2006), lung (Goodman et al. 2003), pancreas (Stolzenberg-Solomon et al. 2009) and prostate cancer (Goodman et al. 2003; Weinstein et al. 2007). Four case-control studies reported that high plasma concentrations of γ-tocopherol were negatively associated with the risk of aerogastric tract cancer (Nomura et al. 1997), cervical neoplasia (Cho et al. 2009) and prostate cancer (Helzlsouer et al. 2000; Weinstein et al. 2007). However, two studies showed γ-tocopherol (Kabat et al. 2009) or both αT and γT levels (Kim et al. 2010) are associated with increased risk of breast cancer. Ingles et al. (Ingles et al. 1998) found negative association between the α-tocopherol/γ-tocopherol ratio and the risk of colorectal cancer, but not with the individual vitamin E forms.

Unlike large double-blind placebo controlled intervention trials that are considered as 'gold standard' for studying drug efficacy, conclusions based correlation data obtained from case-control studies are often weakened by several weaknesses due to the nature of this type of studies. One caveat to be considered in case-control studies is bias. Secondly, a single determination of micronutrients at a single time point may not reflect the long-term exposure to micronutrients. Thirdly, when blood samples are collected at the time of cancer diagnosis or after, it is possible that the associations observed may be due to the disease that could consequently change overall metabolism in the body. In the studies reviewed here, five included analyses from serum of patients already diagnosed with cancer, three of them showing negative association between αT and cancers (Cho et al. 2009; Ingles et al. 1998; Liang et al. 2008), one reporting positive association (Kim et al. 2010), whereas the other one found negative association of the α-tocopherol:γ-tocopherol ratio with decreased risk of cancer (Ingles et al. 1998). In addition, the measured nutrients such as αT or γT might merely serve as a marker of other important factors such as dietary fat contents because both of them are associated with high fat intake. As a result, the associations observed based on case-control studies must be interpreted with considering these limitations.

15.4 Alpha-Tocopherol and Analogs in Various Cancer Models

Like human clinical intervention studies, most early animal studies on vitamin E and cancer exclusively focused on αT. Potential protective effects of αT supplementation have been investigated in broad ranges of cancer models including skin, prostate, colon and breast cancer. These studies, however, have revealed inconsistent results regarding the beneficial effects of αT on cancer risk. For instance, although many studies have reported protective effects of αT when administered alone (Ichikawa et al. 1993; McVean and Liebler 1997; Mizumoto et al. 1994; Moore et al. 1987; Yano et al. 1994) or in combination with other compounds (Battalora et al. 1993; Bissett et al. 1990; Burke et al. 2000; Chen et al. 2000; Factor et al. 2000; Hirose et al. 1986, 1993; Kakizaki et al. 2001; Limpens et al. 2006; Nakadate et al. 1984; Perchellet et al. 1985, 1987; Sarna et al. 2000; Shamberger and Rudolph 1966; Trickler and Shklar 1987; Wang et al. 1989; Weber et al. 2002; Yam et al. 2001; Yu et al. 2008, 2009), there are plenty of studies also reporting no protective effects (Al-Johar et al. 2008; Berton et al. 1998; Chen et al. 2000; Chung et al. 2003; Hirose et al. 1986, 2002; Hirose et al. 1995; Masui et al. 1986; McCormick et al. 2010; Nakamura et al. 1991; Ogasawara et al. 2007; Ozten et al. 2010; Wenger et al. 2001). In addition, several groups have also reported tumor-promoting activity by αT (Hirose et al. 1993; Kolaja and Klaunig 1997; Mitchel and McCann 1993; Miyauchi et al. 2002; Moore et al. 1987).

Besides naturally occurring RRR-αT, several derivatives from this vitamin E form have been shown to have anticancer effects. For instance, α-tocopheryl succinate (α-TOS) is a redox-inactive αT derivative and can be hydrolyzed in vivo to αT and succinate. Recently, several non-hydrolyzable ether acetic acid derivatives from αT including αTEA (2,5,7,8-tetramethyl-2R-(4R,8R,12-trimethyltridecyl)chroman-6-yloxyacetic acid) have been shown to have potent anticancer effects. In addition, distinctive features between synthetic αT which is composed of mixed stereoisomers of αT (*dl*-α-tocopherol acetate, or *all-rac*-α-tocopheryl acetate) and naturally occurring RRR-αT have also been suggested.

15.4.1 RRR-α-Tocopherols

Skin cancer – Shamberger in 1966 (Shamberger and Rudolph 1966) reported for the first time that topical application of αT reduced skin tumor formation induced by with 3,2′-dimethyl-4-aminobifenyl (DMBA) in mice. Similarly, in a two-stage mouse skin carcinogenesis model, topical application of 40 μmol of *d*-α-tocopherol reversed the effect of the tumor promoter on ornithine decarboxylase and glutathione peroxidase activities, with the concomitant reduction of the incidence of skin tumors (Battalora et al. 1993; Nakadate et al. 1984; Perchellet et al. 1985, 1987). On the other hand, when 80 μmol of topical αT used in the same skin carcinogenesis model, αT acted as a tumor promoter, with similar efficiency as 12-O-tetradecanoylphorbol-13-acetate (TPA) (Mitchel and McCann 1993, 2003).

The extent of topical application of αT in photodamage prevention has also been investigated. αT dispersion (1% in neutral vehicle cream) inhibited the formation of thymine dimers with greater efficacy than α-tocopherol acetate, α-tocopherol methyl ester, γ-tocopherol and δ-tocopherol (McVean and Liebler 1997). In addition, αT inhibited UV irradiation induced DNA damage and p53 expression, but was not effective in preventing UV-induced proliferation and tumor formation (Berton et al. 1998). Interestingly, topical administration of αT (5% solution) reduced UVB-radiation induced skin wrinkling, skin tumor incidence and tumor onset (Bissett et al. 1990).

Prostate cancer – Based on the hypothesis that αT may have potential anti-cancer effect against prostate cancer, Nakamura et al. (1991) studied the effect of dietary αT (1% by weight) on 3,2′-dimethyl-4-aminobifenyl (DMAB)-initiated prostate carcinogenesis in rats. However, these investigators found no significant effect of αT on the incidence of tumors in the prostate or any other organs analyzed, including small and large intestines, pancreas, skin, subcutis, preputial and zymbal glands. Ozten et al. (Ozten et al. 2010) examined the effect of selenomethionine and *dl*-α-tocopherol acetate on prostate cancer in estradiol-treated NBL rats. In this study, αT at 0.2 and 0.4% by weight did not show any effect on the development of prostate carcinomas. Similarly, McCormick et al. (2010) did not find beneficial effect of the same dietary treatments (αT at 2000 and 4000 mg/kg diet) on prostate cancer incidence in rats where prostate epithelial cell proliferation was stimulated by sequential administration of oral cyproterone acetate (for 21 consecutive days), subcutaneous injection of testosterone propionate (for 3 days), followed by a single dose of the carcinogen N-methyl-N-nitrosurea and subcutaneous implantation of testosterone capsules during the study for chronic androgen stimulation.

Unlike αT alone, combination of αT with lycopene seems to show some beneficial results. In the human PC346-C prostate xenograft model in nude mice, αT (*all-rac*-α-tocopheryl acetate) in combination with lycopene (5 mg/kg body weight of each component by oral gavage) suppressed the growth of the prostate xenograft by 75%, and increase median survival by 40% (Limpens et al. 2006). Consistently, in Copenhagen rats injected with MatLyLu Dunning prostate cancer cells, dietary αT and lycopene increased prostate tumor necrotic areas to 36.3, and 35.97%, respectively. On the other hand, αT/lycopene co-treated group had a non-significant increase on the percentage of tumor necrotic area (Siler et al. 2004).

Colon cancer – Most studies regarding the effects of αT on colon cancer revealed no beneficial effects. In F344 male rats which were injected with azoymethane (AOM) to induce colon cancer, dietary vitamin E did not have any effect on colon carcinogenesis, as measured by aberrant crypt foci (ACF, a pre-cancer lesion) (Yao et al. 1996) or tumor incidence or multiplicity (Reddy and Tanaka 1986). Similarly, in Sprague Dawley rats (Maziere et al. 1998), Swiss mice (Temple and el-Khatib 1987), or CD-1 (ICR) BR mice (Chester et al. 1986) injected with 1,2-dimethylhydrazine to initiate colon carcinogenesis, αT did not have inhibitory effect on colon tumor development. In addition, dietary treatments of *dl*-α-tocopheryl acetate at 30 mg/kg or 500 mg/kg diet before induction of colon tumorigenesis by i.p. injection of AOM, did not have any effect on the formation of ACF in young or old C57L/6 mice (Chung et al. 2003). Similarly, in Sprague Dawley rats, dietary treatment of *dl*-α-tocopherol at 100 mg/kg diet and vitamin A at 1.2 mg/kg diet did not show significant effect on ACF formation ($p > 0.05$) in AOM-induced tumorogenesis (Al-Johar et al. 2008). In addition, dietary αT at 0.5% diet did not suppress colon carcinogenesis induced by 2-amino-1-methyl-6-phenylimidazol[4,5-b]pyridine (PhIP) in rats (Hagiwara et al. 1999).

Despite being ineffective in most studies with colon cancer models, supplementation of αT appeared to be capable of reducing colon cancer risk associated with vitamin E deficiency or high fat plus low fiber intake. Thus, dietary vitamin E (90 mg/kg diet) decreased the incidence of AOM-induced colonic tumors and tumor multiplicity in Fischer-344 rats fed low fiber/high fat diet (Shivapurkar et al. 1995). Cook et al. showed that in LACA mice, compared with animals fed a low vitamin E diet (10 mg/kg diet), dietary vitamin E at 600 mg/kg diet reduced the incidence of 1,2-dimethyl hydrazine-induced adenomas and the number of invasive carcinomas in the colon (Cook and McNamara 1980).

In contrast, *dl*-α-tocopheryl acetate at 4% in diet enhanced the tumorigenicity induced by 1,2-dimethylhydrazine dihydrochloride in Swiss mice, as indicated by increased incidences of tumors in the duodenum, cecum, colon, rectum, and anus (Toth and Patil 1983).

Recently, Ogasawara et al. tested whether antioxidants including αT can modulate lung metastasis of colon cancer cells (Ogasawara et al. 2007). In this study, αT was administered via 5 consecutive i.p. injections of 20 μl, 100 mM stock solution,

3 days before tumor inoculation. This treatment did not have inhibitory activity against lung tumor metastasis of murine colon 26-L5 carcinoma cells. Similarly, β-carotene and ascorbic acid were also tested, but had not inhibitory effect on tumor lung metastasis. On the other hand, epigallocatechin gallate, gallocatechin gallate, and genistein reduced tumor nodules in the lungs by 77, 46, and 44%, respectively.

Lung cancer – The effects of αT on lung cancer varied with animal models. In urethane-induced lung carcinogenesis in A/J mice, αT administered via i.p. at 1000 mg/kg body weight did not affect tumor development (Witschi et al. 1981). Consistently, αT did not inhibit tumor growth in nude mice implanted with human lung cancer cells (Li et al. 2011). However, inhaled αT aerosol but not inhaled αT acetate, decreased lung inflammation markers in rats with inflammation caused by bacterial lipopolysaccharide (Hybertson et al. 2005). α-Tocopherol (100 mg/kg) decreased concentrations of thiobarbituric acid reactive substances (TBARS), hydroperoxides, and conjugated dienes in liver, lungs and hearts of nicotine-treated male albino rats (Helen et al. 2003). Similarly, αT administered in diet (at 550.9 mg/kg diet) inhibited TBARS and DNA single strand breaks in lungs of mice treated with 4-nitroquinoline 1-oxide (Ichikawa et al. 1993; Yano et al. 1994). Interestingly, this dietary treatment also reduced lung tumor incidence and multiplicity in spontaneous lung tumorigenesis in A/J mice (Yano et al. 1994). Similarly, dietary αT combined with fish oil and vitamin C led to slower rate of tumor growth and lower metastatic load in mice inoculated with a highly metastatic clone of the 3LL Lewis lung carcinoma cells (Yam et al. 2001).

In addition, the combination of β-carotene, αT and ascorbic acid protected against 4-(methylnitrosamino)-1-(3-pyridyl)-1-butanone-induced lung carcinogenesis in smoke-exposed ferrets (Kim et al. 2006, 2007). A combination of αT and ascorbic acid prevented the smoke-induced lung squamous metaplasia in ferrets (Kim et al. 2011).

Breast cancer – Dietary αT at 1.5 or 1% diet did not inhibit rat mammary carcinogenesis induced by 7, 12-dimethylbenz[a]anthracene (DMBA) (Hirose et al. 1986) or 2-Amino-1-methyl-6-phenylimidazo[4,5-b]pyridine (PhIP) (Hirose et al. 2002), respectively. At 0.5% diet, αT did not reduce the incidence of mammary tumors (the number of rats bearing tumors) induced by injection of PhIP, but decrease the number of tumors per rat (multiplicity) (Hagiwara et al. 1999). Interestingly, in the daunorubicin-induced mammary tumor model in Sprague-Dawley rats, i.p. injection of 1.8 g of α-tocopheryl acetate/m^2/day lowered the incidence of mammary tumors and delayed the onset of tumor formation (Wang et al. 1989). Yu et al. (2008) found that only the synthetic forms of αT (*all-rac*-α-tocopherol and *all-rac*-α-tocopheryl acetate), but not RRR-αT inhibited mammary tumor growth and lung metastases using the transplantable mouse 66c1-4-GFP mammary cancer cells in BALB/c mice.

Liver and other cancers – Although several studies have found that dietary αT exerts antitumor activities in chemically-induced hepatocarcinogenesis (Hirose et al. 1995; Kolaja and Klaunig 1997; Mizumoto et al. 1994; Moore et al. 1987; Tsuda et al. 1994), and in transgenic mice models (Factor et al. 2000; Kakizaki et al. 2001), others report no effect of dietary αT on chemically-induced liver cancer (Lii et al. 1999; Masui et al. 1986).

α-Tocopherol administration has been reported to inhibit chemically-induced oral and esophageal carcinogenesis (Chen et al. 2000; Odukoya et al. 1984; Trickler and Shklar 1987), as well as the incidence and multiplicity of kidney atypical tubules (Hirose et al. 1993), but had no effect on chemically-induced pancreatic adenocarcinoma (Wenger et al. 2001). On the other hand, the administration of αT induced hyperplastic and papillomatous lesions in the forestomach (Hirose et al. 1993; Miyauchi et al. 2002; Moore et al. 1987), and enhanced tumor growth and metastasis in retrovirus-induced cancers (Kline and Sanders 1989).

15.4.2 α-Tocopherol Derivatives

Both redox-active and redox-inactive αT derivatives have been investigated regarding their anticancer effects. α-Tocopheryl succinate (α-TOS), a redox-inactive analogue of vitamin E, has been shown to be a stronger inducer of apoptosis than αT in cell-based studies. Potential anticancer efficacy of α-TOS has been tested in some animal models, which was recently reviewed (Neuzil et al. 2007; Tomasetti and Neuzil 2007). Weber et al. (2002) found that α-TOS is a potent antitumor agent in a xenograft model implanted with human HCT116 colon cancer cells in nude mice. These investigators found that α-TOS and αT (50 μL of 200 mM every 3rd day) resulted in inhibition of tumor growth by 80 and 35% respectively. In addition to the antiproliferative action, α-TOS also has pro-apoptotic activity that may explain its higher efficiency when compared to αT. Other xenograft studies have reported that α-TOS suppressed the growth of tumors implanted from breast cancer cells (Malafa and Neitzel 2000), lung cancer cells (Dong et al. 2009; Quin et al. 2005), prostate cancer cells (Basu et al. 2007; Yin et al. 2009), head and neck squamous cell carcinoma (Gu et al. 2008), and bladder cancer cells (Kanai et al. 2010). Studies in allograft models also support the anticancer effects of α-TOS (Barnett et al. 2002; Hahn et al. 2006; Hrzenjak et al. 2004; Kogure et al. 2005; Malafa et al. 2002; Ramanathapuram et al. 2005). Moreover, antitumor activity of α-TOS has also been reported in chemically-induced tumors (Wu et al. 2001) and protective effect against γ-radiation (Singh et al. 2011).

Besides the hydrolyzable αT derivatives, several non-hydrolyzable αT derivatives have recently been developed and shown to have anticancer properties, such as the non-hydrolyzable RRR-αT ether acetic acid analog (α-TEA) (Hahn et al. 2006; Lawson et al. 2004), α-tocopheryl malonate (Kogure et al. 2005), RRR-α-tocopheryloxybutyl sulfonic acid (Ni et al. 2009), α-tocopheryl melamide (Turanek et al. 2009), and amphiphilic α-tocopherol oligochitosan conjugates (Noh et al. 2011).

Yu et al. (2008, 2009) compared antitumor activity of naturally occurring tocopherols with synthetic αT, i.e., *all-rac*-αT and *all-rac*-α-tocopheryl acetate (*all-rac*-αTAc) that contain a mixture of eight stereoisomers and are commonly used in supplements. In two mammary cancer models, these investigators also compared naturally occurring αT (RRR-αT) and γ-tocopherol (RRR-γT). In these studies, RRR-αT ether-linked acetic acid analog (αTEA), the non-hydrolyzable ether analog of αT, was included as a positive control. In one of the mammary cancer models, murine 66c1-4 GFP mammary cancer cells were inoculated into BALB/c mice, after 10 days of oral administration of 6 mg of the synthetic forms of vitamin E/day and 5 mg of the natural forms of vitamin E/day (Yu et al. 2008). Compared with controls, the synthetic forms of vitamin E (*all-rac*-αT and *all-rac*-α-TAc) and the positive control (αTEA) reduced tumor volume. αTEA and *all-rac*-αT also reduced macroscopic lung tumor metastasis, and the number of macroscopic lung tumor foci. As to the naturally occurring RRR-αT and RRR-γT, only γT reduced tumor growth in comparison with control. In a follow-up study, these investigators examined these vitamin E related compounds in another xenograft breast cancer model where human breast cancer MDA-MB 231-GPF cells were subcutaneous injected into nude mice. The supplementation regime included 378 mg RRR-αT/kg diet; 358 mg RRR-γT/kg diet; 400 mg *all-rac*-αT/kg diet, 243 mg α-TEA/kg diet and 456 mg RRR-αT + 506 mg RRR-γT/kg diet. Significant reduction of tumor volume was observed in RRR-γT, *all-rac*-αT and αTEA dietary groups as compared to basal control diet. No differences in tumor volumes in RRR-αT and RRR-αT+RRR-γT groups were found in comparison with control groups (Yu et al. 2009). These results suggest that the natural form of αT does not possess antitumor activity and appears to block the antitumor efficacy of γT.

15.5 γ-Tocopherol and γT-Rich Mixed Tocopherols in Cancer Models

15.5.1 Mechanistic Bases for Potential Anticancer Activities of γT

Despite αT has drawn most attention in most studies in the past, studies by us and others during the last 15 years have demonstrated that γT, the major form of vitamin E in US diet, has unique activities that are not shared by αT but are potentially important for cancer prevention and therapy (Jiang and Ames 2003; Jiang et al. 2000, 2001). We have found that γT and its terminal metabolite γ-CEHC, unlike αT, exhibit anti-inflammatory effects by inhibition of cyclooxygenase (COX)-catalyzed formation of prostaglandin E2 (PGE_2) in LPS-treated macrophages and IL-1β activated epithelial cells, as well as in carrageenan-induced inflammation model in rats (Jiang and Ames 2003). In this rat inflammation model, γT but not αT also inhibited 5-lipoxygenase (5-LOX)-catalyzed formation of LTB_4 and TNFα (Jiang and Ames 2003). Our recent studies have demonstrated that 13'-carboxychromanol, which is a novel long-chain metabolite of vitamin E forms and is substantially excreted in feces, is a much more potent inhibitor of COX-1, COX-2 and 5-LOX than the unmetabolized vitamin E forms (Jiang et al. 2008; Jiang et al. 2011b).

In addition to its anti-inflammatory properties, γT is better than αT in trapping electrophilic reactive nitrogen oxide species, such as nitrogen dioxide (Cooney et al. 1993, 1995) and peroxynitrite (Christen et al. 1997, 2002), to form a stable adduct, 5-nitro-γ-tocopherol. Thus, γT inhibits methylcholanthrene-induced neoplastic transformation more effectively than αT in C3H/10T1/2 murine fibroblasts, a process believed to be mediated by reactive nitrogen species (Cooney et al. 1993).

We recently showed that γT but not αT inhibits growth and induces apoptosis in prostate cancer cells, but had no effect on healthy prostate epithelial cells (Jiang et al. 2004). This effect appears to stem from interruption of de novo synthesis of sphingolipids by γT, which results in an accumulation of dihydrosphingosine and dihydroceramide (Jiang et al. 2004). Gysin et al. showed that γT is stronger than αT in inhibition of prostate cell proliferation by down-regulation of cyclin D (Gysin et al. 2002). In addition, γT inhibited growth and induced apoptosis in colon cancer cell lines, although the mechanism was not well understood (Campbell et al. 2006).

Based on these exciting mechanistic studies which strongly suggest that γT and possibly other tocopherols may be useful anticancer agents and is likely better than αT, potential anticancer activities of γT have been tested in some animal models. In addition, several groups recently conducted animal studies to investigate whether γT-enriched mixed tocopherols may have chemoprevention activities against various types of cancer, including prostate, colon and breast cancer.

15.5.2 High Pure γ-Tocopherol

As of today, six studies have been conducted to test potential benefits from high-pure γT (>90%) in animal cancer models. Five of these studies indicated beneficial outcomes from γT supplementation against cancer.

Stone et al. (2002) compared the effects of dietary RRR-α-tocopherol and RRR-γ-tocopherol (at 65–66 mg/kg diet) on iron-induced oxidative stress and *ras*-p21 expression in the colon of rats. After 22 weeks on experimental diets, rats fed with γT-containing diet had lower levels of *ras*-p21 in colonocytes, an oncogenic protein that is over-expressed in patients with advanced colorectal cancer, than those fed with αT supplement or αT-deficient diets.

The effects of high pure γT have been studied in three different prostate cancer models. Takahashi et al. used the transgenic rat for adenocarcinoma of prostate (TRAP) model, which is characterized by development of high-grade prostatic intraepithelial neoplasia (PIN) from 4 weeks of age and high incidence of well-moderately differentiated adenocarcinomas by 15 weeks of age (Takahashi et al. 2009). In this model, dietary γT (at 50, 100 or 200 mg/kg diet), but not αT, dose-dependently suppressed tumor progression from prostatic intraepithelial neoplasia to adenocarcinoma in the ventral lobe and led to activation of caspase-3 and 7 in the ventral prostate of rats. Jiang et al. (2011a) recently showed that γT at 125 mg/kg body weight three times a week (540 mg/kg diet daily) decreased the growth of LNCaP xenograft in nude mice, although being less potent than its tocotrienol analog. In contrast, dietary γT at 200 mg/kg diet or its combination with lycopene did not reduce the growth of prostate tumor that was implanted with Dunning R3327H adenocarcinoma in male Copenhagen rats (Lindshield et al. 2010).

In addition, as discussed in 15.4.1, Yu et al. (2008, 2009) reported that γT supplementation suppressed breast cancer development in two xenograft models, whereas αT did not show any protection. Interestingly, the results from these studies suggest that αT appears to block the anticancer capability of γT when these two are co-administered, which warrants future investigation.

15.5.3 γT-Rich Mixed Tocopherols

The use of γT-rich mixed tocopherols (γ-TmT) was in part due to the lack of economic sources of high-pure individual vitamin E forms including γT. On the other hand, the mixed tocopherols are often obtained from a byproduct of soybean and are therefore relatively cheap. The typical tocopherol composition of γ-TmT includes 50–70% γ-tocopherol, 20–25% δ-tocopherol, ~10% α-tocopherol, and ~0.5–1.5% β-tocopherol. Remarkably, all the seven studies conducted to test the effect of γ-TmT on carcinogenesis in different models, including colon, breast, lung and prostate, showed protective effects.

Based on the evidence that γT and its metabolites suppress COX-stimulated PGE_2, Newmark et al. (2006) hypothesized that γ-TmT may show protective effects against colon cancer because targeting COXs and eicosanoids has been recognized as one of the most promising anticancer strategies (Wang and Dubois 2010). These investigators found that compared with control diet (AIN76A), dietary γ-TmT (at 0.1% in AIN76A diet) reduced AOM-induced ACF (a pre-cancer lesion) by 55% in male F344 rats. To further examining the anti-inflammatory activity, these investigators showed that the mixed tocopherols appeared to attenuate TPA-caused inflammation (Newmark et al. 2006). In a follow-up study, γ-TmT was tested in an inflammation enhanced mouse colon cancer model in male CF-1 mice where colon tumorogenesis was induced by AOM and promoted by dextran sulfate sodium (DSS) that is known to caused colon inflammation. The results showed that mice fed AIN93M diets containing γ-TmT at 0.17–0.3% (w/w diet) had reduced number of colon adenomas compared with controls, although the outcomes were somewhat dependent upon the way of AOM injection (Ju et al. 2009). Interestingly, the γ-TmT regimen appeared to suppress DSS-induced inflammation only when mice were also co-injected with AOM, but seemed to worsen the inflammation caused by DSS alone.

Besides colon cancer, the similar supplementation of γ-TmT was also tested in other cancer models. Suh et al. (Lee et al. 2009; Suh et al. 2007) showed that γ-TmT supplementation at 0.1, 0.3 and 0.5% in diet inhibited the development of mammary tumors that were induced by N-methyl-N-nitrosourea injection in female Sprague Dawley rats. These regimens suppressed mammary tumor growth and tumor multiplicity, and increased the expression of p21, p27 caspase-3 and peroxisome proliferator activated receptor-γ. The studies on lung cancer models (Lambert et al. 2009; Lu et al. 2010) also found that γ-TmT containing diets inhibited growth and reduced volume of lung tumors in mice. In addition, the beneficial effect of γ-TmT (at 0.1%) was also found in transgenic murine prostate cancer model (TRAMP) where γ-TmT significantly suppressed the incidence of palpable tumor and prostate intraepithelial neoplasia development (Barve et al. 2009). Interestingly, γ-TmT treatment significantly up-regulated the transcription factor Nrf2 and consequently up-regulated several phase II detoxifying antioxidant enzymes, which provides plausible explanations for the observed tumor suppression effects by the tocopherol mixtures.

15.6 Tocotrienols

15.6.1 Molecular Bases of Tocotrienols as Potential Anticancer Agents

Besides tocopherols, tocotrienols, especially γ-tocotrienol and δ-tocotrienol, respective analogs of γT and δT with an unsaturated side chain and abundant in palm oil, have been reported to exhibit potent anticancer effects in various types of cancer cells (Shah and Sylvester 2004, 2005; Sylvester et al. 2005; Wali et al. 2009; Yap et al. 2008). In cell-based studies, γ-tocotrienol appears to show stronger efficacy than γT in the anti-proliferation and pro-apoptotic activity (Jiang et al. 2011a; Yap et al. 2008). δ-tocotrienol appears to have similar or slightly stronger anticancer efficacy than γ-tocotrienol. Biochemical events associated with γ-tocotrienol-induced anticancer actions have been well characterized, including its activation of caspase-8 or JNK, induction of endoplasmic reticulum (ER) stress and inhibition of PI3K-mediated AKT phosphorylation (Park et al. (2010); Shah and Sylvester 2004, 2005; Sylvester et al. 2005; Wali et al. 2009; Yap et al. 2008). γ-tocotrienol has also been shown to inhibit NFkB in various types of cells (Ahn et al. 2007). Compared with tocopherols, γ-tocotrienol showed similar or stronger anti-inflammatory activity by modulation of COX- and 5-LOX-mediated reactions (Jiang et al. 2008, 2011b). Long-chain metabolites of γ-tocotrienol appears to be potent inhibitor of COXs (Jiang et al. 2008). Recently Jiang et al. (2011a) showed that γ-tocotrienol induces apoptosis and autophagy by causing intracellular accumulation of dihydrosphingosine and dihydroceramide and is more potent than γT in these activities. In addition, combinations of tocotrienols (γ-tocotrienol or δ-tocotrienol) with statins have been shown to synergistically inhibit cancer cell growth in cell based studies (Wali and Sylvester 2007; Wali et al. 2009), which is partially explained by the fact that γ-tocotrienol is capable of suppressing statin-promoted up-regulation HMG-CoA reductase (Yang et al. 2010). These interesting cell-related studies have prompted many groups to investigate potential anticancer effects of tocotrienols in different animal cancer models.

15.6.2 Tocotrienol Mixtures

Dietary palm oil, a rich source of carotenoids, tocotrienols, and tocopherols, appears to have antitumor activity in chemically-induced mammary tumor in rats (Sundram et al. 1989; Sylvester et al. 1986), and attenuates TPA-promoted skin tumors (Kausar et al. 2003). A caveat with these studies using palm oil is that the effects cannot be attributed to a single component. Subsequent studies have therefore investigated potential anti-carcinogenic properties of tocotrienol-enriched fractions from palm oil and found beneficial effects in different cancer models such as chemically-induced hepatocarcinogenesis (Makpol et al. 1997; Ngah et al. 1991; Shamaan et al. 1993), xenograft breast cancer studies in nude mice (Nesaretnam et al. 2004), spontaneous hepatocarcinogenesis and chemically-induced lung cancer (Wada et al. 2005), ultraviolet B damaged-skin (Shibata et al. 2010; Yamada et al. 2008), and angiogenesis (Nakagawa et al. 2007). Since these tocotrienol-enriched products derived from palm oil have varied compositions and amounts of tocotrienols and may also contain other active compounds such as tocopherols, the anticancer effects cannot be attributable to a single tocotrienol form.

15.6.3 γ-Tocotrienol

Six studies have been reported on in vivo anti-cancer effects of high-pure γ-tocotrienol ($\geq$ 95%), all of which used xenograft models. In 1997, He et al. (1997) studied the effect of dietary γ-tocotrienol on the growth of mouse melanoma B16(F10)-implanted in female C57BL mice. Dietary treatments, which included α-tocopherol (97%) and γ-tocotrienol (98%) at 116 and 924 μmol/kg diet levels, were given 10 days prior to and 28 days following tumor-cell implantation. Compared with αT supplemented group, γ-tocotrienol significantly delayed the onset of tumor detection and reduced tumor weight. In addition, the effect of these dietary treatments on the survival of mice bearing implanted melanoma was studied, where mice were given diets containing 2 or 4 mmol γ-tocotrienol/kg diet 14 days after the implantation. Compared with control fed animals, γ-tocotrienol containing diets prolonged the survival of mice bearing implanted melanomas by increasing the mean duration of survival by 30%.

Potential protective effects of γ-tocotrienol on prostate cancer have been investigated. Jiang et al. (2011a) recently showed that γ-tocotrienol (125 mg/kg body weight administered by gavage three times a week during 5 weeks) significantly inhibited tumor development in nude mice implanted with androgen-sensitive human prostate adenocarcinoma (LNCaP) cells. The study also showed that γ-tocotrienol exhibited stronger anticancer activity than γ-tocopherol in the xenograft model, which paralleled with much higher cellular accumulation of γ-tocotrienol. Yap et al. reported that γ-tocotrienol (50 mg/kg /day five times a week for 2 weeks) inhibits androgen-independent prostate cancer (AIPCa) tumor growth in a xenograft model. The antitumor capacity of γ-tocotrienol was enhanced when co-administered with docetaxel (Yap et al. 2010). These investigators also indicated that γ-tocotrienol appeared to be selectively accumulated in tumor tissues, which may account for its high anticancer efficacy in vivo. In an earlier study, Kumar et al. examined the anti-tumor properties of γ-tocotrienol in a model where human prostate cancer bone metastasizing (PC3) cells were injected to athymic male CBy.Cg.*Foxnl^{nu}* mice and γ-tocotrienol at 400 mg/kg body weight was injected subcutaneously in the neck of nude mice (Kumar et al. 2006). Mice were then irradiated

(5 Gy/min for a final dose of 12 Gy) at the rear part of the body including the location of the tumor. The results indicated that the size of the tumors was decreased by almost 40% only in γ-tocotrienol injected and irradiated mice. Lipid peroxidation increased in tumors from mice irradiated and treated with γ-tocotrienol. Surprisingly, although rectum tissue was not affected by the treatments, kidney tissue was equally sensitized to lipid peroxidation as the tumors when both irradiation and γ-tocotrienol were given. The increase in lipid peroxidation in tumors is associated to their destruction, but the mechanism(s) involved is not fully understood. This study suggests that if sensitivity of kidney can be resolved, the combination of irradiation and γ-tocotrienol may be an useful therapy for advanced prostate cancer.

Kunnumakkara et al. (2010) showed that oral administration of γ-tocotrienol (400 mg/kg BW) inhibited the growth of pancreatic tumor that was formed from human pancreatic cancer cells (MIA PaCa2) implanted in athymic nu/nu mice. In addition, γ-tocotrienol treatment enhanced the antitumor properties of gemcitabine, a standard treatment drug for pancreatic cancer.

Hiura et al. (2009) reported that dietary γ-tocotrienol or δ-tocotrienol (0.1% by weight) similarly delayed the growth of hepatoma MH134 cells in C3H/HeN mice. These investigators also found that tocotrienols are accumulated specifically in tumor but not in normal tissues. Kulkarni et al. (2010) showed that γ-tocotrienol appeared to have radioprotective effects on hematopoietic stem and progenitor cells, and therefore may serve as potential adjuvant to radiotherapy for cancer. Specifically, γ-tocotrienol at a dose of 200 mg/kg body weight, which was subcutaneously injected in CD2F1 mice 24 h prior to irradiation, provided protection of hematopoietic tissues from radiotherapy.

15.6.4 δ-Tocotrienol

In most cell-based studies, δ-tocotrienol showed similar or slightly more potent anticancer effects than γ-tocotrienol with respect to the anti-proliferation and pro-death activities (He et al. 1997). Three studies have been carried out using $\geq$ 98% pure δ-tocotrienol to examine its in vivo anticancer activity. Hiura et al. (2009) reported that dietary δ-tocotrienol and γ-tocotrienol (0.1% by weight) similarly delayed tumor growth in C3H/HeN mice implanted with murine hepatoma MH134. Both of these tocotrienols appeared to accumulate specifically in tumor tissues but not other normal tissues.

McAnally et al. (2007) studied the effect of dietary δ-tocotrienol on the growth of mouse melanoma B16(F10) implanted in C57BL female mice. Dietary δ-tocotrienol reduced tumor weight only in combination with lovastatin in the diet (62.5 mg δ-tocotrienol/kg body weight per day + 12.5 mg lovastatin/kg body weight per day), when compared to non-supplemented control group.

Shibata et al. (2009) studied the antiangiogenic potential of δ-tocotrienol as compared to αT in an in vivo mouse angiogenesis assay. δ-Tocotrienol (30 μg) but not α-tocopherol inhibited tumor cell-induced angiogenesis formation.

15.6.5 *Toxicity of Tocotrienols*

Nakamura et al. (2001) reported that in a 13-week feeding study which investigates potential toxicity from a tocotrienol mixture (α-tocotrienol 21.4%, β-tocotrienol 3.5%, γ-tocotrienol 36.5%, δ- tocotrienol 8.6%, α-tocopherol 20.5%, β-tocopherol 0.7%, γ-tocopherol 1.0% and δ-tocopherol 0.5%), the no-observed-adverse-effect level for tocotrienols was daily 120 mg/kg BW, slight adverse effect was seen at doses of 473 mg/kg BW, and more adverse effect including suppression of body weight was observed at 1,895 mg/kg BW. Takaski et al. (2008, 2009) studied potential toxicological effects of long term (1–2 years) exposure to tocotrienol mixture in rats. One-year chronic exposure of rats to 2% tocotrienol mixture diets induced highly proliferative liver lesions, nodular hepatocellular hyperplasia (NHH). However, NHH did not harbor neoplastic characteristics from increased exposure despite sustained high cellular proliferation. The tocotrienol mixture did not induce tumor in any other organ besides the liver. In addition, Yap et al. determined acute toxicity of γ-tocotrienol by single i.p. injection of escalating doses of this compound in C57BL/6 black male mice and found that γ-tocotrienol at 800 mg/kg did not cause any death among five-injected mice, whereas death starts to be seen when 1,000 mg/kg was used (Yap et al. 2010).

15.7 Conclusion Remarks

The large clinical trials and recent animal studies strongly indicate that different forms of vitamin E appear to play distinct roles in cancer prevention and treatment. αT, the major form of vitamin E in tissues and the only vitamin E form known to be required to have adequate dietary intake to prevent nutrient deficiency, may be useful in prevention of cancers that are promoted by nutrient deficiency, increased oxidative stress related to heavy smokers as well as poor diets such as high fat combined with low-fiber diets. On the other hand, αT supplementation may be futile to individuals who have adequate antioxidant levels and non-heavy smokers. In contrast, due to the unique anti-inflammatory and anticancer activities of other forms of vitamin E, γT, δT and tocotrienols are likely better than αT in cancer prevention and may even be useful in chemotherapy. In particular, γT and tocotrienols have been shown to inhibit COX- and 5-LOX-mediated eicosanoid formation and induce cancer cell death by modulating sphingolipid metabolism, whereas αT is much less efficient in these activities. Based on these exciting mechanistic observations, animal studies have been undertaken to examine potential anticancer efficacy of these vitamin E forms in vivo. Emerging evidence from various animal models already indicates promising anticancer effects of these compounds.

In the future, studies using cancer models that bear genetic lesions and/or mimic human cancer development are needed to further evaluate the role of different vitamin E forms in cancer prevention and treatment. Given that long-chain carboxychromanols are even stronger than the unmetabolized vitamin E forms in inhibition of COX- and 5-LOX-catalized reactions and induction of cancer cell death (Jiang Q,

Jang Yumi, Jiang Z, Wang Y and Kuah S, unpublished observations), these vitamin E metabolites and analogs may be more effective than their vitamin E precursors as anticancer agents, which warrants further investigation. Furthermore, combination therapies that include combinations of tocotrienols and statins or other chemotherapeutic agents may represent new promising and effective strategies against relatively advanced cancers.

Acknowledgements This work was in part supported by grants (R21 CA152588, R01AT006882 and R21CA133651) to QJ from National Institutes of Health. SYMC was supported by CONACYT sabbatical scholarship (144665).

References

Ahn KS, Sethi G, Krishnan K et al (2007) Gamma-tocotrienol inhibits nuclear factor-kappaB signaling pathway through inhibition of receptor-interacting protein and TAK1 leading to suppression of antiapoptotic gene products and potentiation of apoptosis. J Biol Chem 282:809–820

Albanes D, Malila N, Taylor PR et al (2000) Effects of supplemental alpha-tocopherol and beta-carotene on colorectal cancer: results from a controlled trial (Finland). Cancer Causes Control 11:197–205

Al-Johar D, Shinwari N, Arif J et al (2008) Role of Nigella sativa and a number of its antioxidant constituents towards azoxymethane-induced genotoxic effects and colon cancer in rats. Phytother Res 22:1311–1323

Ames BN, Elson-Schwab I, Silver EA (2002) High-dose vitamin therapy stimulates variant enzymes with decreased coenzyme binding affinity (increased K(m)): relevance to genetic disease and polymorphisms. Am J Clin Nutr 75:616–658

Barnett KT, Fokum FD, Malafa MP (2002) Vitamin E succinate inhibits colon cancer liver metastases. J Surg Res 106:292–298

Barve A, Khor TO, Nair S et al (2009) Gamma-tocopherol-enriched mixed tocopherol diet inhibits prostate carcinogenesis in TRAMP mice. Int J Cancer 124:1693–1699

Basu A, Grossie B, Bennett M et al (2007) Alpha-tocopheryl succinate (alpha-TOS) modulates human prostate LNCaP xenograft growth and gene expression in BALB/c nude mice fed two levels of dietary soybean oil. Eur J Nutr 46:34–43

Battalora MS, Kruszewski FH, DiGiovanni J (1993) Inhibition of chrysarobin skin tumor promotion in SENCAR mice by antioxidants. Carcinogenesis 14:2507–2512

Berton TR, Conti CJ, Mitchell DL et al (1998) The effect of vitamin E acetate on ultraviolet-induced mouse skin carcinogenesis. Mol Carcinog 23:175–184

Bissett DL, Chatterjee R, Hannon DP (1990) Photoprotective effect of superoxide-scavenging antioxidants against ultraviolet radiation-induced chronic skin damage in the hairless mouse. Photodermatol Photoimmunol Photomed 7:56–62

Blot WJ, Li JY, Taylor PR et al (1993) Nutrition intervention trials in Linxian, China: supplementation with specific vitamin/mineral combinations, cancer incidence, and disease-specific mortality in the general population. J Natl Cancer Inst 85:1483–1492

Brigelius-Flohe R (2005) Induction of drug metabolizing enzymes by vitamin E. J Plant Phys 162:797–802

Brigelius-Flohe R, Traber MG (1999) Vitamin E: function and metabolism. FASEB J 13: 1145–1155

Burke KE, Clive J, Combs GF, Jr et al (2000) Effects of topical and oral vitamin E on pigmentation and skin cancer induced by ultraviolet irradiation in Skh:2 hairless mice. Nutr Cancer 38:87–97

Campbell SE, Stone WL, Lee S et al (2006) Comparative effects of RRR-alpha- and RRR-gamma-tocopherol on proliferation and apoptosis in human colon cancer cell lines. BMC Cancer 6:13

Chen X, Mikhail SS, Ding YW et al (2000) Effects of vitamin E and selenium supplementation on esophageal adenocarcinogenesis in a surgical model with rats. Carcinogenesis 21:1531–1536

Chester JF, Gaissert HA, Ross JS et al (1986) Augmentation of 1,2-dimethylhydrazine-induced colon cancer by experimental colitis in mice: role of dietary vitamin E. J Natl Cancer Inst 76:939–942

Cho H, Kim MK, Lee JK et al (2009) Relationship of serum antioxidant micronutrients and sociodemographic factors to cervical neoplasia: a case-control study. Clin Chem Lab Med 47:1005–1012

Christen S, Woodall AA, Shigenaga MK et al (1997) gamma-tocopherol traps mutagenic electrophiles such as NO(X) and complements alpha-tocopherol: physiological implications. Proc Natl Acad Sci U S A 94:3217–3222

Christen S, Jiang Q, Shigenaga MK et al (2002) Analysis of plasma tocopherols alpha, gamma, and 5-nitro-gamma in rats with inflammation by HPLC coulometric detection. J Lipid Res 43:1978–1985

Chung H, Wu D, Han SN et al (2003) Vitamin E supplementation does not alter azoxymethane-induced colonic aberrant crypt foci formation in young or old mice. J Nutr 133:528–532

Clark LC, Combs GF Jr, Turnbull BW et al (1996) Effects of selenium supplementation for cancer prevention in patients with carcinoma of the skin. A randomized controlled trial. Nutritional Prevention of Cancer Study Group. JAMA 276:1957–1963

Cook MG, McNamara P (1980) Effect of dietary vitamin E on dimethylhydrazine-induced colonic tumors in mice. Cancer Res 40:1329–1331

Cooney RV, Franke AA, Harwood PJ et al (1993) γ-Tocopherol detoxification of nitrogen dioxide: Superiority to α-tocopherol. Proc Natl Acad Sci USA 90:1771–1775

Cooney RV, Harwood PJ, Franke AA et al (1995) Products of γ-tocopherol reaction with NO_2 and their formation in rat insulinoma (RINm5F) cells. Free Rad Biol Med 19:259–269

Dong LF, Freeman R, Liu J et al (2009) Suppression of tumor growth in vivo by the mitocan alpha-tocopheryl succinate requires respiratory complex II. Clin Cancer Res 15:1593–1600

Eidelman RS, Hollar D, Hebert PR et al (2004) Randomized trials of vitamin E in the treatment and prevention of cardiovascular disease. Arch Intern Med 164:1552–1556

Ezzedine K, Latreille J, Kesse-Guyot E et al (2010) Incidence of skin cancers during 5-year follow-up after stopping antioxidant vitamins and mineral supplementation. Eur J Cancer 46: 3316–3322

Factor VM, Laskowska D, Jensen MR et al (2000) Vitamin E reduces chromosomal damage and inhibits hepatic tumor formation in a transgenic mouse model. Proc Natl Acad Sci USA 97:2196–2201

Gann PH (2009) Randomized trials of antioxidant supplementation for cancer prevention: first bias, now chance–next, cause. JAMA 301:102–103

Gaziano JM, Glynn RJ, Christen WG et al (2009) Vitamins E and C in the prevention of prostate and total cancer in men: the Physicians' Health Study II randomized controlled trial. JAMA 301:52–62

Goodman GE, Schaffer S, Omenn GS et al (2003) The association between lung and prostate cancer risk, and serum micronutrients: results and lessons learned from beta-carotene and retinol efficacy trial. Cancer Epidemiol Biomarkers Prev 12:518–526

Gu X, Song X, Dong Y et al (2008) Vitamin E succinate induces ceramide-mediated apoptosis in head and neck squamous cell carcinoma in vitro and in vivo. Clin Cancer Res 14:1840–1848

Gysin R, Azzi A, Visarius T (2002) Gamma-tocopherol inhibits human cancer cell cycle progression and cell proliferation by down-regulation of cyclins. FASEB J 16:1952–1954

Hagiwara A, Boonyaphiphat P, Tanaka H et al (1999) Organ-dependent modifying effects of caffeine, and two naturally occurring antioxidants alpha-tocopherol and n-tritriacontane-16,18-dione, on 2-amino-1-methyl-6-phenylimidazo[4,5-b]pyridine (PhIP)-induced mammary and colonic carcinogenesis in female F344 rats. Jpn J Cancer Res 90:399–405

Hahn T, Szabo L, Gold M et al (2006) Dietary administration of the proapoptotic vitamin E analogue alpha-tocopheryloxyacetic acid inhibits metastatic murine breast cancer. Cancer Res 66:9374–9378

Hartman TJ, Albanes D, Pietinen P et al (1998) The association between baseline vitamin E, selenium, and prostate cancer in the alpha-tocopherol, beta-carotene cancer prevention study. Cancer Epidemiol Biomarkers Prev 7:335–340

He L, Mo H, Hadisusilo S et al (1997) Isoprenoids suppress the growth of murine B16 melanomas in vitro and in vivo. J Nutr 127:668–674

Heinonen OP, Albanes D, Virtamo J et al (1998) Prostate cancer and supplementation with alpha-tocopherol and beta-carotene: incidence and mortality in a controlled trial. J Natl Cancer Inst 90:440–446

Helen A, Krishnakumar K, Vijayammal PL et al (2003) A comparative study of antioxidants S-allyl cysteine sulfoxide and vitamin E on the damages induced by nicotine in rats. Pharmacology 67:113–117

Helzlsouer KJ, Huang HY, Alberg AJ et al (2000) Association between alpha-tocopherol, gamma-tocopherol, selenium, and subsequent prostate cancer. J Natl Cancer Inst 92:2018–2023

Hercberg S, Galan P, Preziosi P et al (2004) The SU.VI.MAX Study: a randomized, placebo-controlled trial of the health effects of antioxidant vitamins and minerals. Arch Intern Med 164:2335–2342

Hercberg S, Ezzedine K, Guinot C et al (2007) Antioxidant supplementation increases the risk of skin cancers in women but not in men. J Nutr 137:2098–2105

Hercberg S, Kesse-Guyot E, Druesne-Pecollo N et al (2010) Incidence of cancers, ischemic cardiovascular diseases and mortality during 5-year follow-up after stopping antioxidant vitamins and minerals supplements: a postintervention follow-up in the SU.VI.MAX Study. Int J Cancer 127:1875–1881

Hirose M, Masuda A, Inoue T et al (1986) Modification by antioxidants and p,p′-diaminodiphenylmethane of 7,12-dimethylbenz[a]anthracene-induced carcinogenesis of the mammary gland and ear duct in CD rats. Carcinogenesis 7:1155–1159

Hirose M, Yada H, Hakoi K et al (1993) Modification of carcinogenesis by alpha-tocopherol, t-butylhydroquinone, propyl gallate and butylated hydroxytoluene in a rat multi-organ carcinogenesis model. Carcinogenesis 14:2359–2364

Hirose M, Hasegawa R, Kimura J et al (1995) Inhibitory effects of 1-O-hexyl-2,3,5-trimethylhydroquinone (HTHQ), green tea catechins and other antioxidants on 2-amino-6-methyldipyrido[1,2-a:3′,2′-d]imidazole (Glu-P-1)-induced rat hepatocarcinogenesis and dose-dependent inhibition by HTHQ of lesion induction by Glu-P-1 or 2-amino-3,8-dimethylimidazo[4,5-f]quinoxaline (MeIQx). Carcinogenesis 16:3049–3055

Hirose M, Nishikawa A, Shibutani M et al (2002) Chemoprevention of heterocyclic amine-induced mammary carcinogenesis in rats. Environ Mol Mutagen 39:271–278

Hiura Y, Tachibana H, Arakawa R et al (2009) Specific accumulation of gamma- and delta-tocotrienols in tumor and their antitumor effect in vivo. J Nutr Biochem 20:607–613

HPSCG (2002) MRC/BHF Heart Protection Study of antioxidant vitamin supplementation in 20,536 high-risk individuals: a randomised placebo-controlled trial. Lancet 360:23–33

Hrzenjak A, Reicher H, Wintersperger A et al (2004) Inhibition of lung carcinoma cell growth by high density lipoprotein-associated alpha-tocopheryl-succinate. Cell Mol Life Sci 61: 1520–1531

Hybertson BM, Chung JH, Fini MA et al (2005) Aerosol-administered alpha-tocopherol attenuates lung inflammation in rats given lipopolysaccharide intratracheally. Exp Lung Res 31:283–294

Ichikawa T, Ishikawa G, Yano T (1993) The prevention of oxy radical-mediated lung tumorigenesis in mice by vitamin E. J Nutr Sci Vitaminol (Tokyo) 39 Suppl:S49–55

Ingles SA, Bird CL, Shikany JM et al (1998) Plasma tocopherol and prevalence of colorectal adenomas in a multiethnic population. Cancer Res 58:661–666

Jenab M, Riboli E, Ferrari P et al (2006) Plasma and dietary carotenoid, retinol and tocopherol levels and the risk of gastric adenocarcinomas in the European prospective investigation into cancer and nutrition. Br J Cancer 95:406–415

Jiang Q, Ames BN (2003) Gamma-tocopherol, but not alpha-tocopherol, decreases proinflammatory eicosanoids and inflammation damage in rats. FASEB J 17:816–822

Jiang Q, Elson-Schwab I, Courtemanche C et al (2000) gamma-tocopherol and its major metabolite, in contrast to alpha- tocopherol, inhibit cyclooxygenase activity in macrophages and epithelial cells. Proc Natl Acad Sci USA 97:11494–11499

Jiang Q, Christen S, Shigenaga MK et al (2001) gamma-tocopherol, the major form of vitamin E in the US diet, deserves more attention. Am J Clin Nutr 74:714–722

Jiang Q, Wong J, Fyrst H et al (2004) {gamma}-Tocopherol or combinations of vitamin E forms induce cell death in human prostate cancer cells by interrupting sphingolipid synthesis. Proc Natl Acad Sci USA 101:17825–17830

Jiang Q, Yin X, Lill MA et al (2008) Long-chain carboxychromanols, metabolites of vitamin E, are potent inhibitors of cyclooxygenases. Proc Natl Acad Sci USA 105:20464–20469

Jiang Q, Rao X, Young Kim C et al (2011a) Gamma-tocotrienol induces apoptosis and autophagy in prostate cancer cells by increasing intracellular dihydrosphingosine and dihydroceramide. Int J Cancer 2011 Mar 11. doi:10.1002/ijc.26054. [Epub ahead of print]

Jiang Z, Yin X, Jiang Q (2011b) Natural forms of vitamin E and 13′-carboxychromanol, a long-chain vitamin E metabolite, inhibit leukotriene generation from stimulated neutrophils by blocking calcium influx and suppressing 5-lipoxygenase activity, respectively. J Immunology 186:1173–1179

Ju J, Hao X, Lee MJ et al (2009) A gamma-tocopherol-rich mixture of tocopherols inhibits colon inflammation and carcinogenesis in azoxymethane and dextran sulfate sodium-treated mice. Cancer Prev Res (Phila) 2:143–152

Kabat GC, Kim M, Adams-Campbell LL et al (2009) Longitudinal study of serum carotenoid, retinol, and tocopherol concentrations in relation to breast cancer risk among postmenopausal women. Am J Clin Nutr 90:162–169

Kakizaki S, Takagi H, Fukusato T et al (2001) Effect of alpha-tocopherol on hepatocarcinogenesis in transforming growth factor-alpha (TGF-alpha) transgenic mice treated with diethylnitrosamine. Int J Vitam Nutr Res 71:261–267

Kanai K, Kikuchi E, Mikami S et al (2010) Vitamin E succinate induced apoptosis and enhanced chemosensitivity to paclitaxel in human bladder cancer cells in vitro and in vivo. Cancer Sci 101:216–223

Kausar H, Bhasin G, Zargar MA et al (2003) Palm oil alleviates 12-O-tetradecanoyl-phorbol-13-acetate-induced tumor promotion response in murine skin. Cancer Lett 192:151–160

Kim YI (2008) Folic acid supplementation and cancer risk: point. Cancer Epidemiol Biomarkers Prev 17:2220–2225

Kim Y, Chongviriyaphan N, Liu C et al (2006) Combined antioxidant (beta-carotene, alpha-tocopherol and ascorbic acid) supplementation increases the levels of lung retinoic acid and inhibits the activation of mitogen-activated protein kinase in the ferret lung cancer model. Carcinogenesis 27:1410–1419

Kim Y, Lian F, Yeum KJ et al (2007) The effects of combined antioxidant (beta-carotene, alpha-tocopherol and ascorbic acid) supplementation on antioxidant capacity, DNA single-strand breaks and levels of insulin-like growth factor-1/IGF-binding protein 3 in the ferret model of lung cancer. Int J Cancer 120:1847–1854

Kim MK, Ahn SH, Son BH et al (2010) Plasma antioxidant concentration, not superoxide dismutase polymorphism, is associated with breast cancer risk in Korean women. Nutr Res 30:705–713

Kim Y, Chongviriyaphan N, Liu C et al (2011) Combined alpha-tocopherol and ascorbic acid protects against smoke-induced lung squamous metaplasia in ferrets. Lung Cancer 2011 Jun 10. [Epub ahead of print]

Kline K, Sanders BG (1989) Modulation of immune suppression and enhanced tumorigenesis in retrovirus tumor challenged chickens treated with vitamin E. In Vivo 3:161–166

Kogure K, Manabe S, Suzuki I et al (2005) Cytotoxicity of alpha-tocopheryl succinate, malonate and oxalate in normal and cancer cells in vitro and their anti-cancer effects on mouse melanoma in vivo. J Nutr Sci Vitaminol (Tokyo) 51:392–397

Kolaja KL, Klaunig JE (1997) Vitamin E modulation of hepatic focal lesion growth in mice. Toxicol Appl Pharmacol 143:380–387

Kulkarni S, Ghosh SP, Satyamitra M et al (2010) Gamma-tocotrienol protects hematopoietic stem and progenitor cells in mice after total-body irradiation. Radiat Res 173:738–747

Kumar KS, Raghavan M, Hieber K et al (2006) Preferential radiation sensitization of prostate cancer in nude mice by nutraceutical antioxidant gamma-tocotrienol. Life Sci 78:2099–2104

Kunnumakkara AB, Sung B, Ravindran J et al (2010) {Gamma}-tocotrienol inhibits pancreatic tumors and sensitizes them to gemcitabine treatment by modulating the inflammatory microenvironment. Cancer Res 70:8695–8705

Lambert JD, Lu G, Lee MJ et al (2009) Inhibition of lung cancer growth in mice by dietary mixed tocopherols. Mol Nutr Food Res 53:1030–1035

Lawson KA, Anderson K, Simmons-Menchaca M et al (2004) Comparison of vitamin E derivatives alpha-TEA and VES in reduction of mouse mammary tumor burden and metastasis. Exp Biol Med (Maywood) 229:954–963

Lee IM, Cook NR, Gaziano JM et al (2005) Vitamin E in the primary prevention of cardiovascular disease and cancer: the Women's Health Study: a randomized controlled trial. Jama 294:56–65

Lee HJ, Ju J, Paul S et al (2009) Mixed tocopherols prevent mammary tumorigenesis by inhibiting estrogen action and activating PPAR-gamma. Clin Cancer Res 15:4242–4249

Li GX, Lee MJ, Liu AB et al (2011) delta-tocopherol is more active than alpha – or gamma -tocopherol in inhibiting lung tumorigenesis in vivo. Cancer Prev Res 4:404–413

Liang D, Lin J, Grossman HB et al (2008) Plasma vitamins E and A and risk of bladder cancer: a case-control analysis. Cancer Causes Control 19:981–992

Liede K, Hietanen J, Saxen L et al (1998) Long-term supplementation with alpha-tocopherol and beta-carotene and prevalence of oral mucosal lesions in smokers. Oral diseases 4:78–83

Lii CK, Chen CW, Liu JY et al (1999) Lack of effect of dietary alpha-tocopherol on chemically induced hepatocarcinogenesis in rats. Nutr Cancer 34:192–198

Limpens J, Schroder FH, de Ridder CM et al (2006) Combined lycopene and vitamin E treatment suppresses the growth of PC-346C human prostate cancer cells in nude mice. J Nutr 136: 1287–1293

Lindshield BL, Ford NA, Canene-Adams K et al (2010) Selenium, but not lycopene or vitamin E, decreases growth of transplantable dunning R3327-H rat prostate tumors. PLoS One 5:e10423

Lippman SM, Klein EA, Goodman PJ et al (2009) Effect of selenium and vitamin E on risk of prostate cancer and other cancers: the Selenium and Vitamin E Cancer Prevention Trial (SELECT). JAMA 301:39–51

Lonn E, Bosch J, Yusuf S et al (2005) Effects of long-term vitamin E supplementation on cardiovascular events and cancer: a randomized controlled trial. JAMA 293:1338–1347

Lu G, Xiao H, Li GX et al (2010) A gamma-tocopherol-rich mixture of tocopherols inhibits chemically induced lung tumorigenesis in A/J mice and xenograft tumor growth. Carcinogenesis 31:687–694

Makpol S, Shamaan NA, Jarien Z et al (1997) Different starting times of alpha-tocopherol and gamma-tocotrienol supplementation and tumor marker enzyme activities in the rat chemically induced with cancer. Gen Pharmacol 28:589–592

Malafa MP, Neitzel LT (2000) Vitamin E succinate promotes breast cancer tumor dormancy. J Surg Res 93:163–170

Malafa MP, Fokum FD, Mowlavi A et al (2002) Vitamin E inhibits melanoma growth in mice. Surgery 131:85–91

Malila N, Virtamo J, Virtanen M et al (1999) The effect of alpha-tocopherol and beta-carotene supplementation on colorectal adenomas in middle-aged male smokers. Cancer Epidemiol Biomarkers Prev 8:489–493

Malila N, Taylor PR, Virtanen MJ et al (2002) Effects of alpha-tocopherol and beta-carotene supplementation on gastric cancer incidence in male smokers (ATBC Study, Finland). Cancer Causes Control 13:617–623

Masui T, Tsuda H, Inoue K et al (1986) Inhibitory effects of ethoxyquin, 4,4′-diaminodiphenylmethane and acetaminophen on rat hepatocarcinogenesis. Jpn J Cancer Res 77:231–237

Maziere S, Meflah K, Tavan E et al (1998) Effect of resistant starch and/or fat-soluble vitamins A and E on the initiation stage of aberrant crypts in rat colon. Nutr Cancer 31:168–177

McAnally JA, Gupta J, Sodhani S et al (2007) Tocotrienols potentiate lovastatin-mediated growth suppression in vitro and in vivo. Exp Biol Med (Maywood) 232:523–531

McCormick DL, Rao KV, Johnson WD et al (2010) Null activity of selenium and vitamin e as cancer chemopreventive agents in the rat prostate. Cancer Prev Res (Phila) 3:381–392

McVean M, Liebler DC (1997) Inhibition of UVB induced DNA photodamage in mouse epidermis by topically applied alpha-tocopherol. Carcinogenesis 18:1617–1622

Miller ER, 3rd, Pastor-Barriuso R, Dalal D et al (2005) Meta-analysis: high-dosage vitamin E supplementation may increase all-cause mortality. Ann Intern Med 142:37–46

Mitchel RE, McCann R (1993) Vitamin E is a complete tumor promoter in mouse skin. Carcinogenesis 14:659–662

Mitchel RE, McCann RA (2003) Skin tumor promotion by Vitamin E in mice: amplification by ionizing radiation and Vitamin C. Cancer Detect Prev 27:102–108

Miyauchi M, Nakamura H, Furukawa F et al (2002) Promoting effects of combined antioxidant and sodium nitrite treatment on forestomach carcinogenesis in rats after initiation with N-methyl-N′-nitro-N-nitrosoguanidine. Cancer Lett 178:19–24

Mizumoto Y, Nakae D, Yoshiji H et al (1994) Inhibitory effects of 2-O-octadecylascorbic acid and other vitamin C and E derivatives on the induction of enzyme-altered putative preneoplastic lesions in the livers of rats fed a choline-deficient, L-amino acid-defined diet. Carcinogenesis 15:241–246

Moore MA, Tsuda H, Thamavit W et al (1987) Differential modification of development of preneoplastic lesions in the Syrian golden hamster initiated with a single dose of 2,2′-dioxo-N-nitrosodipropylamine: influence of subsequent butylated hydroxyanisole, alpha-tocopherol, or carbazole. J Natl Cancer Inst 78:289–293

Nakadate T, Yamamoto S, Aizu E et al (1984) Effects of flavonoids and antioxidants on 12-O-tetradecanoyl-phorbol-13-acetate-caused epidermal ornithine decarboxylase induction and tumor promotion in relation to lipoxygenase inhibition by these compounds. Gann 75:214–222

Nakagawa K, Shibata A, Yamashita S et al (2007) In vivo angiogenesis is suppressed by unsaturated vitamin E, tocotrienol. J Nutr 137:1938–1943

Nakamura A, Shirai T, Takahashi S et al (1991) Lack of modification by naturally occurring antioxidants of 3,2′-dimethyl-4-aminobiphenyl-initiated rat prostate carcinogenesis. Cancer Lett 58:241–246

Nakamura H, Furukawa F, Nishikawa A et al (2001) Oral toxicity of a tocotrienol preparation in rats. Food Chem Toxicol 39:799–805

Nesaretnam K, Ambra R, Selvaduray KR et al (2004) Tocotrienol-rich fraction from palm oil affects gene expression in tumors resulting from MCF-7 cell inoculation in athymic mice. Lipids 39:459–467

Neuzil J, Tomasetti M, Zhao Y et al (2007) Vitamin E analogs, a novel group of "mitocans," as anticancer agents: the importance of being redox-silent. Mol Pharmacol 71:1185–1199

Newmark HL, Huang MT, Reddy BS (2006) Mixed tocopherols inhibit azoxymethane-induced aberrant crypt foci in rats. Nutr Cancer 56:82–85

Ngah WZ, Jarien Z, San MM et al (1991) Effect of tocotrienols on hepatocarcinogenesis induced by 2-acetylaminofluorene in rats. Am J Clin Nutr 53:1076S–1081S

Ni J, Mai T, Pang ST et al (2009) In vitro and in vivo anticancer effects of the novel vitamin E ether analogue RRR-alpha-tocopheryloxybutyl sulfonic acid in prostate cancer. Clin Cancer Res 15:898–906

Noh SM, Han SE, Shim G et al (2011) Tocopheryl oligochitosan-based self assembling oligomersomes for siRNA delivery. Biomaterials 32:849–857

Nomura AM, Stemmermann GN, Lee J et al (1997) Serum micronutrients and prostate cancer in Japanese Americans in Hawaii. Cancer Epidemiol Biomarkers Prev 6:487–491

Odukoya O, Hawach F, Shklar G (1984) Retardation of experimental oral cancer by topical vitamin E. Nutr Cancer 6:98–104

Ogasawara M, Matsunaga T, Suzuki H (2007) Differential effects of antioxidants on the in vitro invasion, growth and lung metastasis of murine colon cancer cells. Biol Pharm Bull 30:200–204

Ozten N, Horton L, Lasano S et al (2010) Selenomethionine and alpha-tocopherol do not inhibit prostate carcinogenesis in the testosterone plus estradiol-treated NBL rat model. Cancer Prev Res (Phila) 3:371–380

Park SK, Sanders BG, Kline K (2010) Tocotrienols induce apoptosis in breast cancer cell lines via an endoplasmic reticulum stress-dependent increase in extrinsic death receptor signaling. Breast Cancer Res Treat 124:361–375

Perchellet JP, Owen MD, Posey TD et al (1985) Inhibitory effects of glutathione level-raising agents and D-alpha-tocopherol on ornithine decarboxylase induction and mouse skin tumor promotion by 12-O-tetradecanoylphorbol-13-acetate. Carcinogenesis 6:567–573

Perchellet JP, Abney NL, Thomas RM et al (1987) Effects of combined treatments with selenium, glutathione, and vitamin E on glutathione peroxidase activity, ornithine decarboxylase induction, and complete and multistage carcinogenesis in mouse skin. Cancer Res 47:477–485

Qiao YL, Dawsey SM, Kamangar F et al (2009) Total and cancer mortality after supplementation with vitamins and minerals: follow-up of the Linxian General Population Nutrition Intervention Trial. J Natl Cancer Inst 101:507–518

Qu CX, Kamangar F, Fan JH et al (2007) Chemoprevention of primary liver cancer: a randomized, double-blind trial in Linxian, China. J Natl Cancer Inst 99:1240–1247

Quin J, Engle D, Litwiller A et al (2005) Vitamin E succinate decreases lung cancer tumor growth in mice. J Surg Res 127:139–143

Ramanathapuram LV, Hahn T, Dial SM et al (2005) Chemo-immunotherapy of breast cancer using vesiculated alpha-tocopheryl succinate in combination with dendritic cell vaccination. Nutr Cancer 53:177–193

Reddy BS, Tanaka T (1986) Interactions of selenium deficiency, vitamin E, polyunsaturated fat, and saturated fat on azoxymethane-induced colon carcinogenesis in male F344 rats. J Natl Cancer Inst 76:1157–1162

Reiter E, Jiang Q, Christen S (2007) Anti-inflammatory properties of alpha- and gamma-tocopherol. Mol Aspects Med 28:668–691

Rexrode KM, Lee IM, Cook NR et al (2000) Baseline characteristics of participants in the Women's Health Study. J Womens Health Gend Based Med 9:19–27

Sarna S, Kumar A, Bhola RK (2000) alpha-Tocopherol enhances tumour growth inhibition by cis-dichlorodiammine platinum (II). Braz J Med Biol Res 33:929–936

Shah S, Sylvester PW (2004) Tocotrienol-induced caspase-8 activation is unrelated to death receptor apoptotic signaling in neoplastic mammary epithelial cells. Exp Biol Med 229:745–755

Shah SJ, Sylvester PW (2005) Gamma-tocotrienol inhibits neoplastic mammary epithelial cell proliferation by decreasing Akt and nuclear factor kappaB activity. Exp Biol Med 230:235–241

Shamaan NA, Wan Ngah WZ, Ibrahim R et al (1993) Effect of tocotrienol on the activities of cytosolic glutathione-dependent enzymes in rats treated with 2-acetylaminofluorene. Biochem Pharmacol 45:1517–1519

Shamberger RJ, Rudolph G (1966) Protection against cocarcinogenesis by antioxidants. Experientia 22:116

Shibata A, Nakagawa K, Sookwong P et al (2009) delta-Tocotrienol suppresses VEGF induced angiogenesis whereas alpha-tocopherol does not. J Agric Food Chem 57:8696–8704

Shibata A, Nakagawa K, Kawakami Y et al (2010) Suppression of gamma-tocotrienol on UVB induced inflammation in HaCaT keratinocytes and HR-1 hairless mice via inflammatory mediators multiple signaling. J Agric Food Chem 58:7013–7020
Shivapurkar N, Tang Z, Frost A et al (1995) Inhibition of progression of aberrant crypt foci and colon tumor development by vitamin E and beta-carotene in rats on a high-risk diet. Cancer Lett 91:125–132
Siler U, Barella L, Spitzer V et al (2004) Lycopene and vitamin E interfere with autocrine/paracrine loops in the Dunning prostate cancer model. FASEB J 18:1019–1021
Singh VK, Parekh VI, Brown DS et al (2011) Tocopherol succinate: modulation of antioxidant enzymes and oncogene expression, and hematopoietic recovery. Int J Radiat Oncol Biol Phys 79:571–578
Stolzenberg-Solomon RZ, Sheffler-Collins S, Weinstein S et al (2009) Vitamin E intake, alpha-tocopherol status, and pancreatic cancer in a cohort of male smokers. Am J Clin Nutr 89: 584–591
Stone WL, Papas AM, LeClair IO et al (2002) The influence of dietary iron and tocopherols on oxidative stress and ras-p21 levels in the colon. Cancer Detect Prev 26:78–84
Suarna C, Wu BJ, Choy K et al (2006) Protective effect of vitamin E supplements on experimental atherosclerosis is modest and depends on preexisting vitamin E deficiency. Free Radic Biol Med 41:722–730
Suh N, Paul S, Lee HJ et al (2007) Mixed tocopherols inhibit N-methyl-N-nitrosourea-induced mammary tumor growth in rats. Nutr Cancer 59:76–81
Sundram K, Khor HT, Ong AS et al (1989) Effect of dietary palm oils on mammary carcinogenesis in female rats induced by 7,12-dimethylbenz(a)anthracene. Cancer Res 49:1447–1451
Sylvester PW, Russell M, Ip MM et al (1986) Comparative effects of different animal and vegetable fats fed before and during carcinogen administration on mammary tumorigenesis, sexual maturation, and endocrine function in rats. Cancer Res 46:757–762
Sylvester PW, Shah SJ, Samant GV (2005) Intracellular signaling mechanisms mediating the antiproliferative and apoptotic effects of gamma-tocotrienol in neoplastic mammary epithelial cells. J Plant Phys 162:803–810
Takahashi S, Takeshita K, Seeni A et al (2009) Suppression of prostate cancer in a transgenic rat model via gamma-tocopherol activation of caspase signaling. Prostate 69:644–651
Tasaki M, Umemura T, Inoue T et al (2008) Induction of characteristic hepatocyte proliferative lesion with dietary exposure of Wistar Hannover rats to tocotrienol for 1 year. Toxicology 250:143–150
Tasaki M, Umemura T, Kijima A et al (2009) Simultaneous induction of non-neoplastic and neoplastic lesions with highly proliferative hepatocytes following dietary exposure of rats to tocotrienol for 2 years. Arch Toxicol 83:1021–1030
Taylor PR, Qiao YL, Abnet CC et al (2003) Prospective study of serum vitamin E levels and esophageal and gastric cancers. J Natl Cancer Inst 95:1414–1416
Temple NJ, el-Khatib SM (1987) Cabbage and vitamin E: their effect on colon tumor formation in mice. Cancer Lett 35:71–77
The Alpha-Tocopherol BCCPSG (1994) The effect of vitamin E and beta carotene on the incidence of lung cancer and other cancers in male smokers. N Engl J Med 330:1029–1035
Tomasetti M, Neuzil J (2007) Vitamin E analogues and immune response in cancer treatment. Vitam Horm 76:463–491
Toth B, Patil K (1983) Enhancing effect of vitamin E on murine intestinal tumorigenesis by 1,2-dimethylhydrazine dihydrochloride. J Natl Cancer Inst 70:1107–1111
Trickler D, Shklar G (1987) Prevention by vitamin E of experimental oral carcinogenesis. J Natl Cancer Inst 78:165–169
Tsuda H, Uehara N, Iwahori Y et al (1994) Chemopreventive effects of beta-carotene, alpha-tocopherol and five naturally occurring antioxidants on initiation of hepatocarcinogenesis by 2-amino-3-methylimidazo[4,5-f]quinoline in the rat. Jpn J Cancer Res 85:1214–1219

Turanek J, Wang XF, Knotigova P et al (2009) Liposomal formulation of alpha-tocopheryl maleamide: in vitro and in vivo toxicological profile and anticancer effect against spontaneous breast carcinomas in mice. Toxicol Appl Pharmacol 237:249–257

Varis K, Taylor PR, Sipponen P et al (1998) Gastric cancer and premalignant lesions in atrophic gastritis: a controlled trial on the effect of supplementation with alpha-tocopherol and beta-carotene. The Helsinki Gastritis Study Group. Scand J Gastroenterol 33:294–300

Virtamo J, Edwards BK, Virtanen M et al (2000) Effects of supplemental alpha-tocopherol and beta-carotene on urinary tract cancer: incidence and mortality in a controlled trial (Finland). Cancer Causes Control 11:933–939

Virtamo J, Pietinen P, Huttunen JK et al (2003) Incidence of cancer and mortality following alpha-tocopherol and beta-carotene supplementation: a postintervention follow-up. Jama 290: 476–485

Vivekananthan DP, Penn MS, Sapp SK et al (2003) Use of antioxidant vitamins for the prevention of cardiovascular disease: meta-analysis of randomised trials. Lancet 361:2017–2023

Wada S, Satomi Y, Murakoshi M et al (2005) Tumor suppressive effects of tocotrienol in vivo and in vitro. Cancer Lett 229:181–191

Wali VB, Sylvester PW (2007) Synergistic antiproliferative effects of gamma-tocotrienol and statin treatment on mammary tumor cells. Lipids 42:1113–1123

Wali VB, Bachawal SV, Sylvester PW (2009) Endoplasmic reticulum stress mediates gamma-tocotrienol-induced apoptosis in mammary tumor cells. Apoptosis 14:1366–1377

Wang D, Dubois RN (2010) Eicosanoids and cancer. Nat Rev Cancer 10:181–193

Wang YM, Purewal M, Nixon B et al (1989) Vitamin E and cancer prevention in an animal model. Ann N Y Acad Sci 570:383–390

Weber T, Lu M, Andera L et al (2002) Vitamin E succinate is a potent novel antineoplastic agent with high selectivity and cooperativity with tumor necrosis factor-related apoptosis-inducing ligand (Apo2 ligand) in vivo. Clin Cancer Res 8:863–869

Weinstein SJ, Wright ME, Pietinen P et al (2005) Serum alpha-tocopherol and gamma-tocopherol in relation to prostate cancer risk in a prospective study. J Natl Cancer Inst 97:396–399

Weinstein SJ, Wright ME, Lawson KA et al (2007) Serum and dietary vitamin E in relation to prostate cancer risk. Cancer Epidemiol Biomarkers Prev 16:1253–1259

Wenger FA, Kilian M, Ridders J et al (2001) Influence of antioxidative vitamins A, C and E on lipid peroxidation in BOP-induced pancreatic cancer in Syrian hamsters. Prostaglandins Leukot Essent Fatty Acids 65:165–171

Witschi HP, Hakkinen PJ, Kehrer JP (1981) Modification of lung tumor development in A/J mice. Toxicology 21:37–45

Wright ME, Virtamo J, Hartman AM et al (2007) Effects of alpha-tocopherol and beta-carotene supplementation on upper aerodigestive tract cancers in a large, randomized controlled trial. Cancer 109:891–898

Wu K, Shan YJ, Zhao Y et al (2001) Inhibitory effects of RRR-alpha-tocopheryl succinate on benzo(a)pyrene (B(a)P)-induced forestomach carcinogenesis in female mice. World J Gastroenterol 7:60–65

Yam D, Peled A, Shinitzky M (2001) Suppression of tumor growth and metastasis by dietary fish oil combined with vitamins E and C and cisplatin. Cancer Chemother Pharmacol 47:34–40

Yamada Y, Obayashi M, Ishikawa T et al (2008) Dietary tocotrienol reduces UVB-induced skin damage and sesamin enhances tocotrienol effects in hairless mice. J Nutr Sci Vitaminol (Tokyo) 54:117–123

Yang Z, Xiao H, Jin H et al (2010) Synergistic actions of atorvastatin with gamma-tocotrienol and celecoxib against human colon cancer HT29 and HCT116 cells. Int J Cancer 126:852–863

Yano T, Obata Y, Ishikawa G et al (1994) Effect of vitamin E on 4-nitroquinoline 1-oxide-induced lung tumorigenesis in mice. Int J Vitam Nutr Res 64:181–184

Yao K, Latta M, Bird RP (1996) Modulation of colonic aberrant crypt foci and proliferative indexes in colon and prostate glands of rats by vitamin E. Nutr Cancer 26:99–109

Yap WN, Chang PN, Han HY et al (2008) Gamma-tocotrienol suppresses prostate cancer cell proliferation and invasion through multiple-signalling pathways. Br J Cancer 99:1832–1841

Yap WN, Zaiden N, Luk SY et al (2010) In vivo evidence of gamma-tocotrienol as a chemosensitizer in the treatment of hormone-refractory prostate cancer. Pharmacology 85:248–258

Yin Y, Ni J, Chen M et al (2009) RRR-alpha-vitamin E succinate potentiates the antitumor effect of calcitriol in prostate cancer without overt side effects. Clin Cancer Res 15:190–200

Yu W, Jia L, Wang P et al (2008) In vitro and in vivo evaluation of anticancer actions of natural and synthetic vitamin E forms. Mol Nutr Food Res 52:447–456

Yu W, Jia L, Park SK et al (2009) Anticancer actions of natural and synthetic vitamin E forms: RRR-alpha-tocopherol blocks the anticancer actions of gamma-tocopherol. Mol Nutr Food Res 53:1573–1581

Yusuf S, Dagenais G, Pogue J et al (2000) Vitamin E supplementation and cardiovascular events in high-risk patients. The Heart Outcomes Prevention Evaluation Study Investigators. N Engl J Med 342:154–160

Chapter 16
Augmenting the Efficacy of Chemo- and Radio-Therapy by Nutraceuticals: Evidence from Pre-clinical and Clinical Trials

Yiwei Li, Dejuan Kong, Aamir Ahmad, Bin Bao, and Fazlul H. Sarkar

Abstract In recent years, dietary agents such as isoflavone genistein, curcumin, indole-3-carbinol (I3C), 3,3'-diindolylmethane (DIM), (-)-epigallocatechin-3-gallate (EGCG), resveratrol, and lycopene have received increased attention as anti-cancer agents. There has been a growing interest in investigating the effects of these dietary agents known as nutraceuticals on the inhibition of cancer cell growth in combination with chemotherapeutics or radiotherapy. The results from pre-clinical in vitro and in vivo experimental studies have demonstrated that the anti-cancer effects of chemotherapeutics and radiotherapy could be enhanced by combination treatment with nutraceuticals. Experimental evidence have also shown that the enhanced anti-cancer effects of nutraceuticals could in part due to deregulation of NF-κB, Akt, MDR, COX-2, AR, MAPK, and apoptotic signaling pathways that are known to play critical roles in cell survival and therapeutic resistance. In this chapter, we are summarizing the current evidence from pre-clinical and clinical trials demonstrating the effects and the molecular mechanisms of nutraceutical intervention in combination treatments, and we believe that this information would allow researcher to have a fresh look at the potential value of nutraceutical in cancer therapy.

16.1 Introduction

Although significant efforts have been made toward developing different cancer therapeutic strategies over the past several decades, cancer still remains the second leading cause of death in the United States (Jemal et al. 2010). The high mortality of cancer is partly due to therapeutic resistance, which is responsible for tumor recurrence and metastasis. To date, surgery, radiotherapy and chemotherapy still comprise the standard treatment for the majority of cancers. In order to improve the efficacy of these therapies, combination treatments using chemotherapeutics

F.H. Sarkar (✉)
Departments of Pathology and Oncology, Karmanos Cancer Institute, Wayne State University, 740 HWCRC, Detroit, Michigan 48201, USA
e-mail: fsarkar@med.wayne.edu

F.H. Sarkar (ed.), *Nutraceuticals and Cancer*, DOI 10.1007/978-94-007-2630-7_16,

with distinct targeted agents are considered more promising because such strategy yield better survival of patients diagnosed with cancers. However, the combination treatment is associated with certain degree of dose-related toxicity. Therefore, the development of personalized mechanism-based and targeted therapeutic strategies to improve therapeutic efficacy and minimal side effects is considered very important for the successful treatment of cancers. In targeted combination therapy, combined agents with lower toxicity typically target specific cell signaling pathways which play critical roles in the development and progression of cancer. By blocking these important targets that are responsible for cancer cell survival and growth, the targeted combination therapy will more effectively inhibit cancer cell proliferation, tumor progression and recurrence.

To achieve high efficacy and low toxicity in cancer therapy, selecting therapeutic agents is a critical step in designing therapeutic strategy. In recent years, dietary agents such as isoflavone genistein, curcumin, indole-3-carbinol (I3C), 3,3'-diindolylmethane (DIM), (-)-epigallocatechin-3-gallate (EGCG), resveratrol, lycopene, etc, have been recognized as anti-cancer agents (Surh 2003). These agents are known as nutraceuticals, which exert their anti-cancer activities through regulation of different cell signaling pathways that are known to be involved in the development and progression of cancer. By regulating cell signaling transduction, these nutraceuticals can sensitize cancer cells to apoptotic cell death. Importantly, these nutraceuticals are non-toxic, and therefore, conventional cancer therapies combined with these nutraceuticals may exert enhanced anti-cancer activity through synergic action or reversing resistance to apoptotic properties (Sarkar and Li 2006). Thus the combination treatment may also decrease the systemic toxicity caused by chemotherapeutics or radiotherapy because lower doses of chemotherapeutic agents could be useful when combined with nutraceutical whereby systemic toxicity could be minimized. In this chapter, we summarize the state of our current knowledge regarding the molecular effects of nutraceuticals on cancer treatments in pre-clinical and clinical trials.

16.2 Nutraceuticals Enhance Anti-cancer Activities of Chemotherapeutics and Radiotherapy

16.2.1 Isoflavone and Its Derivatives

Isoflavones are mainly found in Leguminosae family. Foods such as soy, lentil, bean, and chickpea are sources of isoflavones. Soybean contains abundant amounts of isoflavones. Three main isoflavones including genistein, daidzein, and glycitein are found in soybeans and most soy-protein products. Evidence from epidemiological and in vivo studies have shown decreased risk of cancer associated with soy consumption (Messina et al. 1994). It has been found that soy isoflavones could have protective effects against various cancers (Messina et al. 1994). Emerging evidence has also indicated that isoflavone and its derivatives could enhance anti-cancer activities of chemotherapeutics or other conventional therapies, suggesting that isoflavone and its derivatives could be very useful in the combination treatment of cancer.

Genistein is the most important isoflavone in cancer research. The experimental studies have shown that isoflavone genistein could enhance the anti-cancer effects of chemotherapeutic agents in various cancers in vitro and in vivo. We have found that isoflavone genistein in vitro increased growth inhibition and apoptotic cell death caused by chemotherapeutic agents such as cisplatin, docetaxel, doxorubicin, and gemcitabine in prostate, breast, pancreas, and lung cancers (Banerjee et al. 2005, 2007; El-Rayes et al. 2006; Li et al. 2004, 2005, 2006). We found that pretreatment of cancer cells with isoflavone genistein prior to treatment with lower doses of chemotherapeutic agents caused a significantly greater degree of growth inhibition and apoptosis, suggesting that combination treatment with isoflavone genistein and conventional chemotherapeutic agents could increase anti-cancer activities of chemotherapeutic agents with lower toxicity to normal cells. To investigate whether similar effect of isoflavone genistein could be demonstrated in vivo, we conducted animal studies and found that dietary isoflavone genistein could potentiate the anti-cancer activities of gemcitabine and docetaxel in an animal tumor model, leading to greater apoptotic cell death and tumor growth inhibition (Banerjee et al. 2005; Li et al. 2006). In addition to solid tumors, we also observed that isoflavone genistein could sensitize diffuse large cell lymphoma to CHOP (cyclophosphamide, doxorubicin, vincristine, prednisone) chemotherapy, resulting in greater inhibition of lymphoma cell growth (Mohammad et al. 2003). More importantly, we also found that anti-tumor, anti-invasion, and anti-metastatic activities of docetaxel could be enhanced by isoflavone genistein through the inhibition of osteoclastic bone resorption and prostate cancer bone metastasis (Li et al. 2006), suggesting that isoflavone genistein could be useful in combination with chemotherapeutic agents for the treatment of metastatic prostate cancer.

Other investigators have reported similar results showing that the anti-cancer effects of chemotherapeutics could be enhanced by isoflavone genistein. It was reported that the combination of genistein and 5-fluorouracil synergistically induced apoptotic cell death in chemo-resistant HT-29 colon cancer cells (Hwang et al. 2005). Isoflavone genistein also potentiated the effect of arsenic trioxide against human hepatocellular carcinoma through the down-regulation of Akt and NF-κB (Ma et al. 2011). It was also found that genistein increased the anti-cancer effect of bleomycin in HL-60 cells, but not in normal lymphocytes in an in vitro study (Lee et al. 2004). Recent report showed that isoflavone genistein could enhance the inhibitory effect of trichostatin A, a novel anti-cancer drug, on the growth of human lung carcinoma cells through the activation of caspase-3 and induction of apoptosis (Shiau et al. 2010). The synergistic action of genistein and cisplatin or carmustine on growth inhibition of glioblastoma and medulloblastoma cells has also been observed (Khoshyomn et al. 2000, 2002). These reports support our findings and suggest that isoflavone genistein could be useful as a potent therapeutic agent in combination with conventional therapeutics for the treatment of human malignancies. It is important to note that most in vitro studies have used pure genistein as opposed to isoflavone, which is used in most human studies. We found that pure genistein has adverse effects (increased nodal metastasis) in prostate cancer animal model; however, such adverse effects was not seen when isoflavone was used during radiosensitization experiments in vivo (Raffoul et al. 2007a), and these results clearly suggest that isoflavones should be the choice for human clinical studies.

A number of phase I and II clinical trials has been conducted to investigate the toxicity and effects of isoflavones in healthy men and the patients with prostate cancer (Busby et al. 2002; Fischer et al. 2004b; Kumar et al. 2004, 2007; Takimoto et al. 2003). The safety of purified unconjugated genistein, daidzein, and glycitein, and the defined pharmacokinetic parameters have been tested in healthy men using a single dose (Busby et al. 2002). It was found that the dietary supplements of purified unconjugated isoflavones administered to humans in single doses exceeding normal dietary intake by many folds resulted in minimal clinical toxicity. Another phase I trial using multiple-dose of isoflavone in men with prostate cancer also showed similar results (Fischer et al. 2004a, b). It has been reported that oral administration of soy isoflavones achieved plasma genistein concentrations that have been associated with anti-metastatic activity in vitro (Takimoto et al. 2003). The observed maximum plasma genistein concentration ranged from 2.7 to 27.4 μM (Busby et al. 2002). These results suggest that isoflavone genistein can be administrated safely with minimal side effect and that the plasma genistein concentration achieved in vivo was comparable to the concentrations used in most in vitro experiments. Importantly, the results from a clinical trial showed that supplementing early stage prostate cancer patients with soy isoflavones altered surrogate markers of proliferation such as serum PSA and free testosterone in a larger number of subjects in the isoflavone supplemented group than the group receiving placebo, suggesting the beneficial effects of isoflavone on early stage prostate cancer (Kumar et al. 2004). This encouraging clinical evidence from phase I/II trials underscore the importance of further consideration in designing clinical trials investigating the efficacy of soy isoflavones alone and/or in combination with conventional therapeutics. Recently, several clinical trials are being conducted using isoflavone genistein or formulated genistein in combination with IL-2 or gemcitabine in the treatment of melanoma, kidney and pancreatic cancers (Table 16.1).

The experimental studies also showed that the efficacy of radiotherapy could be potentiated by isoflavones. It was reported that the combination of isoflavone genistein and radiation enhanced inhibitory effects of radiation on DNA synthesis and cell growth (Hillman et al. 2001). Furthermore, isoflavone genistein combined with radiation led to a greater control of the growth of the primary tumor and metastasis to lymph nodes than either isoflavone genistein or radiation alone, suggesting that isoflavone genistein enhanced the radiosensitivity of prostate cancer cells (Hillman et al. 2004). Genistein combined with radiation also caused greater inhibition in PC-3 colony formation with more cancer cell death compared to either genistein or radiation alone. Mechanistic studies showed that increased cell death by genistein and radiation occurred via inhibition of NF-κB, leading to altered expression of regulatory cell cycle proteins, cyclin B and $p21^{WAF1/Cip1}$, and

Table 16.1 The new or ongoing clinical trials to investigate the effects of nutraceuticals in combination with other therapies in clinic

NCT ID	Title	Interventions	Phases
Isoflavone and derivatives			
NCT00276835	Genistein and interleukin-2 in treating patients with metastatic melanoma or kidney cancer	Interleukin-2, genistein	Phase 0
NCT01182246	AXP107-11 in combination with gemcitabine therapy for treatment in patients with pancreatic cancer	AXP107-11 (crystalline genistein formulation)	Phase I/II
NCT00382811	A Phase III study of weekly carboplatin with and without phenoxodiol in patients with platinum-resistant, recurrent epithelial ovarian cancer	Phenoxodiol, carboplatin	Phase III
NCT00303888	Docetaxel with or without phenoxodiol in treating patients with recurrent advanced ovarian epithelial cancer, fallopian tube cancer, or primary peritoneal cavity cancer	Phenoxodiol, docetaxel	Phase I/II
NCT00091377	Phenoxodiol combined with either cisplatin or paclitaxel in treating patients with recurrent late-stage ovarian epithelial, fallopian tube, or primary peritoneal cancer	Phenoxodiol, cisplatin, paclitaxel	Phase I/II
Curcumin			
NCT01048983	Reducing symptom burden – non small cell lung cancer (NSCLC)	Armodafinil, bupropion, minocycline, curcumin	Phase I/II
NCT00486460	Phase III trial of gemcitabine, curcumin and celebrex in patients with advance or inoperable pancreatic cancer	Gemcitabine, curcumin	Phase III
NCT00113841	Curcumin (diferuloylmethane derivative) with or without bioperine in patients with multiple myeloma	Curcumin, bioperine	
NCT01320436	Curcumin + aminosalicylic acid (5ASA) versus 5ASA alone in the treatment of mild to moderate ulcerative colitis	Curcumin, 5-aminosalicylic acid	Phase III
NCT00745134	Curcumin with pre-operative capecitabine and radiation therapy followed by surgery for rectal cancer	Curcumin, capecitabine, radiotherapy	Phase II

Table 16.1 (continued)

NCT ID	Title	Interventions	Phases
NCT00295035	Phase III trial of gemcitabine, curcumin and celebrex in patients with metastatic colon cancer	Celecoxib, curcumin	Phase III
DIM			
NCT00591305	New therapy of laryngeal papilloma in children	DIM, 585 nm pulsed dye laser	Phase II
EGCG			
NCT01116336	Chemoprevention with green tea polyphenon and erlotinib in patients with premalignant lesions of head and neck	Erlotinib, green tea polyphenon	Phase I
NCT00844792	Study of antioxidants on prostate tumors in men undergoing radical prostatectomy for prostate cancer	Green tea extract, radiotherapy	Phase II
Resveratrol			
NCT00920556	A clinical study to assess the safety and activity of SRT501 alone or in combination with bortezomib in patients with multiple myeloma	SRT501 (resveratrol), bortezomib	Terminated
Lycopene			
NCT00844792	Study of antioxidants on prostate tumors in men undergoing radical prostatectomy for prostate cancer	Lycopene, radiotherapy	Phase II

thereby promoting G_2/M arrest and increased radiosensitivity (Raffoul et al. 2006). Soy isoflavone also enhanced prostate cancer radiotherapy through down-regulation of apurinic/apyrimidinic endonuclease 1/redox factor-1 expression (Raffoul et al. 2007b). Recent findings from our group has also shown similar results in lung cancer (Singh-Gupta et al. 2011). These results suggest that combining isoflavone genistein with radiation could be an important and novel strategy for the treatment of prostate cancer. Similar report also showed that isoflavone genistein enhanced the radiosensitivity of cervical cancer cells through increased apoptosis, prolonged cell cycle arrest and impaired repair of DNA damage (Yashar et al. 2005). Isoflavone genistein also enhanced radiosensitivity in human esophageal cancer cells in vitro (Akimoto et al. 2001), suggesting that the enhancement of radiosensitivity by isoflavone genistein is not cell-type dependent. All of these results demonstrate that radiotherapy combined with isoflavone can lead to enhanced cell growth inhibition and apoptotic cell death of various cancers compared to mono-therapy, which has also been summarized in a recent review article by our collaborator at our institution (Hillman and Singh-Gupta 2011). Our group has reported the results of a phase II clinical trial of isoflavones in prostate cancer patients combined with radiotherapy whereby the side effects of radiotherapy was significantly improved (Ahmad et al. 2010). This pilot study was not powered to assess the clinical benefit, which underscore the need for such a clinical trial.

To enhance the anti-tumor activity of isoflavone, several isoflavone derivatives have been synthesized and used in experiments and in clinical trials. These synthetic isoflavone derivatives inhibited cancer cell growth in vitro with low IC_{50}. Moreover, at low concentration, these synthetic isoflavones could enhance the anti-cancer activity of conventional chemotherapeutic agents, suggesting their potent effects for combination treatment. Phenoxodiol is one of the isoflavone analogues and has shown a broad-spectrum anti-cancer effect. In an animal study, phenoxodiol inhibited dimethylbenz[a]anthracene (DMBA)-induced mammary carcinogenesis in female Sprague-Dawley rats, suggesting that phenoxodiol is an effective chemopreventive agent against DMBA-induced oncogenesis (Constantinou et al. 2003). In clinical trials, phenoxodiol has been used both as a monotherapy and in combination with standard chemotherapeutics. In some cancers, phenoxodiol appears to be strong enough to work on its own as a monotherapy. However, one of the major benefits of phenoxodiol is its ability to sensitize cancer cells to the anti-cancer effects of conventional chemotherapeutics (Alvero et al. 2006). In cancer cells that are susceptible to the effects of standard chemotherapeutics, phenoxodiol increases their sensitivity to those agents. In cancer cells that have become resistant to the effects of conventional chemotherapeutics, phenoxodiol restores chemo-sensitivity (Kamsteeg et al. 2003; Sapi et al. 2004). By exposing chemo-resistant cancer cells to phenoxodiol first, long-standing drug-resistance was reversed, making cancer cells susceptible once again to conventional chemotherapeutics such as cisplatin, carboplatin, taxanes and gemcitabine. Phase I/II clinical trials using phenoxodiol have shown some disease stabilization without severe toxicity (Choueiri et al. 2006). Phenoxodiol is currently undergoing clinical studies in phase II/III trials to investigate the effects of phenoxodiol combined with carboplatin, docetaxel, cisplatin, or paclitaxel in patients diagnosed with ovarian, fallopian tube, or primary peritoneal cavity cancers (Table 16.1).

16.2.2 Curcumin

Curcumin is extracted from *Curcuma longa* (tumeric). Curcumin has received much attention due to its pronounced anti-inflammatory, anti-oxidative, anti-atherogenic, and anti-carcinogenic activities. Curcumin has been shown to inhibit cancer cell growth in vitro and in vivo (Aggarwal et al. 2003; Li et al. 2002; Pereira et al. 1996). Curcumin also showed strong antioxidant and anticancer properties through regulating the expression of genes in multiple signaling pathways.

It was found that curcumin and celecoxib synergistically inhibited the growth of colorectal cancer cells (Lev-Ari et al. 2005). Curcumin also enhanced the anti-cancer activities of cisplatin, doxorubicin, and Taxol in HA22T/VGH hepatic cancer cells, Hela cells, or CAOV3 and SKOV3 ovarian cancer cells (Bava et al. 2005; Chan et al. 2003; Notarbartolo et al. 2005). Experimental studies suggest that curcumin alone could have a beneficial value in the treatment of hormone refractory prostate cancers (HRPC). In combination with taxane, curcumin could enhance cytotoxicity and reverse prostate cancer cell resistance to taxane, suggesting that curcumin in combination with taxane could be useful in HRPC patients (Cabrespine-Faugeras et al. 2010). In addition, curcumin treatment combined with TRAIL increased the number of hypodiploid cells and induced DNA fragmentation in LNCaP cells (Deeb et al. 2003). Curcumin also sensitized TRAIL-resistant xenografts in prostate, suggesting that curcumin in combination with TRAIL could be useful for the prevention and treatment of prostate cancer (Shankar et al. 2008). In pancreatic cancer, curcumin sensitized cancer cells to gemcitabine-induced cell killing (Kunnumakkara et al. 2007; Lev-Ari et al. 2007; Lin et al. 2011), suggesting its beneficial value in the treatment of pancreatic cancer. Recent report showed that curcumin enhanced the sensitivity of cisplatin treatment for lung cancers through the inactivation of ERK1/2 and the down-regulation of thymidine phosphorylase and excision repair cross-complementary 1 (ERCC1) protein levels (Lin et al. 2011; Sreekanth et al. 2011). Moreover, molecular mechanism underlying the chemosensitizing effect of liposomal curcumin in paclitaxel chemotherapy in a mouse model of cervical cancer has been investigated. The results showed that liposomal curcumin augmented the anti-cancer activity of paclitaxel by down-regulation of antiapoptotic factors and survival signals such as NF-κB, Akt and MAPK that play key roles in proliferation, survival, angiogenesis and metastasis (Sreekanth et al. 2011). In addition, curcumin was found to enhance the effects of 5-fluorouracil and oxaliplatin on colon cancer cell growth by modulating EGFR and IGF-1R (Patel et al. 2008).

Activation of multi-drug resistant protein and NF-κB is a major cause leading to drug resistance in cancers. Experimental studies showed that multi-drug resistance-associated protein 5 (MRP5) was a target gene of curcumin. By inhibiting MRP5, curcumin reversed drug resistance and sensitized pancreatic cancer cells to 5-fluorouracil and gemcitabine (Li et al. 2011a). ABCG2/BCRP1 is a multidrug resistance-linked ABC drug transporter and plays an important role in drug resistance. Curcumin has been found to inhibit ABCG2 activity at nanomolar concentrations (Shukla et al. 2009); therefore, the inhibition of ABCG2 could be another mechanism by which curcumin enhance drug sensitivity. Bacillus Calmette-Guerin (BCG) intravesical therapy is a standard treatment for bladder cancer; however, eventual failure of response is a major problem in the treatment of bladder cancer. It was found that curcumin enhanced the up-regulation of TRAIL receptors caused by BCG treatment. More importantly, curcumin suppressed the BCG-induced activation of NF-κB, leading to a significantly greater reduction in the bladder tumor volume (Kamat et al. 2009). These results suggest that combination of curcumin and BCG could be a novel strategy for the treatment of bladder cancer with drug resistance. Similar activation of NF-κB by chemotherapeutics was also observed in breast and colorectal cancers. Curcumin could also inhibit the activation of

NF-κB induced by chemotherapeutics and down-regulate the NF-κB down-stream genes including cyclin D1,c-myc, bcl-2, bcl-xL, cIAP-1, COX-2, ICAM-1, MMP-9, CXCR4 and VEGF, resulting in enhanced cell killing by chemotherapeutics in breast and colorectal cancers (Kang et al. 2009; Kunnumakkara et al. 2009).

In a clinical trial, curcumin has been used in combination with gemcitabine in patients with advanced pancreatic cancer (Epelbaum et al. 2010). Patients received 8000 mg of curcumin by mouth daily; however, such high dose of curcumin caused side effects and patients discontinued or reduced dose of curcumin. One of 11 evaluable patients (9%) had partial response and 4 (36%) had stable disease. These results suggest that other formulations of curcumin with higher bioavailability should be used to enhance the effect of chemotherapy in cancer patients (Epelbaum et al. 2010). In order to further improve the bioavailability of curcumin, synthetic analog of curcumin has been recently developed in our laboratory (Padhye et al. 2009a, b), and such a compound named CDF (curcumin difluorinated) showed to target multiple signaling pathways such as AR/TMPRSS2-ERG/Wnt signaling network, leading to the inactivation of Wnt signaling consistent with inhibition of prostate cancer cell invasion (Li et al. 2011b). Moreover, CDF was found to target cancer stem-like cells and enhanced the activity of gemcitabine in pancreatic cancer (Ali et al. 2010a; Bao et al. 2011).

In cancer radiotherapy, curcumin at a low concentration showed significant enhancement to radiation-induced clonogenic inhibition and apoptosis in PC-3 prostate cancer cells (Chendil et al. 2004). In addition, cervical cancer is highly radioresistant, and it was found that pretreatment of two cervical carcinoma cell lines, HeLa and SiHa, with curcumin before ionizing radiation resulted in a significant dose-dependent radiosensitization of these cells (Javvadi et al. 2008). These results suggest that curcumin is a potent agent in combination treatment with radiotherapy for cancer treatment. Several clinical trials using curcumin in combination treatment with amodafinil, bupropion, minocycline, gemcitabine, celecoxib, capecitabine, or radiotherapy are being conducted to test the effects and toxicity of the combination treatment in patients with multiple myeloma, rectal, colon, and pancreatic cancers (Table 16.1).

16.2.3 Indole-3-Carbinol and 3,3'-Diindolylmethane

Indole-3-carbinol (I3C) is produced from naturally occurring glucosinolates contained in a wide variety of plants including members of the family Cruciferae such as broccoli. 3,3'-diindolylmethane (DIM) is the dimeric product of indole-3-carbinol (I3C). Under the acidic conditions of the stomach, I3C undergoes extensive and rapid self-condensation reactions to form several derivatives. DIM is the major derivative and condensation product of I3C. The evidence from epidemiological studies showed that exposure to indoles through consumption of cruciferous vegetable could decrease cancer risk. Experimental studies demonstrated that DIM could reduce oxidative stress and stimulate the expression of antioxidant response element-driven gene, suggesting the anti-oxidant function of DIM. Animal study showed that DIM was not toxic and had in vivo preventive effect against the development of cancers. Moreover, DIM could inhibit oncogenesis and cancer cell growth, and induce apoptosis in cancer cells in vitro and in vivo, suggesting that DIM could serve as a potent agent for the prevention and/or treatment of cancers.

We and others have found that I3C combined with cisplatin or tamoxifen could inhibit the growth of PC-3 prostate and MCF-7 breast cancer cells more effectively than either agent alone (Cover et al. 1999; Sarkar and Li 2004). We have also investigated the effects of DIM combined with erlotinib or gemcitabine in pancreatic cancer. We found that DIM in combination with erlotinib and gemcitabine showed more potent inhibitory effect on pancreatic cancer growth in vitro and in vivo compared to monotreatment (Ali et al. 2010b). We also observed a significant down-regulation in the expression of COX-2, NF-κB, and EGFR in pancreatic cancer cells treated with combination of DIM, erlotinib and gemcitabine (Ali et al. 2010b).

In colon cancer, DIM could enhance the efficacy of butyrate, which is an inhibitor of histone deacetylase and has been extensively used as a chemoprevention agent for colon cancer. It was found that pretreatment with DIM enhanced butyrate-induced apoptosis in colon cancer cells expressing mutant APC (Bhatnagar et al. 2009). DIM also inhibited survivin mRNA expression, promoted survivin protein degradation, increased expression of Bax and Bak, leading to the enhanced apoptosis (Bhatnagar et al. 2009). Similar effects of DIM were also observed in prostate cancer cells treated with taxotere. It was reported that DIM enhanced taxotere-induced apoptosis and growth inhibition in prostate cancer cells through down-regulation of survivin, AR, and NF-κB (Rahman et al. 2009). The multi-targeted effects of DIM has also been reported in our recent studies showing that DIM (BR-DIM) could effectively targets AR/TMPRSS2-ERG/Wnt signaling network, leading to the inactivation of Wnt signaling consistent with inhibition of prostate cancer cell invasion (Li et al. 2011b). DIM also enhanced anticancer activity of taxotere in human non-small cell lung cancer. The combination treatment resulted in increased apoptotic cells and up-regulated the expression of PARP, Bax, and N-cadherin (Ichite et al. 2009). In breast cancer cells, DIM and paclitaxel synergistically promoted apoptotic cell death of HER2/Neu positive cancer cells with up-regulation of PARP and down-regulation of Bcl-2 and ERK1/ERK2 (McGuire et al. 2006).

A phase I clinical trial using DIM have been conducted by our group in patients with prostate cancers to determine the toxicity profile of DIM and assess its effects on serum PSA and quality of life. The results showed only minimal toxicity; however 225 mg dose twice daily was safe, and thus it was recommended as the dose for subsequent phase II study being conducted by our group. One patient with DIM dose of 225 mg had PSA stabilization. The other ten patients had an initial deceleration of their PSA rise (decrease in slope), suggesting that modest efficacy was achieved (Heath et al. 2010). A phase II clinical trial is being currently conducted using DIM and 585 nM pulsed dye laser in patients with laryngeal papilloma to test new therapeutic strategy in this tumor (Table 16.1).

16.2.4 Epigallocatechin-3-Gallate (EGCG)

Consumption of green tea has been associated with lower incidence of cancers (Jian et al. 2007). Green tea and its constituents have been studied both in vitro and in vivo. Green tea contains several catechins including epicatechin (EC), epigallocatechin (EGC), epicatechin-3-gallate (ECG), and epigallocatechin-3-gallate (EGCG). However, EGCG is the most potent constituent for the inhibition of carcinogenesis and oxidative stress among these catechins. Epidemiologic evidence indicated that consumption of green tea which contained EGCG significantly decreased overall cancer incidence (Nakachi et al. 2000). EGCG promoted cell cycle arrest and apoptosis in cancer cells through the modulations of cyclin/CDK and Bcl-2 family proteins (Nihal et al. 2005). EGCG in vivo also inhibited tumor growth and metastasis in murine melanoma (Taniguchi et al. 1992).

Importantly, it has been found that EGCG combined with tamoxifen significantly induced apoptosis and growth inhibition in MDA-MB-231 human breast cancer cells (Chisholm et al. 2004). EGCG could also chemosensitize resistant tumor cells to doxorubicin in the human carcinoma xenograft model (Zhang et al. 2004), suggesting its effects on cancer therapy in combination with chemotherapeutics. For patients with glioblastoma, temozolomide in combination with surgery and radiation is the standard therapeutic strategy. However, the chemoresistance to temozolomide is present due to elevated expression of endoplasmic reticulum (ER) chaperone GRP78 (glucose-regulated protein 78). EGCG significantly improved the therapeutic effect of temozolomide with decreased expression of GRP78 (Chen et al. 2011). In prostate cancer, EGCG sensitized human prostate cancer cells to TRAIL-mediated apoptosis and synergistically inhibited biomarkers associated with angiogenesis and metastasis including VEGF, uPA, angiopoietin, and MMPs (Siddiqui et al. 2008). EGCG in combination with low dose of doxorubicin (DOX) also exhibited synergistic effects on the inhibition of tumor growth and colony-forming ability of prostate cells (Stearns et al. 2010). Similarly, EGCG combined with low dose of DOX significantly inhibited hepatic cancer cell proliferation in vitro and hepatoma growth in a xenograft mouse model, compared to treatment with either agent alone at the same dose (Liang et al. 2010). Moreover, the administration of DOX in combination with EGCG markedly enhanced intracellular DOX accumulation with the down-regulation of MDR1 and HIF-1α expression (Liang et al. 2010). When EGCG combined with Celastrol derived from the plant 'Thunder God Vine', these natural products augmented the efficacy of conventional chemotherapy in the treatment of leukemia with increased levels of caspases-3 activation and PARP cleavage (Davenport et al. 2010). It was also found that EGCG synergistically sensitized breast cancer cells to paclitaxel in vitro and in vivo with significantly induced apoptosis and decreased GRP78 expression (Luo et al. 2010). EGCG could also sensitize melanoma cells to interferon induced growth inhibition in a mouse model of human melanoma with an increase in Fas protein levels and a decrease in NF-κB activity (Nihal et al. 2009). EGCG together with either cisplatin or tamoxifen also showed enhanced inhibition of cell growth in glioma with decreased expression of telomerase which alters drug sensitivity (Shervington et al. 2009). All of these reports demonstrate that EGCG could enhance the anti-cancer activity of chemotherapeutics in various cancers. Recently, a phase III clinical trial is being conducted using combination of EGCG and Eriotinib to chemoprevent head and neck cancer with premalignant lesion (Table 16.1).

16.2.5 Resveratrol

Resveratrol is a phytoalexin mainly found in grapes. Red wine contains a high level of resveratrol. Resveratrol has been shown to prevent the development of mammary and other tumors in vivo in animal models (Bishayee 2009). Experimental studies also showed that resveratrol exhibited anticancer properties in a variety of cancer cells including lymphoid, myeloid, skin, breast, prostate, and colon cancers (Bishayee 2009). We have recently reported that the biological effects of resveratrol could be enhanced in lower pH (Shamim et al. 2011), suggesting that resveratrol would be effective in cancer in human patient because the pH within the tumor is lower than the overall physiological pH in vivo.

Importantly, resveratrol has been reported to sensitize non-Hodgkin's lymphoma to paclitaxel-mediated apoptosis (Jazirehi and Bonavida 2004). In doxorubicin-resistant AML cell lines, the expression level of the MRP1 gene, which is responsible for drug-resistance, was significantly increased. Resveratrol treatment not only induced cell growth arrest and apoptotic death in doxorubicin-resistant AML cells, but also down-regulated the expression of MRP1 gene (Kweon et al. 2010). Resveratrol also protected against cisplatin-induced cardiotoxicity by alleviating oxidative damage, which is consistent with recent report from our group showing enhanced effects of resveratrol in lower pH (Shamim et al. 2011). It was found that cisplatin treatment caused cardiac-function deterioration, myocardial injury, and increased lactate dehydrogenase activity, which are adverse effects of cisplatin (Wang et al. 2009). However, treatment with resveratrol effectively alleviated these adverse effects of cisplatin and increased the anti-cancer activity of cisplatin in A549 lung cancer cells (Wang et al. 2009). In human pancreatic cancer, resveratrol sensitized pancreatic cancer cells to gemcitabine in vitro and in vivo. The resveratrol-induced sensitization was found to be mediated by the down-regulation of NF-κB, cyclin D1, COX-2, ICAM-1, MMP-9 and survivin (Harikumar et al. 2010). CD133 has recently been proposed as a marker for cancer stem-like cells in brain tumors. Experimental studies showed that resveratrol induced apoptosis and increased radiosensitivity in CD133-positive cells derived from atypical teratoid/rhabdoid tumor (Kao et al. 2009). After resveratrol treatment, the in vitro proliferation rates and in vivo tumor-forming ability of CD133-positive cells was dramatically inhibited with the down-regulation of drug-resistant genes in CD133-positive cells (Kao et al. 2009). Resveratrol also dramatically enhanced 5-Fluoro-Uracil-mediated inhibition of colon cancer cell proliferation (Colin et al. 2009). In human multiple myeloma cells, resveratrol inhibited cell proliferation, induced apoptosis, and overcame chemoresistance through down-regulation of STAT3, Akt, IKK, NF-κB, cyclin D1, cIAP-2, XIAP, survivin, Bcl-2, Bcl-xL, Bfl-1/A1, and TRAF2 (Bhardwaj et al. 2007).

It was reported that medulloblastoma cancer stem-like cells showed significant resistance to radiotherapy compared to the parental medulloblastoma cells. Medulloblastoma cancer stem-like cells could display 3D spheroid formation, enhanced self-renewal, and highly co-expressed 'stem cell' genes such as Oct-4, Nanog, Nestin, and Musashi-1. Resveratrol treatment could effectively inhibit the proliferation of medulloblastoma cancer stem-like cells and significantly enhanced the radiosensitivity of medulloblastoma cancer stem-like cells (Lu et al. 2009). DU145 prostate cancer cells are resistant to ionizing radiation-induced cell death; however, pretreatment with resveratrol significantly increased ceramide and enhanced cell death caused by radiation (Scarlatti et al. 2007). In melanoma cells, the NF-κB pathway, which is involved in the radioprotective response, is highly activated. Resveratrol inhibited STAT3, NF-κB, cFLIP and Bcl-xL expression while it upregulated TRAIL promoter activity and induced TRAIL surface expression in melanoma cells, leading to the dramatic up-regulation of apoptosis caused by radiation (Johnson et al. 2008). Melanoma cells commonly express the death receptors TRAIL-R2/DR5 on cell surface; however, the cells often exhibit resistance to exogenous TRAIL due to up-regulation of STAT3 and NF-κB that control the expression of anti-apoptotic genes including cFLIP and Bcl-xL. Resveratrol also sensitized melanomas to TRAIL through modulation of anti-apoptotic gene expression (Ivanov et al. 2008). These results suggest that resveratrol treatment in combination with TRAIL administration and/or radiotherapy, may have significant efficacy in the treatment of human melanomas. It is important to note that a phase II clinical trial using formulated resveratrol SRT501 combined with bortezomib in patient with multiple myeloma has been terminated because of the failure of kidney function (ClinicalTrial.org), but there was no scientific explanation provided.

16.2.6 Lycopene

Tomatoes are rich source of lycopene, which is the pigment principally responsible for the deep-red color of tomato and its products. Tomato products including ketchup, tomato juice, and pizza sauce, are the richest sources of lycopene in the US diet. Lycopene is a potent antioxidant. It has been shown that lycopene exhibits high physical quenching rate constant with singlet oxygen, suggesting its high activity as antioxidant. Frequent consumption of tomato products is associated with a lower risk of prostate cancer. These findings has been summarized in our recent review article (Sarkar et al. 2010). The inverse associations between plasma lycopene and prostate cancer have also been reported. Experimental studies showed that lycopene inhibited cell growth in breast, prostate, endometrial, and other cancers with regulation of cell cycle-related genes. Animal study showed that lycopene had anti-tumor effects that could be potentiated by vitamin E, an antioxidant that is also present in tomatoes, confirming the anti-cancer activity of lycopene. In a recent review article we have summarized the role of lycopene and its target in human cancer (Sarkar et al. 2010).

Lycopene has been used prior to radical prostatectomy of prostate cancer patients. A phase II trial was performed to evaluate the safety and effect of administering several doses of lycopene to men with clinically localized prostate cancer. Patients with clinically localized prostate cancer were supplemented with lycopene. Plasma lycopene increased from baseline to post treatment in all treatment groups. Serum free testosterone decreased with lycopene supplementation (Kumar et al. 2008), suggesting that steroid hormones related mechanisms are involved. The results from another clinical trial showed that lycopene supplements reduced tumor size and PSA level in localized prostate cancer, suggesting its promising effects on prostate cancer prevention and/or treatment (Kucuk et al. 2001, 2002).

Another clinical study was conducted in men with recurring prostate cancer and rising PSA with dietary intervention rich in tomato products and a soy protein supplement (Grainger et al. 2008). The results showed no grade II, III and IV toxicities. Serum lycopene increased from 0.72 μM to 1.21 μM ($P < 0.0001$) and urinary isoflavone excretion increased from not detectable to 54 μM ($P < 0.05$). Serum PSA decreased in 14/41 men (34%). VEGF was reduced from 87 to 51 ng/ml ($P < 0.05$). These results suggest that consumption of diets rich in tomato products and soy has benefits in prostate cancer prevention or management with excellent compliance and bioavailability of phytochemicals (Grainger et al. 2008). Ongoing clinical trials have been designed to investigate the antioxidant effects of lycopene in men undergoing radiotherapy as combination treatment with lycopene and radiotherapy (Table 16.1).

16.3 Molecular Mechanisms of Cancer Cell Sensitization to Conventional Cancer Therapies by Nutraceuticals

The molecular mechanisms by which nutraceuticals enhance the anti-cancer efficacy of conventional cancer therapies have not been fully elucidated. It is well known that chemotherapy and radiotherapy can induce drug resistance in cancer cells, leading to treatment failure. Experimental evidence has demonstrated that NF-κB, Akt, MDR, AR and some molecules in apoptotic pathway are critically involved in the development of drug resistance. To investigate the molecular mechanism underlying nutraceutical-induced drug sensitivity, in vitro and in vivo experimental studies have been conducted, and showed enhanced anti-cancer effects by nutraceuticals that could in part be due to regulation of NF-κB, Akt, MDR, COX-2, AR and MAPK signaling, which are known to play critical roles in cancer cell survival, invasion and metastasis (Fig. 16.1). Nutraceuticals could also sensitize cancer cells to apoptosis by regulating several important molecules such as Bcl-2, Bcl-X_L, Bax, survivin, XIAP, FLIO, caspases, p21^{WAF1}, and TRAIL in the apoptotic pathway.

It has been well known that many chemotherapeutic agents and radiation induce activity of NF-κB, which causes drug resistance in cancer cells (Chuang et al. 2002; Hillman et al. 2004). From in vitro and in vivo experimental studies, we found that NF-κB activity was significantly increased by cisplatin, docetaxel, gemcitabine, CHOP, and radiation treatment and that the NF-κB inducing activity of these

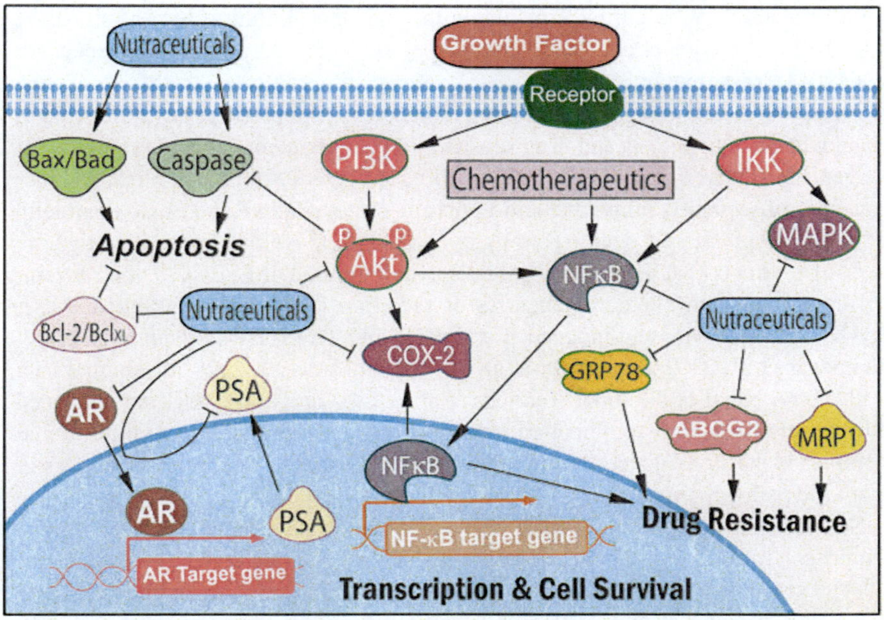

Fig. 16.1 Networks pathway that are involved in chemosensitization by nutraceuticals

agents was completely abrogated by isoflavone genistein, I3C, or DIM treatment in prostate, breast, lung, and pancreatic cancer cells, suggesting that isoflavone, I3C, or DIM pre-treatment inactivate NF-κB, and in turn may contribute to the increased growth inhibition and apoptosis induced by these agents (Ali et al. 2010b; Hillman et al. 2001, 2004; Li et al. 2004, 2005). Other investigators also reported that curcumin, EGCG, and resveratrol enhanced the anti-cancer activity of chemotherapeutics by the inhibition of NF-κB activation (Bhardwaj et al. 2007; Kamat et al. 2009; Nihal et al. 2009; Sreekanth et al. 2011). All of these findings suggest that the inhibition of NF-κB by nutraceuticals is important for chemosensitization and radiosensitization (Fig. 16.1).

The Akt pathway is another important cell signaling pathway which controls cell survival and drug resistance. It has been reported that genistein enhanced necrotic-like cell death with significant inhibition of Akt activity in breast cancer cells treated with genistein and adriamycin, suggesting that the enhanced growth inhibition by genistein and adriamycin is partly due to the inactivation of the Akt pathway (Satoh et al. 2003). Phenoxodiol, one of the synthetic derivatives of genistein in clinical trial, could also inhibit Akt signaling transduction and subsequently activate caspase, leading to the induced apoptosis and increased chemosensitization (Kamsteeg et al. 2003). We and other investigators have also shown that activated Akt was inhibited by isoflavone genistein, curcumin, or resveratrol combined with chemotherapeutics or radiation in pancreatic, cervical, and esophageal cancer cells, suggesting that enhancement of chemotherapeutic or radiation effects by nutraceuticals may be partially mediated through the inhibition of Akt signaling (Fig. 16.1) (Banerjee et al. 2005; Bhardwaj et al. 2007; Ma et al. 2011; Sreekanth et al. 2011; Yashar et al. 2005).

Nutraceuticals also regulate important molecules in apoptotic pathway, leading to the induction of apoptosis and drug sensitization. Experimental studies showed that the genistein derivative phenoxodiol could bind to the tNOX receptor, block its function, and subsequently inhibit the anti-apoptotic proteins XIAP and FLIP, eventually inducing apoptotic cell death (Kamsteeg et al. 2003). We and other investigators have also found that isoflavone genistein, curcumin, DIM, EGCG, or resveratrol combined with chemotherapeutics or radiation significantly inhibited Bcl-2, Bcl-X_L, and survivin, and induced Bax, PARP, and TRAIL (Bhardwaj et al. 2007; Bhatnagar et al. 2009; Davenport et al. 2010; Johnson et al. 2008; Kunnumakkara et al. 2009; Nihal et al. 2005; Rahman et al. 2009), suggesting that the enhanced anti-cancer effect from combination treatment with nutraceuticals and conventional therapies is partly mediated through the regulation of these important molecules in apoptotic pathway (Fig. 16.1).

Several members of multi-drug resistance genes have been involved in the chemosensitization by nutraceuticals. Resveratrol could reverse doxorubicin-induced resistance in acute myeloid leukemia cells via down-regulation of MRP1 expression (Kweon et al. 2010). Curcumin could inhibit the activity of ABCG2, leading to enhanced drug sensitivity (Shukla et al. 2009). EGCG significantly improved the existing therapeutic effect of temozolomide by inhibiting the expression of GRP78 (Chen et al. 2011). EGCG also markedly enhanced intracellular DOX accumulation with the down-regulation of MDR1 (Liang et al. 2010). These results suggest that the inhibition of multi-drug resistance genes by nutraceuticals contributes to enhanced efficacy of cancer combination therapy (Fig. 16.1).

MAPK and other pathways are also involved in chemosensitization by nutraceuticals. Curcumin could inhibit MAPK signaling, causing the decreased drug resistance (Lin et al. 2011; Sreekanth et al. 2011). We reported that the anti-tumor and anti-metastatic activities of docetaxel has been found to be enhanced by isoflavone genistein through the regulation of OPG/RANK/RANKL/MMP-9 signaling in prostate cancer (Li et al. 2006). Other investigators also reported that EGCG and resveratrol could enhance anti-cancer activity of chemotherapeutics by the inhibition of MMPs (Harikumar et al. 2010; Siddiqui et al. 2008). Since DIM, isoflavone genistein, curcumin, and lycopene could inhibit the expression of AR and PSA (Li et al. 2007, 2008; Nakamura et al. 2002; Vaishampayan et al. 2007), these nutraceuticals could be used for the treatment of prostate cancer. It has been reported that the combination of 5-FU and isoflavone genistein enhanced therapeutic effects in colon cancers through the COX-2 pathway (Hwang et al. 2005). We and other investigators have also reported that DIM or resveratrol could potentiate the anti-cancer activity of chemotherapeutics via the down-regulation of NF-κB and COX-2 (Ali et al. 2010b; Harikumar et al. 2010), suggesting the multi-targeted effects of nutraceuticals.

16.4 Conclusion and Perspectives

Emerging evidence from in vitro and in vivo experimental studies along with clinical trials suggest that nutraceuticals may serve as potent agents for enhancing the therapeutic efficacy of chemotherapy, radiotherapy, or other conventional therapies for the treatment of human cancers. However, the limitation of using nutraceuticals in cancer therapy is primarily due to low bioavailability for some nutraceuticals in humans, which limits their utility for cancer treatment. Therefore, structurally-modified synthetic analogues or nanoparticle formulation of nutraceuticals with improved bioavailability are needed for targeted inactivation of signaling pathways that are involved in therapeutic resistance in order to design novel combination therapies for human malignancies. However, further in-depth mechanistic studies and clinical trials are also needed to test the value nutraceuticals in combination treatment of human cancers.

Acknowledgements The authors' work cited in this review article was funded by grants from the National Cancer Institute, NIH (5R01CA083695, 5R01CA108535, 5R01CA132794, and 5R01CA131151 awarded to FHS). We also thank Puschelberg and Guido foundations for their generous contribution to support our research.

References

Aggarwal BB, Kumar A, Bharti AC (2003) Anticancer potential of curcumin: preclinical and clinical studies. Anticancer Res 23:363–398

Ahmad IU, Forman JD, Sarkar FH et al (2010) Soy isoflavones in conjunction with radiation therapy in patients with prostate cancer. Nutr Cancer 62:996–1000

Akimoto T, Nonaka T, Ishikawa H et al (2001) Genistein, a tyrosine kinase inhibitor, enhanced radiosensitivity in human esophageal cancer cell lines in vitro: possible involvement of inhibition of survival signal transduction pathways. Int J Radiat Oncol Biol Phys 50:195–201

Ali S, Ahmad A, Banerjee S et al (2010a) Gemcitabine sensitivity can be induced in pancreatic cancer cells through modulation of miR-200 and miR-21 expression by curcumin or its analogue CDF. Cancer Res 70:3606–3617

Ali S, Banerjee S, Schaffert JM et al (2010b) Concurrent inhibition of NF-kappaB, cyclooxygenase-2, and epidermal growth factor receptor leads to greater anti-tumor activity in pancreatic cancer. J Cell Biochem 110:171–181

Alvero AB, O'Malley D, Brown D et al (2006) Molecular mechanism of phenoxodiol-induced apoptosis in ovarian carcinoma cells. Cancer 106:599–608

Banerjee S, Zhang Y, Ali S et al (2005) Molecular evidence for increased antitumor activity of gemcitabine by genistein in vitro and in vivo using an orthotopic model of pancreatic cancer. Cancer Res 65:9064–9072

Banerjee S, Zhang Y, Wang Z et al (2007) In vitro and in vivo molecular evidence of genistein action in augmenting the efficacy of cisplatin in pancreatic cancer. Int J Cancer 120:906–917

Bao B, Ali S, Kong D et al (2011) Anti-tumor activity of a novel compound-CDF is mediated by regulating miR-21, miR-200, and PTEN in pancreatic cancer. PLoS One 6:e17850

Bava SV, Puliappadamba VT, Deepti A et al (2005) Sensitization of taxol-induced apoptosis by curcumin involves down-regulation of nuclear factor-kappaB and the serine/threonine kinase Akt and is independent of tubulin polymerization. J Biol Chem 280:6301–6308

Bhardwaj A, Sethi G, Vadhan-Raj S et al (2007) Resveratrol inhibits proliferation, induces apoptosis, and overcomes chemoresistance through down-regulation of STAT3 and nuclear factor-kappaB-regulated antiapoptotic and cell survival gene products in human multiple myeloma cells. Blood 109:2293–2302

Bhatnagar N, Li X, Chen Y et al (2009) 3,3′-diindolylmethane enhances the efficacy of butyrate in colon cancer prevention through down-regulation of survivin. Cancer Prev Res (Phila) 2: 581–589

Bishayee A (2009) Cancer prevention and treatment with resveratrol: from rodent studies to clinical trials. Cancer Prev Res (Phila) 2:409–418

Busby MG, Jeffcoat AR, Bloedon LT et al (2002) Clinical characteristics and pharmacokinetics of purified soy isoflavones: single-dose administration to healthy men. Am J Clin Nutr 75:126–136

Cabrespine-Faugeras A, Bayet-Robert M, Bay JO et al (2010) Possible benefits of curcumin regimen in combination with taxane chemotherapy for hormone-refractory prostate cancer treatment. Nutr Cancer 62:148–153

Chan MM, Fong D, Soprano KJ et al (2003) Inhibition of growth and sensitization to cisplatin-mediated killing of ovarian cancer cells by polyphenolic chemopreventive agents. J Cell Physiol 194:63–70

Chen TC, Wang W, Golden EB et al (2011) Green tea epigallocatechin gallate enhances therapeutic efficacy of temozolomide in orthotopic mouse glioblastoma models. Cancer Lett 302:100–108

Chendil D, Ranga RS, Meigooni D et al (2004) Curcumin confers radiosensitizing effect in prostate cancer cell line PC-3. Oncogene 23:1599–607

Chisholm K, Bray BJ, Rosengren RJ (2004) Tamoxifen and epigallocatechin gallate are synergistically cytotoxic to MDA-MB-231 human breast cancer cells. Anticancer Drugs 15:889–97

Choueiri TK, Wesolowski R, Mekhail TM (2006) Phenoxodiol: isoflavone analog with antineoplastic activity. Curr Oncol Rep 8:104–107

Chuang SE, Yeh PY, Lu YS et al (2002) Basal levels and patterns of anticancer drug-induced activation of nuclear factor-kappaB (NF-kappaB), and its attenuation by tamoxifen, dexamethasone, and curcumin in carcinoma cells. Biochem Pharmacol 63:1709–1716

Colin D, Gimazane A, Lizard G et al (2009) Effects of resveratrol analogs on cell cycle progression, cell cycle associated proteins and 5fluoro-uracil sensitivity in human derived colon cancer cells. Int J Cancer 124:2780–2788

Constantinou AI, Mehta R, Husband A (2003) Phenoxodiol, a novel isoflavone derivative, inhibits dimethylbenz[a]anthracene (DMBA)-induced mammary carcinogenesis in female Sprague-Dawley rats. Eur J Cancer 39:1012–1018

Cover CM, Hsieh SJ, Cram EJ et al (1999) Indole-3-carbinol and tamoxifen cooperate to arrest the cell cycle of MCF-7 human breast cancer cells. Cancer Res 59:1244–1251

Davenport A, Frezza M, Shen M et al (2010) Celastrol and an EGCG pro-drug exhibit potent chemosensitizing activity in human leukemia cells. Int J Mol Med 25:465–470

Deeb D, Xu YX, Jiang H et al (2003) Curcumin (diferuloyl-methane) enhances tumor necrosis factor-related apoptosis-inducing ligand-induced apoptosis in LNCaP prostate cancer cells. Mol Cancer Ther 2:95–103

El-Rayes BF, Ali S, Ali IF et al (2006) Potentiation of the effect of erlotinib by genistein in pancreatic cancer: the role of Akt and nuclear factor-kappaB. Cancer Res 66:10553–10559

Epelbaum R, Schaffer M, Vizel B et al (2010) Curcumin and gemcitabine in patients with advanced pancreatic cancer. Nutr Cancer 62:1137–1141

Fischer L, Mahoney C, Jeffcoat AR et al (2004a) Clinical characteristics and pharmacokinetics of purified soy isoflavones: multiple-dose administration to men with prostate neoplasia. Nutr Cancer 48:160–170

Fischer L, Mahoney C, Jeffcoat AR et al (2004b) Clinical characteristics and pharmacokinetics of purified soy isoflavones: multiple-dose administration to men with prostate neoplasia. Nutr Cancer 48:160–170

Grainger EM, Schwartz SJ, Wang S et al (2008) A combination of tomato and soy products for men with recurring prostate cancer and rising prostate specific antigen. Nutr Cancer 60:145–154

Harikumar KB, Kunnumakkara AB, Sethi G et al (2010) Resveratrol, a multitargeted agent, can enhance antitumor activity of gemcitabine in vitro and in orthotopic mouse model of human pancreatic cancer. Int J Cancer 127:257–268

Heath EI, Heilbrun LK, Li J et al (2010) A phase I dose-escalation study of oral BR-DIM (BioResponse 3,3′- Diindolylmethane) in castrate-resistant, non-metastatic prostate cancer. Am J Transl Res 2:402–411

Hillman GG, Singh-Gupta V (2011) Soy isoflavones sensitize cancer cells to radiotherapy. Free Radic Biol Med 51:289–298

Hillman GG, Forman JD, Kucuk O et al (2001) Genistein potentiates the radiation effect on prostate carcinoma cells. Clin Cancer Res 7:382–390

Hillman GG, Wang Y, Kucuk O et al (2004) Genistein potentiates inhibition of tumor growth by radiation in a prostate cancer orthotopic model. Mol Cancer Ther 3:1271–1279

Hwang JT, Ha J, Park OJ (2005) Combination of 5-fluorouracil and genistein induces apoptosis synergistically in chemo-resistant cancer cells through the modulation of AMPK and COX-2 signaling pathways. Biochem Biophys Res Commun 332:433–440

Ichite N, Chougule MB, Jackson T et al (2009) Enhancement of docetaxel anticancer activity by a novel diindolylmethane compound in human non-small cell lung cancer. Clin Cancer Res 15:543–552

Ivanov VN, Partridge MA, Johnson GE et al (2008) Resveratrol sensitizes melanomas to TRAIL through modulation of antiapoptotic gene expression. Exp Cell Res 314:1163–1176

Javvadi P, Segan AT, Tuttle SW et al (2008) The chemopreventive agent curcumin is a potent radiosensitizer of human cervical tumor cells via increased reactive oxygen species production and overactivation of the mitogen-activated protein kinase pathway. Mol Pharmacol 73: 1491–1501

Jazirehi AR, Bonavida B (2004) Resveratrol modifies the expression of apoptotic regulatory proteins and sensitizes non-Hodgkin's lymphoma and multiple myeloma cell lines to paclitaxel-induced apoptosis. Mol Cancer Ther 3:71–84

Jemal A, Siegel R, Xu J et al (2010) Cancer statistics, 2010. CA Cancer J Clin 60:277–300

Jian L, Lee AH, Binns CW (2007) Tea and lycopene protect against prostate cancer. Asia Pac J Clin Nutr 16(Suppl 1):453–457

Johnson GE, Ivanov VN, Hei TK (2008) Radiosensitization of melanoma cells through combined inhibition of protein regulators of cell survival. Apoptosis 13:790–802

Kamat AM, Tharakan ST, Sung B et al (2009) Curcumin potentiates the antitumor effects of Bacillus Calmette-Guerin against bladder cancer through the downregulation of NF-kappaB and upregulation of TRAIL receptors. Cancer Res 69:8958–8966

Kamsteeg M, Rutherford T, Sapi E et al (2003) Phenoxodiol–an isoflavone analog–induces apoptosis in chemoresistant ovarian cancer cells. Oncogene 22:2611–2620

Kang HJ, Lee SH, Price JE et al (2009) Curcumin suppresses the paclitaxel-induced nuclear factor-kappaB in breast cancer cells and potentiates the growth inhibitory effect of paclitaxel in a breast cancer nude mice model. Breast J 15:223–229

Kao CL, Huang PI, Tsai PH et al (2009) Resveratrol-induced apoptosis and increased radiosensitivity in CD133-positive cells derived from atypical teratoid/rhabdoid tumor. Int J Radiat Oncol Biol Phys 74:219–228

Khoshyomn S, Manske GC, Lew SM et al (2000) Synergistic action of genistein and cisplatin on growth inhibition and cytotoxicity of human medulloblastoma cells. Pediatr Neurosurg 33:123–131

Khoshyomn S, Nathan D, Manske GC et al (2002) Synergistic effect of genistein and BCNU on growth inhibition and cytotoxicity of glioblastoma cells. J Neurooncol 57:193–200

Kucuk O, Sarkar FH, Sakr W et al (2001) Phase II randomized clinical trial of lycopene supplementation before radical prostatectomy. Cancer Epidemiol Biomarkers Prev 10:861–868

Kucuk O, Sarkar FH, Djuric Z et al (2002) Effects of lycopene supplementation in patients with localized prostate cancer. Exp Biol Med (Maywood) 227:881–885

Kumar NB, Cantor A, Allen K et al (2004) The specific role of isoflavones in reducing prostate cancer risk. Prostate 59:141–147

Kumar NB, Krischer JP, Allen K et al (2007) A Phase II randomized, placebo-controlled clinical trial of purified isoflavones in modulating steroid hormones in men diagnosed with localized prostate cancer. Nutr Cancer 59:163–168

Kumar NB, Besterman-Dahan K, Kang L et al (2008) Results of a Randomized Clinical Trial of the Action of Several Doses of Lycopene in Localized Prostate Cancer: Administration Prior to Radical Prostatectomy. Clin Med Urol 1:1–14

Kunnumakkara AB, Guha S, Krishnan S et al (2007) Curcumin potentiates antitumor activity of gemcitabine in an orthotopic model of pancreatic cancer through suppression of proliferation, angiogenesis, and inhibition of nuclear factor-kappaB-regulated gene products. Cancer Res 67:3853–3861

Kunnumakkara AB, Diagaradjane P, Anand P et al (2009) Curcumin sensitizes human colorectal cancer to capecitabine by modulation of cyclin D1, COX-2, MMP-9, VEGF and CXCR4 expression in an orthotopic mouse model. Int J Cancer 125:2187–2197

Kweon SH, Song JH, Kim TS (2010) Resveratrol-mediated reversal of doxorubicin resistance in acute myeloid leukemia cells via downregulation of MRP1 expression. Biochem Biophys Res Commun 395:104–110

Lee R, Kim YJ, Lee YJ et al (2004) The selective effect of genistein on the toxicity of bleomycin in normal lymphocytes and HL-60 cells. Toxicology 195:87–95

Lev-Ari S, Strier L, Kazanov D et al (2005) Celecoxib and curcumin synergistically inhibit the growth of colorectal cancer cells. Clin Cancer Res 11:6738–6744

Lev-Ari S, Vexler A, Starr A et al (2007) Curcumin augments gemcitabine cytotoxic effect on pancreatic adenocarcinoma cell lines. Cancer Invest 25:411–418

Li N, Chen X, Liao J et al (2002) Inhibition of 7,12-dimethylbenz[a]anthracene (DMBA)-induced oral carcinogenesis in hamsters by tea and curcumin. Carcinogenesis 23:1307–1313

Li Y, Ellis KL, Ali S et al (2004) Apoptosis-inducing effect of chemotherapeutic agents is potentiated by soy isoflavone genistein, a natural inhibitor of NF-kappaB in BxPC-3 pancreatic cancer cell line. Pancreas 28:e90–e95

Li Y, Ahmed F, Ali S et al (2005) Inactivation of nuclear factor kappaB by soy isoflavone genistein contributes to increased apoptosis induced by chemotherapeutic agents in human cancer cells. Cancer Res 65:6934–6942

Li Y, Kucuk O, Hussain M et al (2006) Antitumor and antimetastatic activities of docetaxel are enhanced by genistein through regulation of osteoprotegerin/receptor activator of nuclear factor-kappaB (RANK)/RANK ligand/MMP-9 signaling in prostate cancer. Cancer Res 66:4816–4825

Li Y, Wang Z, Kong D et al (2007) Regulation of FOXO3a/beta-catenin/GSK-3beta signaling by 3,3′-diindolylmethane contributes to inhibition of cell proliferation and induction of apoptosis in prostate cancer cells. J Biol Chem 282:21542–21550

Li Y, Wang Z, Kong D et al (2008) Regulation of Akt/FOXO3a/GSK-3beta/AR signaling network by isoflavone in prostate cancer cells. J Biol Chem 283:27707–27716

Li Y, Revalde JL, Reid G et al (2011a) Modulatory effects of curcumin on multi-drug resistance-associated protein 5 in pancreatic cancer cells. Cancer Chemother Pharmacol 68:603–610. Epub 2010

Li Y, Kong D, Wang Z et al (2011b) Inactivation of AR/TMPRSS2-ERG/Wnt signaling networks attenuates the aggressive behavior of prostate cancer cells. Cancer Prev Res (Phila) 4: 1495–1506

Liang G, Tang A, Lin X et al (2010) Green tea catechins augment the antitumor activity of doxorubicin in an in vivo mouse model for chemoresistant liver cancer. Int J Oncol 37:111–123

Lin YW, Tsai MS, Weng SH et al (2011) Synergistic effect of curcumin and cisplatin via downregulation of thymidine phosphorylase and ERCC1. Mol Pharmacol 80:136–146

Lu KH, Chen YW, Tsai PH et al (2009) Evaluation of radiotherapy effect in resveratrol-treated medulloblastoma cancer stem-like cells. Childs Nerv Syst 25:543–550

Luo T, Wang J, Yin Y et al (2010) (-)-Epigallocatechin gallate sensitizes breast cancer cells to paclitaxel in a murine model of breast carcinoma. Breast Cancer Res 12:R8

Ma Y, Wang J, Liu L et al (2011) Genistein potentiates the effect of arsenic trioxide against human hepatocellular carcinoma: role of Akt and nuclear factor-kappaB. Cancer Lett 301:75–84

McGuire KP, Ngoubilly N, Neavyn M et al (2006) 3,3′-diindolylmethane and paclitaxel act synergistically to promote apoptosis in HER2/Neu human breast cancer cells. J Surg Res 132:208–213

Messina MJ, Persky V, Setchell KD et al (1994) Soy intake and cancer risk: a review of the in vitro and in vivo data. Nutr Cancer 21:113–131

Mohammad RM, Al-Katib A, Aboukameel A et al (2003) Genistein sensitizes diffuse large cell lymphoma to CHOP (cyclophosphamide, doxorubicin, vincristine, prednisone) chemotherapy. Mol Cancer Ther 2:1361–1368

Nakachi K, Matsuyama S, Miyake S et al (2000) Preventive effects of drinking green tea on cancer and cardiovascular disease: epidemiological evidence for multiple targeting prevention. Biofactors 13:49–54

Nakamura K, Yasunaga Y, Segawa T et al (2002) Curcumin down-regulates AR gene expression and activation in prostate cancer cell lines. Int J Oncol 21:825–830

Nihal M, Ahmad N, Mukhtar H et al (2005) Anti-proliferative and proapoptotic effects of (-)-epigallocatechin-3-gallate on human melanoma: possible implications for the chemoprevention of melanoma. Int J Cancer 114:513–521

Nihal M, Ahsan H, Siddiqui IA et al (2009) (-)-Epigallocatechin-3-gallate (EGCG) sensitizes melanoma cells to interferon induced growth inhibition in a mouse model of human melanoma. Cell Cycle 8:2057–2063

Notarbartolo M, Poma P, Perri D et al (2005) Antitumor effects of curcumin, alone or in combination with cisplatin or doxorubicin, on human hepatic cancer cells. Analysis of their possible relationship to changes in NF-kB activation levels and in IAP gene expression. Cancer Lett 224:53–65

Padhye S, Banerjee S, Chavan D et al (2009a) Fluorocurcumins as cyclooxygenase-2 inhibitor: molecular docking, pharmacokinetics and tissue distribution in mice. Pharm Res 26:2438–2445

Padhye S, Yang H, Jamadar A et al (2009b) New difluoro Knoevenagel condensates of curcumin, their Schiff bases and copper complexes as proteasome inhibitors and apoptosis inducers in cancer cells. Pharm Res 26:1874–1880

Patel BB, Sengupta R, Qazi S et al (2008) Curcumin enhances the effects of 5-fluorouracil and oxaliplatin in mediating growth inhibition of colon cancer cells by modulating EGFR and IGF-1R. Int J Cancer 122:267–273

Pereira MA, Grubbs CJ, Barnes LH et al (1996) Effects of the phytochemicals, curcumin and quercetin, upon azoxymethane-induced colon cancer and 7,12-dimethylbenz[a]anthracene-induced mammary cancer in rats. Carcinogenesis 17:1305–1311

Raffoul JJ, Wang Y, Kucuk O et al (2006) Genistein inhibits radiation-induced activation of NF-kappaB in prostate cancer cells promoting apoptosis and G2/M cell cycle arrest. BMC Cancer 6:107

Raffoul JJ, Banerjee S, Che M et al (2007a) Soy isoflavones enhance radiotherapy in a metastatic prostate cancer model. Int J Cancer 120:2491–2498

Raffoul JJ, Banerjee S, Singh-Gupta V et al (2007b) Down-regulation of apurinic/apyrimidinic endonuclease 1/redox factor-1 expression by soy isoflavones enhances prostate cancer radiotherapy in vitro and in vivo. Cancer Res 67:2141–149

Rahman KM, Banerjee S, Ali S et al (2009) 3,3′-Diindolylmethane enhances taxotere-induced apoptosis in hormone-refractory prostate cancer cells through survivin down-regulation. Cancer Res 69:4468–4475

Sapi E, Alvero AB, Chen W et al (2004) Resistance of ovarian carcinoma cells to docetaxel is XIAP dependent and reversible by phenoxodiol. Oncol Res 14:567–578

Sarkar FH, Li Y (2004) Indole-3-carbinol and prostate cancer. J Nutr 134:3493S–348S

Sarkar FH, Li Y (2006) Using chemopreventive agents to enhance the efficacy of cancer therapy. Cancer Res 66:3347–3350

Sarkar FH, Li Y, Wang Z et al (2010) The role of nutraceuticals in the regulation of Wnt and Hedgehog signaling in cancer. Cancer Metastasis Rev 29:383–394

Satoh H, Nishikawa K, Suzuki K et al (2003) Genistein, a soy isoflavone, enhances necrotic-like cell death in a breast cancer cell treated with a chemotherapeutic agent. Res Commun Mol Pathol Pharmacol 113–114:149–158

Scarlatti F, Sala G, Ricci C et al (2007) Resveratrol sensitization of DU145 prostate cancer cells to ionizing radiation is associated to ceramide increase. Cancer Lett 253:124–130

Shamim U, Hanif S, Albanyan A et al (2011) Resveratrol-induced apoptosis is enhanced in low pH environments associated with cancer. J Cell Physiol (Epub ahead of print)

Shankar S, Ganapathy S, Chen Q et al (2008) Curcumin sensitizes TRAIL-resistant xenografts: molecular mechanisms of apoptosis, metastasis and angiogenesis. Mol Cancer 7:16

Shervington A, Pawar V, Menon S et al (2009) The sensitization of glioma cells to cisplatin and tamoxifen by the use of catechin. Mol Biol Rep 36:1181–1186

Shiau RJ, Chen KY, Wen YD et al (2010) Genistein and beta-carotene enhance the growth-inhibitory effect of trichostatin A in A549 cells. Eur J Nutr 49:19–25

Shukla S, Zaher H, Hartz A et al (2009) Curcumin inhibits the activity of ABCG2/BCRP1, a multidrug resistance-linked ABC drug transporter in mice. Pharm Res 26:480–487

Siddiqui IA, Malik A, Adhami VM et al (2008) Green tea polyphenol EGCG sensitizes human prostate carcinoma LNCaP cells to TRAIL-mediated apoptosis and synergistically inhibits biomarkers associated with angiogenesis and metastasis. Oncogene 27:2055–2063

Singh-Gupta V, Joiner MC, Runyan L et al (2011) Soy isoflavones augment radiation effect by inhibiting APE1/Ref-1 DNA repair activity in non-small cell lung Cancer. J Thorac Oncol 6:688–698

Sreekanth CN, Bava SV, Sreekumar E et al (2011) Molecular evidences for the chemosensitizing efficacy of liposomal curcumin in paclitaxel chemotherapy in mouse models of cervical cancer. Oncogene 30:3139–3152

Stearns ME, Amatangelo MD, Varma D et al (2010) Combination therapy with epigallocatechin-3-gallate and doxorubicin in human prostate tumor modeling studies: inhibition of metastatic tumor growth in severe combined immunodeficiency mice. Am J Pathol 177:3169–3179

Surh YJ (2003) Cancer chemoprevention with dietary phytochemicals. Nat Rev Cancer 3:768–780

Takimoto CH, Glover K, Huang X et al (2003) Phase I pharmacokinetic and pharmacodynamic analysis of unconjugated soy isoflavones administered to individuals with cancer. Cancer Epidemiol Biomarkers Prev 12:1213–1221

Taniguchi S, Fujiki H, Kobayashi H et al (1992) Effect of (-)-epigallocatechin gallate, the main constituent of green tea, on lung metastasis with mouse B16 melanoma cell lines. Cancer Lett 65:51–54

Vaishampayan U, Hussain M, Banerjee M et al (2007) Lycopene and soy isoflavones in the treatment of prostate cancer. Nutr Cancer 59:1–7

Wang J, He D, Zhang Q et al (2009) Resveratrol protects against Cisplatin-induced cardiotoxicity by alleviating oxidative damage. Cancer Biother Radiopharm 24:675–680

Yashar CM, Spanos WJ, Taylor DD et al (2005) Potentiation of the radiation effect with genistein in cervical cancer cells. Gynecol Oncol 99:199–205

Zhang Q, Wei D, Liu J (2004) In vivo reversal of doxorubicin resistance by (-)-epigallocatechin gallate in a solid human carcinoma xenograft. Cancer Lett 208:179–186

Index

F.H. Sarkar (ed.), *Nutraceuticals and Cancer*, DOI 10.1007/978-94-007-2630-7,

D

E

F

G

H

I

L

M

N

O

P

R